PERCUTANE MITRAL VALVOTOMY

System requirement:

Windows:

- Operating System
  - Windows Vista or above.
  - Macintosh OS X or above
- Recommended Web Browser – Google Chrome & Mozilla Firefox
- Essential plugins – Java & Flash player
  - If facing problems in viewing content – enable/re-install Java plugin on your web browser setting.
  - If Videos don't show up – enable/re-install Flash Player or manage Flash setting on your web browser settings.
  - You can test Java and Flash by using the links from the help section of the CD/DVD.

Accompanying CD/DVD Rom is compatible and playable only in Computers and not in DVD player.

CD/DVD has Autorun function (only for Windows based systems). If Autorun feature doesn't works, then follow the steps below to access the contents manually:

Windows:

- Click on My Computer
- Select the CD/DVD drive and click open/explore – this will show list of files in the CD/DVD
- Find and double click file – "launch.html"

Mac:

Double click the file "launch.html" located on the root after inserting the CD/DVD. The Mac OSX operating system does not support an Autorun feature.

For more information about troubleshoot of Autorun click on: http://support.microsoft.com/kb/330135

DVD CONTENTS

1. Cine and Echo Videos
2. Procedural Videos

(List of videos are shown on page no. xxix to xxxi)

PERCUTANEOUS MITRAL VALVOTOMY

SECOND EDITION

Harikrishnan S MD DM FRCP FACC
Professor of Cardiology
Sree Chitra Tirunal Institute for Medical Sciences
and Technology (SCTIMST)
Thiruvananthapuram, Kerala, India

Forewords

Jaganmohan A Tharakan
CN Manjunath

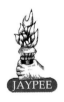

The Health Sciences Publisher

New Delhi | London | Panama

Jaypee Brothers Medical Publishers (P) Ltd

Headquarters

Jaypee Brothers Medical Publishers (P) Ltd
4838/24, Ansari Road, Daryaganj
New Delhi 110 002, India
Phone: +91-11-43574357
Fax: +91-11-43574314
Email: jaypee@jaypeebrothers.com

Overseas Offices

J.P. Medical Ltd
83 Victoria Street, London
SW1H 0HW (UK)
Phone: +44 20 3170 8910
Fax: +44 (0)20 3008 6180
Email: info@jpmedpub.com

Jaypee Brothers Medical Publishers (P) Ltd
17/1-B Babar Road, Block-B, Shaymali
Mohammadpur, Dhaka-1207
Bangladesh
Mobile: +08801912003485
Email: jaypeedhaka@gmail.com

Jaypee-Highlights Medical Publishers Inc
City of Knowledge, Bld. 235, 2nd Floor, Clayton
Panama City, Panama
Phone: +1 507-301-0496
Fax: +1 507-301-0499
Email: cservice@jphmedical.com

Jaypee Brothers Medical Publishers (P) Ltd
Bhotahity, Kathmandu, Nepal
Phone: +977-9741283608
Email: kathmandu@jaypeebrothers.com

Website: www.jaypeebrothers.com
Website: www.jaypeedigital.com

Percutaneous Mitral Valvotomy

First Edition: 2012

Second Edition: **2018**

ISBN: 978-93-86056-82-5

Printed at: Ajanta Offset & Packagings Ltd., Faridabad, Haryana

Dedicated to

The memory of my mother
B Radhamani Amma

REVIEWS

"This book has something for everyone. There is a great deal of useful information for the novice who is interested in adopting percutaneous mitral valvotomy, and there are many pearls for the experienced operator."

Ted Feldman MD
North Shore University Health System, USA
Journal of Interventional Cardiology—Vol 25, 3, June 2012. 319-320

"The book is a nearly complete encyclopaedia on percutaneous balloon mitral valvuloplasty (PBMV) discussing all its aspects covering anatomy, physiology, pathology, procedure details, and all the new gadgets".

K Sarat Chandra
Indian Heart Journal, 2012

"The broad scope of this book, which covers every aspect of mitral stenosis and describes in meticulous detail the techniques and equipment used in mitral valvotomy, are the primary strengths of this book".

Amit Prasad MD
Ochsner Clinic Foundation, USA
Doody's Book Review Service, 2012

CONTRIBUTORS

Ajeet Arulkumar MD DM
Interventional Cardiologist
Frontier Lifeline Hospital
Chennai, India

Amit Kumar Chaurasia MD DM
Consultant Interventional Cardiologist
Hungarian Institute of Cardiology
Budapest, Hungary

Anees Thajudeen MD DM
Additional Professor
Sree Chitra Tirunal Institute for
Medical Sciences and Technology
Thiruvananthapuram, India

Antwon Robinson MD
Interventional Cardiologist
The Jackson Clinic
Tennessee, USA

Arun Gopalakrishnan MD DM
Assistant Professor
Sree Chitra Tirunal Institute for
Medical Sciences and Technology
Thiruvananthapuram, India

Arun SR MD DM
Consultant Cardiologist
General Hospital
Thiruvananthapuram, India

BC Srinivas MD DM
Professor, Sri Jayadeva Institute of
Cardiovascular Sciences and Research
Bengaluru, India

Bhavesh Harivadan MD DM
Interventional Cardiologist
Zydus Hospital
Gujarat, India

Biju Soman MD DPH
Additional Professor
Achutha Menon Centre for Health Science
Studies, SCTIMST
Thiruvananthapuram, India

Boonjong Saejueng MD
Cardiologist
Chest Disease Institute, Nonthaburi
Thailand

Carlo de Asmundis MD PhD
Professor of Cardiology
UZ Brussel, Vrije Universiteit Brussel
Brussels
Belgium

Chandrasekharan C Kartha MD FRCP
Professor of Eminence
Rajiv Gandhi Centre for Biotechnology
Thiruvananthapuram, India

Col. Subroto Kumar Datta MD DM
Professor
Army College of Medical Sciences
Delhi, India

CN Manjunath MD DM
Director, Sri Jayadeva Institute of
Cardiovascular Sciences and Research
Bengaluru, India

Dale Murdoch MBBS FRACP MPhil
Interventional Cardiologist
The Prince Charles Hospital
Brisbane
Australia

Darragh Moran MD
Cardiology Specialist Registrar
Royal College of Physicians of Ireland
Ireland

Darren Walters MBBS MPhil FRACP
Interventional Cardiologist
The Prince Charles Hospital
Brisbane, Australia

Dash PK MD DM
Senior Consultant Cardiologist
Sri Sathya Sai Institute of Higher
Medical Sciences
Anantapur, India

Diego Chemello MD
Associate Professor
Universidade Federal de Santa Maria-RS
Brazil

Dinesh Choudhary MD DM
Associate Professor
Sardar Patel Medical College
Bikaner, India

Gadage Siddharth MD DM
Consultant Cardiologist
Ruby Hall Clinic
Pune, India

Gian-Battista Chierchia MD
Professor of Cardiology
UZ Brussel-Vrije Universiteit Brussel
Brussels, Belgium

Harikrishnan S MD DM FRCP
Professor of Cardiology
Sree Chitra Tirunal Institute for
Medical Sciences and Technology
Thiruvananthapuram, India

Hosam Hasan-Ali MD PhD
Associate Professor
Assiut University Hospitals
Assiut, Egypt

Jagdish Dureja MD
Professor, Department of Anesthesiology
Bhagat Phool Singh Mahila
Medical College
Haryana, India

Jayakeerthi Yoganarasimha Rao
MD DM
Consultant Cardiologist
Apollo Health City Jubilee Hills
Hyderabad, India

Kiron Sukulal MD DM
Consultant Cardiologist
Sree Mookambika Institute of Medical
Sciences, Kulasekharam
Kanyakumari, India

Krishnakumar M MD DM
Assistant Professor
Sree Chitra Tirunal Institute for
Medical Sciences and Technology
Thiruvananthapuram, India

Krishnakumar Nair MD DM
Program Director and Consultant
Electrophysiologist
Cardiac Electrophysiology
University of Toronto
Toronto General Hospital
Canada

KS Ravindranath MD DM
Professor
Sri Jayadeva Institute of Cardiovascular
Sciences and Research
Bengaluru, India

Mahesh Kumar S MD DM
Consultant Pediatric Cardiologist
Velammal Medical College
Madurai, India

Mamtesh Gupta MD DM
Senior Consultant
Department of Cardiology
Dhanvantri Jeevan Rekha Heart
Care Hospital
Meerut, India

María C Saccheri MD
Department of Cardiology
Hospital del Gobierno de la Ciudad
de Buenos Aires "Dr. Cosme Argerich"
Buenos Aires, Argentina

Meera R MD DM
Consultant Cardiologist
Kerala Institute of Medical Sciences
Thiruvananthapuram, India

Mohammad A Sherif MD
Cardiology Department
Rostock University Clinic
Rostock, Germany

P Shanmuga Sundaram MD DM
Senior Consultant Cardiologist
Devadoss Multispeciality Hospital
Madurai, India

Pedro Brugada MD PhD
Heart Rhythm Management Center
UZ Brussel
Vrije Universiteit Brussel
Belgium

Prabhavathi MD DM
Professor
Sri Jayadeva Institute of Cardiovascular
Sciences and Research
Bengaluru, India

Pranav Bansal MD
Associate Professor
Department of Anesthesiology
Teerthanker Mahaveer Medical College
Moradabad, India

Prasenjit Das MD DNB
Assistant Professor
Department of Pathology
All India Institute of Medical Sciences
New Delhi, India

Praveen Kerala Varma MS MCh
Clinical Professor and Head
Cardiovascular and Thoracic Surgery
Amrita Institute of Medical Sciences and
Research Center, Kochi, India

Praveen Kumar Neema MD
Professor and Head
Department of Anesthesiology
All India Institute of Medical Sciences
Raipur, India

Praveen Reddy Bayya MS MCh
Consultant Pediatric Cardiac Surgeon
Amrita Institute for Medical Sciences
and Research Center
Kochi, India

Rachel Daniel MD DM
Consultant Cardiologist
NS Hospital
Kollam, India

Raghuram A Krishnan MD DM
Interventional Cardiologist
Al-Shifa Hospital
Malapuram, India

Raja Selvaraj MD DCH DNB
Associate Professor
Jawaharlal Institute of Postgraduate
Medical Education and Research
Puducherry, India

Rajesh Muralidharan MD DM
Consultant Interventional Cardiologist
Baby Memorial Hospital
Kozhikode, India

Ramalingam Vadivelu MD DM
Consultant Cardiologist
Postgraduate Institute of Medical
Education and Research
Chandigarh, India

Randeep Singla MD DM
Assistant Professor
U N Mehta Institute of Cardiology and
Research Centre
Ahmedabad, India

Ravi S Math MD DM
Associate Professor
Sri Jayadeva Institute of Cardiovascular
Sciences and Research
Bengaluru, India

Rohan Vijay Ainchwar MD DM
Consultant Cardiologist
CHL Multispeciality Hospital and
Research Centre
Chandrapur, India

Ruma Ray MD FRCPath
Professor
Cardiac Pathology
All India Institute of Medical Sciences
New Delhi, India

S Venkiteshwaran MD DM
Consultant Pediatric Cardiologist
Lakeshore Hospitals
Kochi, India

Sajith Sukumaran MD DM
Additional Professor
Neurology Department
Sree Chitra Tirunal Institute for
Medical Sciences and Technology
Thiruvananthapuram, India

Sajy Kuruttukulam MD DM
Consultant Cardiologist
Medical Trust Hospital
Kochi, India

Sanjay G MD DM
Additional Professor
Sree Chitra Tirunal Institute for
Medical Sciences and Technology
Thiruvananthapuram, India

Santhosh KG Koshy MD DM
Professor of Medicine
University of Tennessee Health
Sciences Center, USA

Saujatya Chakraborty MD DM
Senior Resident, Postgraduate Institute
of Medical Education and Research
Chandigarh, India

Sethu Parvathy VK BSc DCLT
Cardiac Technologist
Sree Chitra Tirunal Institute for
Medical Sciences and Technology,
Thiruvananthapuram, India

Shiv Bagga MD DM
Consultant Cardiologist
Postgraduate Institute of Medical
Education and Research
Chandigarh, India

Shomu R Bohora MD DM
Cardiac Electrophysiologist
Baroda Heart Institute and Research
Centre, Vadodara, India

Shyam Sundar Reddy MD DM
Interventional Cardiologist
Krishna Institute of Medical Sciences
Hyderabad, India

Sivasubramonian Sivasankaran
MD DM
Professor, Sree Chitra Tirunal Institute
for Medical Sciences and Technology
Thiruvananthapuram, India

Sonny P Jacob MD DM
Consultant Cardiologist
Atlas Star Hospital
Muscat, Oman

Stigimon Joseph MD DM
Senior Consultant
Little Flower Hospital
Ernakulam, India

Suchith Majumdar MD DM
Consultant Cardiologist
Rabindranath Tagore International
Institute of Cardiac Sciences
Kolkata, India

Sudaratana Tansuphaswadikul MD
Chief of Cardiology
Chest Disease Institute
Nonthaburi, Thailand

Suji K BSc DCLT
Scientific Officer
Cardiology Department
Sree Chitra Tirunal Institute for
Medical Sciences and Technology
Thiruvananthapuram, India

Syamkumar Menon MD DM
Associate Professor of Medicine
Division of Cardiology
McMaster University
Hamilton, Canada

Thomas Koshy MD
Professor of Cardiac Anesthesiology
Sree Chitra Tirunal Institute for
Medical Sciences and Technology
Thiruvananthapuram, India

Tomás F Cianciulli MD
Director of Echocardiography Laboratory
Hospital of the Government of the City
of Buenos Aires "Dr. Cosme Argerich"
Buenos Aires, Argentina

Yoav Turgeman MD
Head of Department
Heart Institute
HaEmek Medical Centre
Afula, Israel

FOREWORD TO THE FIRST EDITION

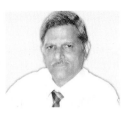

Rheumatic fever and its sequel, chronic rheumatic valvular heart disease, have been recognized for over a century. Its vast impact on societal health, can be measured by the fact that it affects otherwise healthy children and adolescents in the prime of their life and often leaves them crippled forever, despite our understanding that it is a completely preventable disease. Regardless of the major advancements in technology for diagnosis, evaluation and therapy, a heart once afflicted by rheumatic process can rarely be brought back to normalcy and all treatment modalities can at best be described as palliative. However, morbidity and mortality from the disease can be greatly ameliorated with the present-day therapeutic interventions.

The fact that a significant proportion of patients with rheumatic valvular heart disease present with isolated mitral stenosis, often with leaflet fusion along the valve closure line as the only abnormality or as the dominant abnormality, constricting the valve orifice but leaving it competent, lead to innovative treatment strategies like closed mitral commissurotomy, open mitral commissurotomy, and more recently percutaneous mitral valvotomy. All these treatment strategies ensured splitting the fused valve along the natural cleavage line – the valve closure line (commissurotomy) thus ensuring preserved competence of the valve after restoring the orifice area to acceptable levels - so to say, the valve pathology best suited the intervention. Rapid advances in techniques and gadgets and further improvisations have made percutaneous mitral valvotomy, a very safe, effective and durable procedure for relief of mitral stenosis.

In this scenario, when percutaneous mitral valvotomy has largely supplanted surgical commissurotomy, except in specific situations, it is apt that a compendium on the present art, craft and science of the technique of percutaneous mitral valvotomy is brought out under one cover and the contributors to this compendium have made excellent effort in the exposition of the technique of percutaneous mitral commissurotomy, indications, procedural details, the available gadgets and hardware, their merits and pitfalls, complications, results and short- and long-term outcomes.

This compendium will remain a "must read" reference text for all cardiology fellows in training and cardiologists performing mitral commissurotomy procedures.

Prof Jaganmohan A Tharakan MD DM
Former Director and Head of Department of Cardiology
Sree Chitra Tirunal Institute for Medical Sciences and Technology
Thiruvananthapuram, India

FOREWORD TO THE SECOND EDITION

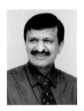

Balloon mitral valvuloplasty is the most common non-coronary intervention done in India and developing countries. Although there is declining trend in the prevalence of rheumatic heart disease, it continues to affect the low socioeconomic strata in adolescent–middle age groups. Rheumatic mitral stenosis is the most common valvular lesion which accounts for nearly 40% of rheumatic valve cases.

Mortality and morbidity is substantially reduced recently because of better awareness, early detection and timely application of modern technology in the form of balloon valvuloplasty and surgical therapy. A lot depends on the mitral valve morphology - so case selection based on echocardiographic assessment assumes paramount importance. Evaluation includes assessment of commissural pathology, calcification and subvalvular disease. In addition to morphology, assessment of mitral regurgitation and profiling the interatrial septum will have direct impact on procedural success and complications.

Transthoracic echo assistance will also be useful in situations of difficult septal puncture. Over-the-wire technique improves the success rate in patients who have difficulty in LV entry, this technique can also be adopted in the presence of LA thrombus limited to appendage. As expertise has grown, indications also have been rapidly expanding. The journey of Balloon Mitral Valvuloplasty (BMV) has undergone significant evolution over these years and travelled through gadgets like Mansfield balloon, double balloon, Inoue balloon, and metal commissurotomy. Accura balloon is evolved from its prototype Inoue balloon. Ever since Inoue balloon is in usage (1994), BMV is the interventional procedure of choice for symptomatic and eligible patients of mitral stenosis. Technically BMV is more demanding than coronary intervention. Experience and expertise will yield good results with less complications. There are not many comprehensive books on BMV. Dr Harikrishnan and his contributors have done an awesome job in conglomerating chapters about basics, hardware, various techniques, complications, tips/tricks across wide spectrum of BMV procedures. Pictures/Video clip illustrations are impressive which can guide the readers for an easy understanding. The book also reviews experiences of various high volume centres from India and abroad.

My hearty congratulations to Dr Harikrishnan and other contributors for their efforts and time in bringing out this excellent comprehensive book which provides A-Z information about mitral valvuloplasty for interventional cardiologists and trainees in cardiology.

Prof CN Manjunath MD DM
Director
Sri Jayadeva Institute of Cardiovascular Sciences and Research
Bannerghatta Road, Bengaluru (Karnataka), India

PREFACE TO THE SECOND EDITION

Since the publication of the first edition of our book, *Percutaneous Mitral Valvotomy*, we got feedback from people from different corners of the world.

The comments we have received included requests for including a few more topics, like 3-D echocardiography and for adding more details about the double balloon technique.

Since the publication of the first edition in 2012, many articles on percutaneous mitral valvotomy (PMV) have got published. Some of them explain new techniques and other few describe new gadgets. We have tried to incorporate all those information into this edition.

Sri Jayadeva Institute of Cardiology, Bengaluru and Sri Sathyasai Institute of Cardiology, Puttaparthi, India, are the two centres having enormous experience in PMV. Highly experienced operators from both centres have contributed in this edition. I am sure that this has enriched this book.

Rheumatic fever and rheumatic heart disease have shown declining trends even in the developing world. It has become a very rare entity in the developed world. Hence, the experience of interventional cardiologists in PMV is coming down and this is a real problem in many countries in Europe and North America. A book like this will be helpful in this regard to brush up their knowledge about the practical aspects.

A DVD is also published along with this edition, where we have included a full video recording of the procedure being done in cath lab, including the preparation of the hardware. This was done following the request from many of the readers of the first edition of the book. The procedural DVD will help in brushing up the skills for those who do the procedure occasionally. We hope this will help the cath lab personnel also.

Seventy-two experts in this field from 14 countries are sharing their expertise and experience in this book. We hope that we have included all major aspects related to this procedure in this new improved edition. We are open to any comments or suggestions which will help to improve this book further.

Harikrishnan S
drharikrishnan@outlook.com

PREFACE TO THE FIRST EDITION

Rheumatic heart disease (RHD) is one of the major problems affecting many developing countries. The lowest estimate of RHD in India reveals that the number of patients is about 2.8 million. The mean age of death being 24.4 years, the affected get taken away at the dawn of their lives. Mitral valve is the most commonly affected valve and mitral valve stenosis (MS) the most common diagnosis.

Medical management can control the symptoms for only a limited period of time. As the disease becomes severe, some form of intervention may be required. The problem is usually mechanical, i.e. either regurgitation or stenosis of the valve.

For MS, the first intervention which came into clinical practice was closed mitral valvotomy (CMV). Lots of patients have been saved by CMV, following which most of them are leading a symptom free, productive life years after the procedure.

The advent of percutaneous catheter techniques has led to the development of different gadgets to open pliable mitral valves. Different types of balloons were developed to open pliable rheumatic mitral valves. The first technique of percutaneous mitral valvotomy (PMV) which gained popularity was the double balloon technique.

But the gadget which changed the face of PMV was the Inoue balloon, which made the procedure simple and safe. Percutaneous mitral valvotomy with Inoue balloon gained worldwide acceptance and is currently the most widely practiced percutaneous mitral valvotomy technique worldwide.

Cribier's metallic commissurotome, Jomiva™ balloon and Multitrack™ balloons are some of the other gadgets that followed. Many patients have benefitted from these techniques too.

With more and more cardiologists and centers performing PMV in India and abroad, the need of a textbook describing the various aspects of this procedure came to our mind. This book is a humble attempt in this regard.

Fifty-seven contributors from 11 countries are sharing their expertise and experience. We have tried to cover all the aspects of the procedure starting from patient selection to long-term follow-up. We hope that we have succeeded at least partly in this venture. We are open to any comments or suggestions which will help to improve this book further.

Harikrishnan S
drharikrishnan@outlook.com

ACKNOWLEDGEMENTS

First and foremost, I am indebted to my Institute, The Sree Chitra Tirunal Institute for Medical Sciences and Technology, Thiruvananthapuram (www. sctimst.ac.in), in bringing out this book. I am profusely grateful to our former Director, Prof K Radhakrishnan, and Prof Jaganmohan Tharakan, the Head of Department of Cardiology who gave me the permission and all the encouragement to bring out this book.

Prof Jaganmohan Tharakan, a teacher par-excellence kindly agreed to write Foreword to the first edition of this book, which I consider a great honour. I am indebted to my other teachers in SCTIMST, Prof Thomas Titus, Prof VK Ajithkumar, Prof V Ramakrishnapillai, Dr Anil Bhat, Dr Bimal Francis and Prof S Sivasankaran whose wisdom and skills helped me in learning this procedure—PMV. Prof CC Kartha was always an inspiration, I thank him.

Prof CN Manjunath, Founder Director of the Jayadeva Institute of Cardiovascular Sciences and Research, Bengaluru which is the centre with maximum experience in PMV globally, has agreed to write the Foreword to the second edition of the book. My sincere thanks are due to him. Few of his colleagues have contributed chapters in this book. My sincere thanks to the Jayadeva team.

My colleagues in SCTIMST-faculty and senior residents, have helped me from the conceptual stage to proofreading. I am grateful to them. My other colleagues - cath lab technologists, cath lab nurses, and staff in the medical records department and computer department of SCTIMST played a major part in bringing out this book.

I am thankful to Mr Suji, Scientific Officer, Cath Labs, SCTIMST who has been immensely helpful in preparing the chapters on hardware. I would also like to thank Subrahmanya HR, Resmy PV, Rasmy S, and Sethuparvathy, our cardiac technologists for their help.

M/s Toray Inc, Vascular concepts, Medtronic Inc, Cook Inc and Lifetechmed, India were quite helpful in giving permissions to use the figures and information from their websites.

I am indebted to Ms Vasanthy, Senior artist and Mr Lijikumar, Senior Technician, both from our medical illustration department for the drawings and the photographs which are used in this book. I also thank Dr Syamkumar Menon, faculty at Mc Master University, Canada for some of the figures.

Mr Thampi NG, Senior Medical Records Officer and Mr Suresh Kumar, Systems Manager provided the data from our computer patient database which is used in this book.

My sincere thanks to Mr Anilbabu, Athiras Communications, Thiruvananthapuram for the video recording and editing of the live recording of the procedure performed in the cath lab. I also thank Dr Sanjay G, Additional Professor, SCTIMST for his help in recording the hemodynamic tracings.

I thank all the contributors for the wonderful job of compiling the chapters in this book.

M/s Jaypee Brothers Medical Publishers did a great job in bringing out this job with such a great lay out. I am extremely thankful to Shri Jitendar P Vij (Group Chairman), Mr Ankit Vij (Group President), Ms Ritu Sharma (Director-Content Strategy) and Ms Sunita Katla (PA to Group Chairman and Publishing Manager) for taking personal interest. Mr Rajesh Sharma (Production Coordinator), Ms Seema Dogra (Cover Visualizer), Mr Arun and others from Kochi Branch helped a lot in bringing out this book, thanks are due to them too.

Mr Manas Chacko, my project staff did an excellent work in compiling the second edition. My thanks are due to him.

I am indebted to those patients whom we had the fortune to treat here in SCTIMST, without whose data, this book would not have materialized.

I thank the Almighty God for all his blessings.

Lastly, I cannot forget the help and encouragement provided by my wife, Resmy and my sons, Vignesh and Vyskah. They have sacrificed a lot in the last few years to make this dream of mine come true.

Harikrishnan S

CONTENTS

DVD CONTENTS

Chapter 35
Video 1—Fig. 35.2: Post PMV severe MR TEE images
Video 2—Fig. 35.2: Post PMV MR medial commissure LA wire seen
Video 3—Fig. 35.2: Cineangiogram Post PMV MR medial commissure LA wire seen

Chapter 39
Video 1—Fig. 39.2.1: Venogram IVC1
Video 2—Fig. 39.2.2: Venogram IVC2
Video 3—Fig. 39.2.3: Venogram IVC3
Video 4—Fig. 39.3: Transjugular PA angio levophase
Video 5—Fig. 39.5: Transjugular balloon dilatation
Video 6—Fig. 39.5: Transjugular
Video 7—Video-1: Transjugular LA angio post-puncture
Video 8—Video-2: Transjugular septal puncture
Video 9—Video-3: Transjugular RA angio (5)
Video 10—Video-4: Transjugular septal dilatation

Chapter 41
Video 1—Video-1: Transthoracic echocardiography showing severe subvalvular
          thickening
Video 2—Video-2: Severe subvalvar disease producing multiple inflow jets
Video 3—Video-3A: Impact of measuring MVA at proper plane
Video 4—Video-3B: Impact of measuring MVA at proper plane
Video 5—Video-4A: Balloon impasse sign
Video 6—Video-4B: Balloon impasse sign
Video 7—Video-5A: Abnormal shape of balloon due to subvalvar disease
Video 8—Video-5B: Normal shape of balloon
Video 9—Video-6A: Severe submitral stenosis
Video 10—Video-6C: Severe submitral stenosis
Video 11—Video-7A: Submitral release from antegrade approach
Video 12—Video-7B: Submitral release from antegrade approach
Video 13—Video-7C: Submitral release from antegrade approach
Video 14—Video-7D: Submitral release from antegrade approach
Video 15—Video-8A: Submitral release from retrograde approach
Video 16—Video-8B: Submitral release from retrograde approach
Video 17—Video-8C: Submitral release from retrograde approach
Video 18—Video-8D: Submitral release from retrograde approach
Video 19—Video-9: Balloon dilatation of subvalvar stenosis

Chapter 42
Video 1—Additional videos
Video 2—Additional videos
Video 3—Additional videos
Video 4—Additional videos
Video 5—Additional videos

Chapter 43
Video 1—Fig. 43.7: BPV with accura balloon pigtail wire in LPA

Chapter 44
Video 1—Fig. 44.3: BTV dilatation RAO
Video 2—Fig. 44.3: BTV entry RAO 30° view

LIST OF PROCEDURAL VIDEOS

Section 1

Introduction

Chapter 1

Prelude

Harikrishnan S

Rheumatic heart disease (RHD) continues to be endemic in developing countries where it still remains as a major cardiovascular problem. Among RHD, isolated mitral valve stenosis occurs in 40% of all patients.[1-3] The data from SCTIMST, one of the tertiary cardiac care centres in India, also showed that the predominant diagnosis among patients with RHD was MS and it constituted 31% of the total RHD burden during 1995-2012 (Fig. 1.1).

Mitral stenosis (MS) is an obstruction to left ventricular (LV) inflow at the level of the mitral valve as a result of a structural abnormality of the mitral valve (MV) apparatus. This prevents proper opening of the valve during diastolic filling of the left ventricle. The normal MV area is 4.0 to 5.0 cm^2. Narrowing of the valve area to less than 2.5 cm^2 typically occurs before the development of symptoms.

Most common cause of MS is rheumatic heart disease. A history of rheumatic fever can be elicited from approximately up to 50% of patients presenting with pure MS. The ratio of women to men presenting with isolated MS is 2:1.[1-3]

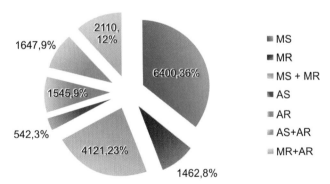

Fig. 1.1: Split-up diagnosis of RHD patients attending SCTIMST, Trivandrum 1995-2015 (Number, Percentage) (Ref. Computer data base SCTIMST accessed 23/06/2017, *Courtesy:* Mr. N J Thampi, Medical Records Officer and Computer Division)

The concept of mitral commissurotomy was first proposed by Brunton in 1902 and the first successful surgical closed mitral commissurotomy was performed in 1923 by Elliot Cutler.[4] But the technique was established and popularized by Harken[5] and Bailey[6] in the 1940s. By the late 1940s and early 1950s, both transatrial and transventricular closed surgical commissurotomies were considered as accepted clinical procedures.

With the development of cardiopulmonary bypass in the 1960s, open mitral commissurotomy (OMV) and replacement of the mitral valve (MV) became the surgical procedures of choice for treatment of MS.

Inoue[7] who is a cardiovascular surgeon from Japan, began to design and develop a new balloon catheter system in 1976. It was first used to create an atrial septal defect (ASD) in children with transposition of great arteries. It was also used to treat membranous obstruction in inferior vena cava and stenotic lesions in the iliofemoral arteries. In 1979, the ability of the balloon to separate fused commissures was evaluated under direct vision as an auxiliary means of open mitral commissurotomy. The fused commissures were found to be separated precisely along their natural lines without injury to leaflets, tearing of chordae tendinae, or creation of significant mitral regurgitation (MR). This led to several trials of inserting the balloon catheter across the mitral valve orifice without open surgery by transseptal catheterization first in canines and then in humans. The balloon was finally perfected in 1980.[7]

In 1982, the first clinical application of the prototype Inoue balloon catheter was successfully achieved in a 33-year-old man with severe rheumatic MS and the initial report was published in 1984.[7] In 1985, Lock et al[8] used cylindrical polyethylene balloon in 8 children with rheumatic mitral stenosis to perform percutaneous mitral valvotomy (PMV) via transseptal approach. Following Lock's report, AL-Zaibag et al.[9] in 1986 introduced the use of a double balloon technique (DBT) for treating rheumatic MS.

Initial reports of Inoue et al.,[7] Lock et al.[8] and Al-Zaibag et al.[9] were essentially limited to young patients who were free of calcific mitral valve disease or MR at baseline. Palacios et al.[10] in 1987 using a single 25 mm balloon, made the first report of successful PMV in adult patients with calcific MS.

Several modifications of PMV technique have been introduced over the years. The use of transarterial retrograde approach for PMV was reported by Babic et al.[11]

CMV, BMV and OMV was compared in a randomized fashion and has found to give comparable long term and short term results.[12] With reports from different centers around the world about the safety and efficacy of Inoue balloon it was granted FDA approval in 1994. Since then Inoue Balloon or balloons with the same principle are the most widely used gadgets for PMV worldwide (Fig. 1.2).

A simplified DBT called the Multi-Track system was developed in Paris by Philip Bonhoeffer and his colleagues, as a valid user-friendly and cost-effective alternative for the treatment of MS.[13] The early experience of 12 patients were reported in 1995, and later on, in 1999 some improvement in the catheter system was made and the first 100 consecutive cases (worldwide) were reported.[13]

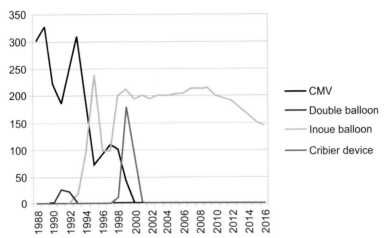

Fig. 1.2: Chart showing the different procedures performed for Mitral Stenosis in SCTIMST, one of the tertiary cardiac care centers in India 1988 – 2016. (Ref. Computer data base SCTIMST accessed 28/02/2017)

In 1997, Cribier et al.[14] introduced a new device featuring a metallic valvulotome instead of a balloon for opening the mitral valve. The success of dilatation with the valvulotome was maintained even in patients with high echo scores and in patients with commissural calcification.[15] The advantage of the system is that the metallic commissurotome can be re-used multiple times after re-sterilization. This is reported as a cost-effective alternative to the Inoue balloon.[16]

Balloons utilizing the same principle as Inoue balloon also came into the market. The Accura™ balloon system is a double lumen balloon catheter similar to the Inoue balloon. Compared to the triple lumen Inoue balloon, the double lumen Accura balloon catheter is reported to be equally effective[17,18] and easy to re-sterilize for multiple re-use.

In a recent large cross-sectional study of balloon mitral valvuloplasty in USA, the authors reported trends of decreasing overall utilization and increasing procedural complication rates (corresponding to increasing age and burden of comorbidities) and cost over a period of 13 years.[19] This report points to the challenges faced by the operators in performing PMV in the modern era.

■ REFERENCES

1. Wood P. An appreciation of mitral stenosis. I. Clinical features. Br Med J. 1954;1(4870):1051–63.
2. Rowe JC, Bland EF, Sprague HB, White PD. The course of mitral stenosis without surgery: ten- and twenty-year perspectives. Ann Intern Med. 1960;52:741–9.
3. Olesen KH. The natural history of 271 patients with mitral stenosis under medical treatment. Br Heart J. 1962;24:349–57.
4. Beck CS, Cutler EC. A cardiovalvulotome. J Exp Med. 1924;40(3):375–9.
5. Harken DE, Ellis LB. The surgical treatment of mitral stenosis; valvuloplasty. N Engl J Med. 1948;239(22):801–9.

6. Bailey CP. The surgical treatment of mitral stenosis (mitral commissurotomy). Dis Chest. 1949;15(4):377–97.
7. Inoue K, Owaki T, Nakamura T, Kitamura F, Miyamoto N. Clinical application of transvenous mitral commissurotomy by a new balloon catheter. J Thorac Cardiovasc Surg. 1984;87(3):394–402.
8. Lock JE, Khalilullah M, Shrivastava S, Bahl V, Keane JF. Percutaneous catheter commissurotomy in rheumatic mitral stenosis. N Engl J Med. 1985;313(24):1515–8.
9. Al Zaibag M, Ribeiro PA, Al Kasab S, Al Fagih MR. Percutaneous double-balloon mitral valvotomy for rheumatic mitral-valve stenosis. Lancet. 1986;1(8484):757–61.
10. Palacios I, Block PC, Brandi S, Blanco P, Casal H, Pulido JI, et al. Percutaneous balloon valvotomy for patients with severe mitral stenosis. Circulation. 1987;75(4):778–84.
11. Babic UU, Vucinic M, Grujicic SM. Percutaneous transarterial balloon valvuloplasty for end-stage mitral valve stenosis. Scand J Thorac Cardiovasc Surg. 1986;20(2):189–91.
12. Ben Farhat M, Ayari M, Maatouk F, Betbout F, Gamra H, Jarra M, et al. Percutaneous balloon versus surgical closed and open mitral commissurotomy: seven-year follow-up results of a randomized trial. Circulation. 1998;97(3):245–50.
13. Bonhoeffer P, Piéchaud JF, Sidi D, Yonga G, Jowi C, Joshi M, et al. Mitral dilatation with the Multi-Track system: an alternative approach. Cathet Cardiovasc Diagn. 1995;36(2):189–93.
14. Cribier A, Rath PC, Letac B. Percutaneous mitral valvotomy with a metal dilatator. Lancet. 1997;349(9066):1667.
15. Eltchaninoff H, Koning R, Derumeaux G, Cribier A. Percutaneous mitral commissurotomy by metallic dilator. Multicenter experience with 500 patients. Arch Mal Coeur Vaiss. 2000;93(6):685–92.
16. Harikrishnan S, Nair K, Tharakan JM, Titus T, Kumar VKA, Sivasankaran S. Percutaneous transmitral commissurotomy in juvenile mitral stenosis--comparison of long term results of Inoue balloon technique and metallic commissurotomy. Catheter Cardiovasc Interv Off J Soc Card Angiogr Interv. 2006;67(3):453–9.
17. Manjunath CN, Gerald Dorros, Srinivasa Kikkeri, Hemanna Setty, Patil Chandrakanth. Experience of percutaneous transvenous mitral commissurotomy: comparison of the triple lumen (Inoue) and double lumen (Accura) variable sized single balloon with regard to procedural outcome and cost savings. J Interv Cardiol. 1998;11107–112.
18. Nair KKM, Pillai HS, Thajudeen A, Tharakan J, Titus T, Valaparambil A, et al. Comparative study on safety, efficacy, and midterm results of balloon mitral valvotomy performed with triple lumen and double lumen mitral valvotomy catheters. Catheter Cardiovasc Interv Off J Soc Card Angiogr Interv. 2012;80(6):978–86.
19. Badheka AO, Shah N, Ghatak A, Patel NJ, Chothani A, Mehta K, et al. Balloon mitral valvuloplasty in United States: A 13 year perspective. Am J Med. 2014.

Chapter 2

Rheumatic Heart Disease—
An Epidemiological Mystery

Biju Soman

Rheumatic heart disease (RHD) is a late sequel of acute rheumatic fever (ARF), which is an autoimmune response (Fig. 2.1) to throat infection with Group A beta hemolytic streptococcus (GABHS).[1] The overall prevalence of ARF has come down in the world, particularly in the developed nations, but the gap between demand and supply of surgical intervention of RHD continues to rise over the last few decades, more so in the developing nations.[2] Recent advances in immunology have brought out interesting information that will have an impact on the way we look at its control strategies.[3]

Magnitude

Rheumatic heart disease is still one of the major public health problems in developing countries like India.[4] Quoting earlier studies, Marion et al. in their

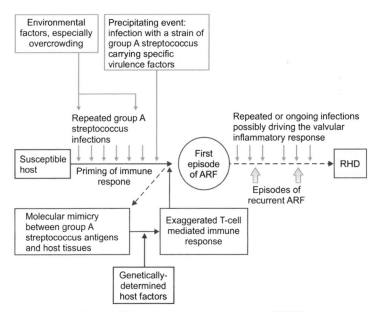

Fig. 2.1: The etiopathological pathway of RHD
(Published with permission from Lancet[2])

recent review article in the Lancet, reiterate that there would be 15.6–19.6 million people with RHD in the world.[2] The authors caution that the true prevalence of RHD as getting revealed in echocardiography-based screening, that detects clinically unapparent cases as well, would be even higher. A recent multicentric study in India done among school children using conventional methods, estimated prevalence of RHD at 0.13 to 1.5 per 1000 children in 5-9 age group and 0.13 to 1.1 per 1000 among children aged 10–14 years of age.[5] However, quoting recent echocardiography-based screening studies, including one from India, Kumar and Tanden in their review article claims that the magnitude of sub-clinical cases of RHD could be as high as 10–20 times that of manifest RH.[6,7] The highest prevalence of ARF in the developed world is seen among the school age children of the aboriginal population in Australia (245–351 per 100,000) and the pacific islanders in New Zealand (80–100 per 100,000).[2] These are the highest documented prevalence in the world, as there are not many systematic prevalence estimates for most countries in the developing world which might have more prevalence of the disease. Similarly highest reported prevalence estimates for RHD among children is from Sub-Saharan Africa (5.7 per 1000) followed by indigenous populations in Australia and New Zealand (3.5 per 1000).[1]

Recent studies from southern states like Kerala in India, report a reduction in prevalence of RHD, from 4.5/1000 (2000) among school aged children to just 0.12/1000 (2006) especially in its southern states like Kerala.[8] The reducing trend is plausible, but the true rate could be much higher if we include the subclinical cases too. For addressing the problem of RHD, we need to put these subclinical cases also under antibiotic prophylaxis as they also have the potential for progressive destruction of heart valves and resultant complications. Add to this is the frequently increasing outbreaks of ARF infections occurring in the western world, as in the case from middle class societies in the Lake Salt city in USA and the Gilia in Italy, etc.[9,10] Thus, RHD continues to be an enigma in the clinical and public health arenas of medicine.

Issues with Disease Estimation

Only 3–10% of ARF will progress towards RHD.[11] Revised Jones criteria, which has five major and four minor criteria, is widely used for diagnosing ARF in the clinical setting.[12] The presence of two or more of the major criteria like carditis, polyarthritis, chorea, erythema marginatum or subcutaneous nodules or one major criteria and two of the minor criteria like arthralgia, fever, raised erythrocyte sedimentation rate (ESR) or C–reactive protein or prolonged PR interval on electrocardiogram are suggestive of ARF in the event of antecedent GABHS infection. The presence Sydenham's chorea, indolent carditis and recurrent ARF make the diagnosis more robust. However, detection of substantial numbers of subclinical cases through echocardiographic screening by recent studies calls for a revision of the diagnostic criteria.[2,5,13-15] Inclusion of subclinical RHD as a diagnostic criteria will increase the prevalence by 10–20 fold, and that could result in changes in strategy for control and prophylaxis.[6]

Acute RF calls for long-term prophylactic medication with penicillin over varying periods of time depending on the age and the presence and sequela of carditis.[15]

Risk Factors and Contextual Determinants

The most important determinant of occurrence of rheumatic fever (RF)/RHD is the prevalence of throat infection with Group A streptococcal (GAS) infection, which is closely linked with overcrowding and compromised living conditions. This partially explains why ARF showed a definite decline even before the antibiotic era in the West.[2] The global load of significant GAS infection is around 18.1 million and these form 15–30% of all pharyngitis in children and around 5–10% of pharyngitis in adults which results in 1–2% of all hospital visits.[11] Major complications of GAS infections are ARF, RHD, Acute Post Streptococcal Glomerulonephritis (APSGN) and invasive infections, all of which except APSGN, can be considerably reduced by prompt treatment of GAS infection. As the majority of pharyngitis is caused by viral infections, it is important to restrict antibiotic treatment to bacterial infections like GAS infections.[16]

Centor criteria (tonsillar exudates, tender anterior cervical lymphadenopathy, and absence of cough and history of fever) with limited sensitivity and specificity (75%) have been widely used in developing countries to estimate ARF, although newer guidelines are being made available in the developed world.[16] Usually only less than 3% of GAS throat infections lead to ARF and this occurrence will depend on the rheumatogenicity of the organism and the genetic composition of the host. Except for a few outbreaks which occurred among the middle class sections in the West, RHD is mainly a disease of poverty and overcrowding.[17] In the West, due to improvement in living conditions, rheumatogenic strains of GAS has nearly disappeared from the community, which had brought significant reduction in the number of cases of RF.[17] It is a known fact that RF and RHD runs in families, to an extent that is over and above the influence of socioeconomic status and similarities in life events.[13] This led to the exploration of genetic basis of RF susceptibility.[2,18–20] The genes that code the human leucocyte antigen (HLA), namely HLA-DR7 and HLA-DR4 are found to be the major genetic determinants of RF/RHD in differing parts of the world.[18] Figure 2.2 shows the distribution of the HLA Class II alleles that are associated with RF/RHD.

Certain major histocompatibility complex (MHC) antigens are increasingly being linked with immune responses to GAS. It is postulated that molecular mimicry of exchanging genetic materials between host and pathogen is important in the initiation of RF/RHD as it is true in many autoimmune diseases.[21,22] Genetically susceptible persons, when exposed to streptococci with M protein antigens that have similarity with heart valve and endocardial tissues, produces excess amount of antibodies that bind with normal tissue and initiate a cascade of complement reactions, resulting in tissue distortion. (Fig. 2.3). The concept of Molecular mimicry or cross reactivity says that at the time of infection (initial infection or in subsequent subclinical infections), host cells

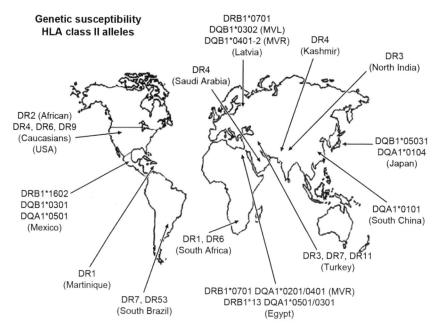

Fig. 2.2: Geographic distribution of genetic susceptibility genes. (Published with permission from Guilherme L, Köhler KF, Postol E, Kalil J. Genes, autoimmunity and pathogenesis of rheumatic heart disease. Ann Pediatr Cardiol. 2011;4:13–21)

acquired certain epitopes (groups of amino acids) from streptococci and will act as permanent antigens that continue to produce excess antibodies which in turn attack the heart valve tissues.[19,21,22]

A Mistakenly Neglected Disease

RF/RHD continues to be a neglected disease because of our real ignorance on its pathophysiology, as rightly highlighted by the Drakensberg declaration in Africa.[23,24] Although conventional school based surveys point to a global reduction in the incidence of RF/RHD, echocardiography based population screening studies in India and many other parts of the world are reporting higher rates of sub-clinical RHDs, to the extent of 10–20 times the figures of school surveys.[2,5,6] These have the potential to develop as florid clinical cases within next one-two decades, causing great suffering to people and huge economic burden to the society. Prompt treatment of GAS infections and secondary prophylaxis using very simple and cost-effective medications are sufficient to avoid the malice.[6] The African consortium had called for a population-based registry approach to tackle the issue of RF/RHD and the President of the World Heart Foundation has called for consorted action against RF/RHD as their World Heart Day message on 29 September 2013.[25,26]

Prompt health care seeking and use (even misuse) of antibiotics in the community has resulted in reduction in ARF complications of GAS infections

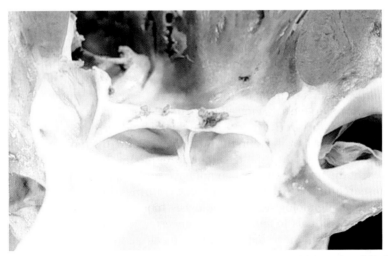

Fig. 2.3: Aortic valve showing active valvulitis. The valve is slightly thickened and displays small vegetations – verrucae (Published with permission from Binotto MA, Guilherme L, Tanaka AC. Rheumatic Fever. Images, Paediatr Cardiol. 2002;11:12-31)

in many parts of the world. A positive correlation between poverty reduction efforts in lowering the prevalence of RF and RHD (after around 2–3 decades of reduction in ARF) is evident from studies in the aboriginal populations of Australia.[1]

Control Strategies

At present there is no definite treatment modalities by which progression of RF to RHD can be prevented. Primordial prevention by way of controlling the environment by better housing and hygiene to limit the occurrence of GABHS infections is the ideal option.[25,27-30] Knowingly or unknowingly that is being done in most of the developed nations and some of the best performing developing situations like Kerala state in India. But blind adaptation of this strategy to other situations would be enormously difficult, if not utopian.

Primary prevention by way of prompt treatment of every potential GAS infections within nine days of onset of symptoms is the second best strategy; the feasibility of which also is questionable in the developing country scenario.[31] Secondary prevention by giving penicillin prophylaxis for all potential cases of RF is considered the most cost effective and practical approach in the control of RHD in the developing world.[32-34] Injectable Benzathine penicillin is the most effective method in terms of efficacy and compliance.[35,36] But the reluctance of physicians due to the scare of anaphylaxis has shifted the majority of RF/RHD patients to shift to oral penicillin with inherent problems of non-compliance and failure of therapy. Establishment of ARF/RHD registries shall enable us to the prompt adoption of these control strategies.[23,25,32] As RHD continue to be the leading cardiac ailment in developing countries, it is crucial to earmark sufficient funds to establish and maintain proper RF/RHD registries in these countries for focused and efficient control measures.[25,37,38]

Development of a rheumatic fever vaccine is another option, although it might not be feasible in the near future.[39,40] The strains of GABHS vary in different parts of the world, even within countries; for example the strains in the northern parts of India are different from those in the southern parts.[41] WHO in its report feels that the efforts to develop a vaccine may not bear fruit in the recent future due to lack of research and fund issues.[42]

Since RHD is a problem in the developing world, the developed nations are not interested to invest huge amounts of money into RF/RHD research. At present the needy countries do not have sufficient infrastructure to carry out research on RF/RHD. The southern countries should form a team of clinicians, epidemiologists, microbiologists, biomedical engineers and public health professionals to spearhead a concerted action against the disease, rather than leaving it to hapless clinicians alone to tackle the problem of RHD. The team should provide leadership for research on newer methods of prevention, potential vaccines, better diagnostics, more durable artificial heart valves, transarterial methods of valve repair, etc. WHO and governments in the developing world should realise the importance of this issue and should develop effective primary and secondary prevention strategies which will help in controlling this major cardiac problem which is a disease primarily affecting the young population.

▦ REFERENCES

1. Carapetis JR, McDonald M, Wilson NJ. Acute rheumatic fever. The Lancet. 2005;366(9480):155–68.
2. Marijon E, Mirabel M, Celermajer DS, Jouven X. Rheumatic heart disease. The Lancet. 2012;379(9819):953–64.
3. Guilherme L, Kalil J. Rheumatic heart disease: molecules involved in valve tissue inflammation leading to the autoimmune process and anti-S. pyogenes vaccine. S. pyogenes. 2013;4:352.
4. Misra M, Mittal M, Singh RK, Verma AM, Rai R, Chandra G, et al. Prevalence of rheumatic heart disease in school-going children of Eastern Uttar Pradesh. Indian Heart Journal. 2007;59(1):42.
5. Shah B, Sharma M, Kumar R, Brahmadathan KN, Abraham VJ, Tandon R. Rheumatic heart disease: progress and challenges in India. Indian J Pediatr. 2013;80 Suppl 1:577–86.
6. Kumar RK, Tandon R. Rheumatic fever & rheumatic heart disease: the last 50 years. Indian J Med Res 2013;137(4):643–58.
7. Saxena A, Ramakrishnan S, Roy A, Seth S, Krishnan A, Misra P, et al. Prevalence and outcome of subclinical rheumatic heart disease in India: the RHEUMATIC (Rheumatic Heart Echo Utilisation and Monitoring Actuarial Trends in Indian Children) Study. Heart. 2011;97(24):2018–22.
8. Kumar RK, Paul M, Francis PT. RHD in India: are we ready to shift from secondary prophylaxis to vaccinating high-risk children. Current Science. 2009;97(3):405.
9. Pastore S, Cunto AD, Benettoni A, Berton E, Taddio A, Lepore L. The resurgence of rheumatic fever in a developed country area: the role of echocardiography. Rheumatology. 2011;50(2):396–400.

10. Veasy LG, Wiedmeier SE, Orsmond GS, Ruttenberg HD, Boucek MM, Roth SJ, et al. Resurgence of acute rheumatic fever in the intermountain area of the United States. New England Journal of Medicine. 1987;316(8):421–7.
11. Assanasen S, Bearman G. Group A streptococcal disease. In: Wallace R, editor. Maxey-Rosenau-Last Public Health and Preventive Medicine, 15 edition. New York: McGraw-Hill Medical; 2007.
12. WHO. Rheumatic fever and rheumatic heart disease. World Health Organ Tech Rep Ser. 2004;923:1–122.
13. Maurice J. Rheumatic heart disease, back in the limelight. The Lancet. 2013;382(9898):1085–6.
14. Marijon E, Celermajer DS, Tafflet M, El-Haou S, Jani DN, Ferreira B, et al. Rheumatic heart disease screening by echocardiography: the inadequacy of World Health Organization criteria for optimizing the diagnosis of subclinical disease. Circulation. 2009;25;120(8):663–8.
15. Bhaya M, Panwar S, Beniwal R, Panwar RB. High prevalence of rheumatic heart disease detected by echocardiography in school children. Echocardiography. 2010;27(4):448–53.
16. Bisno AL. Landmark perspective: The rise and fall of rheumatic fever. J Jama. 1985;254(4):538–41.
17. Carapetis JR. Rheumatic heart disease in developing countries. New England Journal of Medicine. 2007;357(5):439–41.
18. Guilherme L, Köhler KF, Postol E, Kalil J. Genes, autoimmunity and pathogenesis of rheumatic heart disease. Ann Pediatr Cardiol. 2011;4(1):13–21.
19. Guilherme L, Faé KC, Oshiro SE, Tanaka AC, Pomerantzeff PMA, Kalil J. Rheumatic Fever: How S. pyogenes-Primed Peripheral T Cells Trigger Heart Valve Lesions. Annals of the New York Academy of Sciences. 2005;1051(1):132–40.
20. Rashid T, Ebringer A. Autoimmunity in Rheumatic Diseases Is Induced by Microbial Infections via Crossreactivity or Molecular Mimicry. Autoimmune Diseases. 2012;2012:e539282.
21. Cunningham MW. Streptococcus and rheumatic fever. Curr Opin Rheumatol. 2012;24(4):408–16.
22. Rashid T, Ebringer A. Autoimmunity in rheumatic diseases is induced by microbial infections via crossreactivity or molecular mimicry. Autoimmune Dis. 2012;2012:539282.
23. Mayosi B, Robertson K, Volmink J, Adebo W, Akinyore K, Amoah A, et al. The Drakensberg declaration on the control of rheumatic fever and rheumatic heart disease in Africa. S Afr Med J. 2006;96(3 Pt 2):246.
24. Watkins DA, Zuhlke LJ, Engel ME, Mayosi BM. Rheumatic fever: neglected again. Science. 2009;324(5923):37.
25. Robertson KA, Volmink JA, Mayosi BM. Towards a uniform plan for the control of rheumatic fever and rheumatic heart disease in Africa--the Awareness Surveillance Advocacy Prevention (A.S.A.P.) Programme. S Afr Med J. 2006;96 (3 Pt 2):241.
26. Bhaumik S. Doctors call for countries to step up the fight against rheumatic heart disease. BMJ. 2013;346:f3504.
27. Karthikeyan G, Mayosi BM. Is primary prevention of rheumatic fever the missing link in the control of rheumatic heart disease in Africa? Circulation. 2009;120(8):709–13.
28. Ramsey LS, Watkins L, Engel ME. Health education interventions to raise awareness of rheumatic fever: a systematic review protocol. Syst Rev. 2013;2:58.

29. Nordet P, Lopez R, Dueñas A, Sarmiento L. Prevention and control of rheumatic fever and rheumatic heart disease: the Cuban experience (1986-1996-2002). Cardiovasc J Afr. 2008;19(3):135–40.

30. Millard-Bullock D. The Rheumatic Fever and Rheumatic Heart Disease Control programme--Jamaica. West Indian Med J. 2012;61(4):361–4.

31. Cunningham MW. Streptococcus and rheumatic fever. Curr Opin Rheumatol. 2012;24(4):408–16.

32. McDonald M, Brown A, Noonan S, Carapetis JR. Preventing recurrent rheumatic fever: the role of register based programmes. Heart. 2005;91(9):1131–3.

33. Pelajo CF, Lopez-Benitez JM, Torres JM, de Oliveira SK. Adherence to secondary prophylaxis and disease recurrence in 536 Brazilian children with rheumatic fever. Pediatr Rheumatol Online J. 2010;8:22.

34. Manyemba J, Mayosi BM. Penicillin for secondary prevention of rheumatic fever. Cochrane Database Syst Rev. 2002;(3):CD002227.

35. Manyemba J, Mayosi BM. Intramuscular penicillin is more effective than oral penicillin in secondary prevention of rheumatic fever--a systematic review. S Afr Med J. 2003;93(3):212–8.

36. Manji RA, Witt J, Tappia PS, Jung Y, Menkis AH, Ramjiawan B. Cost-effectiveness analysis of rheumatic heart disease prevention strategies. Expert Rev Pharmacoecon Outcomes Res. 2013;13(6):715–24.

37. Bhaumik S. Doctors call for countries to step up the fight against rheumatic heart disease. BMJ. 2013;346:f3504.

38. Ramsey LS, Watkins L, Engel ME. Health education interventions to raise awareness of rheumatic fever: a systematic review protocol. Syst Rev. 2013;2:58.

39. Steer AC, Batzloff MR, Mulholland K, Carapetis JR. Group A streptococcal vaccines: facts versus fantasy. Curr Opin Infect Dis. 2009;22(6):544–52.

40. Dale JB. Current status of group A streptococcal vaccine development. Adv Exp Med Biol. 2008;609:53–63.

41. Steer AC, Carapetis JR. Prevention and treatment of rheumatic heart disease in the developing world. Nat Rev Cardiol. 2009;6(11):689–98.

42. WHO. WHO | Group A streptococcal vaccine development: current status and issues of relevance to less developed countries [Internet]. WHO. 2005 [cited 2014 Jul 4]. Available from: http://www.who.int/maternal_child_adolescent/documents/ivb_05_14/en/.

Chapter 3

Anatomy of the Mitral Valve

Yoav Turgeman, Hosam Hasan-Ali,
Syamkumar Menon, Raghuram A Krishnan

The mitral valve (MV) is a funnel shaped structure attached proximally to the junction of the left atrium (LA) and left ventricle (LV) and distally to the chordae tendineae which is anchored to the LV cavity. It resembles the Bishop's mitre, hence the name.

The mitral valve apparatus is a complex structure. It consists of 6 components: annulus fibrosus, leaflets, chordae tendineae, papillary muscles, posterior left atrial wall and left ventricular wall (Fig. 3.1). These six components should be considered functionally as a unit, since derangement of any one component can cause MV dysfunction.[1]

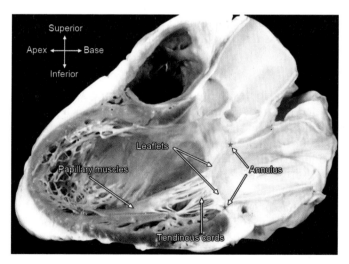

Fig. 3.1: As shown in this section of the human heart taken to simulate the parasternal long axis, echocardiographic cut, the mitral valve is a complex structure made up of the annulus, the leaflets, the tendinous cords, and the papillary muscles. Note that the superior leaflet of the valve, in fibrous continuity with the leaflets of the aortic valve, has greater depth than the inferior leaflet, which is hinged from the atrioventricular junction (Reproduced with kind permission from Robert H. Anderson and Mazyar Kanani; Mitral valve repair: critical analysis of the anatomy discussed. Multimedia Manual of Cardiothoracic Surgery doi:10.1510/mmcts.2006.002147)

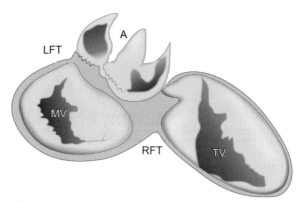

Fig. 3.2: The fibrous skeleton of the heart. Note the D shaped mitral annulus. *Abbreviations*: LFT, left fibrous trigone; RFT, right fibrous trigone; A, aortic valve; TV, tricuspid valve; MV, mitral valve (Image Courtesy: Dr Syamkumar Menon MD, McMaster University, Canada)

Mitral Annulus

The MV is attached proximally to the fibrous skeleton of the heart. The fibrous skeleton of attachment of mitral valve is D shaped and is called the mitral annulus (Fig. 3.2). The straight portion of the D is attached to the area below the aortic valve—subaortic part of mitral orifice. The curved portion (ventricular portion) is attached to the ventricular wall. During systole, the curved portion shortens while the straight part remains the same. Thus, the MV is not planar in shape as always assumed, but it is saddle shaped.[2,3]

Left Atrium

The left atrium contributes to the functioning of the MV by its contraction and relaxation.[4] The force of atrial contraction produces a jet stream across the mitral orifice. The jet stream creates an area of negative pressure, which exerts a suction effect on the valves pulling them together. In addition, eddy currents produced by the sudden movement imparted to the ventricular blood by atrial jet, exerts a force on the ventricular surface of the leaflets further aiding valvular closure.[5]

Although it has been confirmed that atrial contraction and relaxation influence MV closure in man, loss of effective atrial contraction (for example atrial fibrillation) does not necessarily cause mitral regurgitation.[4]

Mitral Valve Leaflets

The MV has 2 leaflets, anterior and posterior leaflets, connected together at junctions called commissures, which are junctions of continuous leaflet tissue.[6] This is in distinction to the semilunar valve commissures, which represent spaces between cusps. The anterior mitral leaflet (AML) occupies roughly one-third of the annular circumference and is wider than the posterior leaflet. Due to its relationships with the aortic valve and septal structures, the term "*aortic leaflet*" will be more suited.

The posterior mitral leaflet (PML) is longer, less mobile and encircles 2/3rd of the circumference of the MV orifice.[7] On the other hand, the height of the anterior mitral leaflet (AML) measured from apex to basilar attachment is almost twice the height of the posterior leaflet.[5]

Although the basal to margin length and the basilar attachment of each mitral leaflet are quite different, the surface area of each leaflet is virtually identical. The area of the leaflets is about 2.5 times the area of the mitral orifice at the level of the mitral annulus[7] permitting a large area of coaptation between their vertically directed lower borders. Although the contribution to valve closure differs between the 2 leaflets, improper function or loss of substance of either leaflet may allow severe mitral regurgitation.[5]

The posterior mitral leaflet shows considerable variation in its sub-divisions into one to three scallops; lateral, middle and medial (96% of posterior leaflets are triscalloped with the middle scallop being the largest).[8] Starting from the anterolateral commissure, towards the opposite postero-medial one, the scallops of the PML can be designated as: P1, P2, and P3 respectively. The corresponding areas of the AML (in spite of the fact that the AML is an undivided structure) are designated as A1, A2 and A3. The three scallops need not be of the same size (Fig. 3.3).

The ends of the closure line of the leaflets are referred to as commissures. The two commissures are designated as the anterolateral and postero-

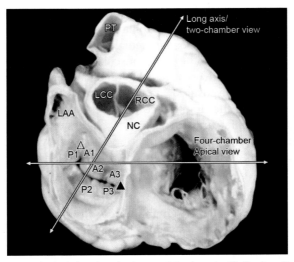

Fig. 3.3: Specimen picture showing the base of the heart with the location of two- and four-chamber echocardiographic views superimposed (double-headed arrows). (1) Base of the adult heart specimen showing the mitral valve with double-headed arrows superimposed demonstrating the two- and four-chamber echocardiographic approach. *Abbreviations:* Triangle, anterolateral commissure; black triangle, posteromedial commissure; A1–A3, divisions of the aortic mitral leaflet; P1–P3, divisions of the mural leaflet of the mitral valve; LAA, left atrial appendage; PT, pulmonary trunk; NC, noncoronary cusp of the aorta; LCC, left coronary cusp of the aorta; RCC, right coronary cusp of the aorta (Reproduced with permission from McCarthy, et al. *European Journal of Echocardiography* (2010) 11, i3–i924)

medial commissures (Fig. 3.3). Each leaflet has an atrial and a ventricular surface. The chordae tendineae are attached to the underside of the leaflets and the area of attachment of the chordae on the leaflet is called the rough zone. The area on the leaflet which is devoid of chordal attachments is called the clear zone. In normal valve closure, the two leaflets meet each other snugly along the rough zone and free edge in apposition but at an angle to the smooth zone.

Microscopic Structure of the Valve Leaflets

On microscopic examination, the leaflets have a fibrous skeleton (the fibrosa), covered towards the atrial side by a layer of myxomatous connective tissue (the spongiosa). The atrial and ventricular endocardium are continued over the leaflet surface, the so-called "atrialis" being a thin layer of collagen and elastic tissue covering the atrial aspect of the leaflets.[3]

■ MITRAL SUBVALVULAR APPARATUS

Left ventricular free wall, two papillary muscles and chordae tendineae constitute the subvalvular apparatus.

Papillary Muscles

Different from the tricuspid valve, there is no direct attachment of the mitral valve to the ventricular septum. Both the anterolateral and posteromedial papillary muscles are attached to the left ventricular free wall near the apex and its mid-third. The anterolateral papillary muscle consists of a single large trunk (and head), whereas the posteromedial papillary muscle consists of one to three heads.[9,10] They have the same muscular volume and are innervated by the left His bundle network. The posteromedial papillary muscle receives its blood supply from the posterior descending branch of the right coronary artery (depending on the dominance of the coronary artery system), and the anterolateral papillary muscle receives its blood supply from the diagonal branches of the left anterior descending artery and often by marginal branches of the left circumflex artery as well.[10]

Chordae Tendineae

They are fibrous strings which emanate from the tip of the two papillary muscles and insert into their overlying commissures and into both adjacent leaflets (Fig. 3.4).

Although the chordae tendineae system has been extensively investigated, its physiologic and functional assessment remains controversial, mainly due to large variations in number, origin, length, direction and point of insertion to the mitral leaflets. From each papillary muscle head, chordae tendineae originate and insert into the corresponding half of the two mitral leaflets. After a variable course and division (Fig. 3.4), each chordae tendineae branches into two to four small digits termed the *functional unit* that are attached to the ventricular aspect of the leaflet. Points of chordal insertion

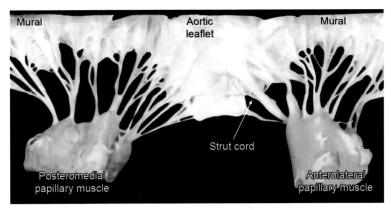

Fig. 3.4: View of the ventricular surface of an adult mitral valve. The chords extend not only from the free edge of the leaflet to the papillary muscles but also from the ventricular surface. This difference in chordal attachment, such as the stabilizing strut chords connecting the ventricular surface to the papillary muscles, demonstrates that the thickness and morphology of the leaflet varies from the annular attachment to the free edge (Reproduced with permission from McCarthy, et al. European Journal of Echocardiography (2010) 11, i3–i924)

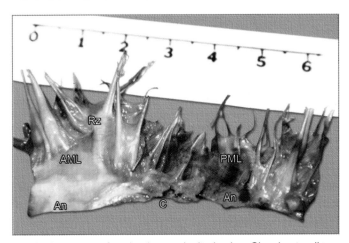

Fig. 3.5: Ventricular aspect of excised normal mitral valve. Chordae tendineae directed to the anterior mitral leaflet are inserted in the rough zone. Chordae tendineae directed to the posterior mitral leaflet inserted all along the leaflet body.
Abbreviations: AML, anterior mitral leaflet; PML, posterior mitral leaflet; An, annulus; Rz, rough zone; C, commissure

vary among the two leaflets. Most of the chordae tendineae directed to the anterior mitral leaflet terminate at the edge of the ventricular aspect (called the *rough zone),* whereas chordae tendineae directed to the posterior leaflet are inserted from the edge back along the leaflet body (called the *clear zone)* to the annular area (Fig. 3.5).

Until 1970, the most commonly used classifications of chordae tendineae were those suggested by Tandler[11] and later by Quain.[12] This classification

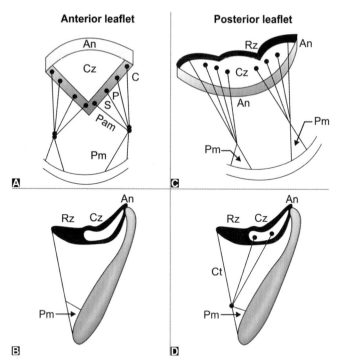

Figs 3.6A to D: A schematic of the classification of Lam et al11 showing course and point of insertion of chordae tendineae directed to the anterior and posterior mitral leaflets. Top left, A, and top right, C, present a ventricular view of the anterior and posterior mitral leaflets, respectively. Bottom left, B, and bottom right, D, present a lateral view, respectively. *Abbreviations*: An, annulus; Cz, clear zone; Rz, rough zone; Pm, papillary muscle; Ct, chordae tendineae; C, commissural; P, paracommissural; Pam, paramedian; S, strut

divides the chordae tendineae into three orders: The first order chordae tendineae insert into the leaflet's edge, the second-order chordae tendineae insert 6 to 8 mm beyond the free margins and the third- order chordae tendineae insert into the basal portion of the ventricular aspect of the posterior leaflet. Although the classification of Tandler[11] and Quain is simple to use, it neither emphasizes the morphologic differences between chordae tendineae nor relates their sites of insertion to their function.

In 1970, Lam et al[13] introduced a new classification that distinguish commissural and leaflet chordae tendineae and relates chordae tendineae function to their morphology and location (Figs 3.6A to D). As presented in Figure 3.5, according to the classification of Lam et al.[13] four types of chordae tendineae terminate at the rough zone of each half of the anterior mitral leaflet: Strut (main), commissural, paracommissural and paramedian. The strut chordae tendineae are the thickest and constitute the "skeleton" of the chordal system directed to the anterior leaflet. The average length and thickness (± SD) of chordae tendineae of the anterior leaflet are 17.5 ± 2.5 mm and

Table 3.1: Anatomic classifications of the chordae tendineae

*Tandler and Quain classification**	*Lam classification*[+]
First order	1. Commissural chordae
	2. Rough zone chordae of the anterior and posterior leaflets that insert into the free margin of both leaflets.
Second order	Rough zone chordae of the anterior and posterior leaflets that insert 6 to 8 mm beyond the free margin (strut chordae of anterior and cleft chordae of the posterior leaflets).
Third order	Basal chordae of the posterior leaflet.

* Taken from—Tandler et al[11] and Walmsley et al[12]

+ Taken from—Lam et al[13]

0.84 ± 0.28 mm) respectively.[13] The posterior mitral leaflet has three types of chordae tendineae: The basal (annular region), the cleft (indentations between scallops), and the rough zone. The average length and thickness of the rough zone chordae tendineae of the posterior leaflet is 14 ± 0.8 mm and 0.65 ± 0.24 mm, respectively.[13] Table 3.1 compares the classification of Lam et al[13] with the classification of Tandler[11] and Quain.[12] From a practical point of view, a classification based on the point of insertion has a greater advantage for both the surgeon and the interventional cardiologist.

Function of the SVA

Until two decades ago, the closure and opening of the atrioventricular valves were considered to be a passive consequence of dynamic pressure gradients between the atria and ventricles throughout the cardiac cycle; however, it has been shown by Marzilli et al[14] that opening and closing of the atrioventricular valves is an active process involving a synchronous function of all mitral structural components including the SVA. In fact, all subvalvular structures, including left ventricular free wall, papillary muscles and chordae tendineae have an important role in opening and closure of the mitral valve leaflets.[1]

During ventricular systole, the main role of papillary muscles and chordae tendineae is to prevent mitral leaflets prolapse into the left atrium. Maximal shortening and elongation of the papillary muscles occurs 65 ± 6 ms after peak shortening and elongation of the muscular wall fibers.[14] This time delay leads to active separation of both mitral leaflets during early diastole and approximation between left ventricular free wall and mitral leaflets during early systole, enabling the "keystone" mechanism of the mitral valve to happen.[15] The major contribution of the chordae tendineae to the closure of the mitral valve is by ensuring proper position of the rough zones of the two leaflets in order to maintain valve competence. Rough zone chordae tendineae are more important in preventing mitral valve prolapse than commissural chordae tendineae, whereas the strut (main) chordae tendineae are particularly the pillars of the keystone mechanism of the mitral valve.[16]

In 1983, Hetzer et al.[17] revived the concept that preservation of chordae tendineae integrity contributes to preservation of left ventricular contractility after mitral valve surgery. Studies[17,18] have shown that left ventricular function was higher in patients who underwent mitral valve replacement without resection of chordae tendineae compared to the classic operation with chordae tendineae resection. This is most probably related to preservation of left ventricular geometry.[1,17]

Left Ventricle

The last component of the mitral valve apparatus is the left ventricle. It also contributes significantly to the integrity and functioning of the mitral valve apparatus. The papillary muscles are attached to the free wall of the LV. Normal contractility and normal geometry of the left ventricle is essential for the normal functioning of the mitral valve apparatus.

■ MITRAL VALVE ORIFICE

Obviously, the major orifice of the mitral valve is the area between the leaflets but much blood passes between the interchordal spaces. The major orifice between the leaflets is called the primary mitral valve orifice. The spaces between the chordae are called secondary orifices. Since there is fusion of the chordae tendineae in rheumatic processes, it can narrow the secondary mitral orifice.

Pathological Anatomy in Rheumatic Mitral Stenosis

Rheumatic activity results in four forms of pathology of the mitral valve described by Rusted et al. who examined 70 hearts of patients with mitral stenosis; commissural (30%), cuspal (15%), chordal (10%) and combined (45%) (Table 3.2). The most commonly affected part is the area of the commissures 76%.[19]

Table 3.2: Pathological findings in 70 patients with rheumatic mitral stenosis[9]

Type of mitral stenosis	Number of cases
Commissural	22
Cuspal	11
Chordal	6
Combined:	
Cuspal + commissural	10
Chordal + commissural	10
Chordal + cuspal + commissural	11

Anatomically, the rheumatic process converts the MV into either a leathery contracted cusp (diaphragm like) or the typically funnel shaped MV, the former being twice as common as the latter. The orifice of the MV becomes fish-mouthed or buttonhole-like.[20] The maximum obstruction of this funnel shaped valve occurs at its apex, which is within the left ventricular cavity. The primary orifice located at the level of the annulus will be far less narrowed. When only one commissure is fused or one is fused more than the other, the stenotic orifice is eccentrically located. A centrally located orifice indicates symmetrical commissural fusion.[21]

Calcification may occur in any part of the MV or its associated structures but, it is found most frequently in the leaflets and in the commissural regions.[22]

The various anatomic forms of mitral stenosis affect atrioventricular filling in a similar manner. The degree of stenosis is often fixed due to commissural fusion and possibly to chordal abnormalities. However, in pure cuspal form of mitral stenosis the degree of apparent valve narrowing as evidenced clinically and hemodynamically appears more severe than that found anatomically. This physiologic anatomic dissociation is likely related to stiffened and possibly calcific valve cusps. These cusps while potentially mobile, may fail to open in response to given left atrial pressure regardless whether the commissures are fused or not. It is therefore possible to have the MV wide open on surgical or pathological inspection and yet have the valve remain severely stenotic under in vivo conditions.[21] This is not uncommon in mitral restenosis.

In rheumatic mitral stenosis the chordae tendineae are occasionally retracted such that the leaflets appear to be inserted directly into the papillary muscles. When this occurs, mitral stenosis is severe because the interchordal spaces are almost entirely obliterated. Sometimes chordae inserting into one papillary muscle are well preserved, whereas those inserting into the other papillary muscle are partially or completely fused. Such severe pathology is difficult to treat with percutaneous mitral valvotomy.

▨ REFERENCES

1. Perloff JK, Roberts WC. The mitral apparatus. Functional anatomy of mitral regurgitation. Circulation. 1972;46(2):227–39.
2. Levine RA, Triulzi MO, Harrigan P, Weyman AE. The relationship of mitral annular shape to the diagnosis of mitral valve prolapse. Circulation. 1987;75(4):756–67.
3. Muresian H, Diena M, Cerin G, Florin Filipoiu. The mitral valve: New insights into the clinical anatomy. Medica J Clin Med. 2006;80–7.
4. Williams JC, Sturm RE, Wood EH, Vandenberg RA. Effect of varying ventricular function by extrasystolic potentiation on closure of the mitral valve. Am J Cardiol. 1971;28(1):43–53.
5. Silverman ME, Hurst JW. The mitral complex. Interaction of the anatomy, physiology, and pathology of the mitral annulus, mitral valve leaflets, chordae tendineae, and papillary muscles. Am Heart J. 1968;76(3):399–418.
6. Waller BF, Schlant RC. Anatomy of the heart. In: Alexander RW, Schlant RC, Fuster V, O'Rourke RA, Roberts R, Sonnenblick EH (Eds). Hurst's "The heart." 9th ed. 19-80: New York: McGrow-Hill, health profession division; 1998.

7. Roberts WC. Morphologic features of the normal and abnormal mitral valve. Am J Cardiol. 1983;51(6):1005–28.
8. Ranganathan N, Lam JH, Wigle ED, Silver MD. Morphology of the human mitral valve. II. The value leaflets. Circulation. 1970;41(3):459–67.
9. Duplessis La, Marchand P. The anatomy of the mitral valve and its associated structures. Thorax. 1964;19:221–7.
10. Ranganathan N, Burch GE. Gross morphology and arterial supply of the papillary muscles of the left ventricle of man. Am Heart J. 1969;77(4):506–16.
11. Tandler J. Anatomie des herzens: Handbuch des anatomie des menschen. Bandelben Gustav Fish. 3:1913;84.
12. Walmsley T. Quain's anatomy: The Heart, Part III. 2nd ed. London, UK: Longman, Groen; 1929;p. 81.
13. Lam JH, Ranganathan N, Wigle ED, Silver MD. Morphology of the human mitral valve. I. Chordae tendineae: a new classification. Circulation. 1970;41(3):449–58.
14. Marzilli M, Sabbah HN, Lee T, Stein PD. Role of the papillary muscle in opening and closure of the mitral valve. Am J Physiol. 1980;238(3):H348–354.
15. Antunes MJ. Functional anatomy of the cardiac valves. In: Acar J, Bodnar E (Eds). Textbook of Acquired Heart Valve Disease. London, UK: ICR Publishers, 1995, pp. 1-37.
16. Pocock WA, Lakier JB. Mitral stenosis. In: Barlow JB (Eds). Perspective on The Mitral Valve. Philadelphia, PA: FA. Davis, 1987, pp. 151-80.
17. Hetzer R, Bougioukas G, Franz M. Mitral valve replacement with preservation of papillary muscle and chordae tendineae: revival of a seemingly forgotten concept; I. Preliminary clinical report. Thorac Cardiovasc Surg. 1983;291–6.
18. Okita Y, Miki S, Kusuhara K, Ueda Y, Tahata T, Yamanaka K, et al. Analysis of left ventricular motion after mitral valve replacement with a technique of preservation of all chordae tendineae. Comparison with conventional mitral valve replacement or mitral valve repair. J Thorac Cardiovasc Surg. 1992;104(3):786–95.
19. Edwards Je, Rusted Ie, Scheifley Ch. Studies of the mitral valve. II. Certain anatomic features of the mitral valve and associated structures in mitral stenosis. Circulation. 1956;14(3):398–406.
20. Waller B. Rheumatic and non-rheumatic conditions producing valvular heart disease. In: Fankl WS, Bnest AN (Eds). Valvular Heart Disease: Comprehensive Evaluation and Management. Philadelphia FA Davis. 1986;p.3.
21. Selzer A, Cohn KE. Natural history of mitral stenosis: a review. Circulation. 1972;45(4):878–90.
22. Lackman AS, Roberts WC. Calcific deposits in stenotic mitral valves. Extent and relation to age, sex, degree of stenosis, cardiac rhythm, previous commissurotomy and left atrial body thrombus from study of 164 operatively- excised valves. Circulation 1978;57(4):808-15.

Chapter 4

Pathological Aspects of Rheumatic Mitral Stenosis

Ruma Ray, Prasenjit Das

▓ NORMAL MITRAL VALVE

The mitral valve, so named because of its resemblance to a bishop's mitre, is a bicuspid valve, comprising of a triangular anteromedial leaflet, which is stretched diagonally from posterior-medial aspect of muscular ventricular septum and gets attached to the anterolateral wall of left ventricle. The anterior leaflet occupies one-third of the valve circumference. The longer, less mobile and quadrangular posterolateral leaflet encircles two-third of the circumference of the mitral valve leaflet.[1] The valve cusps are anchored to the myocardium by means of two fibroelastic slings, which are the extension of the subendothelial fibroelastic layers of both atria and ventricles. At the mitral valve ring these fibroelastic layers converge and unite together to form the dense collagenous skeleton of the mitral valve leaflets, the lamina fibrosa (Figs 4.1A and B). The lamina fibrosa forms the main backbone of the valve and is particularly condensed at the peripheral attached margin of the valve leaflets, called the valve annulus. On both sides of lamina-fibrosa there are narrow zones of relatively loose fibroelastic tissue, rich in proteoglycans. Both the atrial and ventricular free surfaces of valve leaflets are covered by a single layer of

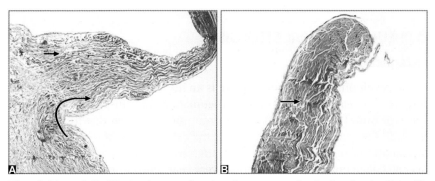

Figs 4.1A and B: Photomicrographs showing a normal mitral valve leaflet with convergent fibroelastic slings from both the atrial and ventricular surfaces to the valve annulus (A, H&E x 40). The converged fibroelastic layers form the fibrous backbone of leaflet, the lamina fibrosa (B, H&E x 40)

endothelial cell. The annular structures of all the four cardiac valves together form the central cardiac skeleton that is anchored to the collagenous tissue of endocardium, myocardium and epicardium. At the free margin, the lamina fibrosa of valve leaflets connect with the tubular fibrous chordae tendinae, which bridges the leaflets to the papillary muscles.[2]

On ultrastructural examination the endocardial cells are seen to possess many basal protrusions towards the underlying valve matrix.[3] The valve interstitial cells (VICs), that are present in the subendocardial matrix, have been shown to contain different candidate genes in normal valves, in comparison to the diseased mitral valves by affymetrix gene chip assays. Depending on the activity of these different genes, there may be 18-20 fold increase of extra-cellular matrix production in disease conditions.[4] Cardiac VICs are fundamentally tissue-specific myofibroblasts and are present in all the layers of valve tissue, although they tend to be more superficial in location than fibroblasts, keeping company with smooth muscle cells. Previously viewed more simply as cellular factories of valvular extracellular matrix, myofibroblasts are now thought to be multifunctional, playing pivotal roles in processes like cell–cell communication, regulated matrix secretion, migration, repair and contractility. These VICs can be activated by platelet derived growth factor (PDGF) and basic fibroblast growth factor (bFGF) released from the activated endocardial cells. Thus these cells are crucial in maintaining normal valvular microenvironment, as proteoglycans are thought to play an important role in the assembly of collagen fibrils and, consequently, in the maintenance of valve structure. Apart from these a few other cells are also identified in the mitral valve; however their identification requires special techniques, like immunohistochemistry against specific antigenic epitopes on these cell surfaces; e.g. CD117 positive mast cells or CD34 positive stem cells, etc.[5]

Normal mitral valve function thus requires integrity and coordinated interactions between all these cellular and structural components, namely ventricular and atrial myocardium, valve annulus, mitral valve leaflets, valve commissures and the subvalvular apparatus, including papillary muscles and chordae tendinae.[5]

■ RHEUMATIC MITRAL STENOSIS

Introduction

In the developing nations where there is an inherent shortage of health care resources, repeated episodes of acute rheumatic fever (ARF) is the commonest cause of mitral stenosis (MS). The current mortality rate due to rheumatic heart disease has, however, declined in the developed countries due to wide availability of prophylactic penicillin thereby.[6] Mitral valve disease affects over 80,000 people in North America every year, with a prevalence of 5 out of 10,000 people.[4] Screening with echocardiography reveals a higher prevalence of rheumatic heart disease as compared to clinical screening.[7]

According to a publication in 2005, the prevalence of rheumatic heart disease (RHD) is approximately 1 to 5 cases per 1000 among school-age children in developing countries, the highest prevalence being in sub-Saharan Africa. Around 15 million people are affected by RHD in the developing nations.[8] Whereas pure mitral stenosis (MS) is highly suggestive of rheumatic heart disease, MS associated with mitral regurgitation (MR) or MS with aortic stenosis may also be of rheumatic origin.[7] Only about 50% of cases of classical RHD are associated with a history of ARF. It has been estimated that 233,000 to 492,000 deaths per year occur worldwide due to RHD, of which in the developing countries the mortality is around 95 percent.[9,10]

Mitral stenosis (MS) is a condition in which the flow of oxygenated blood from left atrium to left ventricle faces resistance due to non-pliability of mitral valve leaflets as the valve leaflets become distorted, thickened, puckered and calcified with commissural fusion along with thickening and shortening of the chordae tendinae. Unless proved otherwise, MS commonly occurs due to RHD. Other rare causes of MS include congenital MS, left atrial myxoma with obstruction of the mitral valve orifice, mediastinal irradiation, intake of drugs like methysergide, infective endocarditis with obstructive vegetations, systemic lupus erythematosus, antiphospholipid antibody syndrome, rheumatoid arthritis, gout, amyloidosis, Whipple disease, carcinoid heart disease, mucopolysaccharidosis, Fabry's disease, massive calcification of mitral annulus and pseudoxanthoma elasticum.[9]

In adults non-rheumatic MS is extremely rare.[11] Roberts WC (1983) conducted an autopsy study on 1,010 patients with severe cardiac dysfunction secondary to primary valvular heart disease of which 434 (43%) had MS with or without MR. All these 434 cases of MS (100%) were rheumatic in origin.[9] Another such study by Olson and colleagues revealed that out of 452 stenotic mitral valves, 450 (99%) were classified under post-inflammatory disease (the great majority being rheumatic) and only the remaining 2 patients (0.5%) had congenitally stenotic mitral valves.[12] According to the reports from some developing countries like South Africa, the prevalence of pure rheumatic mitral stenosis (38%) was higher than either rheumatic mitral regurgitation (30.6%) or mixed group (30%).[13]

Mitral valve is the commonest valve affected in ARF. This is probably because among the four cardiac chambers, pressure difference between the left atrium and the left ventricle is the highest. In 25% cases the mitral valve is affected in an isolated manner; while in other 40% cases MS is associated with MR.[14] It has been seen that only 3% of the individuals affected by group A beta haemolytic streptococcal upper respiratory tract infection develop acute rheumatic fever. The exact etiology behind the valvular involvement in ARF is enigmatic. The proposed theories include injury by liberated oxygen labile streptolysin O,[15] abnormal immunogenic reactions due to antigenic mimicry, autoimmune reactivity due to cross reactivity of the antibodies directed against carbohydrate moiety in the streptococcal cell membrane[16] and genetic predisposition.[1] In industrialized countries, the interval between the occurrence of ARF and the onset of symptoms from MS is usually 15 to 40 years, resulting in usual clinical presentation in the third to fifth decade of life.[17] However in the developing and the under developed nations MS can occur below 20 years of age, a condition that is also known as juvenile MS.[18]

There is a recent study that has identified some possible associated factors like nanobacteria that contribute in rheumatic valve calcification. In a study by Hu YR et al. (2009) nanobacteria like particles have been detected in the calcified material of rheumatic mitral valve disease by using monoclonal antibody 8D10. They are Gram-negative bacteria that range in size from 80 to 500 nm.[19] They can produce carbonate hydroxyapatite crystals and form a hard coat surrounding themselves at pH 7.4 under physiological phosphate and calcium concentrations. The black particles of carbonate hydroxyapatite crystals in nanobacteria can be detected with TEM negative staining and appear as high density images without uranyl-acetate staining, while the rest of the proteins require uranyl-acetate staining.[19]

Valvular calcification in RHD is not a random passive process. It is a dynamic and finely regulated inflammatory cellular process that involves expression of osteoblast markers like osteopontin and osteocalcin along with neoangiogenesis.[20]

Pathophysiology

Acute rheumatic fever (ARF) leads to pancarditis of which it is the valvular endocarditis that plays a key role in the pathogenesis of MS. In valvular endocarditis the valve becomes oedematous, swollen and small fibrin rich vegetations are seen along with the line of contact of the valve leaflets, i.e. 1–2 mm away from the free edge. Collagen beneath the vegetations shows degenerative changes and an occasional Aschoff's nodule. Following an episode of ARF healing occurs by fibrosis. With repeated bouts of ARF there is progressive fibrosis of the valve leaflets. Fibrosis is not anatomically confined within a single leaflet and it encroaches from one leaflet to the other through the commissures that finally results in commissural fusion. Progressive fibrosis leads to thickening of valve leaflet that becomes less pliable and finally stenosis ensues.

The normal area of the mitral valve orifice is 4–6 sq. cm. When it is reduced to 2 sq.cm, there is increased left atrial pressure as the flow from left atrium is obstructed. Increased left atrial pressure results in pulmonary arterial hypertension. Critical MS occurs when the opening is reduced to 1 sq. cm. The left atrial pressure then reaches to such a level that leads to hyperplasia and hypertrophy of pulmonary vein and capillaries, resulting in elevated pulmonary pressure.[1] Longstanding elevated pulmonary artery pressure leads to pulmonary incompetence, hypertrophy and dilatation of right ventricle. The tricuspid valve ring dilates and eventually there is right sided cardiac failure along with functional tricuspid regurgitation.[21,22] Symptoms of heart failure (orthopnoea, paroxysmal dyspnoea and occasionally haemoptysis) develop as the mitral valve orifice decreases to less than 1.0–1.5 cm.

Progressive left atrial enlargement and residual blood in left atrium leads to dilatation of left atrial appendage and mural thrombus formation due to blood stasis; in 9–20% of the affected older patient's these mural thrombi may embolize.[1,22] Up to 40% of patients with MS may develop atrial fibrillation.[22] Fibrosis of the left atrial wall and disorganization of atrial musculature lead to alteration of normal conduction velocity and refractory period. There is premature atrial activation, resulting in atrial fibrillation. Atrial fibrillation leads to inefficient filling of the left ventricle; resulting in decreased cardiac output. A vicious cycle is thus created as low cardiac output may increase the heart rate and further causes inefficient cardiac filling. However, mostly the left ventricular function itself is usually well maintained in pure MS.[23]

Pathology

Though traditionally the whole diseased mitral valve is removed; nowadays there is a trend to excise the anterior leaflet of mitral valve during valve replacement surgery or only a part of the posterior mitral valve leaflet is removed for reparative procedures.[24] Before starting the embedding procedure the excised leaflets are kept in 4% neutral formal buffer saline for proper fixation. Then the leaflets are photographed both from the atrial and the ventricular surfaces and examined closely under a hand-lens for presence of any vegetation. Then the valves are examined in terms of transparency, color, pliability, hard calcified foci, any hemorrhagic focus, commissural fusion, appearance and length of chordae tendinae and appearance of papillary muscles. In addition, the annular diameter is measured using valve sizers to determine the extent of stenosis. If valve sizers are not available threads may be used to determine the total annular area with the aid of a scale. All these parameters can be semi-quantified.[25] Several sections are taken for histopathological examination including the free edges and from macroscopically visible abnormal areas. If the specimen includes chordae tendinae and tip of the papillary muscles, then the subvalvular apparatus (SVA) should be sectioned for microscopic examination. The SVA includes the left ventricular free wall, two papillary muscles and chordae tendinae. The anterior mitral valve leaflet can be sectioned from the inter-chordal space at the free margin to the base of its attachment, while the posterior mitral valve leaflet can be taken in a similar manner through the center of the leaflet component closest to the posteromedial commissure. Removal of an entire diseased valve is presently a rare surgical procedure.

Macroscopic Features

Grossly only one or both valve cusps may be received for histopathological examination depending on the requirements and surgical procedures performed. In any of these conditions the mitral leaflets are opaque and may show foci of whitish dots of calcification. On palpation the leaflets are stiff and hard at areas owing to calcification. The valves may show retraction of free edges. Vegetations may be seen on the atrial surface of the cusps. The chordae are thickened, firm, shortened and adherent to each other. The sub-valvular inter-chordal space may disappear in up to 40% cases of rheumatic MS as seen in autopsy series, with short thick chords attached almost directly to the papillary muscles. This impedes the interchordal blood flow and causes subvalvular stenosis. There is commissural fusion and at the commissures

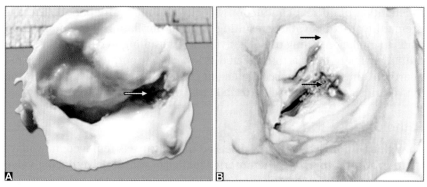

Figs 4.2A and B: (A) Pearly white calcified nodules are seen focally. Near the valve closure line, there are erosion and microthrombi (white arrow); (B) Gross photomicrograph of surgically excised mitral valves showing thickened, opaque and scarred valve leaflets with commissural fusion (black arrows)

of mitral valves, there is often loss of surface endothelium with erosion and overlying small thrombus formation (Figs 4.2A and B). Severe deformity of SVA has been shown to impact the outcome of percutaneous balloon mitral vulvoplasty adversely and if present valve replacement surgery becomes a better option.[26] It is so because in absence of active SVA, mitral valve is characteristically retracted. Retraction of MV also leads to mitral regurgitation (MR).

Sometimes the specimen of the heart can be received for histopathological examination after an autopsy procedure. Rarely, the pericardium shows features of fibrinous 'bread and butter' pericarditis, which is more commonly seen in hearts with ARF (Fig. 4.3A). Grossly the left auricle and the left atrium are dilated. The left ventricular shape is usually normal. In severe MS the left ventricle can be atrophic and appear smaller. In long standing MS, there can be dilatation of the root of pulmonary artery and right ventricle. Right atrial dilatation associated with a thrombus is an extremely rare finding. In 3-8% of cases the free thrombus in dilated left atrial cavity behaves as a 'ball thrombus' and aggravates the stenosis. Thrombosis may often be seen inside the atrial appendage or it may protrude into the atrial cavity. In a few cases of severe MS there may be calcification of the left atrial endocardium. On opening the left side of heart, the mitral valve may attain a typical 'fish mouth' or 'button hole' appearance when visualized from the atrial aspect (Fig. 4.3B). There is usually marked fibrosis of the mitral valve leaflets with commissural fusion. Calcification may occur either in the form of nodules or plaques (Fig. 4.3C) and are mostly seen towards commissures. Annular circumference is usually normal; however, the commissures are usually deformed and show fusion with the adjacent valve leaflet. The attached chordae tendineae are short (defined by a reduced length, measuring half of the normal length) and stout/thickened (defined as increased thickness of >3 times the normal thickness). The adjacent chordae are commonly fused. The scarring and contraction along with shortening of the chordae causes the inter-adherent leaflets giving

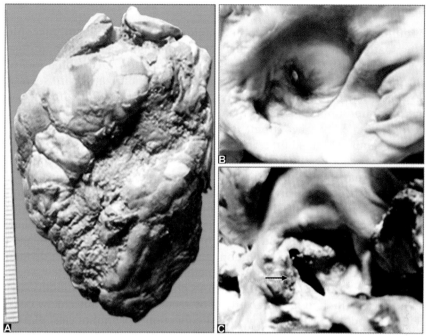

Figs 4.3A to C: (A) The pericardial surface of the heart show thickening and opacity of the pericardium with numerous ragged fibrinous tags hanging from its surface, commonly called the "bread and butter" pericarditis; (B) Gross photograph of a severely stenotic mitral valve seen through the left atrial cavity show a typical 'fish mouth' mitral orifice; (C) Photograph of another severely stenotic mitral valve show numerous small calcified nodules (black arrow), as seen along the closure line of fused valve leaflets

a funnel-like appearance; where the inlet of the funnel is at the level of mitral annulus and the tip is in the inlet of the left ventricular cavity. Sometimes the chordal shortening may be so severe that the valve appears to sit directly on the tip of the papillary muscles. Though these chordal abnormalities are common, they are not imperative for a diagnosis of a rheumatic mitral valvular disease.[6] Papillary muscles on cross section may show focal or diffuse fibrosis, in contrast to the hypertrophied papillary muscles in mitral regurgitation.[25-29] In the deformed mitral valve leaflets, occasionally there may be 'Lambl's excrescences', which may mimic as a papillary tumor on the atrial surface of the deformed mitral valve cusp.[30,31] Grossly the presence of 'bread and butter' pericarditis and vegetations of ARF implies activity. These vegetations are small and seen along the line of closure of the valve leaflets.

Hence morphologically, rheumatic involvement of the mitral valve is defined as diffuse fibrous thickening of the margins of closure; where one or both the valve commissures are fused, resulting in either an eccentric or centrally located stenotic mitral valve orifice.[6] Rusted et al (1956) described four types of stenosis. These types were classified as: commissural, cuspal, chordal and combined. The latter group is the most common and accounts for more than 50% of the cases.[31]

Microscopic Features

Rheumatic MS is a macroscopic diagnosis. However on microscopic examination, the leaflet substance shows collagen degeneration, diffuse fibrosis with hyalinization and areas of calcification. Occasional foci of chronic inflammatory cell infiltrate and neovascularization are seen. A rare case may reveal presence of amyloid. However, according to a study the commonest finding in a rheumatic mitral valvular lesion is the myxoid degeneration of the valve stroma that occurs due to excessive accumulation of glycosaminoglycans in the valve stroma produced by the VIC cells[7] (Fig. 4.4). Neovascularization is another common finding in RHD[27-29] (Fig. 4.5). Rarely one may encounter presence of Aschoff nodule which is the diagnostic hallmark of rheumatic heart disease. First described by Aschoff in 1904, Aschoff nodule is formed by collection of lymphocytes, plasma cells, histiocytes with caterpillar cells having single or multiple nuclei (Anitschkow's or Aschoff cells) and giant cells around a focus of fibrinoid necrosis of the collagen (Fig. 4.6). According to its evolution, an Aschoff nodule has been divided into: (i) an acute phase (fibrinoid degeneration), that occurs after few weeks of an attack of ARF and, (ii) granulomatous phase occurring 3–6 months after an attack of ARF and is characterized by recruitment of Anitschkow cells[6] (Figs 4.6 and 4.7). Hence even a focal collection of lymphocytes, plasma cells, fibrinoid material and histiocytes in an appropriate clinical setting may indicate an early Aschoff nodule formation.[32] In the granulomatous phase, the Anitschkow cells and the Aschoff giant cells, which commonly express HLA-DR antigen, form relatively well recognized nodules. Presence of such nodules is pathognomonic of rheumatic valvular heart disease; however it does not necessarily indicate an ongoing rheumatic fever or activity.[6] They are commonly seen in the interstitial spaces of myocardium, especially at posterior

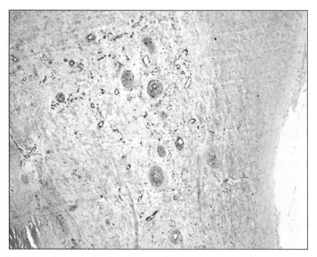

Fig. 4.4: Photomicrograph of a rheumatic mitral valve leaflet showing myxoid degeneration of the stroma and neovascularization (H&E × 100)

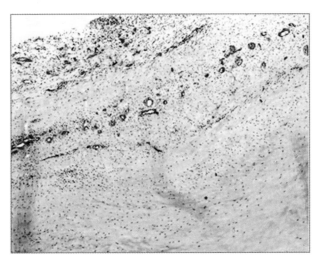

Fig. 4.5: A rheumatic mitral valve leaflet showing prominent neovascularization and subendothelial collection of moderately dense chronic inflammatory cell infiltrate (H&E × 100)

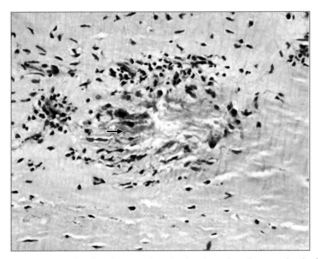

Fig. 4.6: Photomicrograph of a rheumatic mitral valve showing an Aschoff nodule in granulomatous phase, with fibrinoid necrosis in the center of the nodule (black arrow), surrounded by lymphocytes, plasma cells and histiocytes with typical caterpillar like nuclear chromatin (H&E × 200)

wall of left atrium and ventricles, as well in the inter-ventricular septum and in endocardium. They are rarely seen in the valve substance. Valvular involvement in ARF also includes aggregation of fibrin and platelets forming small (1-3 mm) vegetations sometimes called "verrucae" along the lines of closure of the valve leaflets. Organization of these verrucae or the thrombi at the commissures or the chordae is the main cause of mitral cusp deformity or sub-valvular stenosis in the absence of rheumatic activity.[30]

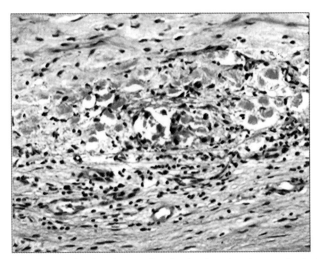

Fig. 4.7: Photomicrograph of a rheumatic mitral valve showing an Aschoff nodule in acute phase with inflammatory cell infiltrate around the lamina fibrosa with fibrinoid necrosis (H&E × 400)

Among the chronic changes of rheumatic carditis, there may be calcification of the mitral valve cusps or the annulus that depends on the patient's age, sex, severity of the valve damage and the pressure gradient between the left atrium and the ventricle. Calcification occurs following degeneration of the valve components. Lesser or minimal calcium deposition, as identified by bowing of the leaflets in 2 dimensional echocardiogram (2D echo) may still be an indication of surgical or balloon valvoplasty; severe calcium deposition on the other hand, as identified by no/minimum valve movement on 2D echo, is unsuitable for valvoplasty. Extensive calcium deposition is usually noted in older male patients with higher pressure gradient across the mitral valve.[11,6] The process of calcification usually starts at the leaflet tip and gradually extends towards the annulus. The calcific nodules may erode the endocardial layer and result in thrombus formation. The atrial appendage is often biopsied during correction of mitral stenosis and is seen to be affected in 50% of the rheumatic mitral valvular diseases. It shows hypertrophy of muscle fibers in form of pleomorphism and anisonucleosis.[7]

In an interesting study by Leão1 SC et al. (2012), the authors have demonstrated high expression of endothelin receptor A (ETr-A) and ETr-B in stenotic MV. While the ETr-A causes vasoconstriction, along with stimulation of fibroblasts and release of pro-inflammatory cytokines leading to deposition of type 1 collagen and inflammation of MV; the ETr-B receptor causes vasodilatation and counteracts the effects of Etr-A. The latter may be responsible for vascularity and calcification of the valve cusps. These findings are interesting in view that if validated further, these receptors can be selectively targeted to reduce the pathological deformity in RF.[33] On the other hand in other studies it has been shown that the cross reactivity of streptococcal antigens and MV components are noted due to binding of streptococcal cell wall components to HLA-DR, mannose binding lectins (MBL) or toll like receptors (TLR) present on the MV. These receptors-ligand binding lead to release of TNF-α and other pro-inflammatory cytokines, leading to inflammatory deformity.[34] In contrast some authors had suggested an autoimmune link to development of rheumatic MS, in view of their finding of reduced circulating CD4+CD25+ immune regulatory FoxP3 cells.[35] These theories though seem to be diverse but may be inter-linked, which need to be established further.

Mitral Valve with Previous Mitral Valvoplasty/Valve Replacement

Often mitral valve leaflets may be excised and submitted for evaluation following re-stenosis after a previous valvoplasty or commissurotomy due to MS. On microscopical examination the valve leaflets, in addition to the changes of rheumatic MS show healed commissurotomy fracture lines and calcification or thrombi along these lines. Restenosis occurs either due to rheumatic activity, inadequate surgical excision or cicatrization of valvotomy lesion. It may also result due to organization of thrombi. In mechanical dysfunction of the prosthetic valve, usually adherent antemortem clot is identified on the prosthetic valve. In autopsied cases with prosthetic valve implantation, the specimen should be carefully examined for valvular dehiscence with paravalvular leak, pannus formation, thrombosis and presence of infective vegetations.

Pathology of Complications of Rheumatic Mitral Valve Stenosis

As already discussed, pulmonary hypertension (PHT) develops in about 70% of patients with RHD. The morphological findings in PHT following rheumatic MS include mascularization of the interalveolar septae along with intraalveolar deposit of hemosiderin laden macrophages and moderate medial hypertrophy of the medium sized branches of pulmonary arteries.[36]

Massive left atrial ball thrombus may develop in 3–8% of cases. Atrial fibrillation, endocardial calcification or calcification of the free atrial wall may be identified in severe mitral stenosis, as a complication of rheumatic endocarditis. Single chordae may rupture and the ruptured end of the chordae may lie free or may adhere to the adjacent chordae.

Giant cell myocarditis like lesion with small multinucleated cells in the left atrial wall or atrial appendage may be seen as a non-specific lesion to myocardial stress of severe mitral stenosis.[29] Postsurgical myocardial dysfunction may develop due to rheumatic coronary vasculitis. Due to the rheumatic vasculitis of renal arteries the patients may develop systemic hypertension.[30]

ACKNOWLEDGEMENT

We thankfully acknowledge the contribution of Shiv K Chowdhury, MS, MCh, Professor of Cardiovascular Surgery for providing the excised valve specimens.

▓ REFERENCES

1. Rahimtoola SH, Enriquez-Sarano M, Schaff HV, Frye RL. Mitral valve disease. Editor in chief: Hurst JW; Editors: Fuster V, Alexander RW, O'Rourke RA; Associate editors: Roberts R, King III SB, Wellens HJJ. Hurst's the Heart, 10th edition. McGraw-Hill, New Delhi. 2001. pp 1687–729.
2. Young B. Heath JW (Eds). Wheater's Functional Histology. A Text and Colour Atlas. Chapter 8. Circulatory System, 4th Edition. Churchill Livingstone, Spain. 2000;pp146–7.
3. Minshall RD, Tiruppathi C, Vogel SM, Malik AB. Vesicle formation and trafficking in endothelial cells and regulation of endothelial barrier function. Histochem Cell Biol. 2002;117:105–12.
4. Cruz RP, Rezai N, Walinski H, Luo Z, Triche T, McManus BM, et al. Granville. Mitral valve disease: a genomic comparison of valvular interstitial cells from normal, floppy and rheumatic valves. Cardiovascular Pathology. 2004;13:S17–S79.
5. Prunotto M, Caimmi PP, Bongiovanni M. Cellular pathology of mitral valve prolapsed. Cardiovascular Pathology. doi:10.1016/j.carpath.2009.03.002.
6. Marcus RH, Sareli P, Pocock WA, Barlow JB. The Spectrum of Severe Rheumatic Mitral Valve Disease in a Developing Country: Correlations among Clinical Presentation, Surgical Pathologic Findings, and Hemodynamic Sequelae. Ann Intern Med. 1994;120:243–45.
7. Marifon E, Ou P, Celemafer DS, Ferreira B, Mocumbi AO, Jani D, et al. Prevalence of rheumatic heart disease detected by Echocardiographic screening. N Eng J Med. 2007;357:470–6.
8. Carapetis JR, Steer AC, Mulholland EK, Weber M. The global burden of group A streptococcal diseases. Lancet Infect Dis. 2005;5:685–94.
9. Schoen FJ, Edwards WE. Valvular heart disease: general principles and stenosis. In: Silver MD, Gotlieb AI, Schoen FJ (Eds). Cardiovascular Pathology. USA. Churchill Livingstone; 2001:402–42.
10. Carapetis JR, Steer AC, Mulholland EK, Weber M. The global burden of group A streptococcal diseases. Lancet Infect Dis. 2005;5:685–94.
11. Rowe JC, Bland EF, Sprague HB, White PD. The course of mitral stenosis without surgery: Ten and twenty years perspectives. Ann Intern Med. 1960;52:741–49.
12. Olson LJ, Subramanian R, Ackermann DM, Orszulak TA, Edwards WD. Surgical pathology of the mitral valve. A study of 712 cases spanning 21 years. Mayo Clin Proc. 1987;62:22–34.
13. Marcus RH, Sareli P, Pocock WA, Barlow JB. The spectrum of severe rheumatic mitral valve disease in a developing country. Correlations among clinical presentation, surgical pathologic findings, and hemodynamic sequelae. Ann Intern Med. 1994;120:177–83.
14. Hortskotte D, Niehues R, Strauer BE. Pathomorphological aspects, aetiology and natural history of acquired mitral valve stenosis. Eur Heart J. 1991;12(5 suppl B) 5–60.
15. Ginsburg I. Mechanism of cell and tissue injury induced by group A streptococci: Relation to past streptococcal sequelae. J Infect Dis. 1972;126:419–39.
16. Goldstein I, Halpern B, Robert L. Immunogenic relationship between streptococcus A polysaccharide and the structural glycoproteins of heart valve. Nature. 1967;213:44.
17. Horstkotte D, Niehues R, Strauer BE. Pathomorphological aspects, aetiology and natural history of acquired mitral valve stenosis. Eur Heart J. 1991;12(suppl B):55–60.

18. Yonga GO, Bonhoeffer P. Percutaneous transvenous mitral commissurotomy in juvenile mitral stenosis. East African Medical Journal. 2003;80:172–74.
19. Hu YR, Zhaoa Y, Suna YW, Lüb YD, Liua ZL, Lia JM, et al. Detection of nanobacteria-like material from calcified cardiac valves with rheumatic heart disease. Cardiovascular Pathology. doi:10.1016/j.carpath.2009.06.004.
20. Rajamannan NM, Nealis TB, Subramanian M, Panolya S, Stock SR, Ignatiev CI, et al. Calcified rheumatic valve neoangiogenesis is associated with vascular endothelial growth factor expression and osteoblast like bone formation. Circulation. 2005;111:3296–3301.
21. Waller BF. Rheumatic and non rheumatic conditions producing valvular heart disease. In Frankl WS, Brest AN (Eds). Cardiovascular clinics. Valvular Heart Disease: Comprehensive evaluation and management. Philaedelphia, F.A. Davis, 1986, pp. 3–104.
22. Meisner JS, Keren G, Pajaro OE, Mani A, Strom JA, Frater RW, et al. Atrial contribution to ventricular filling in mitral stenosis. Circulation. 1991;84:1469–80.
23. Gaasch WH, Folland ED. Left ventricular function in rheumatic mitral stenosis. Eur Heart J. 1991;12 (suppl B):66-69.
24. Roberts WC, Morrow AG. Cardiac valves and the surgical pathologist. Arch Pathol. 1966;82:309-13.
25. Rosai J. Rosai and Ackerman's Surgical Pathology. 9th edition (Vol. 2). Mosby, India. 2004;pp 2422-24.
26. Turgeman, Atar S, Rosenfeld T. The subvalvular apparatus in rheumatic mitral stenosis; Methods of assessment and therapeutic implications. Chest. 2003; 124:1929-36.
27. Olson LJ, Subramanian R, Ackermann DM, Orszulak TA, Edwards WD. Surgical pathology of the mitral valve. A study of 712 cases spanning 21 years. Mayo Clin Proc. 1987;62:22-34.
28. Dare AJ, Veinot JP, Edwards WD, Tazelaar HD, Schaff HV. New observations on the etiology of aortic valve disease. A surgical pathologic study of 236 cases from 1990. Hum Pathol. 1993;24:1330-8.
29. Hanson TP, Edwards BS, Edwards JE. Pathology of surgically excised mitral valves. One hundred consecutive cases. Arch Pathol Lab Med. 1985;109:823-8.
30. Pomerance A. Chronic rheumatic and other inflammatory valve disease (Chapter 11). In Pomerance A, Davis MJ (eds). The Pathology of the Heart. Blackwell Scientific Publications. London. 1975. pp 307-25.
31. Rusted IE, Scheiflay CH, Edwards JE. Studies of the mitral valve: certain anatomic features of the mitral valve and associated structures in the mitral stenosis. Circulation. 1956;14:398–405.
32. Love GL, Restrepo C. Aschoff bodies of rheumatic carditis are granulomatous lesions of histiocytic origin. Mod Pathol. 1988;1:256–61.
33. Leão1 SC, Souto FMS, da Costa RV, Rocha TFA, Pacheco YG, Rodrigues TMA. Gene expression of endothelin receptors in replaced rheumatic mitral stenotic valves. Rev Bras Cir Cardiovasc. 2012;27(4):512–9.
34. Artola RT, Mihos CG, Santana O. The immunology of mitral valve stenosis. Int J Interferon, Cytokine and Mediator Research 2011;3:1-8.
35. Yildiz A, Ozeke1 O, Aras D, Balci M, Deveci B, Ergun K, et al. Circulating CD4+CD25+ T cells in rheumatic mitral stenosis. The Journal of Heart Valve Disease 2007;16:461–7.
36. Tandon HD, Kasturi J. Pulmonary vascular changes associated with isolated mitral stenosis in India. Br Heart J. 1975;37:26–36.

Chapter 5

Pathophysiology, Natural History and Hemodynamics of Mitral Stenosis

Krishnakumar M, Mahesh Kumar S, Arun SR

Rheumatic fever and RHD is a sequelae of beta hemolytic streptococcal throat infection triggering an autoimmune reaction in the human body. The autoimmune response is both cell and humoral immunity mediated. There is evidence to show that the development of valvular pathology is an ongoing process.[1,2]

The orifice area of normal mitral valve is about 4 to 6 cm². The chronic rheumatic activity results in one or more of the following pathological processes after a variable latent period:

1. Fusion of commissures.
2. Thickening, fibrosis, retraction of edges of valve leaflets.
3. Calcification of leaflet tissue.
4. Shortening, thickening and fusion of chordae.

These pathological processes results in a funnel-shaped mitral apparatus in which the orifice of the mitral opening is narrowed. Interchordal fusion obliterates the secondary orifices, and commissural fusion narrows the principal orifice.[3,4] When the valve area reduces to < 2.5 cm² blood can flow from left atrium (LA) to left ventricular (LV) only if propelled by a pressure gradient. Obstruction to mitral valve flow occurs due to:

1. Reduced leaflet opening due to the above-mentioned factors (reduction of primary orifice).
2. Subvalvular obstruction (reduction in secondary orifice).
3. Rarely, mitral annular calcification.[3-6]

■ NATURAL HISTORY OF MITRAL STENOSIS

The above-mentioned pathophysiological changes gradually develop over several years. There is usually a time interval of several years between the initial attack of carditis and the clinical evidence of mitral stenosis (MS).

Bland and Jones,[7] in their 20 years follow-up study of children with acute rheumatic fever, showed that in the majority of cases the process of development of MS takes longer than a decade.

The majority of patients with fully developed MS remain asymptomatic for a varying length of time. Thus, there is a "latent" period of MS, which might be subdivided into two stages: first, the stage of formation of MS, and second, the asymptomatic stage of fully developed MS.[8] Wood's[9] series showed that the latent period lasted over an average of 19 years: the mean age for the attack of carditis was 12 years and the age at the appearance of symptoms, 31 years. Wood[9] also estimated that from the onset of symptoms to the stage of total disability, an average of 7 years elapsed.

There is significant difference in the age of onset of symptoms among patients in developing and developed countries.[10-13] In developing countries 25–40% of the patients with MS developed significant symptoms before the age of 20 years,[11-13] while this was at fourth or fifth decade in developed countries.[10]

Roy et al[13] coined the term Juvenile MS to this entity where the patients present before the age of 20 years. The early presentation may be due to the increased virulence of the *Streptococcus* organism causing a more severe primary rheumatic insult or the repeated subclinical streptococcal infections these patients are exposed to.

Development of pulmonary hypertension is a major event in the natural history of MS. Pulmonary hypertension is a prognostic variable affecting the natural history of MS.[14,15]

About 50% of patients have one or more episodes of acute deterioration due to one of the complications of MS. Atrial fibrillation is the most common complication of MS (40%).[9] Atrial fibrillation often starts in a paroxysmal form; later, it may appear in persistent form, but usually responds to antiarrhythmic therapy, and finally, it becomes permanent and therapy resistant form.

Systemic emboli are among the most dreaded complications of MS. The incidence of systemic embolism is 9–14% in patients with MS, 65–70% of these will be cerebral embolism.[16-18]

Causes of death: It is reported that 62% of patients died of CHF or pulmonary edema, 22% due to thromboembolic complications and 8% due to infections. So a total of 92% of the patients died due to direct effect of MS.[16]

The above-mentioned data is based on the natural history studies done in the preintervention era. This definitely must have been altered with the advent of closed mitral valvotomy, open mitral valvotomy and mitral valve replacement and the facilities for early diagnosis and treatment.

■ PATHOPHYSIOLOGY OF MITRAL STENOSIS

Subsequent to the above-mentioned pathophysiological processes, the mitral valve orifice becomes progressively smaller, and leads to at least three distinct and important circulatory changes.

The first is the development of a pressure gradient across the mitral valve. While the LV mean diastolic pressure remains at its normal level of about 5 mm Hg, the left atrial mean pressure rise progressively and can reach even up to about 25 mm Hg or more.

A second major circulatory change is reduction of blood flow across the mitral valve, i.e. reduction of the cardiac output. The flow is determined not only by cardiac output, but also by the duration of time for diastolic flow (diastolic filling period).

The third hemodynamic sequelae of MS is the stagnation of blood in the LA. Peak LV inflow velocities across the normal mitral valve may reach 0.8–1.2 m/s. But in severe MS, velocities reach 3 m/s or more. The transmitral flow velocities which increase during exercise may reach up to 3.5 m/s. When the LA pressure increases to >25 mm Hg imbalance between hydrostatic and oncotic pressures occur in the pulmonary vasculature leading to pulmonary edema.

Severity of Mitral Stenosis (ACC-AHA)[6]

	Mild	*Moderate*	*Severe*
Mean gradient (mm Hg)	<5	5–10	>10
PASP (mm Hg)	<30	30–50	>50
Valve area (cm²)	>1.5	1–1.5	<1.0

But in the 2014 Guidelines, ACC-AHA has proposed a different classification. Stages A–D. [Stage A is doming of mitral valve with normal hemodynamics. Progressive MS (Stage B is MVA >1.5 cm² and PHT <150 ms and normal pulmonary pressure). Severe and very severe MS (asymptomatic – stage C and symptomatic – stage D)] are as in Table 5.1

Table 5.1: Classification of MS – Based on 2014 ACC-AHA guidelines			
	Progressive MS	*Severe MS*	*Very severe MS*
Mitral valve area (cm²)	>1.5	<1.5	<1
Pulmonary artery systolic pressure (mm Hg)	<30	>30	
Pressure half time (ms)	<150	>150	>220

In MS, the stenosis occur serially at two levels: first at the mitral valve level and then in the arterioles of the lung, when pulmonary vascular disease develops.

The following are the different clinical and hemodynamic syndromes in patients with significant MS (Fig. 5.1).

1. Patient with mild/moderate MS, normal pulmonary vascular resistance and normal sized heart (symptomatic only when stressed hemodynamically).
2. Acutely decompensated patient with severe MS, normal pulmonary vascular resistance and normal sized heart in acute pulmonary edema.
3. Relatively asymptomatic patient with severe MS, increase in pulmonary vascular resistance and RV hypertrophy.
4. Severe MS, extreme degree of pulmonary vascular resistance, pulmonary hypertension, RV dilatation and right ventricular failure.

When both heart rate and cardiac output increase in situations such as exercise, the rise in left atrial pressure is dramatic. Due to the elevated venous pressure, there will be intra-alveolar edema. In the initial stages the extruded fluid will be cleared by the increased lymphatic drainage. When the LA pressure

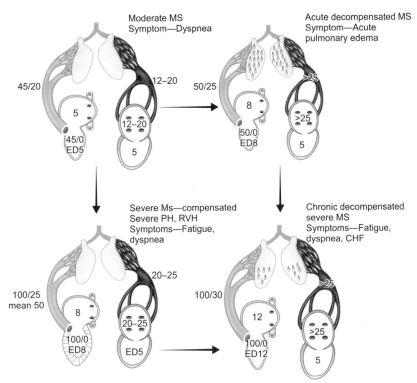

Fig. 5.1: Different hemodynamic stages of mitral stenosis (MS—mitral stenosis, PH—pulmonary hypertension, RVH—right ventricular hypertrophy, CHF—congestive heart failure)

increases to >25 mm Hg, the imbalance between hydrostatic and oncotic pressures in the pulmonary vasculature overwhelms all the compensatory mechanisms resulting in acute pulmonary edema.

The bronchial veins become dilated consequent to the increased venous pressure. Hemoptysis may occur due to the rupture of these bronchial veins.

The increased pulmonary vascular resistance and the resultant low cardiac output protect the patient from developing pulmonary congestion by avoiding surge of blood from PA into the pulmonary capillary bed.

The decreased lung compliance and vital capacity because of the above-mentioned effects underlie dyspnea on exertion which is the predominant symptom in MS.

OBSTRUCTIVE PHYSIOLOGY OF MITRAL STENOSIS

The transmitral pressure gradient depends on the valve area and the flow rate. As we know, doubling of the flow rate quadruples the pressure gradient.

Many patients with MS will go on without symptoms unless they face a physiological or pathological situation which results in hemodynamic stress.

The first bouts of dyspnea in patients with MS are usually precipitated by tachycardia (exercise, pregnancy, infection, hyperthyroidism, sexual activity) which causes an increase in rate of transmitral flow and decrease in the diastolic filling time. In some patients, the symptoms may be gradual in onset, but in some patients, the disease may be unmasked when the patients develop atrial fibrillation (AF).

One important point to remember is that the rate of valve narrowing is not predicted by initial mitral valve area (MVA) or mitral valve gradient (MVG). Mitral valve obstruction leads to adaptive changes in LA, LV, pulmonary vasculature and right heart resulting in the clinical manifestations of MS.

Influence of Heart Rate

The blood flow across the mitral valve is pulsatile and intermittent. Usually, the pressure gradient is greatest in early diastole. A long diastole, from a low heart rate, may cause the complete decompression of the engorged LA. In such a case, the transvalvular pressure gradient will be trivial. Atrial contraction, in a patient in sinus rhythm, increases the pressure gradient and results in high velocity inflow of blood through the stenotic valve.

The duration of the diastolic filling period is critical in the assessment of the clinical impact of a given degree of MS. Mitral stenosis actually increases the diastolic filling period at a given heart rate, due to earlier opening and late closure of the mitral valve caused by the elevation of the left atrial pressure.

But, when the heart rate is increased, the hemodynamics of MS dramatically worsen because the diastolic filling period is reduced. The increase in mean gradient and the rise in mean left atrial pressure are also apparent with short cycle lengths during atrial fibrillation.

The reduction in cardiac output is related not only to the severity of the stenosis, but also to secondary circulatory alterations, such as pulmonary vascular disease. In severe MS, the resting cardiac output is frequently reduced. Resting cardiac output averaging 4.1 ± 1.3 L per minute are described in patients needing balloon mitral valvuloplasty compared to a normal value of about 6 L per minute. Cardiac output in patients with MS complicated by severe pulmonary hypertension is still low and is reported to be in the order of 3.2 ± 0.7 L per minute.[19]

■ CHAMBER DYNAMICS IN MITRAL STENOSIS: ■ LEFT ATRIUM AND LEFT VENTRICLE

In response to the chronic hemodynamic effects of MS, remodeling occurs in LA and LV. This remodeling affects not only the clinical features of MS, but also influences the cardiac output and the pressure wave forms.

Left Atrium

The combination of the hemodynamic effects of MS and atrial inflammation due to the rheumatic processes lead to progressive LA dilation, fibrosis and disorganization of muscle bundles. Large 'a' wave in LA pressure tracing in MS reflects the kinetic energy dissipated in overcoming the resistance across the valve.[20]

In a highly compliant LA a known increase in volume will produce a small change in pressure, generating a small *v* wave. In contrast, when atrial compliance is reduced, the same volume of blood entering the LA will produce greater increase in pressure and a large *v* wave.

Pattern of blood flow in LA is altered with acceleration of blood flow velocity just proximal to the obstructed valve. Pulmonary vein flow is reduced in systole with increased flow reversal.[21,22]

In mild MS, total filling volume is usually normal, because the increased pressure in the left atrium pseudonormalizes the filling pattern.

With more severe stenosis, moderate to severe elevation in left atrial pressure occurs along with the following important alterations in filling dynamics:[21-25]

1. The atrial reservoir function is modified, and it extends throughout diastole. The elevated and slowly decaying left atrial pressure becomes the major driving force for the transmitral flow. Even at normal resting heart rate the LA does not decompress, filling continues, and diastasis is not present.
2. Active atrial pump function is reduced with more severe stenosis. Whereas in mild MS, atrial contraction accounts for $29 \pm 5\%$ of the total filling volume, in severe MS this contribution falls to $9 \pm 5\%$.[12] Loss of atrial contraction would dramatically reduce the transvalvular flow if the dilated LA did not maintain the high driving pressure throughout diastole. The chronically dilated, relatively thin walled fibrosed LA will not be able to act effectively as a pressure pump which normally enables adequate LV filling.

Atrial Fibrillation

The onset of atrial fibrillation with loss of atrial contraction often leads to a hemodynamic/clinical decompensation (decrease in cardiac output and increase in left atrial pressure). This seems to be due to the effect of accelerated ventricular rate on diastolic filling time, rather than to the loss of atrial booster function. The shortened diastole further compromises the reservoir function, the major mechanism of LV filling.

Changes in the LA lead to disparate conduction velocities and non-homogeneous refractory periods. Premature atrial activation caused either by automatic focus/re-entry may precipitate AF. Predictors of AF in patients with MS include age (strongest predictor), severity of MS, degree of LA dilation and height of LA pressure.[26,27] The initial episodes of AF leads to atrophy of atrial muscles, further atrial enlargement and further inhomogeneity of refractoriness and conduction—all these will lead to irreversible AF.

Development of AF leads to:
1. Reduction of cardiac output by 20%.
2. Worsening of TMG leading to onset/worsening of symptoms.
3. Thrombus formation in the LA.

Effect of Mitral Stenosis on Left Ventricle

Patterns of diastolic filling of LV are altered with prolonged early diastolic filling and loss of diastasis period. Abnormal LV geometry also occurs due to tricuspid valve regurgitation (TR) causing volume overload of RV, pulmonary hypertension causing pressure overload of RV and more rapid filling of RV compared to LV.[28]

Left ventricular end diastolic pressure (LVEDP) is usually normal in patients with isolated MS. It can be elevated with coexisting MR, aortic valve disease, systemic hypertension, coronary artery disease and cardiomyopathy. In chronic RHD, LV diastolic properties can also be altered due to rheumatically mediated interstitial fibrosis and restriction caused by attachment to the thickened and immobile mitral apparatus.[29] So the elderly can develop symptoms earlier than younger patients with the same degree of valve stenosis and gradients.

LV end diastolic volume is within normal range in 85% of patients and reduced in others. LV mass is usually normal but slightly reduced in 10% of the patients with MS.

Twenty five to thirty percent of patients with MS have ejection fraction (EF) and indices of systolic performance below normal due to:
a. Reduction in preload.
b. Systemic vasoconstriction leading to increase in afterload.
c. Extension of scarring from the MV into the adjacent posterior basal myocardium.[30]
d. Valvular cardiomyopathy.
e. Coexisting coronary artery disease.[21,22]

■ PULMONARY CIRCULATION

See Chapter 47 pulmonary hypertension and PMV.

Right Ventricle

With moderately elevated pulmonary artery systolic pressures (up to 60 mm Hg) RV function is usually maintained in patients with MS. Further elevation in PA pressure can lead to initial hypertrophy and later dilatation and eventual failure of RV. Rheumatic involvement of the tricuspid valve and annular dilation contributes to TR which in turn worsens the RV failure.[31] Failure of RV adaptation and subsequent failure results in signs and symptoms of right heart failure like elevated jugular venous pressure, hepatomegaly, pedal edema and intestinal congestion which are common features in the late stages of MS.

■ HEMODYNAMICS OF MITRAL VALVE STENOSIS

Echocardiography is the preferred modality to assess hemodynamics of MS. This is detailed in Chapter 11. Presently hemodynamic measurements are obtained in the cardiac catheterization laboratory when the patient is taken up for a percutaneous mitral valvotomy. Simultaneous measurements of LV end diastolic pressure, LA pressure [either directly or with pulmonary capillary wedge pressure (PCWP) as a surrogate], cardiac output, heart rate and diastolic filling period are required to accurately assess the hemodynamics. Preferably LV pressure and pulmonary capillary wedge pressure or LA pressure tracings are to be recorded simultaneously using two pressure transducers with identical sensitivity.

The PCWP tracing ideally should be realigned by 50 to 70 ms to the left (with tracing paper or electronically by the recording device itself) to account for the time delay in transmission of LA pressure to pulmonary venous bed. The detailed description of assessment of hemodynamics in the cathlab is described elsewhere.

Left Atrial Pressure Waveform

The *a* wave is the first positive wave recorded from the LA, which is due to the contraction of the atria (this is seen after the P wave on the electrocardiogram). The second positive wave appearing on the downslope of the *a* wave is the *c* wave of ventricular contraction. The *c* wave may not be visible in some cases. The third positive wave, the *v* wave, is due to atrial filling occurring during ventricular systole. The peak of *v* wave usually corresponds to the electrocardiographic T wave.[32] The negative slopes of the *a* and *v* waves are the *x* and *y* descents, respectively. The *x* descent may be interrupted by the positive "*c*" wave and the descent.

In patients with normal sinus rhythm and MS, the "a" wave may be quite large, and values as high as 50 mm Hg may be seen occasionally. A prominent *v* wave may also be observed in pure MS because left atrial volume and pressure are already high, and any additional increase in volume that occurs during passive atrial filling results in a greater increase in pressure, generating a prominent *v* wave (Fig. 5.2).[33] There also may be a contribution of reduced

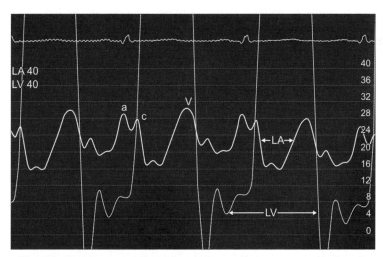

Fig. 5.2: Simultaneous left atrial and left ventricular pressure tracings in a patient with hemodynamically significant mitral stenosis

left atrial compliance from fibrosis. The presence of a large v wave correlates strongly with diminished exercise tolerance and is a significant predictor of pulmonary hypertension.[34,35] Furthermore, because MS delays emptying of the LA, the slope of they descent, representing the phase of early and rapid ventricular filling, is delayed (Fig. 5.2) compared to the rapid descent seen in mitral regurgitation.

The existence of a pressure gradient between the LA and left ventricle during diastole defines MS. Even in patients without any obstruction at the mitral valve level, a very small gradient must normally exist to allow blood to flow into the left ventricle, but this is usually not appreciable by the clinically used, fluid-filled transducers.

In general, the PCWP correlates well with left atrial pressure, which is particularly true when the PCWP is low (<25 mm Hg), with no significant difference noted between left atrial and the PCWP.[36,37] When PCWP is >25 mm Hg, considerable error may exist (variance in excess of 10 mm Hg).

Although a good correlation exists between the mean left atrial pressure and PCWP, the transmitral gradient using the PCWP does not correlate as well with the gradient obtained using the left atrial pressure.[38-40] Major sources of error exist; first, the PCWP introduces a time delay (40–160 msec), depending on the position of the catheter; and second, dampening is present of the post–v wave descent, intrinsic to the generation of a PCWP waveform that will add to the gradient. In addition, in the presence of pulmonary hypertension (a common occurrence in patients with MS), it may not be possible to obtain a true PCWP from the pulmonary artery position, and instead represent a hybrid between the two pressures and falsely elevate the "wedge."[40] These factors conspire to elevate the mean diastolic gradient compared to that obtained with left atrial pressure. Adjustment for the time delay by phase shifting the tracing relative to the LV pressure provides a more accurate reflection of the left-atrial-left-ventricular pressure gradient.[39]

However, several experts believe that these inaccuracies make the use of the PCWP an unreliable gauge of the transmitral gradient, and thus this method should not be used to make major decisions such as referral for mitral balloon valvuloplasty.[38,40] Such cases should be considered for transseptal catheterization to confirm the gradient with a left atrial pressure measurement before making a major decision related to the mitral valve stenosis.

The most important precaution to be taken in measuring transmitral gradients in the cathlab are the hemodynamic artefacts resulting in inaccurate measurements. Pressure transducers should first be carefully levelled, calibrated, and zeroed. The lengths and diameters of the connecting tubes should be identical in both the transducers. Because the pressures under consideration are relatively low, small errors in zeroing, transducer levels or differences in frequency response between the two transducers may cause errors in assessment of the transmitral gradient.[41]

HEMODYNAMICS OF PERCUTANEOUS BALLOON MITRAL VALVOTOMY

The hemodynamic improvements of PMV are apparent immediately.[42-46] Both the left atrial pressure and the transmitral gradient fall and the cardiac output increases. Mitral valve orifice area increases on average from a baseline of 1.0–2.2 cm^2 and is similar to the results of open surgical commissurotomy.[42] There may be a slight elevation in the LV end-diastolic pressure as the chronically under-filled LV is now filling almost normally. Also we know that there is some amount of fibrosis of the LV in rheumatic disease.

The fall in pulmonary hypertension happens acutely and there is a progressive fall even up to a year.[47-51] The detailed discussion on PH is in Chapter 57.

Significant regression of tricuspid regurgitation and right ventricular function has been reported even in the presence of a structural abnormality of the tricuspid valve.[52]

The long-term results following PMV are favorable with most of the patients maintaining symptomatic benefit over many years, the detailed discussion on long term outcomes following PMV is given in Chapter 58.

REFERENCES

1. Carapetis JR, McDonald M, Wilson NJ. Acute rheumatic fever. Lancet. 2005;366(9480):155–68.
2. Guilherme L, Faé KC, Oshiro SE, Tanaka AC, Pomerantzeff PMA, Kalil J. Rheumatic fever: how S. pyogenes-primed peripheral T cells trigger heart valve lesions. Ann N Y Acad Sci. 2005;1051:132–40.
3. Roberts WC, Perloff JK. Mitral valvular disease. A clinicopathologic survey of the conditions causing the mitral valve to function abnormally. Ann Intern Med. 1972;77(6):939–75.
4. Edwards JE, Rusted IE, Scheifley CH. Studies of the mitral valve. II. Certain anatomic features of the mitral valve and associated structures in mitral stenosis. Circulation. 1956;14(3):398–406.
5. Lachman AS, Roberts WC. Calcific deposits in stenotic mitral valves. Extent and relation to age, sex, degree of stenosis, cardiac rhythm, previous commissurotomy and left atrial body thrombus from study of 164 operatively-excised valves. Circulation. 1978;57(4):808–15.
6. Bonow RO, Carabello BA, Chatterjee K, de Leon AC Jr, Faxon DP, Freed MD, et al. 2008 Focused update incorporated into the ACC/AHA 2006 guidelines for the management of patients with valvular heart disease: a report of the American College of Cardiology/American Heart Association Task Force on Practice Guidelines (Writing Committee to Revise the 1998 Guidelines for the Management of Patients With Valvular Heart Disease): endorsed by the Society of Cardiovascular Anesthesiologists, Society for Cardiovascular Angiography and Interventions, and Society of Thoracic Surgeons. Circulation. 2008;118(15):e523–661.
7. Bland EF, Duckett Jones T. Rheumatic fever and rheumatic heart disease; a twenty year report on 1000 patients followed since childhood. Circulation. 1951;4(6):836–43.
8. Selzer A, Cohn KE. Natural history of mitral stenosis: a review. Circulation. 1972;45(4):878–90.

9. WOOD P. An appreciation of mitral stenosis. I. Clinical features. Br Med J. 1954;1(4870):1051–63.

10. Rowe JC, Bland EF, Sprague HB, White PD. The course of mitral stenosis without surgery: ten- and twenty-year perspectives. Ann Intern Med. 1960;52:741–9.

11. Cherian G, Vytilingam Ki, Sukumar Ip, Gopinath N. Mitral valvotomy in young patients. Br Heart J. 1964;26:157–66.

12. Al-Bahrani IR, Thamer MA, al-Omeri MM, al-Naaman YD. Rheumatic heart disease in the young in Iraq. Br Heart J. 1966;28(6):824–8.

13. Roy SB, Gopinath N. Mitral stenosis. Circulation. 1968;38(1 Suppl):68–76.

14. Rothenberg AJ, Clark JG, Muenster JJ, Carleton RA. The natural history of mitral stenosis. Dis Chest. 1969;55(1):3–6.

15. Fawzy ME, Hassan W, Stefadouros M, Moursi M, El Shaer F, Chaudhary MA. Prevalence and fate of severe pulmonary hypertension in 559 consecutive patients with severe rheumatic mitral stenosis undergoing mitral balloon valvotomy. J Heart Valve Dis. 2004;13(6):942–947; discussion 947-48.

16. Olesen KH. The natural history of 271 patients with mitral stenosis under medical treatment. Br Heart J. 1962;24:349–57.

17. Ellis LB, Harken DE. Arterial embolization in relation to mitral valvuloplasty. Am Heart J. 1961;62:611–20.

18. Casella L, Abelmann WH, Ellis LB. Patients with mitral stenosis and systemic emboli; Hemodynamic and clinical observations. Arch Intern Med. 1964;114: 773–81.

19. Ribeiro PA, Al Zaibag M, Abdullah M. Pulmonary artery pressure and pulmonary vascular resistance before and after mitral balloon valvotomy in 100 patients with severe mitral valve stenosis. Am Heart J. 1993;125(4):1110–4.

20. McDonald M, Brown A, Noonan S, Carapetis JR. Preventing recurrent rheumatic fever: the role of register based programmes. Heart Br Card Soc. 2005;91(9):1131–3.

21. Stott DK, Marpole DG, Bristow JD, Kloster FE, Griswold HE. The role of left atrial transport in aortic and mitral stenosis. Circulation. 1970;41(6):1031–41.

22. Carleton RA, Graettinger JS. The hemodynamic role of the atria with and without mitral stenosis. Am J Med. 1967;42(4):532–8.

23. Stojnić BB, Radjen GS, Perisić NJ, Pavlović PB, Stosić JJ, Prcović M. Pulmonary venous flow pattern studied by transoesophageal pulsed Doppler echocardiography in mitral stenosis in sinus rhythm: effect of atrial systole. Eur Heart J. 1993;14(12):1597–601.

24. Lee MM, Park SW, Kim CH, Sohn DW, Oh BH, Park YB, et al. Relation of pulmonary venous flow to mean left atrial pressure in mitral stenosis with sinus rhythm. Am Heart J. 1993;126(6):1401–7.

25. Meisner JS, Keren G, Pajaro OE, Mani A, Strom JA, Frater RW, et al. Atrial contribution to ventricular filling in mitral stenosis. Circulation. 1991;84(4):1469–80.

26. Diker E, Aydogdu S, Ozdemir M, Kural T, Polat K, Cehreli S, et al. Prevalence and predictors of atrial fibrillation in rheumatic valvular heart disease. Am J Cardiol. 1996;77(1):96–8.

27. Acar J, Michel PL, Cormier B, Vahanian A, Iung B. Features of patients with severe mitral stenosis with respect to atrial rhythm. Atrial fibrillation in predominant and tight mitral stenosis. Acta Cardiol. 1992;47(2):115–24.

28. Gaasch WH, Folland ED. Left ventricular function in rheumatic mitral stenosis. Eur Heart J. 1991;12 Suppl B:66–9.

29. Lee YS, Lee CP. Ultrastructural pathological study of left ventricular myocardium in patients with isolated rheumatic mitral stenosis with normal or abnormal left ventricular function. Jpn Heart J. 1990;31(4):435–48.

30. Mohan JC, Chutani SK, Sethi KK, Arora R, Khalilullah M. Determinants of left ventricular function in isolated rheumatic mitral stenosis. Indian Heart J. 1990;42(3):175–9.

31. Iskandrian AS, Hakki AH, Ren JF, Kotler MN, Mintz GS, Ross J, Kane SA. Correlation among right ventricular preload, afterload and ejection fraction in mitral valve disease: radionuclide, echocardiographic and hemodynamic evaluation. J Am Coll Cardiol. 1984;3:1403–11.

32. Musser BG, Bougas J, Goldberg H. Left heart catheterization II. With particular reference to mitral and aortic valvular disease. Am Heart J 1956;52:567–80.

33. Morrow AG, Braunwald E, Haller JA, Sharp EH. Left atrial pressure pulse in mitral valve disease: A correlation of pressures obtained by transbronchial puncture with the valvular lesion. Circulation. 1957;16:399–405.

34. Park S, Ha JQ, Ko YG, et al. Magnitude of left atrial v wave is the determinant of exercise capacity in patients with mitral stenosis. Am J Cardiol 2004; 94:243–5.

35. Ha JW, Chung N, Jang Y, et al. Is the left atrial v wave the determinant of peak pulmonary artery pressure in patients with pure mitral stenosis? Am J Cardiol. 2000;85:986–91.

36. Braunwald E, Moscovitz HL, Amram SS, et al. The hemodynamics of the left side of the heart as studied by simultaneous left atrial, left ventricular, and aortic pressures; particular reference to mitral stenosis. Circulation. 1955;12:69–81.

37. Walston A, Kendall ME. Comparison of pulmonary wedge and left atrial pressure in man. Am Heart J. 1973;86:159–64.

38. Hildick-Smith DJ,Walsh JT, Shapiro LM. Pulmonary capillary wedge pressure in mitral stenosis accurately reflects mean left atrial pressure but overestimates transmitral gradient. Am J Cardiol. 2000;85:512–15.

39. Lange RA, Moore DM, Cigarroa RG, Hillis LD. Use of pulmonary capillary wedge pressure to assess severity of mitral stenosis: Is true left atrial pressure needed in this condition? J Am Coll Cardiol. 1989;13:825–31.

40. Schoenfeld MH, Palacios IF, Hutter AM, et al. Underestimation of prosthetic mitral valve areas: Role of transseptal catheterization in avoiding unnecessary repeat mitral valve surgery. J Am Coll Cardiol. 1985;5:1387–92.

41. Hammer WJ, Roberts WC, de Leon AC. "Mitral stenosis" secondary to combined "massive" mitral annular calcific deposits and small, hypertrophied left ventricles. Hemodynamic documentation in four patients. Am J Med. 1978;64:371–6.

42. Gorlin R, Gorlin G. Hydraulic formula for calculation of the area of the stenotic mitral valve, other cardiac valves, and central circulatory shunts. Am Heart J 1951;41:1–29.

43. Cohen MV, Gorlin R. Modified orifice equation for the calculation of mitral valve area. Am Heart J. 1972;84:839–40.

44. Hakki AH, Iskandrian AS, Bemis CE, et al. A simplified formula for the calculation of stenotic cardiac valve areas. Circulation. 1981;63:1050–5.

45. Brogan WC, Lange RA, Hillis LD. Simplified formula for the calculation of mitral valve area: Potential inaccuracies in patients with tachycardia. Cathet Cardiovasc Diagn. 1991;23:81–83.

46. Klarich KW, Rihal CS, Nishimura RA. Variability between methods of calculating mitral valve area: Simultaneous Doppler echocardiographic and cardiac catheterization studies conducted before and after percutaneous mitral valvuloplasty. J Am Soc Echo. 1996;9:684–90.

47. Wang A, Ryan T, Kisslo KB, et al. Assessing the severity of mitral stenosis: Variability between non-invasive and invasive measurements in patients with symptomatic mitral valve stenosis. Am Heart J. 1999;138:777–84.

48. Rayburn BK, Fortuin NJ. Severely symptomatic mitral stenosis with a low gradient: A case for low technology medicine. Am Heart J. 1996;132:628–32.

49. Feldman T. Core curriculum for interventional cardiology: Percutaneous valvuloplasty. Catheter Cardiovasc Intcrv. 2003;60:48–56.

50. Reyes VP, Raju S, Wynne J, et al. Percutaneous balloon valvuloplasty compared with open surgical commissurotomy for mitral stenosis. N Engl J Med. 1994;331:961–67.

51. Iung B, Garbarz E, Michaud P, et al. Late results of percutaneous mitral commissurotomy in a series of 1024 patients. Analysis of late clinical deterioration: frequency, anatomic findings and predictive factors. Circulation. 1999; 99(25):3272–8.

52. Hannoush H, Fawzy ME, Stefadouros M, et al. Regression of significant tricuspid regurgitation after mitral balloon valvotomy for severe mitral stenosis. Am Heart J. 2004;148:865–70.

Section 2

Evaluation Prior to Percutaneous Mitral Valvotomy

Chapter 6

Mitral Stenosis— Evaluation and Medical Management

Harikrishnan S, Stigimon Joseph

The aim of management of mitral stenosis (MS) is to control symptoms and to prevent the complications of mitral stenosis. The major complications of mitral stenosis are acute pulmonary edema, pulmonary hypertension, systemic thromboembolism and right heart failure. The management should also aim to prevent progression of the valve lesions, by preventing recurrences of rheumatic fever.

■ CLINICAL HISTORY

Patients with hemodynamically significant mitral stenosis will have initially left heart symptoms of dyspnea, orthopnea and paroxysmal nocturnal dyspnea (PND). They go on to develop pulmonary hypertension and pulmonary vascular disease, and ultimately develop right heart failure and systemic venous congestion.

The chance of sudden cardiac death (SCD) in patients with MS is rare. But they go on to develop acute pulmonary edema, which can be life-threatening. Unless they get treated at the correct time, they occasionally succumb to an episode of pulmonary edema. This is important in developing countries where the access to medical facilities are limited and also the facilities to diagnose and manage heart diseases are limited. So, the early identification and early referral and intervention in patients with hemodynamically significant MS is very important.

Worsening of symptoms in patients occur when they face some form of hemodynamic stress like a pneumonia, when they are challenged with increased heart rates. This also happens when they develop atrial fibrillation (AF) or become pregnant when there may be a sudden increase in heart rate. The hemodynamics of MS is described in detail in the chapter on hemodynamics and natural history (Chapter 5).

Recent worsening of symptoms is an indication to have a detailed evaluation in patients with MS. Orthopnea and PND usually signifies a hemodynamically significant MS. An episode of acute pulmonary edema is a definite indication to advice PMV in a patient with significant MS. Onset of AF or the presence of AF signifies usually an advanced stage of the disease and is a pointer towards a hemodynamically significant MS. American Heart Association (AHA) recommends PMV to patients who have even moderate MS and in AF.

Physical Examination

Patients with severe MS usually have low cardiac output. Due to the low stroke volume, the pulse volume may be low in these patients. The Jugular venous pressure (JVP) usually has a prominent *a* wave in patients in sinus rhythm and who have significant pulmonary hypertension.

A readily palpable, tapping first heart sound suggests that the anterior mitral valve leaflet is pliable. A diastolic thrill may be palpable at the apex. Features like right ventricular (RV) lift palpable in the left parasternal region and a loud and palpable P2 in the 2nd left intercostal space will be seen in patients with MS and pulmonary hypertension.

Auscultatory signs of MS are loud first heart sound, an opening snap (OS), and a middiastolic murmur (low pitched, decrescendo diastolic murmur) with pre-systolic accentuation (in patients in SR). These signs may be better appreciated when auscultated with the patient in the left lateral decubitus position.

Murmur of Mitral Stenosis

Importantly, murmurs are helpful in assessing the severity of the MS and also assessing the pliability of the valve. As the MS becomes severe, the A2-OS interval is shortened and the length of the mid-diastolic rumble is increased. The interval between A_2 and OS varies from 40 to 120 milliseconds. In mild MS, the A2-OS interval is long and the diastolic murmur is short. In severe MS, the A2-OS is short (usually 40 to 60 milli-seconds) and the diastolic murmur is long.

Pliability of the valve (valve suitability for PMV/CMV) is indicated clinically by the following—presence of OS and a loud S1. In the presence of a rigid mitral valve (with or without calcification), OS is usually not heard. In the presence of significant mitral regurgitation, a holosystolic murmur of mitral regurgitation may be present. A well-audible murmur of mitral regurgitation is usually a contraindication to PMV (Fig. 6.1).

Echocardiography and Radiological Evaluation

This is detailed in Chapter 9 and 10 respectively.

Echocardiography

For the patient who have clinical evidence of mitral stenosis, the investigation of choice is echocardiography (ECG), which confirms the diagnosis and estimates the hemodynamic severity. The detailed echocardiographic evaluation of patients with MS is dealt with in the chapter on Echocardiography (Chapter 11).

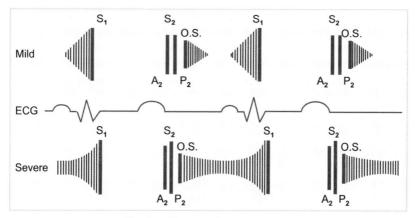

Fig. 6.1: Murmur of mitral stenosis

▓ MEDICAL MANAGEMENT

ACC AHA recommendations 2014 recommends the following as part of medical management of patients with MS.[1] (Modified with permission)

Class I
Anticoagulation (oral anticoagulants - vitamin K antagonists or heparin) is indicated in patients with (1) Mitral stenosis and atrial fibrillation (AF) (paroxysmal, persistent, or permanent), (2) MS and a prior embolic event, or (3) MS and a left atrial thrombus. *(Level of Evidence: B)*

Class IIa
Heart rate control can be beneficial in patients with MS and AF and fast ventricular response. *(Level of Evidence: C)*

Class IIb
Heart rate control may be considered for patients with MS in normal sinus rhythm and symptoms associated with exercise. *(Level of Evidence: B)*

Control of Symptoms

Control of heart rate: The initial symptoms of mitral stenosis are owing to pulmonary venous hypertension due to the elevated left atrial pressure. The symptoms can be managed to some extent by controlling the heart rate which will increase the diastolic filling period and thereby reducing the left atrial pressure.[2]

Beta blockers are the drug of choice in this situation. If the patient cannot tolerate beta blockers, calcium channel blockers like verapamil or diltiazem may be given. The drugs should be started at a low dose and then titrated according to the heart rate. A target heart rate of 50 to 60/bpm is acceptable.[2]

Digoxin can also be given to patients to control heart rate, but beta blockers are preferred. If the patient has pulmonary hypertension or right ventricular failure or atrial fibrillation, digoxin is indicated. Digoxin will control the ventricular rate especially in patients with atrial fibrillation.

There are recent reports on the use of ivabradine in heart rate control in mitral stenosis. Parakh et al. in an open-label, randomized, crossover trial study compared atenolol and Ivabradine in symptomatic mild-moderate mitral stenosis in normal sinus rhythm. They found that ivabradine significantly reduced the heart rate and increased the effort tolerance when compared to atenolol.[3]

Rajesh et al. randomized 82 patients with moderate MS and put them on atenolol or ivabradine and found that heart rate reduction and improvement in exercise capacity was the same with both the drugs.[4]

Dhanger et al. in another randomized comparison of 100 patients, found that ivabradine (mean dose 6.05±1.25 mg) and atenolol (mean dose 60±26.7 mg at 12 weeks) had equal effectiveness but adverse events were more with atenolol.[5]

Diuretics

Diuretics can be given to patients with pulmonary venous hypertension or to patients with symptoms or signs of right heart failure. Potassium sparing diuretic or a combination of loop diuretic and a potassium sparing diuretic may be preferred. Careful watch on potassium levels should be done, as hypokalemia may lead to arrhythmias which can be dangerous in case of digoxin toxicity, not uncommon in these patients.

Rheumatic Fever Prophylaxis

Prophylaxis against recurrence of rheumatic fever is a must in patients with mitral stenosis. It is shown that rheumatic penicillin prophylaxis prevents progression of valve lesions even after a successful intervention. Penicillin is the drug of choice for rheumatic prophylaxis. Injectable benzathine penicillin has the lowest failure rate compared to other modes of penicillin administration and other drugs recommended for prophylaxis.

Even though there is recommendation to discontinue prophylaxis at 45 years of age, in the developing world, physicians tend to continue the prophylaxis life long, even following a successful intervention like valve replacement surgery or PMV.

Infective Endocarditis Prophylaxis

Discussed in Chapter 58.

Anticoagulation

Anticoagulation is recommended in patients with MS and AF and also for patients in SR who had a history of thromboembolism (Vide Supra). The details are given in the chapter on long-term follow-up of patients (Chapter 58).

Follow-up

In the asymptomatic patient, yearly re-evaluation is recommended (ACC 2006). It is recommended to obtain detailed history, do physical examination, get a chest X-ray, and ECG during each evaluation. Clinical findings like shortening of the A2-OS interval, longer duration of the mid diastolic murmur (MDM), and the appearance of findings of pulmonary hypertension indicates the valve lesion has progressed.

We do echocardiographic evaluation yearly especially when there is a change in clinical status or on a clinical suspicion of severe MS. Holter ECG monitoring to detect paroxysmal atrial fibrillation is indicated in patients with history of palpitations.

Patients who are symptomatic should undergo detailed evaluation with a history, physical examination, ECG, chest X-ray, and echocardiogram. Two-dimensional, Doppler and color Doppler echocardiography is indicated to evaluate MV morphology, valve gradients, valve area and pulmonary artery pressure.

Transthoracic echocardiography (TTE) should be performed to re-evaluate asymptomatic patients with MS and stable clinical findings to assess pulmonary artery pressure and valve gradient (very severe MS with mitral valve area <1.0 cm^2 - every year, severe MS with mitral valve area ≤1.5 cm^2 every 1 to 2 years; and progressive MS with mitral valve area >1.5 cm^2 every 3 to 5 years)[1] (ACC – AHA 2014) (Table 6.1).

Table 6.1: Frequency of echocardiograms in asymptomatic patients with MS and normal left ventricular function

Stage	Mitral stenosis
Progressive (Stage B)	Every 3–5 year (MVA >1.5 cm^2)
Severe (Stage C)	Every 1–2 year (MVA 1.0–1.5 cm^2) Once every year (MVA <1.0 cm^2)

Abbreviation: MVA, mitral valve area

Interventions

When the symptoms worsen and cannot be controlled by drugs, some form of intervention is required in symptomatic mitral stenosis. Special situations like pregnancy, left atrial thrombus and the management of MS in the presence of other valve lesions are described elsewhere in this book.

Depending on the morphology of the valve, mitral regurgitation and presence or absence of left atrial thrombi, the patient is sent for either mitral valve replacement or for mitral valvotomy. Nowadays percutaneous mitral valvotomy has almost replaced surgical closed mitral valvotomy as the procedure of choice for pliable mitral stenosis. The indications, contra-indications and mechanism of PMV is described in the next Chapter 7.

Patients with New York Heart Association (NYHA) functional class II symptoms and moderate or severe MS (MV area less than 1.5 cm^2 or mean gradient greater than 5 mm Hg) may be considered for intervention, mostly PMV, if they have pliable valves.

There is a subset of patients who have significant symptoms, but clinical and Doppler echocardiographic evaluation do not indicate significant MS. In such patients, stress testing is required. Formal exercise testing or dobutamine stress may be useful to assess these patients. The detailed description of stress testing is given in Chapter 8.

A small subset of patients will need cardiac catheterization to decide on the need for PMV. It should be done preferably with the patient and the physician prepared for PMV in case it is indicated, so that one more procedure can be avoided.

Diagnostic Testing in MS-Cardiac Catheterization

In the current era, majority of patients with MS can be evaluated with TTE, supplemented in some cases with TEE. In few patients where there is discrepancy between echocardiographic findings and clinical scenario (mostly symptoms) we have to proceed with cardiac catheterization.

This may be either for assessing mitral regurgitation or assessing pulmonary artery pressures or assessing the severity of aortic valve disease. ACC-AHA says "Catheterization is the only method available to measure absolute pressures inside the heart, which may be important in clinical decision making".

Such catheterization studies must be carried out by personnel experienced with catheterization laboratory hemodynamics with simultaneous pressure measurements in the left ventricle and LA, ideally via trans-septal catheterization. Although, a properly performed mean pulmonary artery wedge pressure is an acceptable substitute for mean LA pressure, the LV to pulmonary wedge gradient will overestimate the true transmitral gradient due to phase delay and delayed transmission of pressure changes. The Gorlin equation is applied for calculation of mitral valve area, using cardiac output obtained via thermodilution (when there is no significant TR) or the Fick method. Ideally, measured oxygen consumption should be used in this calculation, but this facility is not available in most of the developing world. Full right-heart pressures should be reported. In cases where exertional symptoms seem out of proportion to resting hemodynamic severity, hemodynamic data may be obtained during exercise.

The details of cardiac catheterization in MS is described in Chapter 18.

▓ MIXED VALVE LESIONS

Patients with mixed valve disease may sometimes become pose clinical challenges. There are no definite guidelines for the management of multi-valvar disease which is very common among patients with Rheumatic heart disease (RHD). So the treating physician has to take an informed decision after discussing with the patient. For example in a patient with severe MS and moderate aortic regurgitation, we may opt for PMV and keep the aortic valve lesion on follow-up. These patients require serial evaluations at intervals earlier than recommended for single valve lesions.

REFERENCES

1. Nishimura RA, Otto CM, Bonow RO, Carabello BA, Erwin JP, Guyton RA, et al. 2014 AHA/ACC guideline for the management of patients with valvular heart disease: executive summary: a report of the American College of Cardiology/ American Heart Association Task Force on Practice Guidelines. J Am Coll Cardiol. 2014;63(22):2438–88.
2. Desai PA, Tafreshi J, Pai RG. Beta-blocker therapy for valvular disorders. J Heart Valve Dis. 2011;20(3):241–53.
3. Parakh N, Chaturvedi V, Kurian S, Tyagi S. Effect of ivabradine vs atenolol on heart rate and effort tolerance in patients with mild to moderate mitral stenosis and normal sinus rhythm. J Card Fail. 2012;18(4):282–8.
4. Rajesh GN, Sajeer K, Sanjeev CG, Bastian C, Vinayakumar D, Muneer K, et al. A comparative study of ivabradine and atenolol in patients with moderate mitral stenosis in sinus rhythm. Indian Heart J. 2016;68(3):311-5.
5. Dhanger MK, Isser HS, Bansal S, Chakraborty P, Gupta P, Sharma N. Comparative study of Ivabradine versus atenolol in symptomatic mitral stenosis patients. Indian Heart J. 2014;66, Suppl 2:S133.

Chapter 7

Percutaneous Mitral Valvotomy— Indications, Contraindications and Mechanism

Harikrishnan S

When the symptoms worsen and cannot be controlled by drugs, some form of intervention is required in symptomatic mitral stenosis. Special situations like pregnancy, left atrial thrombus and the management of MS in the presence of other valve lesions are described elsewhere in this book.

Depending on the morphology of the valve, mitral regurgitation and presence or absence of left atrial thrombi, the patient is sent for either mitral valve replacement or for mitral valvotomy. Nowadays percutaneous mitral valvotomy has almost replaced surgical closed mitral valvotomy as the procedure of choice for pliable mitral stenosis.

The outcome following PMV reportedly depends on the morphology of the valve.[1] So the selection of cases becomes very important in PMV.[2]

▣ MECHANISM OF PERCUTANEOUS BALLOON MITRAL VALVOTOMY

Percutaneous mitral valvotomy (PMV) should perhaps more appropriately be called percutaneous mitral commissurotomy, as the balloon dilatation improves the valve orifice by opening the fused mitral commissures. In some cases, splitting of the subvalvular apparatus might be also seen. As shown by echocardiographic, fluoroscopic and anatomic studies, the expanding balloon splits fused commissures in much the same way as in surgical commissurotomy. The potential of balloon catheters, by application of circumferential tension, to relieve mitral stenosis is inherent in the pathologic process underlying valve obstruction and the previous success of closed surgical commissurotomy.[3]

Al Zaibag et al.[4] showed that the mechanism of dilatation of the valve by using single balloon is mainly by splitting of one or both commissures. He also noticed the splitting of commissures by using the double balloon technique. Reid et al.[5] suggested stretch of mitral annulus as an additional mechanism for the increase in mitral valve area (MVA). Two dimensional echocardiography showed slight reduction in MVA within 24 hours after PMV but no significant change after at least one month of this reduction, suggesting that stretching of the annulus is a mechanism of valve dilatation. In addition to commissural splitting, the balloon dilatation may result in fracture of nodular calcium within the leaflet substance.[6]

Waller et al.[7] studied the mitral valve in operatively excised and necropsy specimens. They showed that single balloon resulted in superficial cracking, double balloon in deeper splitting of one or more fused commissures, while over-sized balloons resulted in injury to the annulus and the left atrial wall. Valves with previous commissurotomies showed splitting adjacent to or at the site of healed cracks.

Ribeiro et al.[8] concluded that commissural splitting occurred preferentially in calcified (81%) as opposed to only 65% of noncalcified commissures and that commissural splitting is the main mechanism by which MVA increases after successful balloon dilation with either single or double balloon.

◼ INDICATIONS AND CONTRAINDICATIONS FOR PMV

In patients with favorable valve morphology as evidenced by noncalcified pliable valves and mild subvalvular fusion, the procedure can be performed with a high success rate (greater than 90%), low complication rate (less than 3%), and a sustained improvement in 80% to 90% over a 3- to 7-year follow-up period.[1,9-11]

Since, the mechanism of PMV is by splitting the fused commissures, the presence of marked fusion and severe calcification of commissures is associated with an increased complication rate. Patients with valvular calcification, thickened fibrotic leaflets with decreased mobility, and subvalvular fusion have a higher incidence of acute complications and a higher rate of restenosis on follow up.[1,10,11] PMV requires lot of expertise and the learning curve is steep. ACC recommends that it is of utmost importance that this procedure be performed in centers with skilled and experienced operators.[9]

Indications for PMV

ACC-AHA in its latest guidelines[2] recommend PMV in selected cases of MS with suitable valve morphology in the absence of left atrial thrombus or moderate to severe MR (Table 7.1).

Table 7.1: Summary of Recommendations for Intervention in mitral stenosis.

Recommendations	*COR*	*LOE*
PMV is recommended for symptomatic patients with severe MS (MVA $\leq$ 1.5 cm^2, stage D) and favorable valve morphology in the absence of contraindications	I	A
Mitral valve surgery is indicated in severely symptomatic patients (NYHA class III/IV) with severe MS (MVA $\leq$ 1.5 cm^2, stage D) who are not high risk for surgery and who are not candidates for or failed previous PMBC	I	B
Concomitant mitral valve surgery is indicated for patients with severe MS (MVA $\leq$1.5 cm^2, stage C or D) undergoing other cardiac surgery	I	C

Contd...

Contd...

Recommendations	COR	LOE
PMBC is reasonable for asymptomatic patients with very severe MS (MVA $\leq$1.0 cm², stage C) and favorable valve morphology in the absence of contraindications	IIa	C
Mitral valve surgery is reasonable for severely symptomatic patients (NYHA class III/IV) with severe MS (MVA $\leq$1.5 cm² stage D), provided there are other operative indications	IIa	C
PMBC may be considered for asymptomatic patients with severe MS (MVA $\leq$ 1.5 cm², stage C) and favorable valve morphology who have new onset of AF in the absence of contraindications	IIb	C
PMBC may be considered for symptomatic patients with MVA > 1.5 cm² if there is evidence of hemodynamically significant MS during exercise	IIb	C
PMBC may be considered for severely symptomatic patients (NYHA class III/IV) with severe MS (MVA $\leq$ 1.5 cm², stage D) who have suboptimal valve anatomy and are not candidates for surgery or at high risk for surgery	IIb	C
Concomitant mitral valve surgery may be considered for patients with moderate MS (MVA 16–2.0 cm²) undergoing other cardiac surgery	IIb	C
Mitral valve surgery and excision on the left atrial appendage may be considered for patients with severe MS (MVA $\leq$1.5 cm², stages C and D) who have had recurrent embolic events while receiving adequate anticoagulation	IIb	C

Abbreviations: AF, atrial fibrillation; CDR, class of recommendation; LOE, level of evidence; MS, mitral stenosis; MVA, mitral valve area; NYHA, New York Heart Assocation; PMBC, percutaneous mitral balloon commissurotomy
Source: Published with permission from JACC[2]

Contraindications for PMV

More than moderate MR, left atrial thrombi and commissural calcium are generally considered as contraindications for PMV. But there are exceptions to this as described in detail below.

■ PMV—SPECIAL CONSIDERATIONS

When to Perform PMV? Earlier the Better?

Some studies indicate that doing PMV when the valve area is around 1.2 cm² is better than doing it when the valve area is less than 1 cm².[3,12] Kang et al. did a prospective study on the outcome of 244 patients with moderate asymptomatic MS who were kept on medical therapy versus those who underwent PMV. The estimated actuarial 11-year event-free survival rate was 89 ± 4% in the PMV group and 69 ± 5% in the conservatively managed group (P < 0.001) but not significantly different in those without atrial fibrillation and previous embolism (86 ± 5% in the PMV group and 79 ± 6% in the Conservative group at 11 years, P = 0.28).[13]

The authors recommended randomized trials to test the hypothesis of early intervention in moderate MS.

Planning Pregnancy

There will be situations when a patient planning pregnancy with moderate MS may come for evaluation. In such situations we will be forced to perform PMV even if the valve area is between 1.1 to 1.3 cm² or even more.

Left Atrial Thrombus

In selected patients with thrombus localized and organized, PMV can be performed using over-the-wire techniques (See the Chapter on LA thrombus and the Chapter on "Over the wire techniques").

Mitral Regurgitation

Moderate or severe MR is a contraindication for performing PMV.[9] Audible MR usually indicates significant regurgitation and the valve may not be amenable to PMV. In borderline cases, TEE may be helpful in assessing MR. Left ventricular angiography is another technique to assess MR, especially in the cathlab, prior to PMV. Left atrial or PCWP wave form showing prominence of "V" wave may not be indicative of significant MR as "V" may be prominent in MS itself. One point we have to remember is that MR in rheumatic MS is due to restriction of leaflet movement. In some cases there may be improvement in MR following PMV. So if the MR is producing a central jet and is 2-3+, the valve may be considered for PMV.

Calcification of the Valve

When there is bicommissural calcification, BMV is contraindicated, because there is high probability of leaflet tear with resultant acute severe mitral regurgitation. There are few reports of successful PMV in patients with severe calcific MS.[14-17] Recently, there was a report describing the successful performance of PMV in a patient with unicommissural calcium.[16] Dreyfus et al. in a recent article compared the outcomes of patients with commissural calcium and reported that the incidence of MR is not different from valves which don't have commissural calcium. They recommended that "though a procedural success was obtained less frequently in patients with calcified commissure but a successful PMV could still be safely achieved in a large proportion of patients. Our results support the use of PMC as a first-line treatment of patients with severe MS even in the presence of significant commissural calcifications with otherwise favorable clinical characteristics".[18] Severe calcification seen on fluoroscopy (graded 1–4) is an indicator of poor outcome following PMV.[8] Even if the leaflet belly shows calcium, when the commissure are relatively free of calcium, PMV can be considered, though the results may not be as good as seen in the case of a noncalcified valve (More detailed description of PMV in calcific valves is given in Chapter 43).

PRACTICAL APPROACH IN THE DEVELOPING WORLD

Even though ACC-AHA recommends intervention in all patients with a valve area </= 1.5 cm², countries with limited resources in the developing world may not be able to follow the recommendations. If the symptoms are well-controlled and the patients have a reasonable effort tolerance (> 7 Mets), they can be closely followed up till the valve area is less than 1.1 cm².

We in SCTIMST are following the protocol which is given in Figure 7.1 for the last many years. We are able to get a good follow-up and reasonable outcomes in such patients.[19-22]

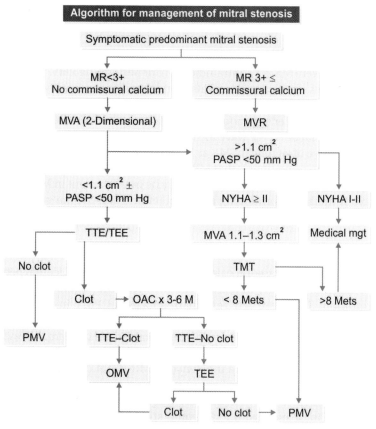

Fig. 7.1: Proposed algorithm for the management of symptomatic mitral stenosis *Abbreviations*: MR, mitral regurgitation; MVR, mitral valve replacement; TMT, tread mill excercise testing; TTE, trans-thoracic echocardiography; TEE, trans-esophageal echocardiography; MVA, mitral valve area; PMV, percutaneous mitral valvotomy; OMV, open mitral valvotomy; NYHA, New York Heart Association; PASP, pulmonary artery systolic pressure; MS, mitral stenosis; OAC, oral anticoagulants

■ REFERENCES

1. Fatkin D, Roy P, Morgan JJ, Feneley MP. Percutaneous balloon mitral valvotomy with the Inoue single-balloon catheter: commissural morphology as a determinant of outcome. J Am Coll Cardiol. 1993;21(2):390-7.

2. Nishimura RA, Otto CM, Bonow RO, Carabello BA, Erwin JP, Guyton RA, et al. 2014 AHA/ACC guideline for the management of patients with valvular heart disease: executive summary: a report of the American College of Cardiology/American Heart Association Task Force on Practice Guidelines. J Am Coll Cardiol. 2014;63(22):2438-88.

3. Herrmann HC. Acute and chronic efficacy of percutaneous transvenous mitral commissurotomy: implications for patient selection. Cathet Cardiovasc Diagn. 1994;Suppl 2:61-8.

4. Al Zaibag M, Ribeiro PA, Al Kasab S, Al Fagih MR. Percutaneous double-balloon mitral valvotomy for rheumatic mitral-valve stenosis. Lancet. 1986;1(8484):757-61.

5. Reid CL, McKay CR, Chandraratna PA, Kawanishi DT, Rahimtoola SH. Mechanisms of increase in mitral valve area and influence of anatomic features in double-balloon, catheter balloon valvuloplasty in adults with rheumatic mitral stenosis: a Doppler and two-dimensional echocardiographic study. Circulation. 1987;76(3):628-36.

6. McKay RG, Lock JE, Safian RD, Come PC, Diver DJ, Baim DS, et al. Balloon dilation of mitral stenosis in adult patients: postmortem and percutaneous mitral valvuloplasty studies. J Am Coll Cardiol. 1987;9:723-31.

7. Waller BF, VanTassel JW, McKay C. Anatomic basis for and morphologic results from catheter balloon valvuloplasty of stenotic mitral valves. Clin Cardiol. 1990;13(9):655-61.

8. Ribeiro PA, Al Zaibag M, Rajendran V, Ashmeg A, Al Kasab S, Al Faraidi Y, et al. Mechanism of mitral valve area increase by in vitro single and double balloon mitral valvotomy. Am J Cardiol. 1988;62(4):264-9.

9. Bonow RO, Carabello BA, Chatterjee K, de Leon AC Jr, Faxon DP, Freed MD, et al. 2008 Focused update incorporated into the ACC/AHA 2006 guidelines for the management of patients with valvular heart disease: a report of the American College of Cardiology/American Heart Association Task Force on Practice Guidelines (Writing Committee to Revise the 1998 Guidelines for the Management of Patients With Valvular Heart Disease): endorsed by the Society of Cardiovascular Anesthesiologists, Society for Cardiovascular Angiography and Interventions, and Society of Thoracic Surgeons. Circulation. 2008;118(15):e523-661.

10. Iung B, Cormier B, Ducimetiere P, Porte JM, Nallet O, Michel PL, et al. Functional results 5 years after successful percutaneous mitral commissurotomy in a series of 528 patients and analysis of predictive factors. J Am Coll Cardiol. 1996;27(2):407-14.

11. Cannan CR, Nishimura RA, Reeder GS, Ilstrup DR, Larson DR, Holmes DR, et al. Echocardiographic assessment of commissural calcium: a simple predictor of outcome after percutaneous mitral balloon valvotomy. J Am Coll Cardiol. 1997;29(1):175-80.

12. Herrmann HC, Feldman T, Isner JM, Bashore T, Holmes DR Jr, Rothbaum DA, et al. Comparison of results of percutaneous balloon valvuloplasty in patients with mild and moderate mitral stenosis to those with severe mitral stenosis. The North American Inoue Balloon Investigators. Am J Cardiol. 1993;71(15):1300-3.

13. Kang D-H, Lee CH, Kim D-H, Yun S-C, Song J-M, Lee C-W, et al. Early percutaneous mitral commissurotomy vs. conventional management in asymptomatic moderate mitral stenosis. Eur Heart J. 2012;33(12):1511-7.

14. Dugal JS, Jetley V, Sabharwal JS, Sofat S, Singh C. Life-saving PTMC for critical calcific mitral stenosis in cardiogenic shock with balloon impasse. Int J Cardiovasc Intervent. 2003;5(3):172–4.

15. Palacios IF, Lock JE, Keane JF, Block PC. Percutaneous transvenous balloon valvotomy in a patient with severe calcific mitral stenosis. J Am Coll Cardiol. 1986;7(6):1416–9.

16. Khandenahally Shankarappa R, Dwarakaprasad R, Karur S, Bachahally Krishnanaik G, Panneerselvam A, Cholenahally Nanjappa M. Balloon mitral valvotomy for calcific mitral stenosis. JACC Cardiovasc Interv. 2009;2(3):263–4.

17. Tuzcu EM, Block PC, Griffin B, Dinsmore R, Newell JB, Palacios IF. Percutaneous mitral balloon valvotomy in patients with calcific mitral stenosis: immediate and long-term outcome. J Am Coll Cardiol. 1994;23(7):1604–9.

18. Dreyfus J, Cimadevilla C, Nguyen V, Brochet E, Lepage L, Himbert D, et al. Feasibility of percutaneous mitral commissurotomy in patients with commissural mitral valve calcification. Eur Heart J. 2014;35(24):1617–23.

19. Harikrishnan S, Bhat A, Tharakan J, Titus T, Kumar A, Sivasankaran S, et al. Percutaneous transvenous mitral commissurotomy using metallic commissurotome: long-term follow-up results. J Invasive Cardiol. 2006;18(2):54–8.

20. Harikrishnan S, Nair K, Tharakan JM, Titus T, Kumar VKA, Sivasankaran S. Percutaneous transmitral commissurotomy in juvenile mitral stenosis--comparison of long term results of Inoue balloon technique and metallic commissurotomy. Catheter Cardiovasc Interv Off J Soc Card Angiogr Interv. 2006;67(3):453–9.

21. Nair K, Sivadasanpillai H, Sivasubramonium P, Ramachandran P, Tharakan JA, Titus T, et al. Percutaneous valvuloplasty for mitral valve restenosis: Postballoon valvotomy patients fare better than postsurgical closed valvotomy patients. Catheter Cardiovasc Interv. 2010;76(2):174–80.

22. Nair KKM, Pillai HS, Titus T, Varaparambil A, Sivasankaran S, Krishnamoorthy KM, et al. Persistent pulmonary artery hypertension in patients undergoing balloon mitral valvotomy. Pulm Circ. 2013;3(2):426–31.

Chapter 8

Stress Testing Prior to Percutaneous Mitral Valvotomy

P Shanmuga Sundaram, Harikrishnan S

There is a subset of patients, who have significant symptoms, but clinical and Doppler echocardiographic evaluation do not indicate significant mitral stenosis (MS). In such patients, stress testing is required. Different stress testing modalities have been tried. Formal exercise testing or dobutamine stress may be useful to assess these patients.

Stress Testing in the Assessment of Patients with Mitral Stenosis

Clinical clues and a transthoracic echocardiography (TTE) is usually sufficient to guide management in asymptomatic patients with mild to moderate MS and in symptomatic patients with severe MS who are candidates for either PMV or surgical mitral valve repair or replacement. Management protocols are less clear in asymptomatic patients with severe MS and in symptomatic patients with only mild to moderate MS. In these two groups of patients exercise testing can provide critical information of functional capacity and exercise-induced symptoms which will aid in decision making.

In asymptomatic patients with severe MS (mean gradient >10 mm Hg and MVA <1.0 cm^2), or symptomatic patients with moderate MS (mean gradient 5 to 10 mm Hg and MVA 1 to 1.5 cm^2), stress testing can provide useful information. The measurement of pulmonary artery pressure during exercise or dobutamine stress echocardiography can help distinguish those who could benefit from valvuloplasty or valve replacement from those who should be maintained on medical therapy.[1]

Stress echocardiography provides added value when more detailed assessment of valve function and its hemodynamic consequences is needed, particularly in the asymptomatic patient and the patient in whom symptoms and Doppler findings at rest are discordant.

The current ACC/AHA guidelines[1] have given a class I recommendation (C) for stress Doppler echocardiography in patients with MS and discordance between symptoms and stenosis severity. The threshold values proposed by the ACC/AHA guidelines 2008[2] for consideration for intervention are a mean transmitral pressure gradient >15 mm Hg during exercise or peak pulmonary artery systolic pressure >60 mm Hg during exercise. In patients with pulmonary artery pressures or valve gradients above these values, PMV or surgical intervention is recommended, even for patients with apparently moderate MS at rest.

TREADMILL EXERCISE TESTING IN PATIENTS WITH MITRAL STENOSIS

Three major studies have evaluated the role of treadmill exercise testing (TMT) in patients with MS.[3-5] In patients with mitral stenosis an excellent correlation was found to exist between mitral valve area (obtained at cardiac catheterization) and duration of exercise.[3,4] The inability to reach stage III of Bruce protocol was associated with critical mitral stenosis. A hypotensive response to exercise though frequent in mitral stenosis, bore no relation whatsoever to the severity of lesions as seen in cases of aortic stenosis.[2] Hsu et al. concluded that limiting symptoms and complex ventricular arrhythmias are the proper endpoints in evaluating the exercise capacity of patients with mitral stenosis after prior echocardiographic exclusion of those with potentially risky floating thrombus.[3]

It is suggested that exercise testing employing the Bruce protocol is a valuable adjunct to other noninvasive tests in the initial evaluation of selected patients with mitral stenosis (Figs 8.1 and 8.2). By virtue of being easily repeated at low-risk, exercise testing may also be useful in long-term follow-up of medically treated patients with mitral stenosis.[5]

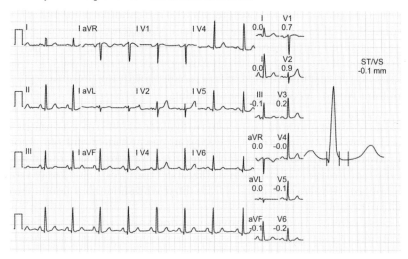

Fig. 8.1: Treadmill exercise test in a patient with MS (Pre-exercise tracing)

DOBUTAMINE STRESS ECHOCARDIOGRAPHY

Dobutamine stress echocardiography (DSE) is useful for risk stratification in patients with rheumatic MS. The absolute increase in the mean diastolic mitral valve gradient at peak DSE (DSE-MG) allowed identification of subgroups with a high or low incidence of significant clinical events at follow-up.

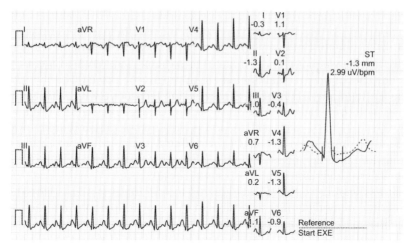

Fig. 8.2: Treadmill exercise test in a patient with MS (Peak exercise tracing—note the good effort tolerance at a reasonably high heart rate)

Dobutamine infusion seems to have advantages over exercise in the setting of mitral valve inflow obstruction. Through its beta$_1$-agonist action, dobutamine increases the heart rate and contractility with a resultant increase in cardiac output, whereas pulmonary and peripheral vascular resistance may fall due to its beta$_2$-agonist effects. The net hemodynamic effect of DSE in patients with MS is similar to that of exercise but it is associated with lower LV end-diastolic, systolic pulmonary artery and pulmonary wedge pressures than exercise at similar degrees of hemodynamic stress, as shown by Hwang et al.[6] This is associated with lower incidence of dyspnea during DSE.

Dobutamine Stress Echocardiography Protocol

Patients are advised not to stop any medications before the test, including beta-adrenergic antagonists. After obtaining a 12-lead ECG at rest, dobutamine is administered by a continuous infusion pump, starting at 10 µg/kg/min for 5 min. The infusion rate is then increased by 10 µg/kg/min every 3 min to a maximum of 40 µg/kg/min. Throughout the test, the 12-lead ECG, transcutaneous oximetry, and vital signs are monitored continuously. The 2-D echocardiographic and Doppler images of mitral and tricuspid inflow are continuously monitored. End points—maximum protocol dose, heart rate > 75% of the age-adjusted maximum heart rate, dyspnea, or a mean diastolic mitral valve gradient at peak DSE (DSE-MG) ≥25 mm Hg obtained at any dose.

In a study conducted by Gilmar Reis et al. a DSE-MG ≥18 mm Hg was found to have a sensitivity of 90%, specificity of 87%, and overall accuracy of 90% in detection of clinical events at follow-up. In this study, DSE added no incremental prognostic information over a standard clinical work-up for patients with MVA <1.0 cm². However, in patients with MVA >1.0 cm², DSE has consistently demonstrated incremental prognostic power, compared to classic cardiac evaluation, correctly classifying an additional 22% of patients in this subgroup (n = 40) as high risk (p = 0.003). Indeed, the best performance of DSE for the identification of high-risk patients was observed in the subgroup with MVA between 1.0 and 1.5 cm^2. For patients with MVA >1.5 cm^2, the test has shown only a small increment in prognostic power. Doppler stress echocardiography is a feasible stress-testing technique with a low rate of complications in patients with MS. It seems to offer important information, not only by helping to classify the underlying hemodynamic burden of the impending obstruction but also by providing data that adequately allow for correct identification of a subgroup of high-risk patients during follow-up, in whom a more aggressive approach should be advised.

Stress testing is a useful diagnostic tool in many patients who have borderline hemodynamics as evaluated by echocardiography and helps in deciding on a definitive management.

■ REFERENCES

1. Bonow RO, Carabello BA, Chatterjee K, de Leon AC Jr, Faxon DP, Freed MD, et al. 2008 Focused update incorporated into the ACC/AHA 2006 guidelines for the management of patients with valvular heart disease: a report of the American College of Cardiology/American Heart Association Task Force on Practice Guidelines (Writing Committee to Revise the 1998 Guidelines for the Management of Patients With Valvular Heart Disease): endorsed by the Society of Cardiovascular Anesthesiologists, Society for Cardiovascular Angiography and Interventions, and Society of Thoracic Surgeons. Circulation. 2008;118(15):e523–661.

2. Nishimura RA, Otto CM, Bonow RO, Carabello BA, Erwin JP, Guyton RA, et al. 2014 AHA/ACC guideline for the management of patients with valvular heart disease: executive summary: a report of the American College of Cardiology/American Heart Association Task Force on Practice Guidelines. J Am Coll Cardiol. 2014;63(22):2438–88.

3. Hsu TS, Lee YS. Endpoints of treadmill exercise testing for functional evaluation of patients with mitral stenosis. Int J Cardiol. 1991;31(1):81–7.

4. Almendral JM, García-Andoain JM, Sánchez-Cascos A, de Rábago P. Treadmill stress testing in the evaluation of patients with valvular heart disease. Possible role in the assessment of functional capacity and severity of the lesion. Cardiology. 1982;69(1):42–51.

5. Vacek JL, Valentin-Stone P, Wolfe M, Davis WR. The value of standardized exercise testing in the noninvasive evaluation of mitral stenosis. Am J Med Sci. 1986;292(6):335–43.

6. Hwang MH, Pacold I, Piao ZE, Engelmeier R, Scanlon PJ, Loeb HS. The usefulness of dobutamine in the assessment of the severity of mitral stenosis. Am Heart J. 1986;111(2):312–6.

Chapter 9

Electrocardiogram in Mitral Stenosis

Krishnakumar Nair, Diego Chemello, Raja Selvaraj

About 100 years back, Thomas Lewis wrote "the electrocardiograms of mitral stenosis are often so characteristic that the valve lesion may be diagnosed from these curves alone".[1] With the coming of imaging, things have changed. Mitral stenosis (MS) was, in fact, the first disease to be diagnosed by echocardiography.[2] Today, imaging is the mainstay of diagnosis and decisions on management.[2] Although, its importance in patients with mitral stenosis has diminished with time, the electrocardiogram (ECG) offers useful, complementary information. Mitral stenosis, of course, does not produce any changes in the ECG by itself. The ECG, instead, reflects the changes secondary to mitral stenosis including left atrial enlargement, changes due to pulmonary hypertension like right ventricular hypertrophy, and atrial fibrillation. Therefore, the ECG is insensitive for mild MS that is not hemodynamically significant.[3]

Since, permutations and combinations of mixed valvular lesions can produce the entire range of electrocardiographic changes; we will discuss only the electrocardiographic changes of isolated mitral stenosis.

■ TERMINOLOGY

P wave abnormalities associated with disease conditions were traditionally given names such as P mitrale, P congenitale, and P pulmonale. These have mostly been replaced by the generic terms left atrial enlargement and right atrial enlargement, which are more appropriate since P wave abnormalities are not specific for the underlying condition, and because multiple factors may influence the P wave simultaneously.[4] The less specific terms left atrial abnormality and right atrial abnormality are even more accurate since the ECG changes are secondary not just to atrial enlargement, but high atrial pressure and intra-atrial conduction abnormalities also.[5–8]

The major electrocardiographic changes seen in mitral stenosis are left atrial abnormality, right atrial abnormality, combined atrial abnormality, right ventricular hypertrophy, and atrial arrhythmias.

■ LEFT ATRIAL ABNORMALITY

Electrocardiographic criteria for left atrial enlargement have limited sensitivity but high specificity compared to echocardiographic criteria. For example, the presence of wide and notched P wave patterns has a sensitivity of only 20% but a specificity of over 90% for detecting echocardiographically enlarged left atria. As previously alluded to, this reflects the fact the ECG changes are related to atrial stretch and conduction abnormalities in addition to enlargement. In fact, other studies have reported better correlations of these abnormalities with ventricular dysfunction than with atrial pathology.

Criteria for the diagnosis of left atrial abnormality include:

1. **P wave widening:** A widened P wave of > 0.12 seconds (Fig. 9.1) with normal or only slightly increased voltage. Left atrial activation begins and ends later than right atrial activation during P wave inscription. Therefore, left atrial abnormality usually involves prolongation of the P wave duration/total atrial activation time.[4] P wave duration has been shown to decrease after mitral commissurotomy, suggesting that it is an index of left atrial stretch.[9]

2. **P wave notching:** Notching of the P wave (Fig. 9.1), usually most obvious in lead II, with an interval between the peaks of > 40 msec. This is seen because the right and left atrial peaks that are normally nearly simultaneous and fused into a single peak become more widely separated.[4]

3. **Morris' index:** This index is the P terminal force, measured as the product of the amplitude and the duration of the terminal negative component of the P wave in lead V1. It has been the most frequently used of the various criteria for left atrial abnormality. A purely negative P wave in V1 is suggestive but can occur without an increased P terminal force. A P terminal force more negative than –0.04 mm-sec in lead VI[10] (Fig. 9.1) has a sensitivity of 67 to 89% and a specificity of 83 to 94%[11-16] for left atrial enlargement.[5]

4. **Macruz's index:** It is the ratio between the duration of the P wave in lead II and the duration of the PR segment.[17] It was initially described as a ratio useful in discriminating between cardiac lesions likely to cause LA involvement and those likely to cause right atrial abnormalities with a value of >1.6 indicating LA involvement. This criterion has a sensitivity of 50 to 65% and specificity of 50 to 89% for LA enlargement.[12,13,17,18] Other

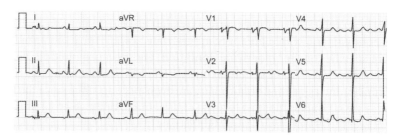

Fig. 9.1: *Sinus rhythm*: P waves in lead II are just greater than 0.12 seconds wide. P waves in leads II, I and aVL show notching with the characteristic "M" pattern. V1 shows typical left atrial abnormality in the form of prominent negative P terminal forces (more negative than 0.04 mm-sec)

than the other limitations common to all electrocardiographic criteria for LA enlargement: an inability to discriminate among LA enlargement, thickening, pressure overload and impaired atrial conduction, drugs that alter the P-R interval may also alter the index.

5. **Left axis of the terminal P wave**: Leftward shift of the mean P wave axis to between –30 and –45 degrees may be significant.

6. **P wave shape**: In one series of patients with mitral stenosis, the shape of the P wave was examined in lead I and II: the abnormal types described were the flat-topped P wave and the pointed P wave. Notching was described separately (Fig. 9.1). Thirty-two cases (61%) with mitral stenosis showed flat-topped P waves in either lead I or II. Pointed P waves were much less common and were found on only six (11%) occasions. Notching was found in sixteen cases (31%) and was nearly always associated with the flat-topped type of P wave.[1]

7. **P wave area**: P wave area more than 24 ms × mV measured from lead II is an indicator of left atrial enlargement.[19]

RIGHT ATRIAL ABNORMALITY

Right atrial abnormality occurs in patients with pulmonary arterial hypertension, or tricuspid valve involvement.

Electrocardiographic Criteria

1. **P wave amplitude**: Peaked P waves with amplitudes in lead II > 0.25 mV (Fig. 9.2) often termed "**P pulmonale**" primarily indicates right atrial abnormality. However, a similar finding may be seen in left atrial abnormality and is termed "**Pseudo P pulmonale**".

2. **P wave axis**: Rightward shift of the mean P wave axis to above +75 degrees.[4]

3. **Initial positive deflection of P wave**: The product of the amplitude and duration of the initial positive deflection of the P wave in lead V1 when > 0.06 mm-sec is a more specific sign of right atrial abnormality. In contrast,

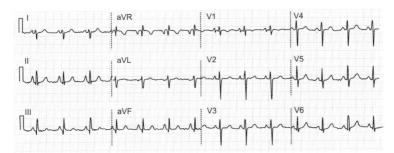

Fig. 9.2: *Pulmonary hypertension in mitral stenosis*: Right axis deviation and R/S ratio in V1 ≥ 1 is seen indicating right ventricular hypertrophy. Right atrial abnormality in the form of prominent peaked P waves in lead II greater than 0.25 mV is seen. Though the P wave is biphasic, prominent initial positivity of the P wave in V1 here indicates right atrial abnormality

as discussed earlier, left atrial abnormality causes more prominent increases in the amplitude of the later P wave forces (**pseudo P pulmonale**). Prominent initial positivity of the P wave in V1 or V2 [1.5 mm (0.15 mV) or more] also indicates right atrial abnormality.

■ COMBINED ATRIAL ABNORMALITY

Combined atrial abnormality is indicated essentially by the presence of some of the features of both right atrial and left atrial abnormality.

■ RIGHT VENTRICULAR HYPERTROPHY

Both moderately severe and severe MS have been associated with severe pulmonary arterial hypertension (PAH).[20,21] However, there is another group of patients with severe MS, with only a mild increase in pulmonary arterial pressure.[22-24] A clear relationship between left atrial size and pulmonary arterial pressure has not been demonstrated.[24] Though PAH has been observed as an indicator of disease severity in patients with MS,[25,26] PAH in patients with rheumatic MS may occur out of proportion to the degree of left atrial hypertension.[22]

Right ventricular dominance indicates presence of pulmonary arterial hypertension, which indicates the severity of mitral stenosis. This could manifest as a displacement of the QRS vector towards right and anterior, as well as delay in the R wave peak onset in right precordial leads.[4] The sensitivity of the ECG to detect RVH is low because only significant RVH can over-ride the dominant vector of left ventricular activation to become manifest on the electrocardiogram.[4] Electrocardiographic changes of right ventricular hypertrophy are more common in patients with juvenile mitral stenosis in whom pulmonary arterial hypertension is most severe.

ECG may show features of right ventricular hypertrophy and right atrial enlargement (Fig. 9.2). Many of the ECG criteria for RVH have been validated with autopsy data.[4,27-30] Some of the common ECG criteria for RVH are:
a. Q waves (especially qR patterns) in the right precordial leads without evidence of myocardial infarction.
b. Low-amplitude (under 600 µV) QRS complexes in lead V1 with a three-fold or greater increase in lead V2.
c. R:S ratio in V1 >1.[31]
d. Tall R in V1 >6 mm.[31]
e. Tall R in aVR >4 mm.[32]

Similar to left ventricular hypertrophy, ST depression and T-wave inversion when seen in right precordial leads with RVH is referred to as "secondary ST-T abnormality" or as "strain".[4]

Prominent left ventricular forces are rarely seen in isolated mitral stenosis. Left ventricular hypertrophy if seen should point suspicion to aortic stenosis, mitral regurgitation or coexistent hypertension.[33]

ATRIAL ARRHYTHMIAS

Thirty to forty percent of patients with mitral stenosis may develop atrial fibrillation.[3,20,21] Atrial fibrillation (Fig. 9.3) and atrial flutter are usually seen in older patients with large left atrium. Depending on the amplitude of the fibrillatory waves, atrial fibrillation has been described as coarse or fine. Coarse AF has been found to be associated with left atrial appendage dysfunction and higher risk of thromboembolism.[34,35]

Arrhythmias occur in mitral stenosis because the electrophysiologic substrate is altered by pressure overload and by the rheumatic process itself.[3,36] Ultrastructural changes resulting in fibrosis in the atria of patients with rheumatic MS[37,38] has been reported earlier suggesting that in patients with RHD, though the electrophysiological mechanism initiating and maintaining AF are not clear, they could be different to that of lone AF.[39]

In a study of MS, following cardioversion of AF, these patients were found to demonstrate significantly shorter ERPs, sinus node dysfunction, and no significant difference in atrial conduction delay to extrastimuli compared with patients in sinus rhythm. At repeat study 3 months following PMV, the ERPs had increased significantly compared with those who were in sinus rhythm.[40] In another study, an acute increase in ERP immediately after PMV was noted. Both these studies did not have normal controls.[41] In a third study, patients with rheumatic MS had significant biatrial remodelling (left atrium more than right atrium) characterized by atrial enlargement, loss of myocardium (areas of low voltage and electrical silence), and areas of electrical scarring associated with conduction abnormalities (fractionated electrograms) and no change or increased refractoriness. As a consequence of these abnormalities, patients with MS may be more susceptible to AF.[42]

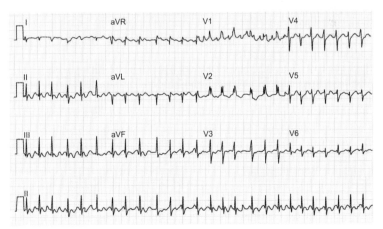

Fig. 9.3: ECG in a patient with severe MS—Shows coarse AF, right axis deviation and incomplete RBBB

MITRAL STENOSIS SEVERITY AND THE ECG

P wave duration and P wave dispersion have been found to correlate with the severity of mitral stenosis.[43] Presence of RBBB also correlates with the severity of MS.[44] It is also mentioned that as the severity of MS increases, the axis shift towards right and once we relieve the obstruction by balloon mitral valvotomy, the axis shifts back.

EFFECTS OF MITRAL VALVOTOMY ON ELECTROCARDIOGRAPHIC CHANGES OF MITRAL STENOSIS

Chandrasekar et al.[45] have reported that the acute hemodynamic changes following balloon mitral valvotomy often produce corresponding electrocardiographic changes. These changes indicated significantly greater hemodynamic benefit than when these changes are not seen. The electrocardiographic changes were mainly in P wave characteristics, and in QRS axis.

CLINICAL SIGNIFICANCE

The electrocardiographic findings of left atrial abnormality are associated with more severe mitral stenosis and with a higher incidence of atrial tachyarrhythmias. In today's world, the electrocardiogram is not as useful as the echocardiogram in the diagnosis and management of mitral stenosis; however, it still remains a useful tool in the armamentarium of the cardiologist mainly in the assessment of rhythm.

REFERENCES

1. Trounce JR. The electrocardiogram in mitral stenosis. Br Heart J. 1952;14(2): 185–92.
2. Chandrashekhar Y, Westaby S, Narula J. Mitral stenosis. Lancet. 2009;374 (9697):1271–83.
3. Bruce CJ, Nishimura RA. Clinical assessment and management of mitral stenosis. Cardiol Clin. 1998;16(3):375–403.
4. Hancock EW, Deal BJ, Mirvis DM, Okin P, Kligfield P, Gettes LS, et al. AHA/ ACCF/HRS recommendations for the standardization and interpretation of the electrocardiogram: part V: electrocardiogram changes associated with cardiac chamber hypertrophy: a scientific statement from the American Heart Association Electrocardiography and Arrhythmias Committee, Council on Clinical Cardiology; the American College of Cardiology Foundation; and the Heart Rhythm Society: endorsed by the International Society for Computerized Electrocardiology. Circulation. 2009;119(10):e251–61.
5. Munuswamy K, Alpert MA, Martin RH, Whiting RB, Mechlin NJ. Sensitivity and specificity of commonly used electrocardiographic criteria for left atrial enlargement determined by M-mode echocardiography. Am J Cardiol. 1984;53(6):829–32.
6. Josephson ME, Kastor JA, Morganroth J. Electrocardiographic left atrial enlargement. Electrophysiologic, echocardiographic and hemodynamic correlates. Am J Cardiol. 1977;39(7):967–71.

7. Di Bianco R, Gottdiener JS, Fletcher RD, Pipberger HV. Left atrial overload: a hemodynamic, echocardiographic, electrocardiographic and vectorcardiographic study. Am Heart J. 1979;98:478-89.

8. Probst P, Hunter J, Gamble O, Cohn K. Investigation of atrial aberration as a cause of altered P wave contour. Am Heart J. 1973;86(4):516-22.

9. John B, Stiles MK, Kuklik P, Brooks AG, Chandy ST, Kalman JM, et al. Reverse remodeling of the atria after treatment of chronic stretch in humans: implications for the atrial fibrillation substrate. J Am Coll Cardiol. 2010;55(12):1217-26.

10. Morris JJ Jr, Estes Eh Jr, Whalen Re, Thompson Hk Jr, Mcintosh HD. P-Wave Analysis In Valvular Heart Disease. Circulation. 1964;29:242-52.

11. Waggoner AD, Adyanthaya AV, Quinones MA, Alexander JK. Left atrial enlargement. Echocardiographic assessment of electrocardiographic criteria. Circulation. 1976;54(4):553-7.

12. Chirife R, Feitosa GS, Frankl WS. Electrocardiographic detection of left atrial enlargement. Correlation of P wave with left atrial dimension by echocardiography. Br Heart J. 1975;37(12):1281-5.

13. Kasser I, Kennedy JW. The relationship of increased left atrial volume and pressure to abnormal P waves on the electrocardiogram. Circulation. 1969;39(3):339-43.

14. Ikram H, Drysdale P, Bones PJ, Chan W. The non-invasive recognition of left atrial enlargement: comparison of electro- and echocardiographic measurements. Postgrad Med J. 1977;53(621):356-9.

15. Perosio AM, Suarez LD, Torino A, Llera JJ, Ballester A, Roisinblit JM. Reassessment of electrovectorcardiographic signs of left atrial enlargement. Clin Cardiol. 1982;5(12):640-6.

16. Rubler S, Shah NN, Moallem A. Comparison of left atrial size and pulmonary capillary pressure with P wave of electrocardiogram. Am Heart J. 1976;92(1):73-8.

17. Macruz R, Perloff JK, Case RB. A method for the electrocardiographic recognition of atrial enlargement. Circulation. 1958;17:882-9.

18. Human GP, Snyman HW. The value of the Macruz index in the diagnosis of atrial enlargement. Circulation. 1963;27:935-8.

19. Zeng C, Wei T, Zhao R, Wang C, Chen L, Wang L. Electrocardiographic diagnosis of left atrial enlargement in patients with mitral stenosis: the value of the P-wave area. Acta Cardiol. 2003;58(2):139-41.

20. Wood P. An appreciation of mitral stenosis. I. Clinical features. Br Med J. 1954;1(4870):1051-63; contd.

21. Wood P. An appreciation of mitral stenosis: II. Investigations and results. Br Med J. 1954;15;1(4871):1113-24.

22. Fawzy ME, Hassan W, Stefadouros M, Moursi M, El Shaer F, Chaudhary MA. Prevalence and fate of severe pulmonary hypertension in 559 consecutive patients with severe rheumatic mitral stenosis undergoing mitral balloon valvotomy. J Heart Valve Dis. 2004;13(6):942-947; discussion 947-48.

23. Ribeiro PA, Al Zaibag M, Abdullah M. Pulmonary artery pressure and pulmonary vascular resistance before and after mitral balloon valvotomy in 100 patients with severe mitral valve stenosis. Am Heart J. 1993;125(4):1110-4.

24. Otto CM, Davis KB, Reid CL, Slater JN, Kronzon I, Kisslo KB, et al. Relation between pulmonary artery pressure and mitral stenosis severity in patients undergoing balloon mitral commissurotomy. Am J Cardiol. 1993;71(10):874-8.

25. Bahl VK, Chandra S, Talwar KK, Kaul U, Sharma S, Wasir HS. Balloon mitral valvotomy in patients with systemic and suprasystemic pulmonary artery pressures. Cathet Cardiovasc Diagn. 1995;36(3):211-5.

26. Krishnamoorthy KM, Dash PK, Radhakrishnan S, Shrivastava S. Response of different grades of pulmonary artery hypertension to balloon mitral valvuloplasty. Am J Cardiol. 2002;90(10):1170-3.

27. Butler PM, Leggett SI, Howe CM, Freye CJ, Hindman NB, Wagner GS. Identification of electrocardiographic criteria for diagnosis of right ventricular hypertrophy due to mitral stenosis. Am J Cardiol. 1986;57(8):639-43.

28. Scott RC. Electrocardiographic-pathologic conference. Right bundle branch block and ventricular hypertrophy. Ohio State Med J. 1967;63(7):916-7.

29. Murphy ML, Hutcheson F. The electrocardiographic diagnosis of right ventricular hypertrophy in chronic obstructive pulmonary disease. Chest. 1974;65(6):622-7.

30. Murphy ML, Thenabadu PN, de Soyza N, Doherty JE, Meade J, Baker BJ, et al. Reevaluation of electrocardiographic criteria for left, right and combined cardiac ventricular hypertrophy. Am J Cardiol. 1984;53(8):1140-7.

31. Myers GB, Klein HA, Stofer BE. The electrocardiographic diagnosis of right ventricular hypertrophy. Am Heart J. 1948;35(1):1-40.

32. Sokolow M, Lyon TP. The ventricular complex in left ventricular hypertrophy as obtained by unipolar precordial and limb leads. Am Heart J. 1949;37(2):161-86.

33. Bruce CJ, Nishimura RA. Newer advances in the diagnosis and treatment of mitral stenosis. Curr Probl Cardiol. 1998;23(3):125-92.

34. Yilmaz MB, Guray Y, Guray U, Cay S, Caldir V, Biyikoglu SF, et al. Fine vs. coarse atrial fibrillation: which one is more risky? Cardiology. 2007;107(3):193-6.

35. Mutlu B, Karabulut M, Eroglu E, Tigen K, Bayrak F, Fotbolcu H, et al. Fibrillatory wave amplitude as a marker of left atrial and left atrial appendage function, and a predictor of thromboembolic risk in patients with rheumatic mitral stenosis. Int J Cardiol. 2003;91(2-3):179-86.

36. Selzer A, Cohn KE. Natural history of mitral stenosis: a review. Circulation. 1972;45(4):878-90.

37. Thiedemann KU, Ferrans VJ. Left atrial ultrastructure in mitral valvular disease. Am J Pathol. 1977;89(3):575-604.

38. Pham TD, Fenoglio JJ Jr. Right atrial ultrastructural in chronic rheumatic heart disease. Int J Cardiol. 1982;1(3-4):289-304.

39. Nair M, Shah P, Batra R, Kumar M, Mohan J, Kaul U, et al. Chronic atrial fibrillation in patients with rheumatic heart disease: mapping and radiofrequency ablation of flutter circuits seen at initiation after cardioversion. Circulation. 2001;104(7): 802-9.

40. Fan K, Lee KL, Chow W-H, Chau E, Lau C-P. Internal cardioversion of chronic atrial fibrillation during percutaneous mitral commissurotomy: insight into reversal of chronic stretch-induced atrial remodeling. Circulation. 2002;105(23):2746-52.

41. Soylu M, Demir AD, Ozdemir O, Topaloğlu S, Aras D, Duru E, et al. Evaluation of atrial refractoriness immediately after percutaneous mitral balloon commissurotomy in patients with mitral stenosis and sinus rhythm. Am Heart J. 2004;147(4):741-5.

42. John B, Stiles MK, Kuklik P, Chandy ST, Young GD, Mackenzie L, et al. Electrical remodelling of the left and right atria due to rheumatic mitral stenosis. Eur Heart J. 2008;29(18):2234-43.

43. Guntekin U, Gunes Y, Tuncer M, Gunes A, Sahin M, Simsek H. Long-term follow-up of P-wave duration and dispersion in patients with mitral stenosis. Pacing Clin Electrophysiol PACE. 2008;31(12):1620-4.

44. Ocal A, Yildirim N, Ozbakir C, Saricam E, Ozdogan OU, Arslan S, et al. Right bundle branch block: a new parameter revealing the progression rate of mitral stenosis. Cardiology. 2006;105(4):219-22.

45. Chandrasekar B, Loya YS, Sharma S, Paidhungat JV. Acute effect of balloon mitral valvotomy on serial electrocardiographic changes and their haemodynamic correlation. Indian Heart J. 1998;50(2):179-82.

Chapter 10

Radiological Evaluation in Mitral Stenosis

Bhavesh Harivadan, Harikrishnan S

Radiological evaluation using chest X-ray and angiography was the major modality to assess mitral stenosis (MS) before the advent of echocardiography. Angiography, as a modality in assessment of MS is now limited to assessment of mitral regurgitation (MR) during percutaneous mitral valvotomy (PMV).

■ CHEST ROENTGENOGRAPHY

The chest X-ray findings in MS are generally a consequence of left atrial enlargement, mitral valve calcification, pulmonary hypertension and right heart failure.[1]

Left Atrial Enlargement

The characteristic radiologic finding of mitral stenosis is selective left atrial enlargement.

An enlarged left atrial appendage will be seen as a convexity at the left upper cardiac border just below the left main bronchus. Left atrial enlargement, alters the left border of the cardiac silhouette so that it becomes straight[2] in contrast to the usual mild concavity evident beneath the pulmonary artery shadow. A double shadow visible through the right atrial shadow indicates LA enlargement. Other indirect evidence of LAE is the elevation of the left main bronchus.

On the lateral chest radiograph, an enlarged LA is seen as a posterior displacement of the upper cardiac border, inferior to the tracheal bifurcation. In fact, a lateral chest radiograph obtained during a barium swallow study may show a large left atrium impinging on the esophagus and displacing it backwards and to the left, in contrast to its usual rightward displacement.

However, aneurysmal enlargement of left atrium favors significant mitral regurgitation either isolated or in association with mitral stenosis. Although, isolated severe MS can cause LA enlargement, aneurysmal enlargement is uncommon. The LV is usually not enlarged in cases of isolated mitral stenosis unless there is clinically significant mitral regurgitation or aortic regurgitation or left ventricular dysfunction (Fig. 10.1).

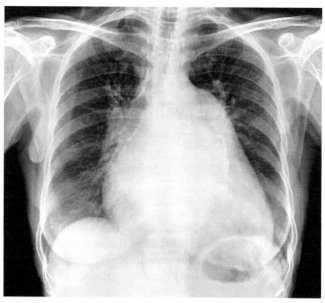

Fig. 10.1: Severe mitral stenosis—note the calcified wall of left atrium. Left atrial enlargement is seen as double shadow. Pulmonary arterial hypertension is evident as dilated central pulmonary arteries

Calcification

Calcification in MS can occur in the following situations:
1. Left atrial wall calcification.
2. Calcified thrombus in the LA appendage or LA roof. This may appear as a curvilinear structure lying fairly high on the cardiac silhouette.
3. Rarely, extensively calcified mitral valves are seen in plain X-ray. Usually, they are seen by fluoroscopy.
4. Mitral annular calcification may be seen in the shape of an ellipse, usually open medially in a J, U, or horseshoe shape.

Pulmonary Hypertension

In the presence of pulmonary arterial hypertension, the main pulmonary artery and central pulmonary vessels appear enlarged. In long standing severe pulmonary hypertension there may be pruning of the peripheral vessels as well (*see* Chapter 57 on PH).

Pulmonary Congestion

As the pulmonary venous pressure increases, it is reflected as a characteristic change in vascularity pattern on the chest X-ray. Normally, in the erect position, pulmonary arterial blood flow is less in the upper zones than in the lower zones. When the mean pulmonary capillary pressure is constantly above 20 mm Hg, vasoconstriction of lower lobe pulmonary arteries will occur and there will

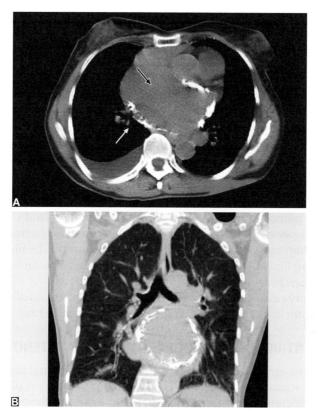

Fig. 10.2: A 71-year-old woman with known mitral stenosis and atrial fibrillation underwent routine preoperative screening for cataract surgery. A follow up non-contrast CT of the chest shows calcifications all along the wall of the left atrium. *Source:* Leacock K, Duerinckx AJ, Davis B. "Porcelain Atrium: A case report with literature review." Case reports in Radiology, vol. 2011, Article ID 501396, 3 pages, 20113.

be equalization of the vascularity, i.e. both upper and lower lobe vascularity will be equal. As the further increase in postcapillary pulmonary hypertension ensues, pulmonary vascular resistance also rises, typically first in the lower zones. At this time, pulmonary blood flow is diverted to the upper lung zones where the resistance initially is unchanged. This results in the "upper lobe diversion" phenomenon observed on the erect chest radiograph also called cephalization. This pattern of cephalization is positively correlated with elevated mean pulmonary wedge pressure, pulmonary artery hypertension and pulmonary vascular resistance.

The horizontal interlobar fissure may be visible, due to collection of edema fluid within the fissure. Pulmonary alveolar edema may appear as confluent pulmonary shadows present mainly in the perihilar region.

The edematous interlobular septa of the lungs associated with high pulmonary venous pressure may be identified on the chest radiograph as opaque lines of different lengths, depending on their location. Kerley et al first described these lines, designated A, B, and C known as Kerley lines.[4]

A lines are 5 to 10 cm long and are non-branching; they fan radially upward and outward from the pulmonary hilum. B lines are best seen in the lower lung zones, perpendicular to the pleural surface; these are shorter than 2 cm. The combination of A and B lines creates a reticular pattern, called C lines, that are transient and difficult to visualize.

All the Kerley lines represent edematous interlobular septa. The pulmonary lobules tend to be large and are oriented obliquely to the pleura in the upper lobes, whereas in the lower lobes, they are shortened and are perpendicular to the pleural surface. This feature results in the characteristic appearance of the B lines, which are the ones most readily identified on the chest radiograph.

Miscellaneous Findings

Pulmonary hemosiderosis develops in long-standing mitral stenosis and pulmonary hypertension. It is seen on the chest image as fine punctuate opacities throughout the lungs (Fig. 10.3). Patients usually give history of hemoptysis in the course of their illness. It is believed to be due to recurrent alveolar hemorrhages leading to iron containing deposits in the pulmonary tissue.

Pulmonary ossified nodules, defined as multiple discrete calcified opacities of up to 10 mm in diameter, may be seen at the bases of the lungs as well.

◾ LEFT VENTRICULAR ANGIOGRAPHY IN MITRAL STENOSIS

Use of LV angiography in mitral stenosis at present is limited to assessment of mitral regurgitation during PMV. However, prior to widespread availability of echocardiography, left ventricular angiography was utilized to assess the severity of mitral stenosis and the severity of subvalvular disease. In mitral stenosis, mitral valve leaflet movement is restricted and leaflets will be visible due to immobility (Fig. 10.4). During left ventricular angiography, hold up of non-opacified blood in the doming mitral leaflet will give a white oval egg like shadow within the black contrast filled LV cavity (white egg sign). Sometimes a narrow jet of contrast entering into LV from LA can be seen, instead of the free flowing puff.

Left Ventricular Function in MS

Some patient with mitral stenosis show impaired left ventricular systolic function.[5,6] Regional and global abnormality of LV myocardial mechanical performance has been reported.[7] 40% of patients were found to have RMWA, 20% each having abnormalities in anterior and posterior territories.[7] Colle et al. has concluded that segmental contraction abnormalities appear to be the main factor involved in the global LVF impairment. "Segmental wall motion abnormalities could be related to subvalvular fibrosis, or LV filling difficulties, or principally, to a possible interplay between the right and the left ventricles."[7]

Fulcrum and Fornix

Fulcrum and fornix are mainly described for showing the mitral valve prolapse in left ventricular angiogram. Fulcrum is the point of attachment of mitral leaflet to

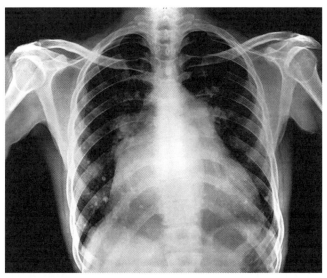

Fig. 10.3: Pulmonary hemosiderosis in MS more prominent in right lower zone. Also note the left and right atrial enlargement, pulmonary venous hypertension (cephalization) and dilated pulmonary arteries suggestive of pulmonary arterial hypertension

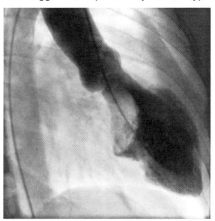

Fig. 10.4: Left ventricular angiogram in severe MS. Note the doming mitral valve

the annulus fibrosus. It is seen in right anterior oblique (RAO) view as the most inferior portion of leaflet attachment to annulus. Fornix is defined as part of LV between the insertion of the mitral leaflets into annulus and base of the papillary muscles (Fig. 10.5).

Assessment of Subvalvar Pathology

Mitral subvalvar pathology can be assessed on left ventricular angiogram and is expressed as the mitral subvalvular distance ratio. This is defined as the ratio of the distance from the mitral valve to the tip of the papillary muscle in end-systole to the distance from the aortic valve to the left ventricular apex in end-diastole as described by Akins et al.[9] Subvalvar distance ratio of <0.2 was

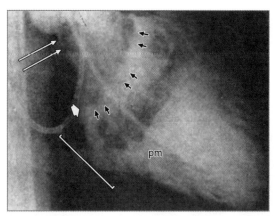

Fig. 10.5: Early diastolic frame of 16 mm cine left ventriculogram from a patient without heart disease. The fulcrum (short wide white arrow) or point of attachment of the mitral leaflets to the mitral annulus is clearly seen. The fornix (white bracket) is the left ventricular wall between the fulcrum and papillary muscles (PM).The papillary muscles are better seen on a systolic frame. The line of attachment of the posterior mitral leaflet (black arrow—heads) sharply outlines the width of the mitral valve. The membranous septum (atrioventricular portion) (long thin white arrows) can be seen in the subaortic region as a smooth straight or minimally curved line beneath the noncoronary leaflet. Nonopacified left atrial blood entering into the left ventricle can be seen as the broad band of lucency encompassing the entire width of the ventricle and immediately in front of the attachment of the posterior mitral leaflet[8]

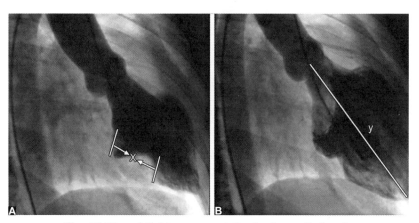

Figs 10.6A and B: Measurement of subvalvar pathology in rheumatic mitral stenosis

considered as severe and >0.2 was mild to moderate subvalvar fibrosis (Figs 10.6A and B).

Assessment of Mitral Regurgitation

The most important use of LV angiography nowadays is the assessment of mitral regurgitation prior to PMV. LV angio is also useful in patients after PMV

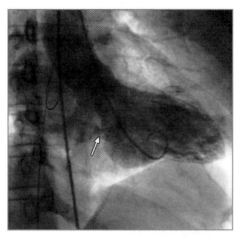

Fig. 10.7: LV angiogram showing moderate commissural MR (arrow) following PMV. See the pigtail shaped guide wire in the left atrium. This patient was followed up and remained stable after one year

for assessment of mitral regurgitation. Caution should be taken in patients who have developed severe MR, as contrast load can precipitate acute pulmonary edema (Fig. 10.7).

REFERENCES

1. Ellis K. Roentgenographic features of mitral valve disease. Ann N Y Acad Sci. 1965;118:490–502.
2. Chadha S, Shetty V, Sadiq A, Hollander G, Shani J. Left heart border straightening in severe mitral stenosis. QJM Mon J Assoc Physicians. 2013;106(8):775-6.
3. Leacock K, Duerinckx AJ, Davis B. Porcelain atrium: a case report with literature review. Case Rep Radiol. 2011;2011:501396.
4. Milne En. Physiological interpretation of the plain radiograph in mitral stenosis, including a review of criteria for the radiological estimation of pulmonary arterial and venous pressures. Br J Radiol. 1963;36:902-13.
5. Holzer JA, Karliner JS, O'Rourke RA, Peterson KL. Quantitative angiographic analysis of the left ventricle in patients with isolated rheumatic mitral stenosis. Br Heart J. 1973;35(5):497–502.
6. Guven S, Sen T, Tufekcioglu O, Gucuk E, Uygur B, Kahraman E. Evaluation of left ventricular systolic function with pulsed wave tissue Doppler in rheumatic mitral stenosis. Cardiol J. 2014;21(1):33-8.
7. Colle JP, Rahal S, Ohayon J, Bonnet J, Le Goff G, Besse P, et al. Global left ventricular function and regional wall motion in pure mitral stenosis. Clin Cardiol. 1984;7(11):573-80.
8. Spindola-Franco H, Bjork L, Adams DF, Abrams HL. Classification of the radiological morphology of the mitral valve. Differentiation between true and pseudoprolapse. Br Heart J. 1980;44(1):30-6.
9. Akins CW, Kirklin JK, Block PC, Buckley MJ, Austen WG. Preoperative evaluation of subvalular fibrosis in mitral stenosis. A predictor factor in conservative vs replacement surgical therapy. Circulation. 1979;60(2 Pt 2):71-6.

Chapter 11

Balloon Mitral Valvotomy— Role of Echocardiography

Hosam Hasan-Ali, Harikrishnan S

■ ANATOMICAL BACKGROUND

The mitral valve (MV) is a complex structure consisting of 6 components; annulus fibrosus, leaflets, chordae tendineae, papillary muscles, posterior left atrial wall and left ventricular wall. These 6 components should be considered functionally a unit, since derangement of any one can cause MV dysfunction.[1] The detailed description of mitral valve anatomy is given in Chapter 3.

Pathological Anatomy in Mitral Stenosis

Rheumatic pathology results in 4 forms of MV pathology—commissural (30%), cuspal (15%), chordal (10%) and combined (45%). The detailed description of the pathological anatomy in mitral stenosis (MS) is given in Chapter 3.

By rheumatic process, the primary orifice of the mitral valve—at the level of the mitral valve annulus gets narrowed due to commissural fusion and valve thickening. The valve orifice which is tubular normally, changes to "funnel-shaped". With the pathology of the leaflets, the orifice becomes fish—mouthed or buttonhole like. The secondary orifices, between the chordal structures also get narrowed due to chordal fusion and chordal shortening. The subvalvar pathology causes the mitral valve opening to become a funnel-shaped structure.

The primary orifice located at the level of the annulus is narrowed mainly due to commissural fusion. When only one commissure is fused or one is fused more than the other the stenotic orifice is eccentrically located. A centrally located orifice indicates symmetrical commissural fusion.[2,3] Though calcification may occur in any part of the MV or its associated structures, it is most frequently found in the leaflets and in the commissural regions.[4,5]

■ PATHOPHYSIOLOGY OF MITRAL STENOSIS

The detailed description of the pathophysiology of MS can be found in Chapter 5. Mitral stenosis leads to obstruction of the left ventricular inflow, leading to raised left atrial (LA) pressure which is passively transmitted to the pulmonary capillary bed. In response to this, there will be pulmonary artery vasoconstriction and the chronically elevated pulmonary venous hypertension will lead to structural changes in the pulmonary arteries. The resultant pulmonary arterial hypertension will lead to right ventricular hypertrophy followed by right ventricular (RV) dilatation and failure.

All the above anatomical and pathophysiological alterations can be evaluated by echocardiography. Henceforth echocardiography is considered as the investigation of choice in the evaluation of patients with mitral stenosis.

ECHOCARDIOGRAPHIC ASSESSMENT IN MS PRIOR TO PERCUTANEOUS MITRAL VALVOTOMY

Echocardiography is the primary modality of evaluation in a patient who is planned for percutaneous mitral valvotomy (PMV). It is essential for the intraprocedural monitoring, the postprocedural assessment and follow-up.

What are the Parameters we Assess for PMV?

To discuss this we should know the indications and contraindications for PMV. The indications are described elsewhere in this book. The absolute contraindications are commissural calcium, left atrial thrombus and ≥ 3+ mitral regurgitation. We get good results following PMV in uniformly thickened valves with no calcium and no significant subvalvar pathology. So, the primary aim of echocardiographic assessment is to find the suitable valve for PMV and identify those valves which will give inadequate results or lead to complications.

EAE-ASE recommendations 2009[6] says that the assessment of severity rheumatic MS should rely mostly on valve area because of the multiple factors influencing other measurements, particularly mean gradient and systolic pulmonary artery pressure.

Parameters Assessed by Echocardiography

A. Preprocedure
1. Severity of MS (Fig. 11.1 and Table 11.1)
2. Pliability (Suitability of the valve for PMV)
   a. Calcification
   b. Valve thickening (uniform/non-uniform)
   c. Subvalvar pathology
   d. Commissural morphology.
3. Mitral regurgitation
4. Left atrial thrombus [Usually performed with transesophageal echocardiography (TEE)]
5. Assessment of the interatrial septum
6. Diseases of the other valves
7. Assessment of pulmonary hypertension.

B. Intraprocedure monitoring
1. Adequacy of commissural splitting (stepwise dilatation)
2. Mitral regurgitation
3. Complications—cardiac tamponade.

C. Postprocedure evaluation

1. Adequacy of commissural splitting
2. Residual stenosis, MR
3. Atrial septal defect (ASD).

Table 11.1: Severity of mitral stenosis modified from ASE/EAE[6]			
Severity	*Mild*	*Moderate*	*Severe*
Mitral valve area (cm²)	>1.5	1–1.5	<1
Pressure half-time (msec)	100–150	150–220	>220
Mean pressure gradient (mm hg)*	<5	5–10	>10

*At heart rates 60–80 bpm in sinus rhythm

M-mode Echocardiography (Figs 11.1 to 11.7)

M-mode echocardiography, the first echocardiographic modality used for the assessment of MS is still widely utilized. The M-mode parameters used to assess the severity of MS are DE amplitude and EF slope.

M-mode Parameters in the Assessment of Severity of MS and Pliability

DE amplitude of more than 18 mm is indicative of a pliable valve. The normal EF slope is 50 to 180 mm/sec. When there is severe MS the EF slope comes down to 10 to 20 mm/sec or can even reach zero (Fig. 11.5). Even though there is correlation between the EF slope and severity of MS, EF slope is found to be altered in left ventricular (LV) diastolic dysfunction. So, it is not found as useful a parameter when we have better techniques like 2D echocardiography.

Two-dimensional Echocardiography

The most important and useful echocardiographic modality in the assessment for PMV is 2D echocardiography. Since the valve morphology is the most

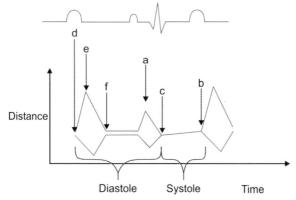

Fig. 11.1: Normal M-mode echocardiography of mitral valve
Courtesy: Edwards F Crooks

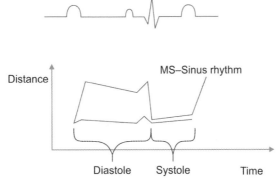

Fig. 11.2: M-mode echocardiography in mitral stenosis in sinus rhythm
Courtesy: Edwards F Crooks

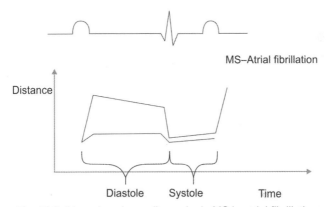

Fig. 11.3: M-mode echocardiography in MS in atrial fibrillation
Courtesy: Edwards F Crooks

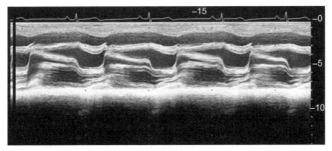

Fig. 11.4: M-mode echo of mitral valve in mitral stenosis.
Note the anterior movement of the PML and thickening of the leaflets

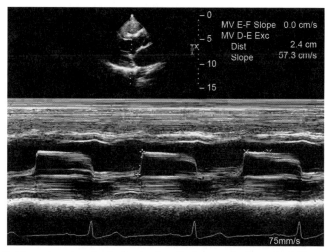

Fig. 11.5: M-mode echo of mitral valve in mitral stenosis. *Note* the DE amplitude of 24 mm and EF slope of 0 cm/sec. This indicates severe and pliable MS

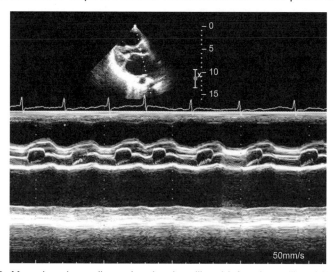

Fig. 11.6: M-mode echocardiography showing dilated left atrium, dilated RV, normal sized aorta and normally opening aortic valve in a patient with tight MS in atrial fibrillation

important predictor of the success of PMV, 2D echocardiographic assessment is very crucial (Figs 11.8 and 11.9).

Due to rheumatic processes, the mitral valve becomes thickened and the mobility of the valve leaflets gets restricted. This will be evident in the parasternal long axis (PLAX) view where the anterior mitral leaflet (AML) shows a "hockey-stick" appearance and the valve appears doming (Fig. 11.8).

The other structures which can be assessed by 2D echo are the aortic and tricuspid valves. The aortic valve is assessed in the PLAX and the parasternal short axis (PSAX) views and also the 5 chamber views. The tricuspid valve is assessed in the apical four chamber (A4C) view.

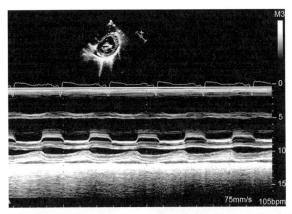

Fig. 11.7: M-mode echocardiography in a patient with severe MS and severe LV dysfunction

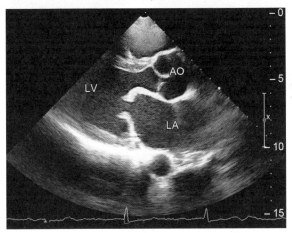

Fig. 11.8: PLAX view showing the grossly thickened mitral valve and anterior mitral leaflet (AML) giving the characteristic "hockey-stick" appearance. Doming of the mitral valve is also seen
Abbreviations: LV, left ventricle; AO, aorta; LA, left atrium

The parameters which are evaluated in the 2D echocardiographic assessment of MS are:
1. Left atrial enlargement.
2. MS severity by planimetry assessment of mitral valve area (MVA).
3. Morphology of the mitral valve
   a. Calcification (especially at the commissure)
   b. Valve thickening (uniform/non-uniform)
   c. Subvalvar pathology
   d. Commissural morphology—fibrosis, fusion
4. LA thrombus (usually performed with TEE, but sometimes detected by TTE itself)
5. Assessment of the interatrial septum
6. Disease of the other valves.

Mitral Valve Area Assessment by Planimetry

Mitral valve area (MVA) measured by planimetry method (Fig. 11.9) has the best correlation with valve area measured on explanted valves.[6] So, this is considered the reference measurement for MVA. Planimetry is the direct measurement of MVA and, unlike other methods, does not involve (1) any hypothesis regarding flow conditions, (2) cardiac chamber compliance, or (3) presence of associated valvular lesions.

The MV in rheumatic MS becomes a funnel-shaped structure that tapers to the primary orifice at its tips. So depending on the area of scanning, the MVA can get altered (Fig. 11.10). The settings of the echo machine also affect the measurement of MVA.

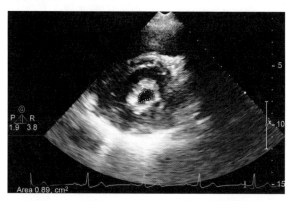

Fig. 11.9: Assessment of MVA by planimetry. The 2D MVA here is 0.894 cm² indicating severe MS. Both the commissures are fused

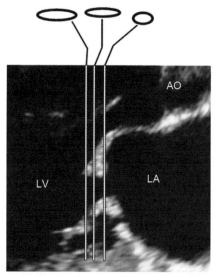

Fig. 11.10: Measurement of 2D MVA by planimetry may be fraught with fallacies if not measured properly. This picture shows significant variation in MVA when measured in three different imaging planes
Abbreviations: LA, left atrium; LV, left ventricle; AO, aorta

How to Ideally Measure MVA by Planimetry

1. The PSAX view—smallest orifice to be identified by scanning from the LA to LV apex.
2. Identification of the orifice at its maximal opening in mid diastole.
3. The measurement plane should be perpendicular to the mitral orifice.
4. Lowest gain settings (increased gain settings lead to "blooming" of echoes, underestimates the MVA).
5. Trace the contour of the inner mitral orifice.
6. Commissures to be included if open.
7. Average of three measurements in SR, 5-10 in AF. (*Ref. EAE ASE guidelines 2009*)[6].

Limitations of Planimetry Measurement

1. Orthogonality of the imaging plane with the mitral orifice is assumed, but not granted.
2. The level at which the 2D plane intersects the funnel formed by the stenotic mitral orifice cannot be controlled by the echocardiographer.
3. Calcium will make the tracing of the contour difficult.
4. Commissures especially the opened commissures will be difficult to be traced accurately.

Mitral Leaflet Separation Index

Another parameter which is useful in assessing the severity of MS is the mitral valve leaflet separation index (Fig. 11.11). It is measured in diastole in PLAX view and apical 4 chamber view, then the average of the two measurements are taken. An index of 0.8 cm or less predicted severe MS. A value of 1.1 to 1.2 cm or more indicates mild MS. This parameter is found to be an independent predictor of success during PMV (with 90% sensitivity and 100% specificity).[7,8]

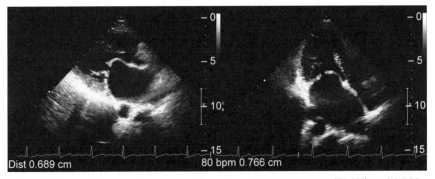

Fig. 11.11: Leaflet separation index. The value obtained is 0.689 (PLAX) and 0.766 (A4C) is averaged to get the value of 0.727 cm which indicates severe MS

Mitral Valve Morphology

As the primary mechanism by which PMV increases MVA is splitting of the fused commissures, commissural morphology is one of the most important factors which influence the outcome of PMV. So, assessment of valve morphology by echocardiography becomes critical.

While assessing the morphology of the valve, mobility, thickening, subvalvar pathology and calcification are the four important parameters which are evaluated. Of these parameters, commissural morphology is the most important.

Various scoring systems are used to grade the morphology of the valve. The details of those are given later in this Chapter.

Mobility of the Valve

Leaflet motion: To assess leaflet motion the MV leaflets are usually imaged in the parasternal long axis view during maximum doming of the anterior leaflet in early diastole. Wilkins scoring system[9] assesses the mobility and grades it into 4. More objective grading of the morphology of the mitral valve is done by the system by Reid et al.[10]

They assess the extent of doming of the anterior mitral leaflet (AML) by drawing a line from the junction of the posterior wall of the aortic root and anterior MV to the tip of the mitral leaflet (xy- H) (Fig. 11.12). From this line, a perpendicular line is drawn to the leading edge of the maximum dome (ab- L). Leaflet mobility is then expressed as a slope by dividing the height of the dome by the length of the dome—H/L[10] (Table 11.2).

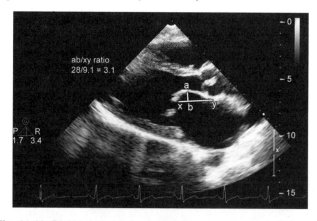

Fig. 11.12: PLAX view demonstrating the measurement of H/L ratio

Table 11.2: Height and length ratio[10]

Height and length ratio (ab/xy)	Grade	Score
< 0.25	Mild	0
0.25–0.44	Moderate	1
> 0.45	Severe	2

Valve Thickening

The normal thickness of the mitral valve is less than 4 mm. Thickness of 5 to 8 mm is considered mildly thickened and >8 mm is considered markedly thickened. Thickening can extend to the whole of the leaflet or it can be localized to the margins.[9] As the thickness increases, the outcome of the procedure becomes worse.

Valve thickening is usually assessed from the 2D image in the PLAX view. A more objective assessment of valve thickening can be obtained by measuring the ratio of the thickness of the valve leaflet to the thickness of the posterior aortic wall (valve thickness/posterior aortic wall thickness— the normal value is <1.4). Ratio up to 2.0 is considered mild thickening, 2 to 5 is moderate and > 5 is considered severe thickening.[10]

Valve Calcification

Even though valve calcification (Figs 11.13 to 11.15) influences the outcome of PMV, it is the calcium in the commissures which mostly influences the outcome. Commissural calcium is analyzed in parasternal short axis view by careful scanning of the MV orifice from the level of the aortic root to the MV leaflets. The echogenicity of the aortic root is used as a point of reference.[11] The severity of commissural calcium is assessed in each commissure as follows (when absent = 0 and when present =1); then the score of both commissures is summed to give a total score – maximum of 2.[12]

Calcification is the most important factor in deciding whether the patient should go for a closed procedure or not. If there is commissural calcium it is a contraindication to a closed procedure (Fig. 11.16). Calcium restricted to the belly of the AML or PML (Fig. 11.14) is not an absolute contraindication to the procedure. Even-though there are reports on PMV in unicommissural calcium, bicommissural calcium (Fig. 11.13) is a contraindication to the procedure.

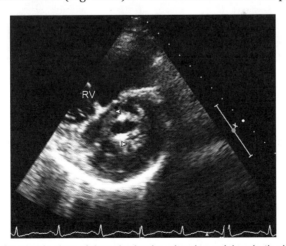

Fig. 11.13: Short axis view of the mitral valve showing calcium in the belly of both AML and PML. This is not a contraindication for PMV
Abbreviations: AML, Anterior mitral leaflet; PML, Posterior mitral leaflet; RV, right ventricle

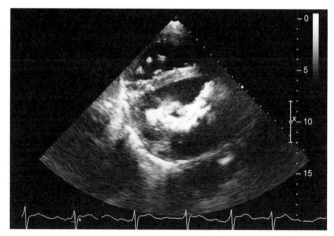

Fig. 11.14: Heavily calcific mitral valve in a patient with severe mitral stenosis (PSAX view)

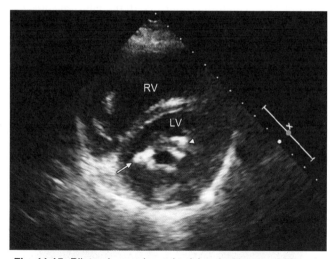

Fig. 11.15: Bilateral commissural calcium in 60-year-old female with severe MS. This is a contraindication of PMV
Abbreviations: LV, left ventricle; RV, right ventricle

Fibrotic valves as evidenced by bright echogenic valve tissue gives inferior results compared to nonfibrotic valves. Fibrotic valves usually yield less to balloon dilatation.

■ SUBVALVAR PATHOLOGY

Subvalvar pathology (SVP) is found to be an important predictor of the outcome of PMV. Higher grades of SVP is associated with poor outcomes after PMV. The subvalvar region is the secondary orifice of the mitral valve, which gets narrowed by rheumatic process.

According to the original description by Wilkins et al[9] subvalvar thickening usually requires a series of modified views to assess it properly. In the parasternal long axis view, the standard alignment should be tilted medially and laterally so that the long axis of each papillary muscle and its attached chordal apparatus can be examined in turn. From the apical window, the extent of subvalvar shortening and scar will be best viewed in a four chamber view with the transducer angled more posteriorly into the left ventricle, or from a foreshortened two chamber view angled medially and laterally.[9]

Detailed description about the assessment of the subvalvar apparatus is given in Chapter 13.

Chambers, Septum and Thrombi

Structures other than mitral valve also need to be assessed while evaluating the patient for PMV. The structures are left atrium including the left atrial appendage and the interatrial septum.

■ LEFT ATRIUM

The left atrium will be dilated in MS (Figs 11.16 and 11.17). The size of the left atrium depends on the severity of the stenosis, duration of obstruction and the presence of mitral regurgitation. The size of the left atrium will increase as the severity of stenosis increases. In some patients with long standing MS as seen in developing countries like India, we may come across very large left atria, called the "aneurysmal LA".

The other structure which needs to be evaluated very closely is the left atrial appendage. It is usually seen in the PSAX view, but it is sometimes difficult to obtain a good image. If we can identify a thrombus in the LAA in transthoracic echocardiography, we can avoid a TEE (Figs 11.17 to 11.19).

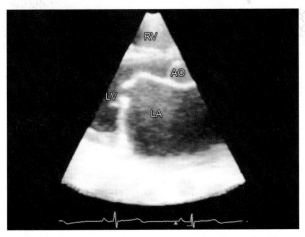

Fig. 11.16: 3D echocardiographic image recorded online using the matrix array probe in PLAX view showing the dilated LA, thickened and doming mitral valve
Abbreviations: RV, right ventricle; AO, aorta; LV, left ventricle; LA, left atrium

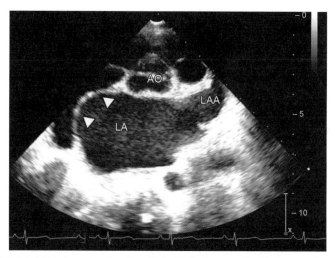

Fig. 11.17: PSAX view showing the dilated left atrium, left atrial appendage which is free of thrombus and bulging IAS towards the right atrium (arrow heads)
Abbreviations: LA, left atrium; AO, aorta; LAA, left atrial appendage

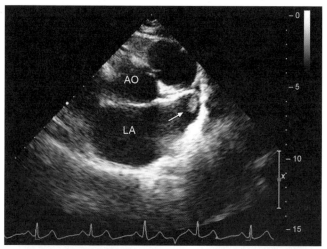

Fig. 11.18: A small thrombus in the apex of the left atrial appendage (PSAX view) 🎥◀
Abbreviations: LA, left atrium; AO, aorta

Left Ventricle

The left ventricle is usually normal in size or slightly smaller in mitral stenosis due to chronic under filling. If the LV is dilated, it may be due to the presence of LV dysfunction (which can be seen in few cases of MS due to extension of the rheumatic pathology into the LV) or most commonly due to the presence of aortic regurgitation or mitral regurgitation. Other uncommon causes are the presence of other diseases like coronary artery disease.

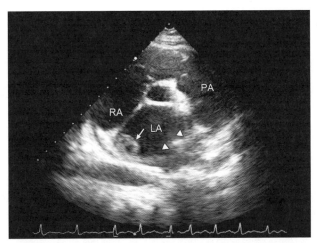

Fig. 11.19: TTE picture showing two thrombi (arrow and arrowheads) in the left atrium. The thrombi shown by the arrow shows partial lysis after initiation of anticoagulation
Abbreviations: RA, right atrium; LA, left atrium; PA, pulmonary artery

Interatrial Septum

The interatrial septum is to be evaluated in detail prior to PMV in order to plan the the transseptal puncture. In severe MS, the IAS may be bulging to the right atrium (Figs 11.17, 11.20 and 11.21) making the transseptal puncture difficult (Figs 11.19 and 11.21). The orientation of the IAS is altered since the LA is dilated and this should be borne in mind while attempting the transseptal puncture. Occasionally, we may come across Lutembacher syndrome which is a combination of rheumatic MS and congenital ASD (Figs 11.22A and B).

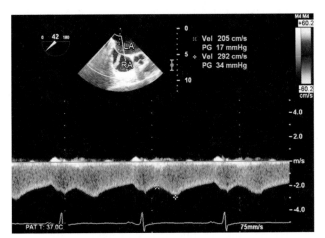

Fig. 11.20: Residual iatrogenic ASD in a patient planned for re-PMV for mitral re-stenosis. *Note* the high gradient of 17 to 32 mm Hg between the left and right atrium, indicative of the high left atrial pressure
Abbreviations: RA, right atrium; LA, left atrium

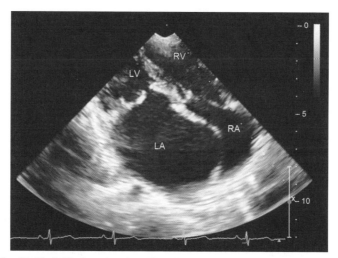

Fig. 11.21: A4C view showing dilated left atrium, thickened and doming
mitral valve and the bulging of the IAS towards the right atrium
Abbreviations: RA, right atrium; LV, left ventricle; LA, left atrium; RV, right ventricle

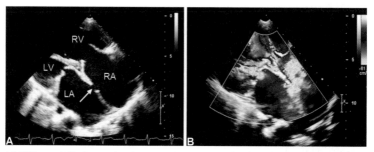

Figs 11.22A and B: Lutembacher syndrome: (A) Showing doming mitral valve and
a defect in the IAS, (B) Color flow mapping showing flow through the ASD and the
turbulence across the MV 📹◀
   Abbreviations: RA, right atrium; LV, left ventricle; LA, left atrium; RV, right ventricle

   Sometimes we may come across patients planned for a re-PMV for mitral
restenosis. Some may have residual ASD which is a remnant of the last
procedure. The flow across the ASD will be of high gradient because of the
very high left atrial pressure (Fig. 11.20).

■ ASSESSMENT OF LESIONS IN OTHER VALVES

Another important use of echocardiography is the assessment of the lesions
in other valves, which even alters the management of the patients (Figs 11.23
to 11.26). For example, a patient with severe MS and significant aortic valve
disease will preferably have double valve replacement than PMV alone.

   A patient having associated aortic stenosis or tricuspid valve stenosis
(Figs 11.23 and 11.24), may be planned for percutaneous aortic valvotomy or
percutaneous tricuspid valvotomy along with PMV.

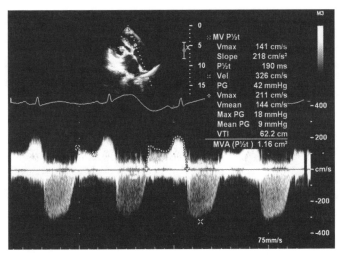

Fig. 11.23: Doppler flow across the tricuspid valve. Shows significant TS with a mean gradient of 9 mm Hg. TR jet peak velocity measured is 36 mm Hg indicating mild PAH

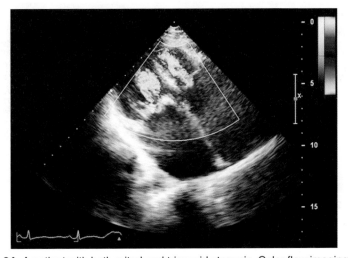

Fig. 11.24: A patient with both mitral and tricuspid stenosis. Color flow imaging shows turbulent flows across mitral and tricuspid valves in diastole

▓ TRANSESOPHAGEAL ECHOCARDIOGRAPHY IN PMV

Transesophageal echocardiography is an essential part of evaluation of the patient prior to PMV. It is useful in the following situations:

1. To rule out left atrial or LA appendage thrombus.
2. Assessment of mitral regurgitation
3. Assess associated lesions like AR
4. Assess the septum, to aid in septal puncture.

Since, the resolution of TTE is poor to image the left atrium and LA appendage, TEE is essential in ruling out thrombi in the left atrium. It is

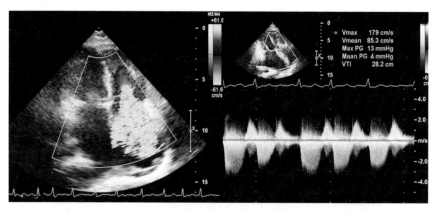

Fig. 11.25: Severe TR in a patient with severe MS and organic tricuspid valve disease. Doppler tracing is seen by the side showing tricuspid valve flow gradient of 4 mm Hg and a RVSP of 50 mm Hg indicating moderate PAH

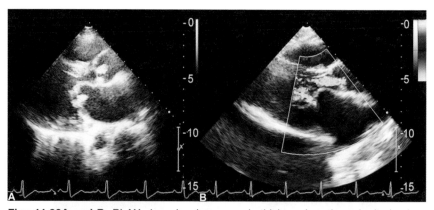

Figs 11.26A and B: PLAX view showing severely thickened aortic and mitral valves in a patient with severe MS and aortic valve disease (A). Color Doppler flow imaging showing aortic regurgitation and mitral stenosis (B)

mandatory to do a TEE and rule out left atrial thrombi before PMV. Images of LA thrombi in TEE are available in Chapter 53. Sometimes pectinate muscles in the left atrial appendage can mimic thrombi. Pectinate muscles are finger like projections which project into the LAA cavity (Fig. 11.27). Usually, they will have the same echotexture as the LAA wall which helps to differentiate them from LA thrombus.

Sometimes in patients with poor TTE windows, TEE can be used to assess the morphology of the valve, the interatrial septum and aortic valve (Figs 11.28 to 11.32).

Mitral regurgitation can be very well-assessed with TEE in multiple views (Fig. 11.33). So when the patient is taken up for TEE prior to PMV, it is always better to assess MR in two views.

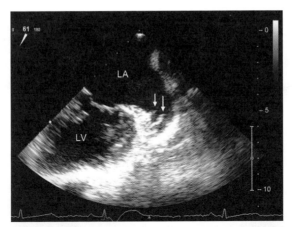

Fig. 11.27: TEE showing LAA, with finger like projections of pectinate muscles
Abbreviations: LV, left ventricle; LA, left atrium

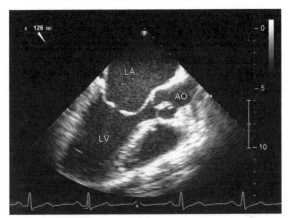

Fig. 11.28: Doming mitral valve—TEE image 📷
Abbreviations: LV, left ventricle; LA, left atrium; AO, aorta

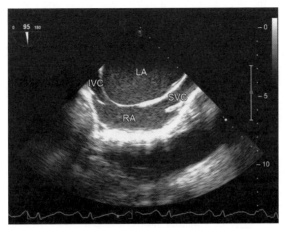

Fig. 11.29: TEE bicaval view showing bulging septum towards the RA; *Abbreviations:*
RA, right atrium; IVC, Inferior vena cava; LA, left atrium; SVC, superior vena cava

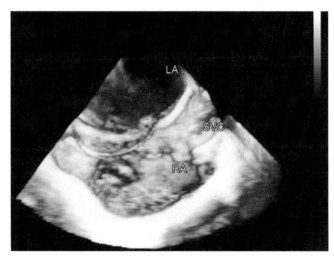

Fig. 11.30: 3D TEE bicaval view showing bulging septum towards the RA
Abbreviations: LA, left atrium; SVC, superior vena cava; RA, right atrium
(*Courtesy*: Dr S Sivasankaran, Dr Anees T, SCTIMST, Trivandrum)

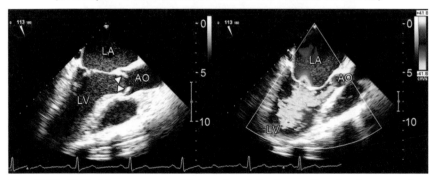

Fig. 11.31: TEE pictures showing thickened and doming aortic valve (arrowheads—panel A) and color flow mapping showing severe turbulence across mitral valve and mild-moderate aortic regurgitation in a patient with aortic and mitral valve disease. Since, the aortic valve disease was mild-moderate, patient underwent successful PMV.
Abbreviations: LA, left atrium; LV, left ventricle; AO, aorta

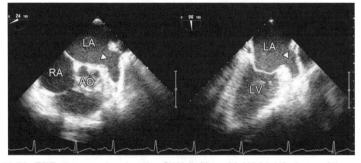

Fig. 11.32: TEE pictures showing the SAX (left) and LAX (right) views of the normal LAA without thrombus or LASEC
Abbreviations: RA, right atrium; LA, left atrium; LV, left ventricle; AO, aorta

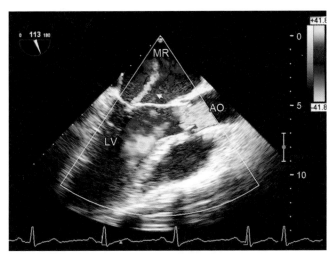

Fig. 11.33: TEE picture (110°) showing thin central jet of MR. This indicates mild MR
Abbreviations: MR, mitral regurgitation; LV, left ventricle; AO, aorta

■ DOPPLER ASSESSMENT OF MITRAL VALVE

Assessment of mitral valve by Doppler is important in assessing the severity of valve lesion, the response to balloon dilatation and also the presence and severity of mitral regurgitation.

The diastolic jet of mitral stenosis (MS) is usually M-shaped (Fig. 11.34). The initial peak is the E wave of early diastole and later peak is the A wave of atrial systole. In mitral stenosis, there is no gap between the two as the pressure gradient is never zero, indicating that there is no diastasis or equalization of atrial and ventricular diastolic pressures. In atrial fibrillation, the A wave will be absent.

The Doppler assessment of MV is usually done in the A4C view, where the flow is aligned to the probe. Color flow can aid in getting a good Doppler signal. Continuous wave Doppler is preferred.

Once the flow signals are obtained, the morphology of the signal and the quantification of the signal gives information about the severity of the valve lesion.

Since, the flow can vary with each cardiac cycle, it is ideal to measure three cardiac cycles and obtain the average even in those patients in sinus rhythm. In AF it is recommended to measure 5 cardiac cycles and average to get the correct gradient and the valve area.

This mean gradient represents the mean of the multiple instantaneous gradients ($p = 4V^2$) and is not calculated from the calculated mean velocity.[15] We have to record the heart rate always, as the mitral valve gradient will increase proportional to the heart rate.

Once the mitral inflow velocity signals are traced out, the integrated software in the echocardiographic equipment will calculate and give the mean and peak velocities. The mean gradient is the most important.

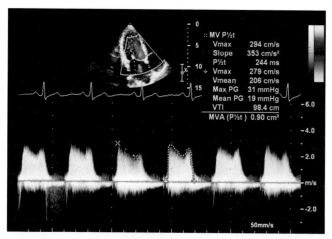

Fig. 11.34: Mitral inflow velocities in a patient in sinus rhythm showing "M" pattern. This shows the measurement mitral valve gradients in a patient with severe MS, the mean gradient here is 19 mm Hg and peak gradient is 31 mm Hg. The picture also shows the calculation of valve area using the pressure half time method. Valve area obtained is 0.9 cm²

Maximal or the peak gradient which is derived from the peak mitral velocity, is influenced by left atrial compliance and LV diastolic function.[6]

In the presence of significant MR or high cardiac output states, there is a significant disproportionate increase in the early transmitral velocity and gradient, compared to the mean gradient. This exaggerated early pressure gradient can be a clue to the presence of unrecognized MR in mitral stenosis.

Even though the mean gradient is considered a more reliable marker, it is also influenced by heart rate, mitral regurgitation and cardiac output.

■ PRESSURE HALF-TIME

Pressure half-time (PHT) analysis is another method used to assess the MVA. PHT is defined as the time interval in milliseconds between the maximum mitral gradient in early diastole and the time point where the gradient becomes half of the peak initial value. Since, it is found that the decline of the velocity of diastolic transmitral blood flow is inversely proportional to mitral valve area, MVA is derived using the empirical formula—MVA = 220/PHT (Table 11.3).

PHT is estimated by tracing the deceleration slope of the E-wave on Doppler spectral display of transmitral flow. Then the valve area is automatically calculated by the software integrated with the echocardiographic equipment. In patients with atrial fibrillation, we should avoid measurement of mitral flow from short diastoles and average at least five different cardiac cycles.[6]

The deceleration slope is sometimes bimodal, the decline of mitral flow velocity being more rapid in early diastole than during the following part of the E-wave (Fig. 11.35). In these cases, it is recommended that the deceleration slope be traced in mid-diastole rather than in early disastole.[6,13]

Table 11.3: Severity of MS based on pressure half-time

Severity of MS	PHT (msec)
Mild	<150
Moderate	150–219
Severe	>220

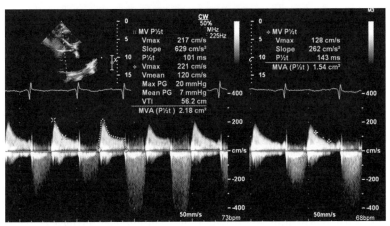

Fig. 11.35: The fallacy in estimating MVA by PHT method. When the initial part of the tracing is used, the MVA is coming as 2.18 cm², but when the middle part of the tracing is used, the MVA is only 1.54 cm²

Advantages of Pressure Half-time

1. Less dependent on heart rate.
2. Less dependent on flow across the valve.
3. Useful in patients with varying R-R intervals like AF or other arrhythmias.
4. In the presence of ASD following PMV.

Disadvantages of Pressure Half-time

1. Diastolic dysfunction of the LV can alter PHT (e.g. LVH). Older patients with MS who have associated systemic hypertension or aortic stenosis may have LVH.
2. Aortic regurgitation: Underestimates the severity of MS. AR increases the left ventricular pressure more quickly in diastole and shortens the PHT.
3. The compliance changes which happens during PMV can affect the PHT. So, it is better to wait for 48–72 hours to calculate the MVA using PHT method as the compliance properties get settled in 2–3 days following PMV.[14]
4. Significant MR underestimates the MVA obtained by PHT. The explanation is the exaggeration of early transmitral flow velocity and gradients across the mitral valve.[15]
5. In some patients with the mitral valve pressure tracing having a concave shape, PHT measurement may not be feasible.

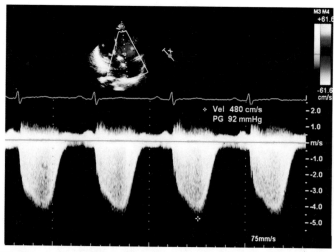

Fig. 11.36: TR velocity being measured to indirectly assess pulmonary hypertension. Here the estimated PA systolic pressure is 92 + 10 = 102 mm Hg

■ PULMONARY HYPERTENSION

Assessment of pulmonary hypertension is important when evaluating a patient for PMV. Presence of pulmonary hypertension influences the decision whether the patient should be sent for PMV or not.

Pulmonary hypertension is usually estimated indirectly from measuring the TR jet velocity and adding the estimated RA pressure to the RV-RA gradient (Fig. 11.36). The details of this measurement is given in Chapter 57. Also the mean PA pressure can be estimated from the PR jet also, by measuring the peak PR and the end PR velocities.

■ PERIPROCEDURAL MONITORING

During PMV, monitoring by echocardiography is a must. TTE is the most commonly used modality since TEE requires intubation and ventilation. TTE is used in the following situations:

1. To see the response to PMV (commissural splitting) with each balloon dilatation and to facilitate graded dilatation.

    Since, the pressure tracings in the laboratory may vary depending on the heart rate or filling pressure, it may not always be reliable to be guided by the pressure data alone. So, imaging by echocardiography helps in choosing the size of the next balloon. 2D imaging and planimetry is the preferred modality as it remains independent of the loading conditions, heart rate and mitral regurgitation.

2. To assess MR. Increase in the grade of MR by two or development of moderate-to-severe MR is an indication to stop the procedure. One grade increase in MR should not deter the operator from using higher balloon diameters and planning further dilatations.

3. To assess complications related to transseptal puncture-pericardial tamponade and pericardial effusion. To detect pericardial effusion, echocardiography is a must in the cathlab. To assess the response to pericardial aspiration also, echocar-diography is essential.
4. To aid in balloon entry into the left ventricle. In patients with very large left atria, entry into the LV may be difficult. TTE aids in such situations where the valve orifice can be located and the balloon directed accurately.
5. To aid in transseptal puncture.

Successful PMV

A successful PMV procedure is defined as a split of one or more mitral valve commissures (Figs 11.37 and 11.38) with:
1. An increase in mitral valve area of at least 50% from the basal
2. A final valve area of >1.5 cm^2
3. Absence of sellers grade of >2 MR.

■ POST-PMV ASSESSMENT (FIGS 11.37 and 11.38)

Echocardiography is the imaging modality of choice immediately following PMV and also on follow-up. Planimetric measurement of MVA using 2D echocardiography is the technique of choice as it is not affected by MR and also shunting through the iatrogenic ASD. Since, stretching of the valve during PMV can overestimate the valve area, it is advisable to measure the valve area on the next day prior to discharge.

If the PMV result is inadequate, the symptoms of the patient should be reassessed and MVR or OMV should be considered as an option.

MR should be assessed and the grade and the mechanism of MR evaluated in detail. This is important in planning management of those patients who

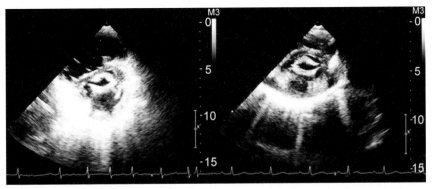

Fig. 11.37: Post-PMV echocardiography. Left picture showing a valve with fully open medial commissure and the right picture showing a valve with a fully open lateral commissure

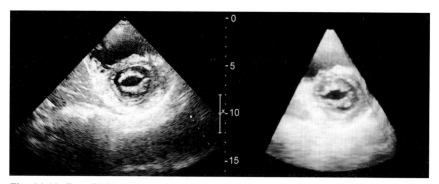

Fig. 11.38: Post-PMV echocardiography. Left picture showing a valve with a fully open commissures and the right picture showing the same valve imaged by 3D matrix array probe, showing both the commissures which are open

develop moderate-to-severe mitral regurgitation after PMV. Commissural MR usually regresses on follow-up. But MR is usually progressive if it is due to either tear of the valve or damage to the chordal structures and needs to be tackled by surgery as early as possible.

■ LEFT ATRIAL FUNCTION (SEE CHAPTER 14)

Assessment of left atrial function is important when evaluating a patient prior to PMV. The detailed description of assessment of left atrial function is provided in Chapter 14.

Mitral Regurgitation

The mechanism of MR in rheumatic mitral stenosis is restriction of leaflet motion. The exception to this is the MR which occurs after percutaneous mitral commissurotomy. It can occur by three mechanisms, tear of the leaflet, damage to the subvalvar structures or excessive split of commissures (Figs 11.39 and 11.40). It is reported that there are three characteristic anatomic features associated with the development of significant MR after PMV: (a) uneven mitral leaflet thickening, (b) severe and extensive subvalvular deformation, and (c) commissural calcification.[16]

■ EXERCISE ECHOCARDIOGRAPHY

Exercise increases the heart rate and the flow across the mitral valve due to increase in cardiac output. Increase in HR reduces the diastolic filling period and increases the gradients. In patients with disproportionate symptoms and low resting gradients, we re-evaluate the gradients after exercise and if the gradients are high, we advise intervention.

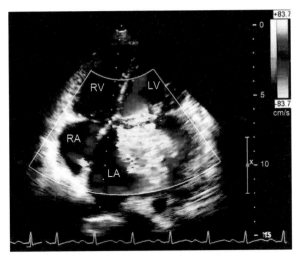

Fig. 11.39: TTE picture showing moderate-to-severe MR following PMV. Iatrogenic ASD following transseptal puncture shunting left to right is also seen
Abbreviations: LA, left atrium; RA, right atrium; LV, left ventricle; RV, right ventricle

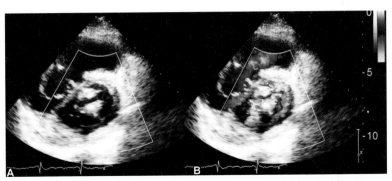

Fig. 11.40: Commissural MR. This echocardiographic image in PSAX view showing a very fibrotic mitral valve following a successful PMV with both commissures open (left). The image on the right shows color flow imaging revealing MR through both the commissures. MR through the commissures are usually benign and will come down on follow-up

Influence of MS in the Assessment of Other Valve Lesions

The severity of AS may be underestimated as the decreased stroke volume due to MS reduces the aortic gradient. By the same principle presence of severe TS can underestimate the severity of MS.

PREDICTIVE VALUE OF ECHOCARDIOGRAPHIC ASSESSMENT OF MV MORPHOLOGY BEFORE PMV

It is a known fact that the outcome of PMV is influenced by the morphology of the valve, the severity of the lesion, the presence of associated lesions and the chamber anatomy and morphology.

Initial reports stressed on the predictive value of valve anatomy on the outcomes, as assessed by echocardiography.[9,17-19] Subsequent publications have been less enthusiastic and found only a weak correlation[20-22] or none at all[23] between echocardiographic scores and the initial increase in mitral valve area (MVA). Also, data concerning the value of anatomy for prediction of severe MR were even more controversial.[24]

This shows that anatomy is only a relative predictor of immediate results. Other factors must be taken into consideration, such as old age, history of previous commissurotomy, higher NYHA class, atrial fibrillation, female gender, small initial MVA, higher degree of MR before PMV or large left atrial size.[25,26]

So, the prediction of immediate results of PMV is multifactorial based on anatomic, clinical and procedural variables.[27] Numerous factors have been studied till now, many of which were found either univariate or multivariate predictors of poor outcome post-PMV.

Echocardiographic Variables and Their Predictive Value

The major echocardiographic variables assessed when a patient is evaluated prior to PMV are:
A. Morphology of the mitral valve
B. Pre-procedural mitral regurgitation (Figs 11.41 and 11.42)
C. Mitral valve area prior to PMV
D. Left atrial size.

Morphology of the Mitral Valve

Several studies were performed to evaluate the echocardiographic parameters by which the outcome of the procedure can be predicted. Reid et al.[10,11] estimated the flexibility of the MV by two-dimensional echocardiography, using a ratio of the angulation of mid leaflet in mid diastole and the leaflet length (Fig. 11.43).

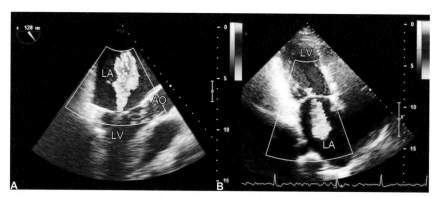

Fig. 11.41: Left-TEE imaging shows central jet, 2-3+ MR. Right-TTE imaging showing central jet of MR. This is not usually a contraindication for PMV since the mechanism of MR is leaflet restriction. This can sometimes decrease following PMV
Abbreviations: LA, left atrium; LV, left ventricle; AO, aorta

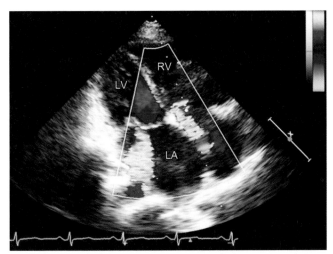

Fig. 11.42: TTE picture showing lateral jet of MR reaching up to the pulmonary veins. This indicates moderate MR and is usually considered a contraindication to PMV. TR jet also is shown indicating moderate TR
Abbreviations: LV, left ventricle; RV, right ventricle; LA, left atrium

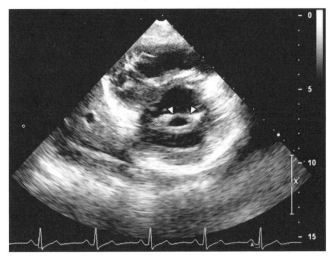

Fig. 11.43: Non-uniform thickening of the valve. In this valve we can see that the middle of the AML is less thickened (between the arrows) than the other areas of the valve and the commissures

Mitral Valve Echocardiographic Scoring Systems

Wilkins scoring system: In 1988, Wilkins' and coworkers[9] from "Massachusetts General Hospital" in Boston (USA), proposed a scoring system to predict the outcome of PMV. They used 4 parameters which were found by previous reports on surgical commissurotomy to predict outcome; MV calcification, thickening, mobility, and subvalvular fibrosis (Table 11.4). A total score is then calculated. They found their score to be the only independent predictor of immediate

Table 11.4: Grading of the mitral valve characteristics from the echocardiographic examination

Grade	Leaflet mobility	Valvular thickening	Subvalvular thickening	Valvular calcification
1	Highly mobile valve with restriction of only the leaflet tips	Leaflets near normal (4–5 mm)	Minimal thickening of chordal structures just below the valve	A single area of increased echo brightness
2	Midportion and base of the leaflet have reduced mobility	Mild leaflet thickening, marked thickening at the margins	Thickening of chordae extending up to one third of chordal length	Scattered areas of brightness confined to leaflet margin
3	Valve leaflets move forward in diastole mainly at the base	Thickening extends through the entire leaflets (5–8 mm)	Thickening extending to the distal third of the chordae	Brightness extending to the midportion of the leaflets
4	No or minimal forward movement of the leaflets in diastole	Marked thickening of all leaflet tissue (>8–10 mm)	Extensive thickening and shortening of all chordae extending to the papillary muscles	Extensive brightness through most of the leaflet tissue

The total echocardiographic score was derived from an analysis of mitral leaflet mobility, valvular and subvalvular thickening, and calcification, which were graded from 0 to 4 according to the above criteria. This gave a total score of 0 to 16 (Wilkins et al, 1988[9])

outcome. These findings were supported by two other reports published by the same group.[19,22]

However, they found that their score could not predict outcome uniformly in all patients. All patients with score <9 had optimal results and those with score >11 had suboptimal results. The score failed to predict outcome in patients with score of 9 to 11.[9]

Reid scoring system: In 1989, Reid and associates,[10] from the University of Southern California in the United States, proposed another scoring system. They used the following 4 parameters; leaflet motion, thickness, subvalvular disease and commissural calcium. A score 0 was assigned to each grade of mild, 1 to moderate and 2 to each grade of severe. Commissural calcium was scored as 0, 1 or 2 based on the number of commissures with calcium (Table 11.5).

Table 11.5: Two-dimensional echocardiographic assessment of mitral valve morphology (Reid et al.1989[10])

Morphologic feature	Definition	Grade	Score
Leaflet motion	H/L ratio: • ≥0.45 • 0.26–0.44 • <0.25	Mild Moderate Severe	0 1 2
Leaflet thickness	MV/PWAo ratio: • 1.5–2 • 2.1–4.9 • ≥5.0	Mild Moderate Severe	0 1 2
Subvalvular disease	• Thin faintly visible chordae tendineae • Areas of increased density equal to endocardium • Areas denser than endocardium with thickened chordae tendineae	Absent-mild Moderate Severe	0 1 2
Commissural calcium	• Homogenous density of mitral valve orifice • Increased density of anterior/posterior • Increased density of both commissures	Absent One commissure Two commissures	0 1 2

H: Height of doming of mitral valve; L: Length of dome of mitral valve; MV: Mitral valve; PWAo: Posterior wall of aorta

Iung and Cormier score: Another scoring system which is popular is the Iung and Cormier score developed by the French interventionists (Table 11.6).

Table 11.6: The French Three – Group Grading (Iung and Cormier score)[27]

Echocardiographic group	Mitral valve anatomy
Group 1	Pliable noncalcified AML and mild subvalvular disease (thin chordae, >=10 mm long)
Group 2	Pliable noncalcified AML and severe subvalvular disease (thick chordae, <10 mm long)
Group 3	Calcification of mitral valve of any extent, as assessed by fluoroscopy, whatever the state of subvalvular apparatus

The Iung and Cormier scoring system is simpler and unique in that it considers the length of the chordae.

Another scoring system which is specific in predicting the development of mitral regurgitation is the MR score.

MR Echocardiographic Score (Padial LR[24]): Thorough examination of surgically excised mitral valves revealed that 3 characteristic anatomic features were associated with the development of significant mitral regurgitation after PMV. They are uneven mitral leaflet thickening, severe and extensive subvalvular deformation, and commissural calcification. The original Wilkins mitral valve echocardiographic score was modified, with special emphasis on these three factors. This MR echocardiographic score could predict the development of severe MR following PMV with high sensitivity and specificity.

Ain Shams Scoring: A group from Ain Shams University in Egypt,[25] in 2008 suggested a novel scoring system for assessing the MV before PMV consisting only of 2 variables:

a. *Scoring of calcification:* Calcification was identified by localized areas of bright echo reflection affecting MV leaflets, seen in parasternal short-axis view at MV level. The absence of calcification was given a score of 0. Calcification localized to leaflet margins was given a score of 2, that extending to leaflet bodies was given a score of 4, while that involving the commissures (whether one or both) was given a score of 6. Calcification score was expressed out of 6.

b. *Scoring of subvalvular involvement:* Subvalvular involvement was identified by thickening of chordae tendineae and/or papillary muscles, seen in parasternal long-axis and apical four chamber views. The absence of subvalvular involvement was given a score of 0. Thickening involving less than half the chordal length was given a score of 2, that involving half or more a score of 4, while that involving the whole chordal length and papillary muscles was given a score of 6. The score of subvalvular involvement was expressed out of 6.

The total novel score is the sum of the calcification score and the score of subvalvular involvement, expressed out of 12.

This score at a cutoff point of 4 compared to Wilkins' score at a cut off value of 8 successfully predicted poor outcome with a higher sensitivity (86.7% versus 60%), higher specificity (82.9 versus 74.3%), and a better positive and negative predictive value (68.4 versus 50%, and 93.5 versus 81.3%, respectively). In multivariate logistic regression analysis it was the only independent predictor of poor outcome.

3D Echocardiographic Scoring System for Mitral Valve: Lastly, another group from Al-Azhar University in Egypt coworking with Erasmus University Medical Center in The Netherlands[28] introduced a real-time three-dimensional echcardiographic score (RT3DE score) for the assessment of MV morphology.

The new RT3DE morphology score (Table 11.7) was derived to include both MV leaflets and the subvalvular apparatus, guided by Wilkins's score. Each leaflet was divided into 3 scallops (anterolateral, A1 and P1; middle, A2 and P2; and posteromedial, A3 and P3) and scored separately (Figs 11.44A and B). The subvalvular apparatus was divided into 3 cut sections of the anterior and posterior chordae at 3 levels: proximal (valve level), middle, and distal (papillary muscle level). Each cut section was scored separately for chordal

Table 11.7: RT3DE score of the mitral valve						
	Anterior leaflet			**Posterior leaflet**		
	A1	**A2**	**A3**	**P1**	**P2**	**P3**
Thickness (0–6) (0 = normal, 1 = thickened)*	0–1	0–1	0–1	0–1	0–1	0–1
Mobility (0–6) (0 = normal, 1 = limited)*	0–1	0–1	0–1	0–1	0–1	0–1
Calcification (0–10) (0 = no, 1–2 = calcified)†	0–2	0–1	0–2	0–2	0–1	0–2

	Subvalvular apparatus†		
	Proximal third	**Middle third**	**Distal third**
Thickness (0–3) (0 = normal, 1 = thickened)	0–1	0–1	0–1
Separation (0–6) (0 = normal, 1 = partial, 2 = no)	0, 1, 2	0, 1, 2	0, 1, 2

*Normal = 0, mild = 1 to 2, moderate = 3 to 4, severe $ 5.
†Normal = 0, mild = 1 to 2, moderate = 3 to 5, severe $ 6.

(Anwar et al. 2010)[55]

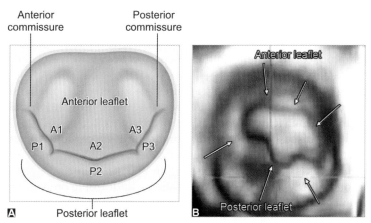

Figs 11.44A and B: (A) Schematic diagram showing the 3 scallops of each leaflet (A1, A2, A3, P1, P2, and P3). (B) Real-time three-dimensional echocardiographic en face view of the MV as seen from the ventricular aspect (Anwar et al. 2010) with permission from Elsevier, J Am Soc Echocardiogr. 2010;23(1):13-22

thickness and the separation in between. Thickness, mobility, and calcification for each MV scallop were assessed qualitatively and scored as follows: normal thickness and mobility were scored as 0 and abnormal thickness or restricted mobility as 1. An absence of calcification was scored as 0, calcification in middle scallop (A2 or P2) was scored as 1, and calcification of the commissural scallops of both leaflets (A1, A3, P1, and P3) was scored as 2. Scoring of the subvalvular apparatus included chordal thickness and the distance of separation between the chordae as follows: normal thickness was scored as 0 and abnormal thickness as 1, normal chordal separation (distance in between >5 mm) was scored as 0, partial separation (distance in between <5 mm) as 1, and absence of separation was scored as 2.

The individual RT3DE score points of leaflets and subvalvular apparatus is summed to calculate the total RT3DE score, ranging from 0 to 31 points. A total score of mild MV involvement is defined as <8 points, moderate MV involvement as 8 to 13 points, and severe MV involvement as ≥14 points.

The limitations of this RT3DE score are the limited availability of RT3DE machines, and the potential complexity of this score compared to the currently used Wilkins' score. Further assessment of this score and prospective validations from multi-institutional studies are needed.[29]

Global Echo-Doppler Scoring System

Another scoring system proposed is the Global Echo-Doppler Scoring System (GEDS).[30] It uses Wilkins score, ratio of leaflet lengths of anterior and posterior mitral leaflets, left atrial diameter, grade of MR, AV compliance, systolic Pulmonary artery pressure (PAP – mmHg)—each scoring from 1 to 2. A score of >7 gives a poor outcome.[30]

Problems Associated with Scoring Systems

The controversy of the published reports regarding the influence of echo-cardiographic scoring systems in the outcome of PMV may be related to the following factors:

1. Grading of the various anatomic features is a subjective, semiquantitative mode of evaluation and is thus exposed to a significant variability, particularly when it involves multiple investigators.[27]
2. Subvalvular disease is an important predictor of successful PMV and risk predictor of MR, and is often underestimated by both TTE and TEE.[27,31]
3. Absence of assessment of commissures in Wilkins' score.[27]
4. Most of the early reports compared patients undergoing procedures with different gadgets, which may have its influence on the outcome.
5. Most of the early reports were on the early learning curve of the technique used, which may have its influence on the outcome.
6. The components of the Wilkins' score may not have the same effect on the outcome, while the total echo score assumes that each of these variables is equally important. Thus, differential weightage of the individual components could result in a more predictive scoring system.[22]

However, some of the more recently published reports still find echocardiographic scoring as an independent predictor of outcome.[27,32]

Also, Stefanadis et al.[33] using the nontransseptal PMV in 441 patients (a multicenter experience), found the echocardiographic score, male gender, preprocedural MR and previous commissurotomy to be significant unfavorable predictors of immediate outcome. Balloon type was also a significant multivariate predictor of outcome. They found that patients with a score ≤8 had significantly higher rates of procedural success, greater final MVA and a lower incidence of significant postprocedural MR, compared to patients with higher scores.

Also, several reports showed that Wilkins' score can predict late outcome; restenosis and event free survival.[32,34]

So, echocardiographic assessment of the MV morphology is now used only as a guide for clinical decision-making, especially for selection of the appropriate balloon catheter size and balloon sizing.[31] In spite of its limitations (Table 11.8), Wilkins' score is still the most widely used score before PMV.

Table 11.8: Limitations of Wilkins' score (Goldstein and Lindsay, 2010 with permission)[29]

1. Echocardiography limited in ability to differentiate nodular fibrosis from calcification

2. Does not assess commissural involvement

3. Does not account for uneven distribution of pathologic abnormalities

4. Does not account for relative contribution of each variable (no weighting of variables)

5. Frequent underestimation of subvalve disease

6. Does not use results from transesophageal echocardiography or three-dimensional echocardiography

Recently, Massachusetts General Hospital coworking with 2 centers in Spain,[32] in a trial to improve the predictive power of Wilkins' score incorporated it in a multifactorial score including clinical, hemodynamic and other anatomic variables. These variables were selected based on multivariate analysis. Score constructed by an arithmetic sum of the number of PMV success predictors (age <55 years, NYHA classes I and II, pre-PMV MVA ≥1 cm², pre-PMV MR grade <2, echocardiographic score ≤8, and male sex) present for each patient. This multifactorial score showed a better sensitivity and specificity compared to Wilkins' score with an incremental ability to predict procedural success (defined as MVA ≥1.5 cm² with final MR grade <3) with a predictive power of 100% with a score of 6.

Preprocedural Mitral Regurgitation

The preprocedural mitral regurgitation was not found to predict the results after PMV in many reports,[19,21-24] but the importance of this factor is increasingly being recognized in many recent reports which evaluated either the univariate[35] or multivariate predictors of outcome.[24]

Iung et al. found that the benefit of using a larger balloon was observed only in the absence of significant initial MR.[35] Zhang et al. found that patients with pre-existing MR have relatively smaller MVA after PMV and higher incidence of later cardiac events.[36] These patients had a lower incidence of bicommissural splitting. The explanation of all these appears to be multifactorial:[37]

1. These patients have more calcified MVs, more incidence of atrial fibrillation[36,37] and more valvular and subvalvular scarring than patients without MR.[27]
2. This cohort of patients has large left atrium.
3. A more conservative approach could have been used when dilating the valves of patients with mild MR in an attempt to prevent worsening of MR.[36]

Preprocedure MVA

Patients with smaller MVA would be expected to have more severe deformities of the MV structure and therefore a poorer result. This was found in most reports, which studied this factor.[27,35]

On the contrary, this variable failed to predict outcome in early reports from Massachusetts General Hospital.[19,22] But the same group in more recent reports found pre-PMV MVA to predict outcomes.[9,17] They explained their findings by the fact that, the patients included in their early studies had severe mitral stenosis with MVA in the range of 0.4 to 1 cm^2, which might obscure the effect of the initial MVA on outcome. They suggested that the effect of the initial MVA on the outcome may appear in reports including patients with larger MVA with less valve pathology who are expected to have more improvement in MVA by PMV.[9]

Left Atrial Size

Left atrial diameter was a significant predictor of outcome in most of the reports either as univariate[18,19] or multivariate.[19] Alfonso et al[20] found that patients with aneurysmally dilated left atrium (> 6 cm) had the following characteristics:
1. They were older, more symptomatic and had atrial fibrillation.
2. They had higher echo score usually as the result of thickened mitral leaflets with more severe subvalvular involvement.
3. They had larger left ventricles and a higher incidence of MR.
4. They had more frequently difficulties in crossing the interatrial septum, and also a higher rate of dilatation failure.

Other less proven factors which could influence the outcome of PMV are the mitral valve annulus diameter and the presence of significant TR.

Other Morphologic Variables Assessed Following PMV

However, not all patients with commissural splitting after the procedure were found to have an optimal MVA.[38] This suggested that the mechanism of successful PMV may be more complex than reported previously. Short-term improvements in MVA and symptoms that occur when commissures are not split may be attributed to other mechanisms, such as improvement of leaflet mobility secondary to disruption of the diseased submitral tissue.[26] The historical obsession of the MVA limited more creative ways of looking at

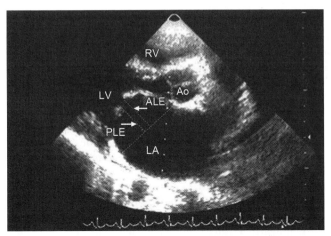

Fig. 11.45: Anterior and posterior leaflets excursion measured in parasternal long axis view

Abbreviations: RV, right ventricle; LV, left ventricle; LA, left atrium; Ao, aorta; ALE, anterior leaflet excursion; PLE, posterior leaflet excursion (Hasan-Ali, et al. 2007, with permission)[12]

the MV. It is assumed that assessment of the other changes produced in MV morphology may have an adjuvant value to the conventional measurement of the MVA.[12] These morphologic measurements are:

Valve mobility: It is assessed by measuring the anterior and posterior leaflets excursion. To measure the excursion; in the parasternal long axis view, at maximum doming in early diastole, a line is drawn at the level of the MV annulus (at the base of the leaflets), and then 2 perpendicular lines were dragged from the tips of the leaflets to that line (Fig. 11.45).

Subvalvular splitting: It is assessed by measuring the area subtended by the papillary muscles and chordae tendineae below the MV, measured at maximum doming of the valve leaflets in early diastole in apical long axis view; where the 2 papillary muscles and the chordae could be seen separated in profile. The subvalvular splitting area was found to increase significantly after PMV.[12]

Degree of commissural splitting: It is assessed in short axis parasternal view as regards the depth score of the splitted commissure. The score is assessed in each commissure as follows (No commissural splitting = 0, partial splitting of the commissure = 0.5, complete splitting of the commissure =1); then the score of both commissures is summed to give a total score of commissural splitting.[12]

CONCLUSION

As we have seen, echocardiographic evaluation is crucial in patient selection for PMV. It is also vital in periprocedural monitoring and also for follow-up of these patients undergoing PMV.

■ REFERENCES

1. Perloff JK, Roberts WC. The mitral apparatus. Functional anatomy of mitral regurgitation. Circulation. 1972;46(2):227–39.
2. Silverman ME, Hurst JW. The mitral complex. Interaction of the anatomy, physiology, and pathology of the mitral annulus, mitral valve leaflets, chordae tendineae, and papillary muscles. Am Heart J. 1968;76(3):399–418.
3. Selzer A, Cohn KE. Natural history of mitral stenosis: a review. Circulation. 1972;45(4):878–90.
4. Lachman AS, Roberts WC. Calcific deposits in stenotic mitral valves. Extent and relation to age, sex, degree of stenosis, cardiac rhythm, previous commissurotomy and left atrial body thrombus from study of 164 operatively-excised valves. Circulation. 1978;57(4):808–15.
5. Harken De, Dexter L, Ellis LB, Farrand RE, Dickson JF 3rd. The surgery of mitral stenosis. III. Finger-fracture valvuloplasty. Ann Surg. 1951;134(4):722–42.
6. Helmut Baumgartner, Judy Hung, Javier Bermejo, et al. Echocardiographic assessment of valve stenosis: EAE/ASE recommendations for clinical practice. Eur J Echocardiography. 2009:10;1-25.
7. Vimal Raj BS, George P, Jose VJ. Mitral leaflet separation index-a simple novel index to assess the severity of mitral stenosis. Indian Heart J. 2008;60(6):563–6.
8. Holmin C, Messika-Zeitoun D, Mezalek AT, Brochet E, Himbert D, Iung B,et al. Mitral leaflet separation index: a new method for the evaluation of the severity of mitral stenosis? Usefulness before and after percutaneous mitral commissurotomy. J Am Soc Echocardiogr. 2007;20(10):1119-24.
9. Wilkins GT, Weyman AE, Abascal VM, Block PC, Palacios IF. Percutaneous balloon dilatation of the mitral valve: an analysis of echocardiographic variables related to outcome and the mechanism of dilatation. Br Heart J. 1988;60(4):299–308.
10. Reid CL, Otto CM, Davis KB, Labovitz A, Kisslo KB, McKay CR. Influence of mitral valve morphology on mitral balloon commissurotomy: immediate and six-month results from the NHLBI Balloon Valvuloplasty Registry. Am Heart J. 1992;124(3):657–65.
11. Reid CL, Chandraratna PA, Kawanishi DT, Kotlewski A, Rahimtoola SH. Influence of mitral valve morphology on double-balloon catheter balloon valvuloplasty in patients with mitral stenosis. Analysis of factors predicting immediate and 3-month results. Circulation. 1989;80(3):515–24.
12. Hasan-Ali H, Shams-Eddin H, Abd-Elsayed AA, Maghraby MH. Echocardiographic assessment of mitral valve morphology after Percutaneous Transvenous Mitral Commissurotomy (PTMC). Cardiovasc Ultrasound. 2007;5:48.
13. Gonzalez MA, Child JS, Krivokapich J. Comparison of two-dimensional and Doppler echocardiography and intracardiac hemodynamics for quantification of mitral stenosis. Am J Cardiol. 1987;60(4):327–32.
14. Harvey Feigenbaum. Fiegenbaum's Echocardiography. 6 Edition P 234, Chapter 8, Hemodynamics.
15. Mohan JC, Mukherjee S, Kumar A, Arora R, Patel AR, Pandian NG. Does chronic mitral regurgitation influence Doppler pressure half-time-derived calculation of the mitral valve area in patients with mitral stenosis? Am Heart J. 2004;148(4):703–9.
16. Hernandez R, Macaya C, Banuelos C, Alfonso F, Goicolea J, Iniguez A, et al. Predictors, mechanisms and outcome of severe mitral regurgitation complicating percutaneous mitral valvotomy with the Inoue balloon. Am J Cardiol. 1992; 70:1169-74.

17. Nobuyoshi M, Hamasaki N, Kimura T, Nosaka H, Yokoi H, Yasumoto H, et al. Indications, complications, and short-term clinical outcome of percutaneous transvenous mitral commissurotomy. Circulation. 1989;80(4):782-92.

18. Vahanian A, Michel PL, Cormier B, Vitoux B, Michel X, Slama M, et al. Results of percutaneous mitral commissurotomy in 200 patients. Am J Cardiol. 1989;63(12):847–52.

19. Herrmann HC, Wilkins GT, Abascal VM, Weyman AE, Block PC, Palacios IF. Percutaneous balloon mitral valvotomy for patients with mitral stenosis. Analysis of factors influencing early results. J Thorac Cardiovasc Surg. 1988;96(1):33–8.

20. Alfonso F, Macaya C, Iniguez A, Banuelos C, Hernandez R, Goicolea J, et al. Comparison of results of percutaneous mitral valvuloplasty in patients with large (greater than 6 cm) versus those with smaller left atria. Am J Cardiol. 1992;69(4):355-60.

21. Herrmann HC, Ramaswamy K, Isner JM, Feldman TE, Carroll JD, Pichard AD, et al. Factors influencing immediate results, complications, and short-term follow-up status after Inoue balloon mitral valvotomy: a North American multicenter study. Am Heart J. 1992;124(1):160–6.

22. Abascal VM, Wilkins GT, O'Shea JP, Choong CY, Palacios IF, Thomas JD, et al. Prediction of successful outcome in 130 patients undergoing percutaneous balloon mitral valvotomy. Circulation. 1990;82(2):448–56.

23. Post JR, Feldman T, Isner J, Herrmann HC. Inoue balloon mitral valvotomy in patients with severe valvular and subvalvular deformity. J Am Coll Cardiol. 1995;25(5):1129–36.

24. Padial LR, Abascal VM, Moreno PR, Weyman AE, Levine RA, Palacios IF. Echocardiography can predict the development of severe mitral regurgitation after percutaneous mitral valvuloplasty by the Inoue technique. Am J Cardiol. 1999;83(8):1210–3.

25. Rifaie O, Esmat I, Abdel-Rahman M, Nammas W. Can a novel echocardiographic score better predict outcome after percutaneous balloon mitral valvuloplasty? Echocardiography. 2009;26(2):119-27.

26. Levin TN, Feldman T, Bednarz J, Carroll JD, Lang RM. Transesophageal echocardiographic evaluation of mitral valve morphology to predict outcome after balloon mitral valvotomy. Am J Cardiol. 1994;73(9):707–10.

27. Iung B, Cormier B, Ducimetière P, Porte JM, Nallet O, Michel PL, et al. Immediate results of percutaneous mitral commissurotomy. A predictive model on a series of 1514 patients. Circulation. 1996;94(9):2124–30.

28. Anwar AM, Attia WM, Nosir YFM, Soliman OII, Mosad MA, Othman M, et al. Validation of a new score for the assessment of mitral stenosis using real-time three-dimensional echocardiography. J Am Soc Echocardiogr Off Publ Am Soc Echocardiogr. 2010;23(1):13–22.

29. Goldstein SA, Lindsay J Jr. Do we need more echo scores for balloon mitral valvuloplasty? J Am Soc Echocardiogr Off Publ Am Soc Echocardiogr. 2010;23(1):23–5.

30. Mahfouz RA, Dewedar A, Elzayat A, Elawady W. Usefulness of the Global Echo-Doppler Score (GEDS) in selection of patients with mitral stenosis for percutaneous balloon mitral valvuloplasty. Cardiol J. 2014;21(2):152–7.

31. Lau KW, Hung JS, Ding ZP, Johan A. Controversies in balloon mitral valvuloplasty: the when (timing for intervention), what (choice of valve), and how (selection of technique). Cathet Cardiovasc Diagn. 1995;35(2):91–100.

32. Cruz-Gonzalez I, Sanchez-Ledesma M, Sanchez PL, Martin-Moreiras J, Jneid H, Rengifo-Moreno P, et al. Predicting success and long-term outcomes

of percutaneous mitral valvuloplasty: a multifactorial score. Am J Med. 2009;122(6):581.e11–19.

33. Stefanadis CI, Stratos CG, Lambrou SG, Bahl VK, Cokkinos DV, Voudris VA, et al. Retrograde nontransseptal balloon mitral valvuloplasty: immediate results and intermediate long-term outcome in 441 cases—a multicenter experience. J Am Coll Cardiol. 1998;32(4):1009–16.

34. Palacios IF, Block PC, Wilkins GT, Weyman AE. Follow-up of patients undergoing percutaneous mitral balloon valvotomy. Analysis of factors determining restenosis. Circulation. 1989;79(3):573–9.

35. Iung B, Garbarz E, Doutrelant L, Berdah P, Michaud P, Farah B, et al. Late results of percutaneous mitral commissurotomy for calcific mitral stenosis. Am J Cardiol. 2000;85(11):1308–14.

36. Alfonso F, Macaya C, Hernandez R, Bañuelos C, Goicolea J, Iñiguez A, et al. Early and late results of percutaneous mitral valvuloplasty for mitral stenosis associated with mild mitral regurgitation. Am J Cardiol. 1993;71(15):1304–10.

37. Zhang HP, Yen GS, Allen JW, Lau FY, Ruiz CE. Comparison of late results of balloon valvotomy in mitral stenosis with versus without mitral regurgitation. Am J Cardiol. 1998;81(1):51–5.

38. Fatkin D, Roy P, Morgan JJ, Feneley MP. Percutaneous balloon mitral valvotomy with the Inoue single-balloon catheter: commissural morphology as a determinant of outcome. J Am Coll Cardiol. 1993;21(2):390–7.

Chapter 12

Three-dimensional Echocardiography in PMV: The Latest Tool

Gadage Siddharth, Sivasubramonian Sivasankaran

▓ INTRODUCTION

The need to identify patients with mitral stenosis who could improve with commissurotomy was the impetus for Edler to work with Hertz to utilise the ultrasound for the generation of pictures of the Mitral valve.[1] Henry in 1975 for the first time planimetered the mitral valve orifice, a measurement hitherto not available without cardiac catheterization.[2] The difficulties in clearly imaging the smallest mitral valve orifice in a diseased valve were partly overcome with the advent of Doppler echocardiography using methods like the continuity equation and the pressure half time.[3] The ability to accurately localise the smallest orifice has essentially made three-dimensional (3D) echocardiography the Gold standard for the assessment of rheumatic mitral stenosis.[4] Though invasive, 3D transesophageal echos (TEE) done simultaneously during pre-procedural evaluation to rule out left atrial thrombi, gives the best pictures to study the mitral valve.[5] The pictures generated by the advanced machines are not only pretty, but have a major role in the management of the mitral valve abnormalities.[6] Though calcification cannot be recognized the 3D TEE, this modality stands as the best measure in calcific highly echogenic valves and in people with poor echo windows.[7] Real-time three-dimensional echocardiography (RT-3DE), now has evolved as the latest tool in evaluation and management of valvular heart disease.[8] It gives a morphologic perspective hitherto not available, for the operator, to decide on the interventional and surgical management and optimise the same. Unlike the conventional echocardiographic techniques where a sector image acquires pixels of data for analysis, the three-dimensional matrix array probes collect volume data as voxels. Obviously the structure if it is perpendicular the direction of interrogation generates the best data sets which can be cropped and analyzed.[9] Transesophageal matrix probes generate the best quality images because of the proximity, higher frequency and frame rates, but may need sedation or general anaesthesia.[9] The major advance that can happen in this field could be the tissue characterization (similar to virtual histology used in intravascular ultrasound), since calcification cannot be precisely estimated by these reflected voxels.[10]

Surgical as well as interventional approaches to management of mitral valve disease also are largely based upon data from transthoracic echocardiography (TTE). Transesophageal echocardiography is a major tool to optimize the outcome of interventions.[11] Graded dilatation of the stenotic mitral valve is now possible by imaging the splitting of the fused commissures at the time of balloon valvuloplasty to optimize results and minimize mitral regurgitation.[12] Sophisticated and precise imaging is needed for a complex dynamic structure like the mitral valve, especially when we embark on a interventional procedure like balloon valvuloplasty and repair, to aid the operator and to optimize the outcome.[13]

The mitral valve apparatus is a complex three-dimensional structure consisting of the leaflets, the mitral annulus, the chordae tendineae, the papillary muscles and the left ventricle itself. Effective performance and interpretation of two-dimensional (2D) echocardiography requires one to mentally integrate the collected images into a three-dimensional (3D) reconstruction of the cardiac anatomy. Two-dimensional echocardiographic reconstruction is limited by the echo window and operator experience. Three-dimensional volume data sets, on the other hand, are less operator dependent. RT-3DE is therefore the best way of assessing cardiac anatomy and plan interventions. The electrocardiographic gating and limitation of respiratory movement needed by the earlier machines are now overcome by volumetric RT-3DE.[3] Commercially available echocardiography systems generally have the following options to work on 3D imaging both for transthoracic as well as Transesophageal probes:[1]

- Full volume acquisition
- Single beat full volume acquisition (Siemens)
- Live 3D echo
- 3D zoom
- Full volume color Doppler acquisition.

Data acquired may be analyzed in using several software platforms such as:

- QLAB (Phillips)
  - Multi plane rendering (MPR)
  - I slice (computer aided slicing of the data set into multi-frame formats)
  - Mitral valve quantification (MVQ).

Three-dimensional Echocardiography in Rheumatic Mitral Stenosis

Mitral Valve Area (MVA)

To identify the best therapeutic strategy in patients with rheumatic mitral valve stenosis, clinical data and accurate measurements of mitral valve area are needed. Doppler based methods are heavily influenced by heart rate, cardiac rhythm, hemodynamic status and angle of incidence. Hence methods based on direct planimetry of the anatomical valve orifice are more reliable.[5] Some workers have concluded that mitral valve area estimated with 3DTEE is significantly less as compared to 2D echo and Doppler methods. Because

2D planimetry tends to overestimate MVA, 3D TOE should be considered for accurate MVA assessment, especially in patients with a large left atrium.[14] Measurement of MVA by planimetry of the orifice on 2D short axis images has several limitations (Fig. 12.1):

- Orthogonality of the imaging plane with the mitral orifice is assumed but not granted.
- Level at which the 2D plane intersects the funnel formed by the stenotic mitral orifice cannot be controlled by the echocardiographer.
- The angle (Mα) between the lines of the true mitral valve (MV) tip and the echo beam-to-MV tip measured in the parasternal long axis view on 2D echo was found to be an independent variable resulting in overestimation of mitral valve area by 2D echo.[14]

Direct planimetry of mitral valve area from 2D echocardiographic images therefore, may overestimate of valve orifice area due to imaging and measurement in an oblique plane. Using the 3D dataset it is possible to obtain sections of the stenotic mitral valve that are exactly orthogonal to the orifice and in its narrowest point. As a result, compared to all other Echo Doppler methods for assessing residual mitral valve orifice area, RT-3DE has the best agreement with invasive methods.[14] Figures 12.2 and 12.3A and B illustrates the planimetry of mitral valve using I slice and MPR planimetry.

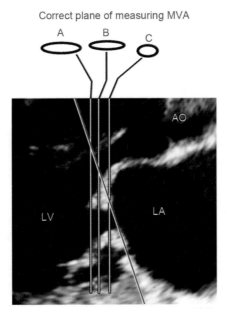

Fig. 12.1: Fallacies of measuring the mitral valve area by 2 dimensional echocardiography. The planimetered valve area could be any of the three values A, B, or C depending on the angle of the ultrasound, whereas the true orifice plane is along the red line

Abbreviations: LV, left ventricle; LA, left atrium; AO, aorta

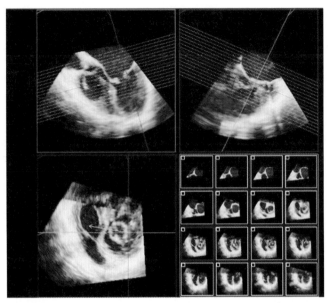

Fig. 12.2: Estimation of mitral valve area by I slice : using computer manipulation in the software provided (Q Lab) multiple planes aligned along the valve can be selected in multiple frame formats of varying thickness and each of these plane can individually, zoomed, reviewed and frozen in diastole to measure the exact valve area

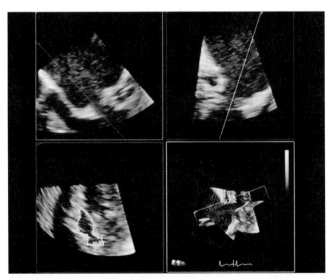

Fig. 12.3A: A Multi-plane rendering of a 3D data set frozen in diastole to measure the smallest mitral valve are. Two orthogonal planes are aligned along the valve orifice so that the third plane measures the exact orifice

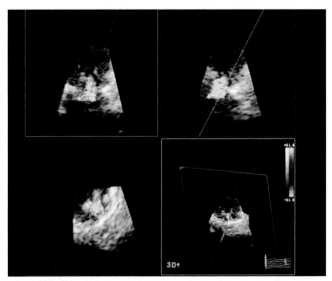

Fig. 12.3B: Multi-plane rendering of the color volume data set of the mitral valve frozen in systole to estimate the regurgitant orifice prior to balloon mitral valvotomy

Mitral Valve Anatomy

Results of percutaneous balloon mitral valvuloplasty are dependent on the mitral valve anatomy.[15] Several prognostic scores are used such as the Wilkins score which rely on anatomical details of mitral valve leaflet such as mobility, thickening, and subvalvular apparatus pathology are better assessed using RT-3DE.[16] Recently, a new RT-3DE based scoring system has also been proposed.[17] Three-dimensional echocardiographic features can differentiate rheumatic from non-rheumatic causes for mitral stenosis as well.[18] Simultaneous assessment of associated other valvular lesions is an integral part of three-dimensional assessment which has a direct influence on the optimal management of the clinical problem.[8]

Procedural 3D TEE in the Interventional Catheterization Laboratory

Real Time Live 3D echocardiography especially 3D TEE may also be used to guide the various steps of the procedure such as transseptal puncture and assess the result of the procedure and the need for additional dilatations.[11] Live 3D echocardiography can be invaluable in early detection and quantification of mitral regurgitation during balloon mitral valvuloplasty and accurately determine its mechanism.

Left Atrial Appendage

Left atrial appendage often is the site of thrombi in rheumatic mitral stenosis especially in atrial fibrillation. Transesophageal echocardiography is generally used to exclude a thrombus in the left atrial appendage prior to a balloon

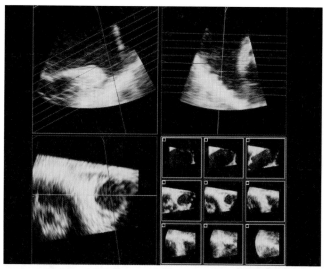

Fig. 12.4: Imaging of the left atrial appendage by I slice in 3 × 3 format

mitral valvuloplasty. Both transthoracic and transesophageal 3D echo has been utilized extensively to understand the appendage pathology.[19,20] The anatomy of the left atrial appendage is variable. RT-3DE is a powerful tool in evaluating the left atrial appendage and is extensively used in planning left atrial appendage device closure procedures. The left atrial appendage can be studied meticulously for thrombi using I slice software in post processing as shown in Figure 12.4. But the procedure needs lot of expertise, since the entire interpretation can be misleading based on the gain settings.

Imaging Protocol

RT3D systems generally have 4 acquisition modes: real time (narrow), zoom (magnified), and wide angle and color Doppler data sets. Three-dimensional scans are usually acquired after adjusting the width and breadth of the data set in the X-plane mode wherein the machine depicts the 2 dimensional orthogonal views of the data set to be acquired.[9] Once optimized the real-time mode displays a pyramidal data set of approximately 50° × 30° for about 45 msec duration. The zoom mode displays a smaller, magnified pyramidal data set of 30° × 30° at a higher resolution. This wide-angle focused mode provides a pyramidal data set of approximately 90° × 90°, which allows inclusion of a larger cardiac volume. But this needs to be manually tilted to see the Mitral valve en face either from the left atrium or ventricle. It is of great use during balloon valvotomy. Using transthoracic matrix array probes color Doppler volume data sets can be acquired, which at present is not possible with the real time and focused modes of interrogation. The funnel shape, commissural fusion and split are best appreciated from the left atrium whereas the chordo-papillary structures from the left ventricle, preferably the transgastric or apical 4 chamber views. The main limitations of the procedure at present are the slow frame rates, lack of color Doppler information in few formats, and prolongation of study time. Finer rapidly moving structures especially at faster heart rates are not clearly imaged and these limitations could be overcome by additional technical advancements in near future. Main limitations of the 3D echocardiography pictures are heavy dependency on the quality of the reflected images, the number of heart beats needed to reconstruct the structure interrogated. Huge amount of data needs to be collected and analyzed by the machine which restricts its ability to limit motion artefacts and to acquire the image at higher frame rates. At present the 3D TEE probe can be used preferably under good sedation or general anesthesia in subjects more than 30 kg of weight.

This wide-angle mode requires ECG gating; because the wide-angle data set is compiled by merging 4 narrower pyramidal scans obtained over 4 to 7 consecutive heart beats. To minimize reconstruction artefacts, data should be acquired during suspended respiration if possible. Although wide angle data sets provide a larger pyramidal scan, this is at the cost of lower resolution, which is decreased compared with the narrow-angle 3D mode. Once a 3D data set is acquired, it must be sliced or "cropped" to visualize the cardiac structures within the pyramid. Multiple cropping methods are available, but a common method displays 2 or 3 imaging planes simultaneously. Each of these imaging planes can be manipulated separately to appropriately align the cardiac structures. Another cropping method involves a single-slice plane that can be manually adjusted to expose and display the cardiac structures of interest. Aligning the smallest diastolic orifice to the interrogation plane provides the best estimate of mitral valve area. Additional 3D images can be reconstructed such as the surgeons view (from the left atrium, Fig. 12.5), the subvalvular apparatus (from the left ventricular aspect, Fig. 12.6) to accurately plan the balloon valvuloplasty. The recent introduction of Volumetric three-dimensional echocardiography, avoids electrocardiographic gating, need for

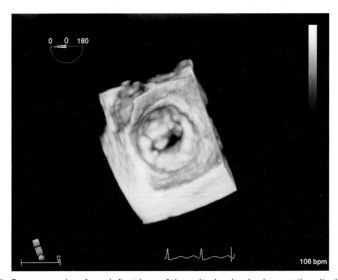

Fig. 12.5: Surgeons view from left atrium of the mitral valve in rheumatic mitral stenosis

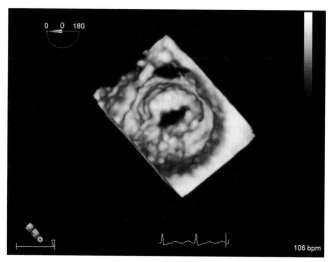

Fig. 12.6: The stenotic mitral valve viewed from the left ventricle

suspending respiration and additional maneuverability of the cross-sectional plane which was hitherto not possible online.[3]

Future Directions[1]

Ongoing developments in 3D echocardiography include technological innovations in transducer technology and expanding clinical applications. Automated surface extraction and quantification, single-heartbeat full-volume acquisition, Transesophageal RT3D imaging, the ability to navigate within the 3D volume, and stereoscopic visualization of 3D images are some of the technological advances that can be expected over the next several years. Combination of the excellent temporal resolution of echocardiography with the excellent spatial resolution of magnetic resonance imaging may herald a new era of "hybrid imaging" in the near future.[21-23]

Standardized and focused 3D protocols will have to be developed refined and rigorously validated so as to optimize clinical application of this technique.

▦ REFERENCES

1. Weyman AE. Assessment of mitral stenosis: Role of real-time 3D TEE. JACC Cardiovasc Imaging. 2011;4(6):589–91.
2. Martin RP. The fish mouth and three-dimensional echocardiography: new technology catches an old problem. J Am Coll Cardiol. 2000;36(4):1362–4.
3. Binder TM, Rosenhek R, Porenta G, Maurer G, Baumgartner H. Improved assessment of mitral valve stenosis by volumetric real-time three-dimensional echocardiography. J Am Coll Cardiol. 2000;36(4):1355–61.
4. Isla LP de, Casanova C, Almería C, Rodrigo JL, Cordeiro P, Mataix L, et al. Which method should be the reference method to evaluate the severity of rheumatic mitral stenosis? Gorlin's method versus 3D-echo. Eur J Echocardiogr. 2007;1;8(6):470–3.

5. Gianstefani S, Monaghan MJ. Accurate assessment of the true mitral valve area in rheumatic mitral stenosis. Heart. 2013;99(4):219–21.
6. Skubas NJ, Shernan SK. Intraoperative 3-dimensional echocardiography for mitral valve surgery: just pretty pictures or ready for prime time? Anesth Analg. 2013;116(2):272–5.
7. Chu JW, Levine RA, Chua S, Poh K-K, Morris E, Hua L, et al. Assessing mitral valve area and orifice geometry in calcific mitral stenosis: A new solution by real-time three-dimensional echocardiography. J Am Soc Echocardiogr. 2008;21(9):1006–9.
8. Zamorano JL, Gonçalves A. Three-dimensional echocardiography for quantification of valvular heart disease. Heart. 2013;1;99(11):811–8.
9. Hung J, Lang R, Flachskampf F, Shernan SK, McCulloch ML, Adams DB, et al. 3D echocardiography: a review of the current status and future directions. J Am Soc Echocardiogr Off Publ Am Soc Echocardiogr. 2007;20(3):213–33.
10. Konig A, Klauss V. Virtual histology. Heart. 2007;93(8):977–82.
11. Zamorano J, Isla LP de, Sugeng L, Cordeiro P, Rodrigo JL, Almeria C, et al. Non-invasive assessment of mitral valve area during percutaneous balloon mitral valvuloplasty: role of real-time 3D echocardiography. Eur Heart J. 2004;1;25(23):2086–91.
12. De Agustin JA, Nanda NC, Gill EA, de Isla LP, Zamorano JL. The use of three-dimensional echocardiography for the evaluation of and treatment of mitral stenosis. Cardiol Clin. 2007;25(2):311–8.
13. Kasliwal RR, Chouhan NS, Sinha A, Gupta P, Tandon S, Trehan N. Real-time three-dimensional transthoracic echocardiography. Indian Heart J. 2005;57(2):128–37.
14. Min S-Y, Song J-M, Kim Y-J, Park H-K, Seo M-O, Lee M-S, et al. Discrepancy between mitral valve areas measured by two-dimensional planimetry and three-dimensional transoesophageal echocardiography in patients with mitral stenosis. Heart. 2013;15;99(4):253–8.
15. Goldstein SA, Lindsay Jr. J. Do We Need More Echo Scores for Balloon Mitral Valvuloplasty? J Am Soc Echocardiogr. 2010;23(1):23–5.
16. Valocik G, Kamp O, Mannaerts HFJ, Visser CA. New quantitative three-dimensional echocardiographic indices of mitral valve stenosis: new 3D indices of mitral stenosis. Int J Cardiovasc Imaging. 2007;23(6):707–16.
17. Anwar AM, Attia WM, Nosir YFM, Soliman OII, Mosad MA, Othman M, et al. Validation of a new score for the assessment of mitral stenosis using real-time three-dimensional echocardiography. J Am Soc Echocardiogr. 2010;23(1):13–22.
18. Krapf L, Dreyfus J, Cueff C, Lepage L, Brochet É, Vahanian A, et al. Anatomical features of rheumatic and non-rheumatic mitral stenosis: Potential additional value of three-dimensional echocardiography. Arch Cardiovasc Dis. 2013;106(2):111–5.
19. Chen O, Wu W-C, Jiang Y, Xiao M-H, Wang H. Assessment of the morphology and mechanical function of the left atrial appendage by real-time three-dimensional transesophageal echocardiography. Chin Med J (Engl). 2012;125(19):3416–20.
20. Kumar V, Nanda NC. Is it time to move on from two-dimensional transesophageal to three-dimensional transthoracic echocardiography for assessment of left atrial appendage? Review of existing literature. Echocardiogr Mt Kisco N. 2012;29(1):112–6.
21. Qamruddin S, Naqvi TZ. Advances in 3D echocardiography for mitral valve. Expert Rev Cardiovasc Ther. 2011;9(11):1431–43.
22. Hlavacek AM, Hamilton Baker G, Shirali GS. Innovation in three-dimensional echocardiography and cardiac computed tomographic angiography. Cardiol Young. 2009;19(Supplement S2):35–42.
23. Valocik G, Kamp O, Mannaerts HFJ, Visser CA. New quantitative three-dimensional echocardiographic indices of mitral valve stenosis. Int J Cardiovasc Imaging. 2007;22;23(6):707–16.

Chapter 13

Subvalvular Apparatus in Rheumatic Mitral Stenosis—Methods of Assessment and Therapeutic Implications

Yoav Turgeman

The diagnosis, evaluation, and treatment of patients with rheumatic mitral stenosis (MS) may involve pediatricians, family practitioners, interventional and noninterventional cardiologists, as well as cardiac surgeons. Treatment of patients with MS should optimally be based on an integration of subjective as well as objective parameters such as functional capacity, compliance, patient age, pulmonary hypertension, cardiac function, and associated valvular abnormalities. However, in common clinical practice, the functional anatomy of the mitral valve is the main parameter that effects the selection of the therapeutic modality.

The subvalvular apparatus (SVA) is an integral part of the mitral valve structural complex and includes the left ventricular free wall, two papillary muscles, and chordae tendineae. Subvalvular deformity was noted in 40% of autopsy specimens of patients with rheumatic MS and in two-third of patients undergoing open mitral commissurotomy.[1-3] It has previously been demonstrated that both immediate and long-term results of percutaneous balloon mitral valvuloplasty (PBMV) are adversely influenced by severe subvalvular deformity.[4,5]

Proper assessment of SVA morphology and function in patients with rheumatic MS is therefore essential for therapeutic decision making— surgery vs palliative PBMV. Several methods and parameters for assessment of SVA are currently available, yet none are easy to use and can be readily used as a "gold standard". Current methods are mainly limited due to difficulties in assessment of the different degrees of pathologic involvement of the various valvular structural components. Moreover, there is no linear correlation between the observed anatomic abnormality and functioning of the mitral valve components.

The aims of this review are to describe anatomic and functional aspects of the SVA, and to define SVA involvement in rheumatic MS. The role of noninvasive and invasive methods for evaluating both the integrity and function of SVA in rheumatic disease, as well as clinical implications and pitfalls in assessment of SVA, will also be discussed.

ANATOMY AND FUNCTION OF SUBVALVULAR APPARATUS

(This is available in the Chapter 3: Anatomy of the mitral valve, which also includes pictures of subvalvular structures).

SVA Involvement in Rheumatic Heart Disease

Subvalvular rheumatic deformity is a result of two closely related mechanisms: (1) a late manifestation of healed inflammation following acute rheumatic valvulitis, and (2) superimposed turbulence that induces fibrosis.[6] Although papillary muscle hypertrophy has been noted by left ventriculography in patients with valvular rheumatic MS more often than in subvalvular MS,[7] it is unusual to find any pathologic involvement of the papillary muscles in rheumatic heart disease.[8] We believe that finding papillary muscle hypertrophy on angiography represents an angiographic pitfall, most probably due to an inability to distinguish between papillary muscle head and the agglutinated bundle of chordae tendineae. However, chordae tendineae involvement in the rheumatic process is not uncommon. Pathologic macroscopic findings such as fusion (agglutination), thickening, retraction, shortening, and calcification are frequently noted. Figures 13.1A and B focusing on posterior mitral leaflet presents normal chordae tendineae and abnormal chordae tendineae with rheumatic involvement. As a consequence of the rheumatic process, the free interchordal space diminishes and the opened "leaflet—chordae tendineae tunnel" available for diastolic flow is limited. This pathologic subtype may be called subvalvular MS.[10]

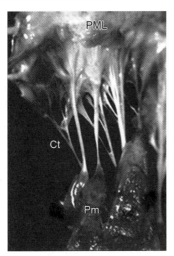

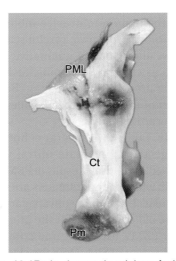

Fig. 13.1A: Posterior mitral leaflet demonstrating thin chordae tendineae with free interchordal space*
Abbreviations: PML, posterior mitral leaflet; Ct, chordae tendineae; Pm, papillary muscle
* Taken from Pocock WA et al[9]

Fig. 13.1B: In rheumatic etiology fusion and agglutination of chordae tendineae with absence of interchordal space leads to the phenomenon of subvalvular stenosis
Abbreviations: PML, posterior mitral leaflet; Ct, chordae tendineae; Pm, papillary muscle

■ METHODS OF ASSESSMENT OF THE SVA

Noninvasive Methods

Cardiac Auscultation

The classical auscultatory features of rheumatic pliable MS are a loud first heart sound, high-pitched opening snap, and presystolic accentuation of the diastolic rumbling murmur. The auscultatory findings are influenced by the anatomy of the valve, the pressure gradient across the valve, as well as the atrioventricular electrical activation (For example, PR interval length in sinus rhythm or the presence of atrial fibrillation).[11,12] Preserved anterior leaflet mobility and normal chordae tendineae length directed to the anterior leaflet are essential to produce these auscultatory findings;[13] however, in the adult Western population, stenotic mitral valves are neither purely pliable nor totally rigid, and a wide range of auscultatory findings representing various levels of pliability may be found.[14]

It is well documented that patients with predominant subvalvular deformity and open commissures, e.g. restenosis after surgical mitral commissurotomy may have auscultatory findings indicating preserved pliability.[9] Thus, the utility of cardiac auscultation for assessment of SVA involvement in rheumatic MS is limited.

Echocardiography

Since the early 1980s, both M-mode and two-dimensional echocardiography are the main noninvasive methods for evaluating subvalvular rheumatic deformity;[15] however, careful scanning of the subvalvular region in multiple views allows only a qualitative assessment of SVA structural components such as chordal thickening, fusion, and calcification. Moreover, measuring chordal length, differentiating chordae tendineae subgroups, and determining point of insertion in each leaflet are extremely limited by two-dimensional echocardiography.[16]

In Table 13.1 several echocardiographic scoring systems have been suggested to evaluate mitral valve anatomy and function and predict immediate and late results of PBMV.[17-19] Most authors use the score of Wilkins et al[17] in which four parameters are semiquantitatively assessed: leaflet mobility, valvular thickening, subvalvular thickening and valvular calcification.[17] The score of Padial et al[18] for the prediction of appearance of mitral regurgitation after PBMV uses the same criteria as in the score of Wilkins et al[17] for the assessment of SVA. Only the classification of Iung et al[19] is more quantitative regarding SVA evaluation, where direct measurements of chordal length are performed. Based on this classification, patients with pliable noncalcified anterior mitral leaflet with thin chordae $\geq$10 mm long have the best chances of achieving optimal immediate and long-term results after PBMV; however, none of the echocardiographic scoring systems have been found to be superior. All scoring systems are limited due to technical factors, difficulty of

Table 13.1: Echocardiographic anatomic classification systems for the assessment of the subvalvular apparatus

Wilkins Score*	Iung Score+
1. Minimal chordal thickening just below the valve	Group 1: Pliable noncalcified anterior mitral leaflet and mild subvalvular disease, i.e. thin chordae ≥10 mm long
2. Chordal thickening to 1/3 of length	Group 2: Pliable noncalcified anterior mitral leaflet and severe subvalvular disease, i.e. thickened chordae <10 mm long
3. Thickening to distal 1/3 of chordae	Group 3: calcification of mitral valve of any extent, as assessed by fluoroscopy, regardless of SVA
4. Extensive thickening and shortening of all chordae extending down to papillary muscle	

*Taken from Wilkins et al[17]; +Taken from Iung et al[19]

reproducibility, as they are only semiquantitative, as well as underestimation of severity, especially regarding the assessment of the SVA.

The advantage of transesophageal echocardiography (TEE) over transthoracic echocardiography (TTE) for SVA evaluation is still controversial. In a study by Hausmann et al,[20] thickening of SVA was graded lower by monoplane TEE than by TTE due to acoustic shadowing of the mitral valve, whereas results of biplane TEE were similar to TTE; the authors conclude that TEE has no clear advantage over TTE for the assessment of the subvalvular apparatus. Levin et al[21] compared the value of monoplane TEE to TTE to predict outcome after PBMV. They found that except for leaflet mobility, TTE scores according to the criteria of Wilkins et al[17] intended to be higher than TEE scores, particularly in the categories of subvalvular disease and valve thickening. Nevertheless, Levin et al[21] conclude that both TEE and TTE have limited ability to accurately identify and evaluate the specific valvular features that influence PBMV outcome, especially subvalvular disease. The additional value of multiplane TEE for the assessment of the mitral valve has been documented by Stewart et al,[22] and is currently the imaging method of choice for the evaluation of the SVA.

In the last decade 3D echocardiography has evolved from research tool to clinical utility in rheumatic MS mainly improving our ability for calculating mitral valve area and monitoring PBMV related complications.[23] The use of 3D for assessing SVA morphology and function is poorly studied.

Invasive Methods

Fluoroscopy and Left Ventriculography

Cardiac fluoroscopy and left ventriculography performed in the right and left anterior oblique projections were the first invasive methods in use for evaluation of both mitral valve morphology and function.[24] Chordal calcification is easily determined by fluoroscopy. In 1979, Akins et al[25] described the "mitral subvalvular distance ratio" by left ventriculography, in order to identify preoperatively patients with significant subvalvular fibrosis who may require valve replacement instead of palliative commissurotomy. This angiographic index compared the maximal length of the chordae tendineae from papillary muscle tip to the mitral valve level in systole with the long axis of the left ventricle (from the apex to the aortic valve) during diastole. An index < 0.14 precluded a good long-term result of mitral commissurotomy alone. Pitfalls in cardiac axis measurements, cardiac rotation due to right ventricular enlargement, electrical instability including the presence of atrial fibrillation, together with the development of echocardiography, have led to abandonment of this index. Fluoroscopy and left ventriculography are currently rarely in use for the assessment of the SVA.

Left Atrial Pressure-Wave Analysis

At the early phase of systole, after the pressure crossing point between the left ventricular and atrial pressure curves, the coapted mitral leaflets continue to ascend into the left atrial cavity, leading to the formation of the left atrial C wave (Fig. 13.2). At the peak of the C wave, the chordae tendineae are fully tensed and elongated while the anterior mitral leaflet is billowing toward the left atrial cavity.[9,26] The absence of left atrial C wave is commonly associated with rigid, short, and thickened chordae tendineae directed to the anterior mitral leaflet;[27] therefore, the presence of left atrial C wave in patients with rheumatic MS indicates a reasonably preserved chordae tendineae length and function.

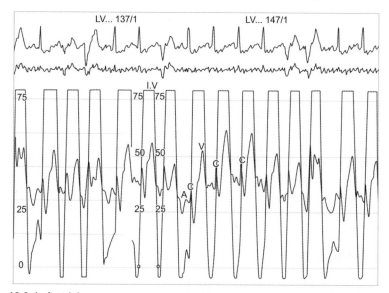

Fig. 13.2: Left atrial pressure-wave recording (a, c and v waves) in a patient with severe pliable MS prior to performing PBMV. The presence of left atrial c wave is a marker for the absence of subvalvular deformity

During PBMV

During the performance of PBMV, two indirect signs have been suggested to indicate the presence of significant subvalvular disease. The "balloon impasse," which, albeit rare, indicates crossing and propagation difficulties of the deflated balloon catheter into the left ventricular apex due to high resistance at the submitral region.[28] The "balloon compression" sign is a result of the distorted inflated balloon configuration at the subvalvular level. As shown in Figures 13.3A and B, the inflated balloon has a distorted contour due to the presence of significant subvalvular deformity, instead of having the typical "hourglass" appearance.[29]

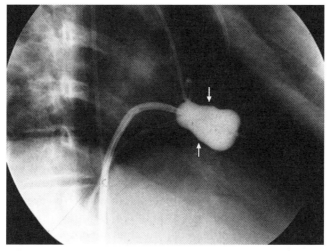

Fig. 13.3A: The balloon compression sign: distortion of the inflated balloon configuration (white arrows) at the subvalvular region

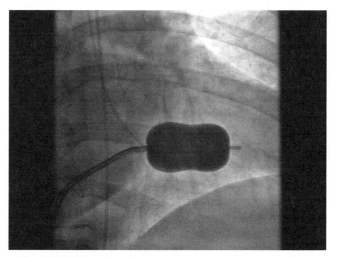

Fig. 13.3B: Typical hourglass appearance of balloon inflation in the absence of significant subvalvular disease

◼ IMPACT OF SVA DEFORMITY ON THE RESULTS OF PBMV

The results of PBMV as well as of surgical closed mitral commissurotomy are mainly determined by the morphologic characteristics of the diseased valve and its supportive structures;[17,30] however, the currently available data and medical literature on PBMV results do not differentiate between deformed mitral valves as a whole, in contrast to valves with fibrosed and distorted SVA only. Palacios et al[31] found the post-dilatation valve area to be significantly lower in patients with greater valve deformity, whereas Feldman and Carroll[32] concluded that valve deformity does not significantly affect the acute results of PBMV. These conflicting studies were performed using two valvuloplasty techniques—conventional double balloon and Inoue balloon—and none of the studies analyzed the data for each of the structural subvalvular components separately; however, several reports[4,33,34] using the Inoue technique emphasize that significant subvalvular deformity, as assessed by noninvasive parameters, cannot be used as a single predictive factor of immediate and long-term results for PBMV in both young and adult patients. In another study,[35] patients with severe SVA deformity were more hemodynamically deranged before PBMV and achieved more hemodynamic benefit, compared to patients with mild-or-moderate SVA involvement; the authors concluded that severe SVA deformity does not have any adverse effect either on immediate results or on intermediate term follow-up. However, severe SVA deformity may impose technical difficulties that may affect procedural immediate results. This is noted with crossing and propagation difficulties such as the balloon impasse, and selection of balloon diameter for the initial inflation.[28]

◼ CLINICAL IMPLICATIONS AND CONCLUSION

In patients with rheumatic heart disease, the advantages of palliation, preservation, and repair of the native mitral valve over valve replacement are well established.[36-38] However, prior to deciding on the preferable therapeutic modality, comprehensive clinical, morphologic, and functional assessment of the diseased valve should be performed with all the parameters taken into consideration.

The SVA is an important constituent of the mitral valve structural complex. Models for ex vivo investigations of the mitral valve and chordae tendineae are currently being developed, and may allow better understanding of the SVA in the near future.[39] Currently, assessment of SVA morphology and functional anatomy in relation to other valvular components remains a clinical challenge. Decisions should only be undertaken by an integration of noninvasive and invasive parameters prior to and also during an interventional therapeutic procedure—either PBMV or surgery.

■ REFERENCES

1. Edwards JE, Rusted IE, Scheifley CH. Studies of the mitral valve. II. Certain anatomic features of the mitral valve and associated structures in mitral stenosis. Circulation. 1956;14(3):398–406.
2. Mullin MJ, Engelman RM, Isom OW, Boyd AD, Glassman E, Spencer FC. Experience with open mitral commissurotomy in 100 consecutive patients. Surgery. 1974;76(6):974–82.
3. Vega JL, Fleitas M, Martinez R, Gallo JI, Gutierrez JA, Colman T, et al. Open mitral commissurotomy. Ann Thorac Surg. 1981;31(3):266–70.
4. Post JR, Feldman T, Isner J, Herrmann HC. Inoue balloon mitral valvotomy in patients with severe valvular and subvalvular deformity. J Am Coll Cardiol. 1995;25(5):1129–36.
5. Bahl VK, Chandra S, Talwar KK, Kaul U, Manchanda SC, Sharma S, et al. Influence of subvalvular fibrosis on results and complications of percutaneous mitral commissurotomy with use of the Inoue balloon. Am Heart J. 1994;127(6):1554–8.
6. Olson LJ, Subramanian R, Ackermann DM, Orszulak TA, Edwards WD. Surgical pathology of the mitral valve: A study of 712 cases spanning 21 years. Mayo Clin Proc. 1987;62(1):22–34.
7. Boucek RJ, Sowton E, Sommer LS. Assessment of ventricular elements of mitral valve by left ventriculography. Br Heart J. 1977;39(10):1088–92.
8. Schoen FJ. Surgical pathology of removed natural and prosthetic heart valves. Hum Pathol. 1987;18(6):558–67.
9. Pocock WA, Lakier JB Mitral stenosis. Barlow JB (Eds). Perspective on the mitral valve. Philadelphia, PA: FA Davis, 1987, pp. 151-80.
10. Schoen EJ, Sutton MJ. Contemporary pathologic consideration in valvular heart disease. In: Cardiovascular pathology. Virmani R, Atkinson JB, Fenoglio JJ (Eds). Philadelphia, PA: WB Saunders, 1991, pp. 334-53.
11. Lakier JB, Pocock WA, Gale GE, Barlow JB. Haemodynamic and sound events preceding first heart sound in mitral stenosis. Br Heart J. 1972;34(11):1152–5.
12. Constant J. Bedside Cardiology, 3rd edn. Boston MA: Little, Brown, 1985;164–86.
13. Cheng TO. Pliability of stenotic mitral valves. N Engl J Med. 1972;286(5):266.
14. Vahanian A, Iung B. Percutaneous mitral balloon commissurotomy: a useful and necessary treatment for the western population. Eur Heart J. 2000;21(20):1651–2.
15. Come PC, Riley MF. M-mode and cross sectional echocardiographic recognition of fibrosis and calcification of the mitral valve chordae and left ventricular papillary muscles. Am J Cardiol. 1982;49:461–66.
16. Reid CL, Chandraratna PA, Kawanishi DT, K.A, Rahimtoola SH. Influence of mitral valve morphology on double-balloon catheter balloon valvuloplasty in patients with mitral stenosis. Analysis of factors predicting immediate and 3-month results. Circulation. 1989;80(3):515–24.
17. Wilkins GT, Weyman AE, Abascal VM, Block PC, Palacios IF. Percutaneous balloon dilatation of the mitral valve: an analysis of echocardiographic variables related to outcome and the mechanism of dilatation. Br Heart J. 1988;60(4):299–308.
18. Padial LR, Freitas N, Sagie A, Newell JB, Weyman AE, Levine RA, et al. Echocardiography can predict which patients will develop severe mitral regurgitation after percutaneous mitral valvulotomy. J Am Coll Cardiol. 1996;27(5):1225–31.
19. Iung B, Cormier B, Ducimetière P, Porte JM, Nallet O, Michel PL, et al. Immediate results of percutaneous mitral commissurotomy. A predictive model on a series of 1514 patients. Circulation. 1996;94(9):2124–30.
20. Hausmann D, Daniel WG, Heublein B, et al. Transesophageal echocardiography in candidates for percutaneous balloon mitral valvuloplasty. Echocardiography. 1994;11:553–9.

21. Levin TN, Feldman T, Bednarz J, Carroll JD, Lang RM. Transesophageal echocardiographic evaluation of mitral valve morphology to predict outcome after balloon mitral valvotomy. Am J Cardiol. 1994;73(9):707-10.

22. Stewart WJ, Griffin B, Thomas JD. Multiplane transesophageal echocardiographic evaluation of mitral valve disease. Am J Card Imaging. 1995;9(2):121-8.

23. Zamorano J, Cordeiro P, Sugeng L, Perez de Isla L, Weinert L, Macaya C, et al. Real-time three-dimensional echocardiography for rheumatic mitral valve stenosis evaluation: an accurate and novel approach. J Am Coll Cardiol. 2004;43(11):2091-6.

24. Ross RS, Criley JM. Cineangiocardiographic studies of the origin of cardiovascular physical Signs. Circulation. 1964;30:255-61.

25. Akins CW, Kirklin JK, Block PC, Buckley MJ, Austen WG. Preoperative evaluation of subvalvular fibrosis in mitral stenosis. A predictor factor in conservative vs replacement surgical therapy. Circulation. 1979;60(2 Pt 2):71-6.

26. Antunes MJ. Functional anatomy of the cardiac valves. In: Acar J, Bodnar E (Eds). Textbook of Acquired Heart Valve Disease. In: Acar J, Bodnar E (Eds). London, UK: ICR Publishers; 1995.pp. 1-37.

27. Turgeman Y, Suleiman K, Freedberg NA, et al. Balloon mitral valvuloplasty and the echocardiographic score: do we have a better alternative [abstract]? Isr J Med Sci 1995;31(suppl):269.

28. Lau KW, Hung JS. Balloon impasse: a marker of severe mitral subvalvular disease and in Inoue-balloon percutaneous transvenous mitral commissurotomy. Cathet Cardiovasc Diagn 1995; 35:310-19.

29. Lau KW, Hung JS. A simple balloon sizing method in Inoue-balloon percutaneous transvenous mitral commissurotomy. Cathet Cardiovasc Diagn 1994; 33:120-29.

30. Iung B, Garbarz E, Michaud P, et al. Late results of percutaneous mitral commissurotomy in a series of 1024 patients: analysis of late clinical deterioration; frequency, anatomic findings and predictive factors. Circulation. 1999; 99:3272-78.

31. Palacios IF, Block PC, Wilkins GT, Weyman AE. Follow-up of patients undergoing percutaneous mitral balloon valvotomy. Analysis of factors determining restenosis. Circulation. 1989;79(3):573-9.

32. Feldman T, Carroll JD. Valve deformity and balloon mechanics in percutaneous transvenous mitral commissurotomy. Am Heart J. 1991;121(6 Pt 1):1628-33.

33. Medeiros CC, de Moraes AV, Cardoso LF, Rati MA, Abensur H, de Azevedo JG, et al. Do mitral valve components have the same predictive value in percutaneous balloon mitral valvuloplasty? Doppler echocardiography study. Arq Bras Cardiol. 1991;57(1):17-20.

34. Law KW, Ding ZP, Koh TH, et al. Percutaneous balloon mitral commissurotomy in patients with coexisting moderate mitral regurgitation and severe subvalvular disease and/or mitral calcification. J Invasive Cardiol. 1996;8:99-106.

35. Sreenivas Kumar A, Kapoor A, Sinha N, Goel PK, Umeshan CV, Tiwari S, et al. Influence of sub valvular pathology on immediate results and follow up events of Inoue balloon mitral valvotomy. Int J Cardiol. 1998;67(3):201-9.

36. Dean LS. Percutaneous transvenous mitral commissurotomy: A comparison to the closed and open surgical techniques. Cathet Cardiovasc Diagn. 1994;Suppl 2:76-81.

37. Cosgrove DM, Chavez AM, Lytle BW, Gill CC, Stewart RW, Taylor PC, et al. Results of mitral valve reconstruction. Circulation. 1986;74(3 Pt 2):182-7.

38. Antunes MJ, Magalhaes MP, Colsen PR, Kinsley RH. Valvuloplasty for rheumatic mitral valve disease. A surgical challenge. J Thorac Cardiovasc Surg. 1987; 94(1):44-56.

39. Katoh T, Ikeda N, Nishi K, Gohra H, Hamano K, Noda H, et al. A newly designed adapter for testing an ex vivo mitral valve apparatus. Artif Organs. 1999;23(10): 920-3.

Chapter 14

Atrial Function in Mitral Stenosis—Effect of Percutaneous Mitral Valvuloplasty

Tomás F Cianciulli, María C Saccheri

▓ INTRODUCTION

Atrial function is an integral aspect of the proper performance of the circulatory system. Anatomical and hemodynamic assessment of left and right atrial function can be performed by two-dimensional echocardiography and tissue Doppler imaging. In recent years, two-dimensional speckle tracking echocardiography is used to assess atrial function. This chapter will discuss the echocardiographic tools for the assessment of atrial function and the effect of percutaneous mitral valvuloplasty on atrial function.

Patients with mitral stenosis who still preserve their sinus rhythm often show left atrial dilatation and systolic dysfunction in the body of the left atrium and left atrial appendage (LAA), a circumstance which may constitute the anatomic-functional substrate for thrombus formation, with the ensuing risk of systemic thromboembolism requiring preventive therapeutic steps.

Since its introduction in 1984 by Inoue,[1] percutaneous mitral valvuloplasty (PMV) has been considered a safe and effective method for the treatment of patients with severe symptomatic mitral stenosis. The resulting increase of the mitral valve area and the consequent decrease in left atrial pressure favor the regression of changes in the left atrium,[2] with an according reduction of thromboembolic risk.

In normal subjects, transesophageal echocardiography (TEE) of the LAA shows a characteristic movement: its apex is highly contractile and is frequently obliterated in systole, whereas the base is poorly contractile. Blood flow velocities can be assessed with pulsed Doppler by positioning the sample volume just inside the LAA at a point where ghost signals due to wall motions were minimal, commonly recorded within the proximal third of the appendage. LAA shows a typical blood flow pattern, consistently of one diastolic forward flow wave (LAA contraction) immediately followed by a systolic backward flow (LAA filling). Following LAA filling, two low positive and negative velocity waves can be seen (systolic reflection wave and early diastolic LAA flow).

Under pathological conditions like mitral stenosis, blood stasis in LAA, generate dynamic swirling smoke-like echoes, known as spontaneous echo contrast (SEC). Numerous studies[2-4] indicate that SEC may be a precursor of thrombus formation and represent a risk factor for the occurrence of thromboembolic events.

The anatomic-functional characteristics of the left atrium after PMV[5,6] has been evaluated in a few studies.

Echocardiographic Assessment of the Left Atrial Size and Function

Images of the LAA should be obtained in the horizontal (0°), vertical (90°), and intermediate imaging planes. LAA dimensions are obtained using the maximal area obtained.[7,8] The following measurements are usually obtained from the TEE:

a. The width of the left atrial appendage is defined in each plane by a line from the confluence of the left upper pulmonary vein and the left atrial appendage to the outermost portion of the mitral annulus (Fig. 14.1). The left atrial appendage length is measured from this confluence to the appendage apex. Left atrial appendage area is measured by manual planimetry. All anatomical measurements are made from cross-sectional images immediately before the QRS complex.

b. Peak late diastolic velocity ("a" wave) of the left upper pulmonary vein (LUPV). It is obtained using the pulsed Doppler sample volume in the pulmonary vein at 1 cm from the left atrium. This measure is used to assess the contractile state of the LA body.[9,10]

c. Peak systolic and diastolic velocity in the left appendage: It is obtained using the pulsed Doppler sample at 1 cm from the base of the LAA. This measure is used to assess the contractile state of the LAA (Figs 14.2A and B).

d. Systolic and diastolic velocity time integrals (VTI) of the LAA: It is the area under the flow curve in the LAA (in cm).

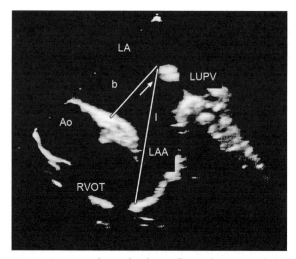

Fig. 14.1: Transverse transesophageal echocardiography, expanded basal short-axis view showing left atrial appendage (LAA) and left upper pulmonary vein.
Abbreviations: LA, left atrium; LUPV, left upper pulmonary vein; Ao, ascending aorta; RVOT, right ventricular outflow tract; b, LAA base; l, LAA length

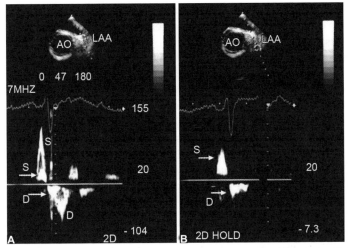

Figs 14.2A and B: Transesophageal echocardiography. Transverse plane of the base at the level of the aortic valve showing the left atrial appendage (LAA) flow velocities and tissue velocities. (A) LAA tissue velocities (S´ and D´) are shown below the spectral wave of LAA flow velocities (S and D); (B) LAA tissue velocities (S´ and D´) are shown expanded due to the decreased Nyquist limit.
Abbreviations: Ao, aorta; S, systolic peak flow velocity; D, diastolic peak flow velocity; S´, systolic peak tissue velocity; D´, diastolic peak tissue velocity

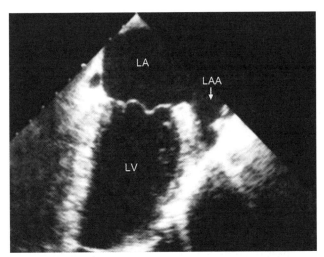

Fig. 14.3: Transesophageal echocardiography: Longitudinal two-chamber view of the left ventricle showing left atrial appendage (LAA)
Abbreviations: LA, left atrium; LV, left ventricle

The longitudinal plane of the two-chamber view at 90° is also used (Fig. 14.3) in order to evaluate the presence of lobes and thrombus in the LAA.

Low wall filter should be used and the cursor of the pulsed Doppler must be placed as parallel as possible to the structure under study in order to avoid the scattering of the ultrasonic signal.

The following definitions of LAA abnormalities are usually used:

a. Systolic dysfunction: When the flow velocity of systolic emptying (Peak S wave) is lower than 50 cm/sec.

b. Spontaneous echo contrast (SEC): It is defined as dynamic intracavitary echoes with a characteristic swirling pattern within the LAA cavity. Particular attention should be given to adjusting the instrument's gain control to differentiate SEC from background noise produced by high gain setting. The intensity of SEC is graded as follow:[9] 1 = no SEC; 2 = faint SEC confirmed by M-mode recordings showing dynamic echoes describing an organized movement that clearly different from "fog" of background noise; and 3 = intense SEC with the classical appearance of "smoke" confirmed on two-dimensional and M-mode recordings.

For the analysis of the LA body the four-chamber view of the transverse mideso-phageal section is employed.

Percutaneous Mitral Valvuloplasty and Atrial Function

Cianciulli et al[6] studied 25 adult patients with symptomatic and pure severe mitral stenosis before and after PMV.

The left atrial (LA) dimension and LA area decreased after PMV (pre 53.8 ± 6 mm, post 48.7 ± 5.2 mm, $p < 0.007$ and pre 32.7 ± 6 cm², post 28.2 ± 4.4 cm², $p < 0.007$, respectively).

After PMV, a significant increase of mitral valve area was observed (pre 0.81 ± 0.1 cm², post 1.85 ± 0.43 cm², $p < 0.0001$), with a significant decrease of trans-mitral mean gradient (pre 13.3 ± 3.6 mm Hg, post 4.9 ± 1.8 mm Hg, $p < 0.0001$).

The pulmonary artery systolic pressure before PMV was 50.2 ± 17.3 mm Hg and decreased significantly after the procedure (36 ± 11.2 mm Hg, $p < 0.004$).

The findings of TEE before and after PMV are summarized in Table 14.1.

No significant differences in the size of the LAA were observed (base: pre 25.1 ± 6.2 mm, post 21.9 ± 5.9 mm, $p = 0.18$; length: pre 50.3 ± 6.4 mm, post 46.1 ± 5.6 mm, $p = 0.09$, and area: pre 7.58 ± 2.4 cm2, post 6.45 ± 1.14 cm2, $p = 0.18$).

Before the PMV, the peak systolic velocity flow of LAA was 18 ± 5 cm/sec and its respective integral was 1.72 ± 0.75 cm (Table 12.1). After PMV, the peak systolic velocity flow of LAA was 24 ± 9 cm/sec and its integral was 2.22 ± 1.02 cm. These values correspond to a significant increase in the anterograde velocity ($p < 0.001$) and its integrals ($p < 0.008$), indicating an increase of 25% and 22%, respectively, with respect to the values previous to the procedure.

Regarding the retrograde component of LAA flow, the peak diastolic velocity before PMV was 25.5 ± 10.2 cm/sec and its integral 2.1 ± 0.7 cm. After PMV, the peak diastolic velocity was 32.9 ± 12.6 cm/sec and its integral 2.8 ± 1.3 cm. A significant difference between the pre and post PMV values of retrograde velocities was observed ($p < 0.006$) and of their integrals ($p < 0.02$), with an increase of 22% and 25%, respectively.

No significant changes were observed in the LUPV dimension after PMV. Before PMV, the peak late diastolic velocity (A wave) of the pulmonary vein was 15 ± 6 cm/sec (Table 14.1), and after the procedure it was 22 ± 12 cm/sec,

Table 14.1: TEE characteristics at baseline and after PMV of the total population (n = 25)			
	Before PMV	*After PMV*	*p-Value*
LAA size			
LAA base (mm)	25.1 ± 6.2	21.9 ± 5.9	0.18
LAA length (mm)	50.3 ± 6.4	46.1 ± 5.6	0.09
LAA Area (cm²)	7.58 ± 2.4	6.45 ± 1.14	0.18
LAA flow velocity			
S wave (cm/sec)	18 ± 5	24 ± 9	< 0.001
D wave (cm/sec)	25.5 ± 10.2	32.9 ± 12.6	< 0.006
Systolic VTI (cm)	1.72 ± 0.75	2.22 ± 1.02	< 0.008
Diastolic VTI (cm)	2.1 ± 0.7	2.8 ± 1.3	< 0.02
LAA tissue velocity			
S′ (cm/sec)	6.92 ± 3.77	11.16 ± 6.61	< 0.002
RAA tissue velocity			
S′ (cm/sec)	16.2 ± 3.7	19.1 ± 4.1	< 0.001
Spontaneous echo contrast			
Faint: n (%)	6 (24%)	19 (76%)	< 0.007
Intense: n (%)	19 (76%)	6 (24%)	< 0.007
Left upper pulmonary vein			
Diameter (mm)	14.7 ± 3	13.6 ± 3.7	0.25
Peak A velocity (cm/sec)	15 ± 6	22 ± 12	< 0.01

Data are expressed as the mean value ± SD or number of patients (%).
TEE—transesophageal echocardiography; PMV—percutaneous mitral valvuloplasty; LAA—left atrial appendage; S wave—peak systolic velocity; D wave—peak diastolic velocity; VTI—velocity time integral; S′—peak systolic myocardial velocity; RAA—right atrial appendage; A—atrial systole.

indicating an average increase of 31.8% of LA body function with respect to previous measurements (p < 0.01).

Before PMV, spontaneous echo contrast (SEC) in LAA was seen in all the patients. It was faint in 6 patients (24%) and intense in 19 patients (76%). After the procedure, SEC in LAA decreased in all the patients. It was faint in 19 patients (76%) and intense in 6 patients (24%), p < 0.007.

The study of Cianciulli et al[6] shows the functional changes of both atria induced by the reduction of afterload after PMV in patients with mitral stenosis and sinus rhythm. Besides, it shows the relevance of TEE as a particularly useful method for evaluating these parameters, which would be impossible to assess with the TTE.

In this study, PMV represented a model of reduction of afterload of both atria, resulting in changes in its global and local systolic function. The improvement of global systolic function of the LA body is expressed by an increase in the peak late diastolic velocity (A wave) of the pulmonary vein flow.[10] The improvement in global and local systolic function of LAA is evidenced by an increase in its flow systolic velocity and tissue systolic velocity respectively.

This study also shows that there is improvement of the local systolic function of the RAA as evidenced by the increase of its tissue contraction velocity.

The most important changes in mitral stenosis are an increase in LA pressure and LA dilatation. Initially, LA dilatation takes place within a physiological range, according to Frank-Starling's law, but in severe mitral stenosis a greater atrial dilatation leads to systolic dysfunction.

In normal subjects, atrial systole contributes 20% of the cardiac output. In mild mitral stenosis, the contribution of the LA to the cardiac index is inversely proportional to its severity, oscillating between 20% and 40% in the mildest cases and decreasing less than 15% in severe mitral stenosis.[11]

In addition to dilatation and systolic dysfunction of the body of LA, patients with mitral stenosis also develop a decrease of the retrograde wave (A) of the pulmonary vein flow, and show dilatation and systolic dysfunction of LAA, as evidenced by an increase of the LAA area and a reduction of its contraction velocity.[12] After PMV, a decrease in the LA pressure occurs with a corresponding increase in the LA pump function, expressed by an increase in the anterograde velocity of LAA flow (S) and in the retrograde flow of the pulmonary vein (A).

In normal subjects,[13] the TEE of the LAA shows systolic flow velocities greater than 50 cm/sec. In this study, the average velocity of LAA systolic flow in patients with mitral stenosis and sinus rhythm was 18 cm/sec. These data suggest the presence of LAA systolic dysfunction.

It is known that LA function is influenced by both atrial and ventricular factors. The atrial factors comprise the LA contractility and relaxation, LA pressure and compliance. The ventricular factors include mitral annular displacement, LV compliance and relaxation. In addition, an increase in LV contractility due to increased LV preload after mitral valve dilation may increase the left atrial performance by mitral annular displacement and an increase of LA reservoir capacity and passive emptying.

Patients with mitral stenosis and sinus rhythm develop contractile dysfunction of the LAA, which is more evident when the SEC is intense. As a result of this contractile dysfunction the risk of thrombus formation increases.[13] Even if the reduction of SEC intensity and the increase of the contractile function of LAA after PMV do not constitute proof for the efficacy of PMV on thromboembolism, they consistently show the beneficial effect of the procedure on the causes of these conditions.[14] Thus, an early intervention might benefit patients with sinus rhythm in order to prevent the development of atrial fibrillation and systemic embolism.[14]

After PMV, there was an increase of RAA myocardial velocities, in relation with the decrease of pulmonary artery systolic pressure ($r = 0.81$, $p < 0.01$). This improvement of RAA function could contribute to prevent the development of atrial fibrillation and pulmonary embolism.

■ CONCLUSION

In patients with mitral stenosis and sinus rhythm who undergo PMV, there is an improvement in the systolic function of LA, LAA and RAA. These results suggest that relief of mitral stenosis may not only confer hemodynamic benefits for the improvement of symptoms but also have a favorable influence on future thromboembolic complications. Thus, an early intervention might benefit patients with sinus rhythm in order to prevent the development of atrial fibrillation and systemic and pulmonary embolism. However, more studies are needed with a greater sample and follow-up for a longer time after PMV to assess the relation of improvement of LAA and RAA systolic function with a possible reduction of the embolic events.

■ REFERENCES

1. Inoue K, Owaki T, Nakamura T, Kitamura F, Miyamoto N. Clinical application of transvenous mitral commissurotomy by a new balloon catheter. J Thorac Cardiovasc Surg. 1984;87(3):394–402.
2. Hernandez R, Bañuelos C, Alfonso F, Goicolea J, Fernández-Ortiz A, Escaned J, et al. Long-term clinical and echocardiographic follow-up after percutaneous mitral valvuloplasty with the Inoue balloon. Circulation. 1999;99(12):1580–6.
3. Pollick C, Taylor D. Assessment of left atrial appendage function by transesophageal echocardiography. Implications for the development of thrombus. Circulation. 1991;84(1):223–31.
4. Pozzoli M, Febo O, Torbicki A, Tramarin R, Calsamiglia G, Cobelli F, et al. Left atrial appendage dysfunction: A cause of thrombosis? Evidence by transesophageal echocardiography-Doppler studies. J Am Soc Echocardiogr Off Publ Am Soc Echocardiogr. 1991;4(5):435–41.
5. Tatani SB, Campos Filho O, Fischer CH, Moisés VA, Souza JAM de, Alves CMR, et al. Functional assessment of the left atrial appendage with transesophageal echocardiography before and after percutaneous valvotomy in the mitral stenosis. Arq Bras Cardiol. 2005;84(6):457–60.
6. Cianciulli TF, Saccheri MC, Lax JA, Sarmiento RA, Bermann AM, Gagliardi JA, et al. Left and right atrial function after percutaneous mitral valvuloplasty in mitral stenosis and sinus rhythm. J Heart Valve Dis. 2008;17(5):492–500.
7. Agmon Y, Khandheria BK, Gentile F, Seward JB. Echocardiographic assessment of the left atrial appendage. J Am Coll Cardiol. 1999;34(7):1867–77.
8. Cianciulli TF, Prezioso HA, Lax JA. Función ventricular. Editorial Médica Panamericana. Cardiología 2.000. Tomo 1. Buenos Aires. Bartolasi C, 1997:433–8.
9. Cormier B, Vahanian A, Iung B, Porte JM, Dadez E, Lazarus A, et al. Influence of percutaneous mitral commissurotomy on left atrial spontaneous contrast of mitral stenosis. Am J Cardiol. 1993;71(10):842–7.
10. Stojnić BB, Radjen GS, Perisić NJ, Pavlović PB, Stosić JJ, Prcović M. Pulmonary venous flow pattern studied by transoesophageal pulsed Doppler echocardiography in mitral stenosis in sinus rhythm: effect of atrial systole. Eur Heart J. 1993;14(12):1597–601.
11. Carleton RA, Graettinger JS. The hemodynamic role of the atria with and without mitral stenosis. Am J Med. 1967;42(4):532–8.
12. Stojnic B, Krajcer Z, Anicic S, Prcovic M. Use of continuous-wave Doppler echocardiography to evaluate the hemodynamic importance of atrial systole in

patients with mitral stenosis. Tex Heart Inst J Tex Heart Inst St Lukes Episcop Hosp Tex Child Hosp. 1990;17(3):219–22.

13. Gölbaşi Z, Ciçek D, Canbay A, Uçar O, Bayol H, Aydogdu S. Left atrial appendage function in patients with mitral stenosis in sinus rhythm. Eur J Echocardiogr J Work Group Echocardiogr Eur Soc Cardiol. 2002;3(1):39–43.

14. Bauer F, Verdonck A, Schuster I, et al. Left atrial appendage function analyzed by tissue Doppler imaging in mitral stenosis: effect of afterload reduction after mitral valve commissurotomy. J Am Soc Echocardiography. 2005;18:934–9.

Section 3

PMV—Procedure, Technical Considerations and Periprocedural Monitoring

Chapter 15

Transseptal Puncture

Harikrishnan S, Krishnakumar Nair

Transseptal puncture is an essential step in performing percutaneous mitral valvotomy (PMV) through the antegrade route.

The knowledge of the anatomy of the interatrial septum is very important in making a safe septal puncture. In mitral stenosis (MS), the left atrium and many a times, the right atrium and right ventricle are dilated distorting the anatomy. Occasionally the patients might have undergone a closed mitral valvotomy (CMV), and rib excision or left atrial appendectomy (LAA) (usually done along with CMV) which further distorts the anatomy. All these make the septal puncture technically demanding and occasionally difficult.

The transseptal puncture technique was developed by Ross, Braunwald and Morrow at the National Heart Institute (now the National Heart, Lung, and Blood Institute), Bethesda in the late 1950s to allow left heart catheterization, principally for the evaluation of valvular heart disease.[1]

The refinements made to the needle and catheter and the development of the combined catheter and dilator set by Mullins, made the procedure safe and easy.[2,3]

▣ ANATOMY OF THE ATRIAL SEPTUM

The interatrial septum is bounded posteriorly by a fold of pericardium between the left and right atria, superiorly by the superior vena cava (SVC), anterosuperiorly by the noncoronary sinus of Valsalva, anteriorly by the septal tricuspid annulus, anteroinferiorly by the coronary sinus os, and inferiorly by the inferior vena cava (Figs 15.1 and 15.2).

The fossa ovalis is the true interatrial portion of the septum, and typically the thinnest portion. It is considered the safe place to create a puncture for entry into the left atrium. The limbus is the pronounced anterosuperior margin of the fossa ovalis within the right side of the interatrial septum (Figs 15.3 and 15.4). It represents the inferior margin of the septum secundum during fetal life. The fossa ovalis appears as a depression in the interatrial septum when viewed from the RA.

The fossa ovalis is surrounded by the muscular septum, the thick portions of the septum secundum and primum composed primarily of atrial muscle.

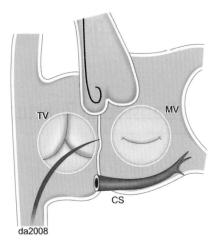

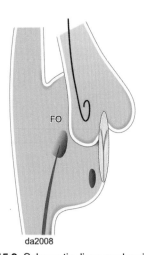

Fig. 15.1: Schematic diagram showing the septum in LAO view. Here the septum is perpendicular to the imaging plane. *Abbreviations:* TV, tricuspid valve; CS, coronary sinus; MV, mitral valve Adapted by permission from BMJ Publishing Group Limited. Mark J Early. How to perform a transseptal puncture. Heart. 2009;95:85–92,[4] copyright 2010

Fig. 15.2: Schematic diagram showing the septum in RAO 40° view. Here the septum is full face to the imaging plane. *Abbreviation:* FO, fossa ovalis Adapted with permission from BMJ Publishing Group Limited. Mark J Early. How to perform a transseptal puncture. Heart. 2009;95:85–92[4]

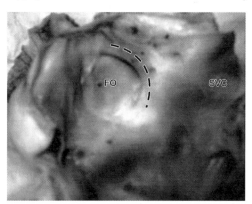

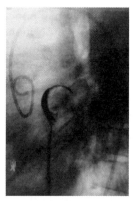

Fig. 15.3: Gross examination of the fossa ovalis from the right atrium. Right atrial view of the atrial septum with limbic ledge seen. *Abbreviations:* FO, fossa ovalis; SVC, superior vena cava (Published with permission from Baballaros et al. Emerging applications for TS catheterization. JACC; 2008:51;2116–22)[5]

Fig. 15.4: Dye in the limbus fossa ovalis. Krishnamoorthy KM. Int J Cardiol. 2001;78:205[6] (Published with permission from Elsevier)

The fossa ovalis is either oval or circular with an average area varying from 1.5 to 2.4 cm² in the adult. It is located posteriorly, at the junction of the mid and lower third of the RA.

In patients with mitral valve disease and a bulging LA, the fossa ovalis can be located more inferiorly.

Since the fossa ovalis has no characteristic radiographic appearance, the placement of catheters in known anatomic locations, such as in the noncoronary sinus of the aortic root, will provide useful landmarks. These landmarks may be helpful in locating the fossa ovalis, and areas where a puncture may be harmful.

The most important structure to avoid injury, is the aortic root. So it is advisable to delineate the position of the aortic root by using a pigtail catheter in the noncoronary sinus which is the lowermost sinus in RAO view.

Placing the fluoroscopy unit in an LAO position between 30 to 45 degrees will provide a perpendicular view of the interatrial septum. Viewed in this plane, the transseptal access device will appear in full profile when the tip is perpendicular to the septum.

The RAO view will enable us to divide the septum into anterior and posterior planes, and allow assessment of the relative anterior and posterior location of the fossa ovalis.

We know that the septum lies between the two atria. The posterior limit of the septum is usually the lateral border of the left atrium. But in patients with MS and large left atria the LA border may be lateral to the RA border ("the shadow out of shadow sign" in fluoroscopy). In such cases the posterior limit of the septum will be the right atrial border, rather than the LA border as there is no septum laterally beyond this point. If the left atrial border is taken as the reference for puncture, it will result in cardiac perforation (Figs 15.5).[7,8]

◼ HOW TO PERFORM TRANSSEPTAL PUNCTURE

Catheters/Instruments Needed
- Mullins sheath (optional) and/or dilator (7F)
- Brockenbrough needle
- Three-way stopcock with saline and contrast.

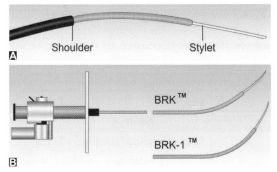

Figs 15.5A and B: (A) Tip of the transseptal needle. The shoulder is designed to stop the needle from advancing too far (approximately 3 mm) beyond the introducer tip; (B) BRK and BRK-1 transseptal needle tips (*Image Courtesy:* St Jude Medical)

Mullins Sheath and Dilator

The Mullins sheath has a 270° curve at the end that is straightened by the dilator, the catheter is available in different shapes with variable radii at its tip. This will allow variable reach within the RA (Table 15.1).

Table 15.1: Specifications and ordering information of Mullins sheath and dilator system

Order	Size	Sheath length	Dilator length	Wire size max
Adult				
EP008591	8 Fr with hemostasis valve	59 cm	67 cm	032 in
EP008552	8 Fr	59 cm	67 cm	.032 in
Pediatric				
EP008532	8 Fr	44 cm	52 cm	.025 in
EP008530	6 Fr	44 cm	52 cm	.024 in

Courtesy: Medtronic Incorporated

Brockenbrough Needle

The needle most commonly used is a Brockenbrough needle (Medtronic) (Fig. 15.6 and Table 15.2). This needle is an 18-gauge hollow tube that tapers distally to 21 gauge. The proximal end has a flange with an arrow that points to the direction of the needle tip (Fig. 15.7).

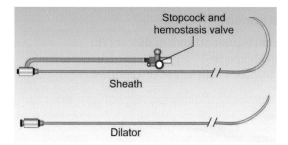

Fig. 15.6: Trans-septal catheter introduction set (Medtronic Inc with permission)

Table 15.2: Specifications and ordering information of Brockenbrough needle

Order number	Size	Length
Adult		
EP003994	18 gauge shaft, 21 gauge tip	71 cm
Pediatric		
EP003997	19 gauge shaft, 22 gauge tip	56 cm

Courtesy: Medtronic Incorporated

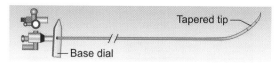

Fig. 15.7: Brockenbrough needle (*Courtesy:* Medtronic Inc.)

St. Jude medicals also are marketing septal puncture needles. They are called BRK needles. There are three curves available two adult curves (BRK, BRK-1) and two pediatric curves BRK-1 and 2. The standard curved BRK needle has a 19° angle between the distal curved segment and the needle shaft. The BRK-1 needle has an accentuated curve (53° angle). The BRK-1 needle is ideal for patients with dilated right atrium. The needle is available in three lengths (71 cm, 89 cm or 98 cm).[9] The pediatric needle is 56 cm long. The new BRK XS transseptal needle features a steeper primary bevel angle and two back bevels that combine to form a distinct point on the tip of the needle. As a result, it requires less puncture force to penetrate the fossa ovalis and can accommodate variances in difficult anatomies.

Septal puncture can be done using Mullins dilator alone (without the sheath) and Brockenbrough needle. Both sheath and dilator are used in the following two situations:

1. When LV entry is planned using a balloon catheter for an over-the wire entry technique, e.g. Cribier's metallic commissurotome, over the wire balloons.
2. Since there are two layers of catheter material (sheath and dilator) it may provide protection during rare occurrence of inadvertent perforation of the dilator catheter by the needle during its manipulation.

Steps in Transseptal Puncture

Step 1: Accessing the left innominate vein (LIV)

Goodale Lubin™/Multipurpose (MPA)™ catheter is introduced into the left innominate vein (Fig. 15.8).

Step 2: An exchange length wire (300 cm) is introduced into the left innominate vein. Exchange length wire will enable easy exchange of the GL/Multipurpose catheter with the Mullins dilator/sheath system. Wire with length of 150 cm can also be used for this purpose and the catheters can be exchanged using the "syringe and saline flushing" technique (Fig. 15.9).

Step 3: Mullins sheath into the left innominate vein

Mullins sheath or dilator is introduced into the innominate vein over the exchange length wire (Fig. 15.10). Check whether the length of the sheath/dilator and the puncture needle, will tally, before selecting the sheath (Fig. 15.11).

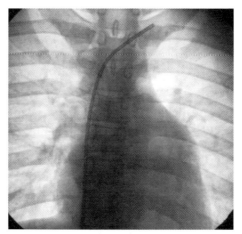

Fig. 15.8: GL catheter in the left innominate vein

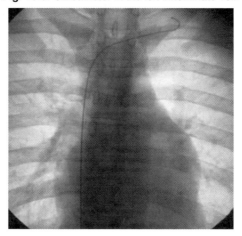

Fig. 15.9: Catheter in the innominate vein replaced by an exchange length (300 cm) wire

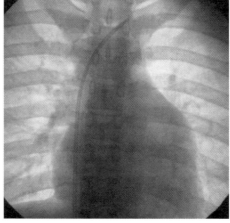

Fig. 15.10: Mullins sheath in the left innominate vein

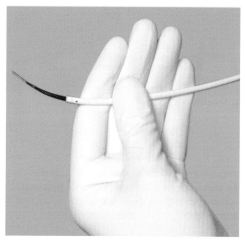

Fig. 15.11: Mullins sheath (white), dilator (gray), needle (silver) assembly

Step 4: Removing the wire from Mullins sheath

Remove the exchange length wire leaving the Mullins sheath/dilator in the innominate vein.

Step 5: Introduction of Brockenbrough needle and making the sheath and needle assembly

The next step in transseptal puncture is the formation of the needle-sheath assembly. For that the Mullins sheath/dilator and the Brockenbrough needle is used. First the length of the needle in relation to the dilator is checked. Ideally the needle should protrude 3-5 mm from the tip of the dilator, when fully inserted.

Once this is confirmed, the Brockenbrough needle attached with three-way stopcock and a syringe filled with saline is introduced through the Mullin's sheath/dilator.

It is better to flush saline continuously while the needle is being tracked as it will smoothen the passage of the needle.

Since the needle system rotates 270° while being introduced, we have to allow free rotation of the needle system. This can be achieved by supporting the needle system in the left palm and pushing the needle with the right hand slowly, allowing free rotation of the needle.

The needle should be parked more than 1 cm (usually two finger breadths, index and middle finger breadths) proximal to the tip of the Mullins sheath (Figs 15.12 and 15.13).

The operator should fix his right index finger between the catheter hub and the direction indicator of the Brockenbrough needle to prevent the needle from moving forward and protruding from the catheter tip (Fig. 15.14A). Usually the direction indicator of the needle is between 4 o'clock and 7 o'clock positions (12 o'clock is the ceiling) (Fig. 15.14B). The thumb and the middle finger should maintain the direction of the needle so that its direction and position

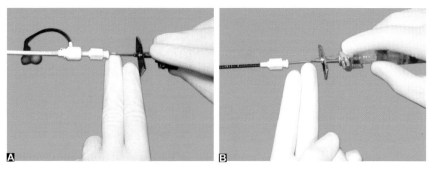

Figs 15.12A and B: Proximal end of the Mullins sheath – dilator – Brockenbrough needle assembly. The needle should be kept 2 finger breadths proximal to the proximal end of hub of the dilator. If we are using the sheath, the dilator should be fully inserted into the sheath (Left – sheath and dilator, right – dilator done)

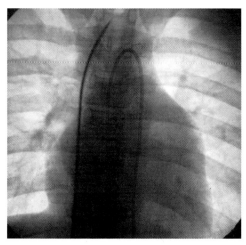

Fig. 15.13: Brockenbrough needle in the Mullins sheath

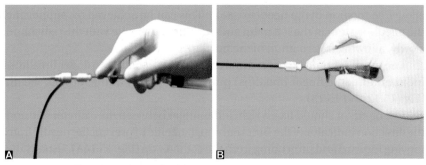

Figs 15.14A and B: Final assembly in position to descent
(Left sheath and dilator, right dilator done)

is not changed. Once the needle is in place, the saline is disconnected and the three-way stopcock is connected to diluted contrast (1:4 dilution) and few ml of contrast is injected through the needle to confirm the flow.

Step 6: Placing the pigtail catheter in aortic sinus
The next step is placing the pigtail catheter in the noncoronary sinus (lowermost) of the aortic root.

Step 7: Descent to the fossa ovalis region
This is done ideally in LAO view where the septum is vertical or it can be done in the the AP view. Keep the pointer in the septal puncture needle pointing to between 3 o'clock and 5 o'clock position, when viewed from the foot-end of the patient. This should put the distal curve of the sheath, dilator and needle perpendicular to the interatrial septum.

Once more confirm that the needle is well inside the dilator by fluoroscopy. Then drag the entire sheath-dilator-needle assembly slowly downward from the SVC to the RA. Be careful that the components of the assembly are not rotating or changing their relative positions to each other.

In the LAO (ideal) or AP view, while descending, observe the tip of the dilator during the drag for any abrupt medial movement. The first movement seen will be the catheter falling into the right atrium (RA) from the SVC and then there will be a second more subtle movement as the catheter falls over the limbic ridge to the fossa ovalis (some authors say that there is a third movement which indicates the aortic root). But since the left atrium is large and pressure overloaded, the "falling forward" motion is often difficult to detect because the fossa ovalis may be shallower.

When the assembly enters the RA there will be few atrial ectopic beats visible in the monitor. The "falling forward" of the catheter can also be mimicked by inadvertent entry into the coronary sinus os if the needle is too far anterior and inferior, or by engaging the membranous septum if even further anterior. Checking the RAO and lateral view will help assess the anteroposterior location of the assembly.

Also, if the needle tip is against the membranous septum or the aortic root, the operator may feel a pulsatile sensation being transmitted through the assembly.

If the transseptal needle is connected to a pressure transducer, as the assembly is pulled down from the superior vena cava to the right atrium and into the fossa ovalis, the pressure tracing gradually dampens and then becomes a straight line to indicate the dilator is abutting the septum. The caudal limit of the descent should not exceed 1/3rd of the distance from the tip of the pigtail to the diaphragm (Fig. 15.15A). If the LA is large we may have to descend more.

■ LANDMARKS FOR SEPTAL PUNCTURE

Transseptal puncture is done usually under fluoroscopic guidance. There are certain fluoroscopic landmarks which are used to identify the location of the fossa ovalis where we usually puncture the septum. The pigtail catheter marks the location of the aortic valve. In the AP view, the tip of the transseptal dilator engages the fossa ovalis inferiorly and medially to the aortic valve.

The cardiac silhouette identifies the posterior and lateral borders of the atria.

To select an optimal transseptal puncture site, there are 2 imaginary reference lines that need to be defined first: (1) the vertical "midline" and (2) the horizontal M-line. The target site for septal puncture is at the intersecting point of the vertical "midline" and the horizontal M-line (Figs 15.15A and B).

Inoue et al described the angiographic method for doing the septal puncture in PMV. Hung et al modified the technique (Hung's fluoroscopic method) and utilized two landmarks: (1) the LA shadow which is visible in most cases of MS and (2) The pigtail catheter kept in the non-coronary sinus of the aortic root.

So as seen in the Figures 15.15A and B, a horizontal line is drawn from the the tip of the pigtail catheter which is kept in the noncoronary sinus of the aortic root and the lateral border of the left atrium. The vertical line drawn from the midpoint of this line is the "vertical midline".

Next step is to get the horizontal M-line. The horizontal "M-line" is the line crossing the center of the mitral annulus. It is derived from a diastolic stop frame of diagnostic left ventriculography obtained in 30-degree RAO projection (Figs 15.15A and B). The plane of the mitral annulus is obtained by joining fulcrum points of the mitral valve. From the midpoint of this line, a horizontal line is drawn towards the vertebral body. This is referenced to a vertebral body. The ideal puncture site is the intersection of the vertical midline and the M-line. Usually the intersection point will be half to one vertebral body below the horizontal line drawn from the aortic root in the vertical midline.

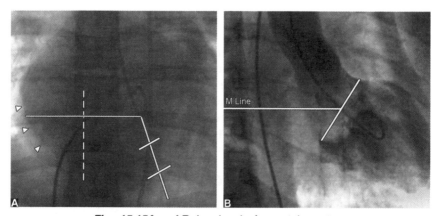

Figs 15.15A and B: Landmarks for septal puncture

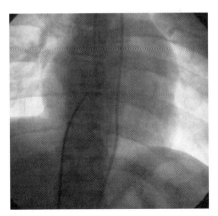

Fig. 15.16: Needle assembly after descent

So if we can have a mental picture of the vertical midline, it will be correct to make the puncture half to one vertebral space below the horizontal plane of the tip of the aortic root catheter (Fig. 15.16).

Needle Orientation

The orientation of the needle which is corresponding to the position indicator is very important.

Usually in a left atrium which is less than 4 cm, the needle will orient in the 4–5 o'clock position itself. When the left atrium is moderately enlarged (40–50 mm) the needle will be between 5 o'clock and 6 o'clock positions. If the left atrium is grossly enlarged, the needle will be at 6 o'clock position.

In our hospital, our practice is to maintain the needle in the correct orientation as far as possible during the descent. Then the needle position will be checked and altered in RAO 40° and lateral (90°) views. If the needle position is altered, then it is rechecked in all the three views (RAO 40, AP and left lateral views).

We may have to adjust and orient the needle especially in cases of large left atrium. This is done routinely in the lateral view and confirmed in other views.

We usually do the puncture in the lateral view while many others do puncture in AP, RAO or in LAO views depending on their practice and experience.

If we are not able to engage the needle in an appropriate position the needle is removed from the catheter and a fresh attempt is made by passing a guidewire through the Mullins sheath and placing it again in the innominate vein.

Shaw et al has described a technique called the "staircase movement" technique, which uses the same needle assembly to be put back into the SVC (Fig. 15.17).

But if there is any resistance during the ascend of the catheter due to the assembly hitting the right atrial appendage or free wall, it is always better to remove the needle and put back the Mullins sheath in the innominate vein.

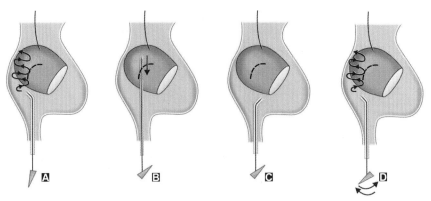

Fig. 15.17: Staircase movement for septal reascend. (A) After the catheter and needle have been placed in the lower half of the right atrium, the curve is rotated to 12 o'clock (as seen from below) and then rotated between 10 o'clock and 2 o'clock as the catheter and needle are advanced to the top of the right atrium. (B) The catheter and needle are rotated posteromedially and drawn down the atrial septum. (C) If they reach the bottom of the atrial septum without a clear movement into the foramen ovale then the movement down the septum is repeated. (D) The catheter and needle are again rotated to 12 o'clock and moved from side to side while being readvanced to the top of the right atrium. TR Shaw. Anterior staircase maneuver for atrial transseptal puncture. Br Heart J. 1994;71: 297-301¹⁰ (Published with permission)

Staining of the Septum

Once we have engaged the needle in the correct position, next step is to flush contrast and stain the septum. If the needle is snuggly fitting the septum, we may not able to flush, but the septum will get stained. Staining the septum is of no major consequence except that it can produce ectopic beats rarely.

Staining will give us an idea about the site of puncture. A vertical septal stain indicates that we are parallel to the septum and actually dissecting it. A more horizontal stain is better. If the puncture site is too low and the needle is facing the thick muscular septum, it will produce a more horizontal septal stain.

If we find a horizontal septal stain and the needle is not entering LA easily, it is advised to bring the needle more caudally and repeat the puncture. If the stain is seen on the aortic sinus or aortic wall (Figs 15.18A and B), the procedure has to be abandoned and the patient should be watched for cardiac tamponade, aortic dissection or aortic regurgitation.

Step 8: Confirmation in RAO view (Figs 15.19A and B)
In this view the septum is fully enface to the operator. The position of Mullins sheath and puncture should anterior to the descending aortic catheter.

Step 9: Confirmation in lateral view (Fig. 15.20)
The needle position is confirmed in lateral view. In the lateral projection, the fossa is usually halfway along the imaginary line from the tip of the

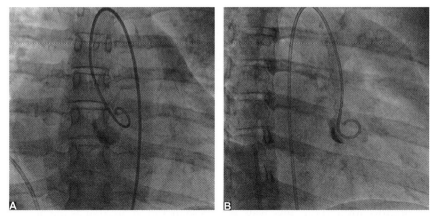

Figs 15.18A and B: Stain in the aortic root during attempted septal puncture: (A) AP view, (B) RAO view ▣◀

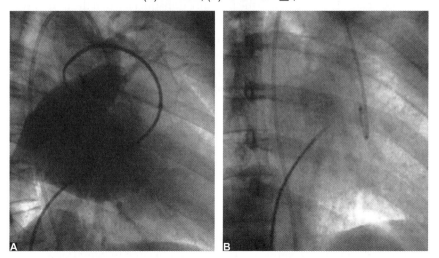

Figs 15.19A and B: LA angiogram in RAO 40° view. In this view the septum is fully 'en-face' to the operator. Note the position of the Mullins sheath and puncture needle—it is anterior to the descending aortic catheter ▣◀

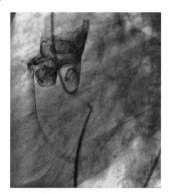

Fig. 15.20: Aortic root injection in lateral view confirming the position of aorta

pigtail catheter to the posterior border of the heart. The needle should face posterosuperomedially towards the LA.

Step 10: Aortic root contrast injection (Fig. 15.20)

Aortic root angiogram: This is to identify the position of the aortic sinuses and aorta. We have to make sure that the needle is away from aortic root. Contrast injection is done usually to make sure that the needle is away and not facing the aortic root.

Step 11: Puncture

Puncture is done by abruptly jerking the needle forwards inside the Mullins sheath maintaining the direction of the needle using the right hand and holding and fixing the sheath with the left hand. This should be observed on fluoroscopy and the "give way" will be seen and (more) felt as the needle suddenly jumps across the septum (Figs 15.21A and B).

If the needle is connected to the pressure transducer, when the puncture is made there is a sudden elevation of pressure as the needle passes through the septum before a definite left atrium pressure wave is seen (Fig. 15.22).

Once left atrial entry via the fossa ovalis is confirmed, advance the sheath/dilator assembly into the left atrium. It is advised to keep the needle in a fixed position and advance the sheath alone into the left atrium. It is better to direct the system posteriorly (3 o'clock position) in the lateral view while advancing the needle-dilator assembly into the left atrium. While advancing, it is better to give puffs of contrast to see the posterior limit of the left atrial wall.

The position of the catheter in the left atrium (Fig. 15.23) can be confirmed by the following methods:

1. Pressure: Will show left atrial pressure
2. Oxygen saturation: Will show bright blood, >95%
3. Position: The catheter tip will be posterior in lateral view
4. The position can be confirmed by contrast injection in lateral view
5. The left main bronchus in LAO view represents the roof of the left atrium.

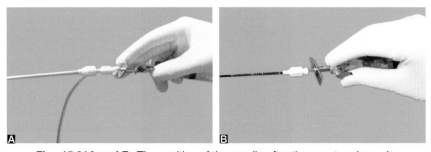

Figs 15.21A and B: The position of the needle after the puncture is made. Note the needle has got fully inserted into the dilator

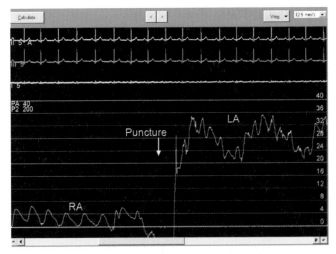

Fig. 15.22: Pressure recording during septal puncture. Note the sudden transition from right atrium to left atrium

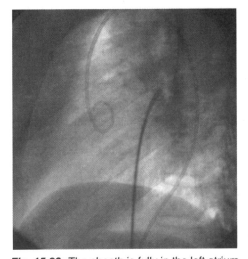

Fig. 15.23: The sheath is fully in the left atrium

■ SEPTAL PUNCTURE WITHOUT ARTERIAL STICK

This strategy is usually employed by electrophysiologists while doing ablation treatment of atrial fibrillation. The major difference is that the aortic pigtail catheter is replaced by an electrode through the femoral venous route at the bundle of His position. The His bundle electrogram is classically recorded immediately inferior to the non-coronary sinus of the aorta, which is the caudal most aspect of the aorta. In LAO view, the tip of the His catheter should point directly to the fluoroscopy screen. In addition, a catheter placed in the coronary sinus indicates the floor of the left atrium. The septal puncture needle in RAO view should either point slightly more posterior than or should be parallel to the coronary sinus catheter.[10]

■ PROBING THE SEPTUM

In 20–25% of adult patients, the fossa ovalis is probe patent [patent foramen ovale (PFO)] and may not require needle puncture.[11,12] In approximately two thirds of patients, the fossa is paper thin, and the catheter can be passed into the LA with gentle pressure and rotation of the dilator.[11] Krishnamoorthy et al. have reported the use of probing entry into the left atrium. They reported that probing the fossa achieves left atrial entry in 90% of patients. This maneuver avoids needle puncture and reduces puncture time as well as fluoroscopy time.[13] They report it as a safe alternative. Mahmoodul Hassan from Pakistan has also reported a success rate of 87% by probing in a series of 500 patients.[14]

The use of the probing method is discussed in detail in the chapter on "PMV in technically challenging situations" (Chapter 49).

■ REFERENCES

1. Ross J Jr, Braunwald E, Morrow AG. Left heart catheterization by the transseptal route: A description of the technique and its applications. Circulation. 1960;22: 927–34.
2. Brockenbrough EC, Braunwald E, Ross J Jr. Transseptal left heart catheterization. A review of 450 studies and description of an improved technic. Circulation. 1962;25:15–21.
3. Mullins CE. Transseptal left heart catheterization: Experience with a new technique in 520 pediatric and adult patients. Pediatr Cardiol. 1983;4(3):239–45.
4. Earley MJ. How to perform a transseptal puncture. Heart Br Card Soc. 2009;95(1):85–92.
5. Babaliaros VC, Green JT, Lerakis S, Lloyd M, Block PC. Emerging applications for transseptal left heart catheterization old techniques for new procedures. J Am Coll Cardiol. 2008;51(22):2116–22.
6. Krishnamoorthy KM. Dye in the limbus fossa ovalis. Int J Cardiol. 2001;78(2):205.
7. Hung JS. Atrial septal puncture technique in percutaneous transvenous mitral commissurotomy: mitral valvuloplasty using the Inoue balloon catheter technique. Cathet Cardiovasc Diagn. 1992;26(4):275–84.
8. Trehan V, Mukhopadhyay S, Yaduvanshi A, Mehta V, Sunil Roy TN, Nigam A. Non-surgical method of managing cardiac perforation during percutaneous transvenous mitral commissurotomy. Indian Heart J. 2004;56:328–32.
9. Tzeis S, Andrikopoulos G, Deisenhofer I, Ho SY, Theodorakis G. Transseptal catheterization: considerations and caveats. Pacing Clin Electrophysiol PACE. 2010;33(2):231–42.
10. Shaw TR. Anterior staircase manoeuvre for atrial transseptal puncture. Br Heart J. 1994;71(3):297–301.
11. Bloomfield DA, Sinclair-Smith BC. The limbic ledge. A landmark for transseptal left heart catheterization. Circulation. 1965;31:103–7.
12. Sweeney LJ, Rosenquist GC. The normal anatomy of the atrial septum in the human heart. Am Heart J. 1979;98(2):194–9.
13. Krishnamoorthy KM, Dash PK. Transseptal catheterization without needle puncture. Scand Cardiovasc J SCJ. 2001;35(3):199–200.
14. Haq M ul, Hafizullah M, Gul AM, Jan HU, Awan ZA. Percutaneous transvenous mitral commissurotomy (PTMC) through patent foramen ovale (PFO) a novel approach. J Postgrad Med Inst. 2008;22(2):148–51.

Chapter 16

Use of Safe-Sept Guidewire in Transseptal Access

Carlo de Asmundis, Darragh Moran, Jayakeerthi Yoganarasimha Rao,
Gian-Battista Chierchia, Pedro Brugada

Transseptal (TS) puncture is a key feature of procedures requiring direct access to the left-sided cardiac chambers, be it interventions on the mitral valve or ablations on the left side. The risk of complications related to transseptal puncture is estimated to be less than 1%,[1] although this is mostly attributed to its long learning curve, and it is considered a relatively safe and straightforward procedure in experienced hands.[2] However, in cases of challenging TS punctures, such as the presence of a thick, aneurysmal or extremely elastic fossa ovalis, the risk of complications increases. As these complications may be disastrous, we are always in search of newer, safer and user-friendly modalities to facilitate TS puncture. The Safe-Sept system is one such modality that fits the bill.

INDICATIONS

- Resistant septum, especially in patients who have had TS procedures prior
- Elastic septum
- Aneurysmal septum.

TECHNICAL ASPECTS

The Safe-Sept guidewire (Safe-Sept, Pressure Products, Inc., San Pedro, CA, USA), is made of nitinol, and is J-shaped at the distal end, with a sharp-tip (Fig. 16.1A). It is 135 cm long and 0.014" in diameter, and allows compatibility with all currently available adult TS introducer systems. As the wire is made of nitinol (nickel-titanium alloy) which is known for its memory, it gives the tensile strength to spring back to the J-shape once the distal part is out of the introducer system. At the distal end just proximal to the curved segment, there is a radiopaque segment that helps to monitor the extent of advancement of the wire in the left atrium and pulmonary vein. This is because the curved J-tip as such, is relatively radiolucent and hence not easily visible. To make the procedure easier and safer, the guidewire has markers on the proximal aspect also, which is 72 cm from the tip. This gives some guidance to the operator to

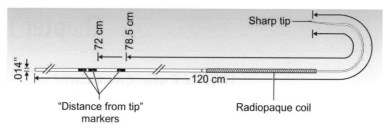

Fig. 16.1A: Illustration of the features of the nitinol J-shaped Safe-Sept guidewire

estimate the position of the guidewire tip within the sheath, as it may not be clearly visible under fluroscopy (Fig. 16.2B).

Once across the septum, we should make sure the radiopaque segment is out of the introducer system to ensure the needle has enough support to cross over the wire. Being a high volume center, especially for atrial fibrillation ablations, where patients require one or two TS punctures each time and multiple times over many years, we come across septa which are very difficult to cross with the usual needles. We use this system in some such cases, especially those who have undergone at least 2 previous TS procedures and the septum is rendered resistant, though this guidewire can be used on a routine basis In the experience of Wadhera et al.[3] a successful TSP was achieved in all but one patient (success rate of 98%) with no complications. A majority of the TSP were achieved with just one pass even though half the TSP were performed by the fellows.

While our use of the guidewire in TS access is based on certain criteria, a recent study defined resistant septum as one which does not yield despite moderate force, and they used the Safe-Sept system in such cases which accounted for about 20% of cases.[4] They found no specific anatomic markers to describe a resistant septum. It is also of significance to note that studies have described presence of muscle fibers in the fossa ovalis area,[5] which could be one reason for the difficult access in some. Success rates are high and the wire provides a measure of security as we avoid greater force to cross the septum, when used in situations mentioned earlier.

We routinely perform transesophageal echocardiography (TEE) during the TS access (Fig. 16.2C), including while using this system which is considered safe. The reasons are:

- As an academic center, TEE helps the fellows to learn the anatomy better.
- Furthermore, when performed under TEE guidance, direct visualization of the septum and the fossa ovalis area helps in more precise positioning of the sheath at the thinnest part before the puncture, minimizing the risk of major complications.[6]
- TEE also visualizes the Safe-Sept wire entry into the LA and helps in its positioning.

The wire's most interesting features are the immediate down curving into a J-shape after crossing the septum and the possibility to advance the TS system 'over the wire' after the placement of the wire in the LSPV similar to the previously described technique by Cheng using an 0.014" angioplasty guidewire inserted into the needle hub and advanced in the LA.[7] This greatly

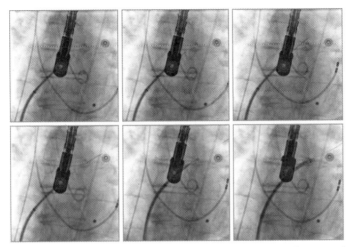

Fig. 16.2B: The different steps in the use of the Safe-Sept guidewire—fluoroscopic images

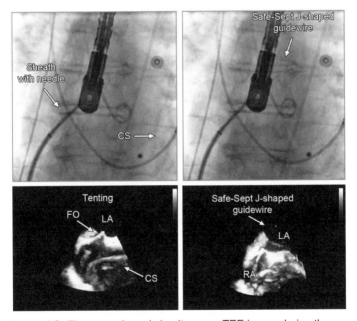

Fig. 16.2C: Fluoroscopic and simultaneous TEE image during the use
of Safe-Sept device for septal puncture
Abbreviations: FO, fossa ovalis; LA, left atrium; CS, coronary sinus; RA, right atrium

diminishes the probabilities of accidental penetration of critical anatomical structures such as the aortic root and the posterior wall of the LA.

With over a thousand TS access per year, we find the need for the Safe-Sept guidewire in about 5% of TS punctures. We also use radiofrequency ablation for the TS puncture and have found this more cost-effective in such circumstances, as we have devised our own method[8] without using the commercially available radiofrequency perforation devices (TorFlex Trans-septal Guiding Sheath,

Baylis Medical Company, Inc.), as we find radiofrequency puncture in difficult cases, a cost-effective and equally safe alternative.

Advantages of Safe-Sept Guidewire

- As the tip is self-folding, it avoids a direct entry of the sharp tip into any tissue ahead of it.
- As less force is required to cross the septum, the puncture is more controlled, and, hence avoids hitting the posterior wall once the septum gives way, the mechanism responsible for effusions in similar scenarios.

Limitations

The sharp tip protrudes outward, a few mm beyond the curve, leaving scope for accidental puncture of tissue around.

Our Suggestions

While in our experience, the use of this novel nitinol J-shaped guidewire has been helpful and has permitted easy and safe 'over the wire' TS access, we follow a few steps to make it safer.

One such, is to make sure that the sharp tip points anteriorly or downwards and not posteriorly (on TEE), while being advanced in the LA. This is important because, it is the natural tendency of the TS system to rotate posteriorly once it crosses the septal resistance. Hence, the visualization of the distal curve enface with its tip pointing down in the AP view on cine, is optimal rather than the curve being in an oblique position or the tip pointing up to avoid inadvertent perforation of the roof or the posterior wall.

Secondly, we advance the wire in the LA a short distance after radiopaque segment is out of the system, so that the distal curve is at or near the ostium of the left superior pulmonary vein but not into it. This gives just enough support for the needle and the system to crossover the wire, while avoiding damage to the pulmonary vein.

In summary, with an established technique like the TS puncture which has been around for several decades, coming back to fore with an increase in indications for direct left atrial access, there has been great progress in developing hardware which make the TS puncture safer and easier. The Safe-Sept guidewire is one such modality, for use in both routine and difficult TS access.

▨ REFERENCES

1. De Ponti R, Cappato R, Curnis A, Della Bella P, Padeletti L, Raviele A, et al. Trans-septal catheterization in the electrophysiology laboratory: data from a multicenter survey spanning 12 years. J Am Coll Cardiol. 2006;47(5):1037-42. Epub 2006 Feb 9.
2. FagundesRL, Mantica M, De Luca L, Forleo G, PappalardoA,AvellaA, et al. Safety of single transseptal puncture for ablation of atrial fibrillation:Retrospective study from a large cohort of patients. J Cardiovasc Electrophysiol. 2007;18:1277-81.

3. Vineet Wadehra, Alfred E. Buxton, Antonios P. Antoniadis, James W. McCready, Calum J. Redpath, Oliver R. Segal, et al. The use of a novel nitinol guidewire to facilitate transseptal puncture and left atrial catheterization for catheter ablation procedures. Europace Oct 2011, 13 (10) 1401-1405; DOI: 10.1093/europace/eur155.

4. De Ponti R, Marazzi R, Picciolo G, Salerno-Uriarte JA. Use of a novel sharp-tip, J-shaped guidewire to facilitate transseptal catheterization. Europace 2010;12(5): 668–73.

5. Platonov PG, Mitrofanova L, Ivanov V, Ho SY. Substrates for intra-atrial and interatrial conduction in the atrial septum: anatomical study on 84 human hearts. Heart Rhythm Off J Heart Rhythm Soc. 2008;5(8):1189–95.

6. Chierchia GB, Capulzini L, de Asmundis C, Sarkozy A, Roos M, Paparella G, et al. First experience with real-time three-dimensional transoesophageal echocardiography guided transseptal in patients undergoing atrial fibrillation ablation. Europace. 2008;10:1325–8.

7. Cheng A, Calkins H. A conservative approach to performing transseptal punctures without the use of intracardiac echocardiography: stepwise approach with real-time video clips. J Cardiovasc Electrophysiol. 2007;18:686–9.

8. Capulzini L, Paparella G, Sorgente A, de Asmundis C,Chierchia GB, Sarkozy A, et al. Feasibility, safety, and outcome of a challenging transseptal puncture facilitated by radiofrequency energy delivery: a prospective single-centre study. Europace. 2010;12:662–7.

Chapter 17

Percutaneous Mitral Valvotomy—Procedure

Harikrishnan S, Sanjay G, Rajesh Muralidharan

Percutaneous mitral valvotomy (PMV) is usually done as an inpatient procedure. Since, there is always a chance of mitral valve replacement (MVR) or surgical intervention being needed due to complications related to septal puncture, surgical standby is usually arranged for.

PREPARATION OF THE PATIENT (SCTIMST PROTOCOL)

1. Fasting overnight
2. TEE usually done on the day of procedure to check for LA thrombus and assess interatrial septum and mitral regurgitation (MR)
3. Premedication
   - Inj. Chlorpheniramine maleate 2 cc IV on call
   - Inj. Hydrocortisone 100 mg IV on call
4. Prophylactic antibiotics
   - Inj. Augmentin (Amoxicillin–Clavulanic acid) 1.2 g IV ATD
   - Inj. Cefotaxime 1 gm IV
   - Inj. Ciprofloxacin 200 mg IV infusion over 30 minutes

   All three are given one hour prior to the procedure and ciprofloxacin infusion will be on flow while the patient is shifted to cathlab.

Antibiotics after procedure (Given parenterally for 48 hours and then continued orally):
- Inj. Augmentin (amoxicillin–clavulanic acid) 1.2 gm 12 hourly.
- Inj. Cefotaxime 1 gm IV eight hourly
- Inj. Ciprofloxacin 200 mg IV infusion over 30 minutes twice daily
- Oral antibiotics for three more days
- Cap. Augmentin 325 mg twice daily × 3 more days
- Tab. Ciprofloxacin 500 mg BD × 3 more days.

OBTAINING THE VASCULAR ACCESS

- Right femoral vein—7 French
- Right femoral artery—6 F or 5 F (To introduce pigtail catheter to locate aorta and to enter LV and obtain left ventricular end-diastolic pressure).

PREPARATION OF THE SEPTAL PUNCTURE SYSTEM AND THE BALLOON

- This process is to be performed taking all aseptic precautions.
- The cardiac technologist should be very cautious and change over to the sterile cathlab dress for preparing the hardware, some of which are 200 to 300 cm long.
- Since many developing countries resterilize and reuse some of the hardware, the preparation of balloon catheter and transseptal puncture set should be very meticulous.
- The Brockenbrough needle is usually EtO (ethylene oxide) sterilized. It has to be checked for its integrity, especially the tip with its welded joint, which can breakaway during reuse.
- The balloon, taken out from the glutaraldehyde (Cidex™) solution is thoroughly cleansed with a sterile cotton gauze soaked in saline. The balloon lumen is also flushed with saline.
- The process is repeated for three or more times.
- The hardware is thoroughly checked for any damage. The tip of the balloon and the knob are specifically looked at, as they can get detached on multiple reuse.
- The pigtail shaped wire is thoroughly checked for the integrity in the welded area (at the junction of the floppy and the straight portion).
- A contrast-saline mixture at 1:4 dilution is prepared.
- The balloon hub is connected to a 20 mL syringe containing the contrast-saline mixture with a 10 mm extension tubing connected with a 3-way stop cock.
- The contrast mixture is pushed into the balloon kept vertically down and the 3-way is locked.
- Tap the balloon properly so that air inside the balloon comes up. Release the 3-way and push out the air.
- Again push the contrast mixture into the balloon, lock the three-way, check for any air inside the balloon again. Once it is made sure that the balloon is completely air free, proceed to the next step.
- Measure the balloon diameter with Vernier calipers provided along with the balloon. Adjust the volume of contrast to get the adequate sized balloon (Fig. 17.1). Usually an addition of around 1 mL of contrast, will increase the size of the balloon by 1 mm, but this varies with the size of the balloon (1 mL = 1 mm in the case of 24 mm balloon).
- Release the 3-way lock letting the contrast-saline mixture come into the syringe by itself. Don't aspirate further. Close the free hub of the 3-way using a stopper, to prevent inadvertent leakage of the contrast.
- Always note the amount of contrast inside the syringe. This will be useful to check whether there was any contrast leak during the handling of the balloon.
- Introduce the straightener into the balloon and slenderize it.
- Now the balloon is ready for introduction into the left atrium.

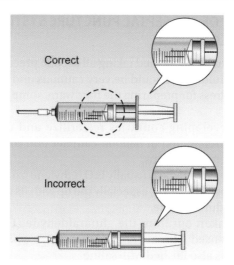

Fig. 17.1: The correct and incorrect methods of filling the syringe during preparation of the balloon system (*Source:* Reproduced with kind permission from Toray Inc.)

■ STEPS OF PERCUTANEOUS MITRAL VALVOTOMY

Assessing Hemodynamics

This is done using a Goodale Lubin™ (GL) or multipurpose (MPA) catheter. These catheters will allow easy access to the SVC and the left innominate vein as the initial step to septal puncture.

Right Atrial Pressure

Right atrial pressure provides an indication of the filling pressure which can influence the hemodynamics. Low filling pressure results in spuriously low left atrial pressure affecting the assessment of the transmitral gradient. If the right atrial pressure is very low, it is advisable to infuse 200–300 mL of non-heparinized saline and recheck the pressures.

Pulmonary Artery Pressure

Assessing the pulmonary artery pressure is important as it indicates the severity of the disease. The response of pulmonary artery pressure to PMV is an indicator of the success of the procedure.

Septal Puncture

This is described in detail in Chapter 15 on transseptal puncture.

Entering the Left Atrium and Balloon Inflation

Step 1: Recording the Pressures in the Left Atrium

After transseptal puncture, we have the Mullins' sheath in the left atrium (LA). We can record the pressure in the left atrium using the Mullins' sheath/dilator.

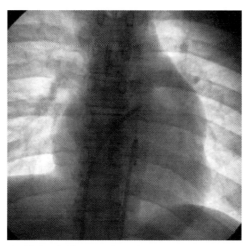

Fig. 17.2: Mullins' dilator in the left atrium. The pigtail catheter
is in the descending aorta

Simultaneously, we can record the left ventricular pressure by advancing the pigtail catheter into the left ventricle (This is usually done in PA view). Before this, withdraw the pigtail catheter which is already in the ascending aorta to the descending aorta, flush it with saline and then reintroduce the catheter into the ascending aorta and then enter LV. (Since, the patient is not heparinized, there is a possibility of having thrombi in the pigtail catheter. So, it is better to flush the catheter in the descending aorta). Then measure the pressure simultaneously in LA and LV. Once the LV pressure is measured, pull back the pigtail catheter again to the descending aorta (Fig. 17.2).

Step 2: Introduction of the Pigtail Shaped Left Atrial Guidewire

The next step is the introduction of the pigtail guidewire into the LA through the Mullins sheath or dilator. Sometimes, the wire may enter one of the pulmonary veins or the LA appendage. In such situations, we have to realign the catheter away from the mouth of the pulmonary vein or LA appendage by rotating it or slightly withdrawing the catheter.

The pigtail guidewire once in the LA cavity forms a nice loop which is freely movable in the left atrium. Once, the pigtail shaped wire is optimally placed in the left atrium, the Mullins sheath/dilator is withdrawn (Fig. 17.3).

Step 3: Dilatation of the Groin Access Site and the Interatrial Septum

Once the pigtail wire is inside the left atrium, the Mullins sheath/dilator is withdrawn and removed from the LA. Then the groin (venous puncture site) is dilated with an artery forceps to allow the passage of the dilator and the balloon. Following this, the 14F dilator is introduced over the pigtail wire and the groin entry point is dilated. Subsequently, the dilator is advanced over the pigtail wire and the septum is dilated (Fig. 17.4). The dilator should be

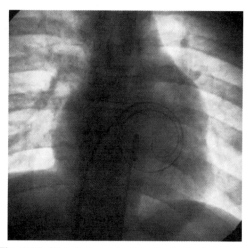

Fig. 17.3: Pigtail-shaped guidewire in the left atrium

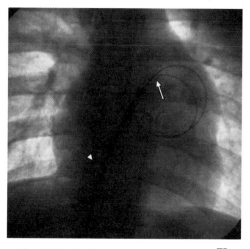

Fig. 17.4: Dilating the interatrial septum 📷

advanced up to the shadow of the left bronchus (arrow) which is supposed to be the superior border of the left atrium. The operator should realize that the catch of the septum is actually much lower and will correspond to the double shadow of the left atrium (arrow head) (Fig. 17.4). Once the interatrial septum is dilated, echocardiography is performed to rule out any pericardial collection. If there is no pericardial collection, heparin is administered (100 U/kg).

Step 4: Introduction of Balloon into Left Atrium (LA)

The slenderized balloon is then inserted into LA. Once the tip of the balloon reaches the left bronchus, we can be sure that the balloon is inside the LA. Once the balloon is in the LA, the inner gold colored hub is removed along with the outer stainless steel hub (straightener). When the straightener is removed, the

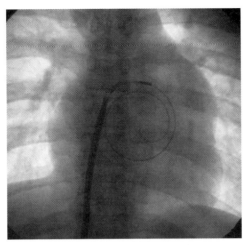

Fig. 17.5: Introduction of the slenderized balloon into the left atrium

balloon is advanced to coil over the LA wire (Fig. 17.5). Then a small inflation is given to the balloon to prevent its slippage into right atrium. Once the balloon is secured in the LA, the pigtail-shaped LA wire is slowly removed. Then the balloon is aspirated and flushed with saline.

Step 5: Crossing the Mitral Valve and Balloon Dilatation

This is carried out in the right anterior oblique (RAO) view. For crossing the mitral valve and entering the LV, we have to use the LV entry stylet. Usually, the stylet is given a slight anterior curve to facilitate LV entry (Fig. 17.6). The stylet is given 2–3 anticlockwise rotations so that the balloon faces the LV (Fig. 17.7). Once the balloon faces the valve it is denoted by the following signs:
1. Bobbing of the balloon
2. Falling of aortic pressure as the balloon partially obstructs the mitral valve.
3. If the ECG shows ventricular ectopics, it indicates that part of the balloon is already in the LV.
   Entry of the balloon into LV can also be confirmed by echocardiography. Once we are sure that the balloon is entering LV, withdraw the stylet and advance the balloon towards the LV apex.
   There are various techniques to cross the mitral valve and enter the LV. These are discussed in detail in Chapter 49.
   Once the balloon reaches the LV apex, the balloon is inflated. On Inflation, the distal balloon expands first. The partly inflated balloon is pulled back so that the waist aligns across the valve orifice. Once this happens, inflate the balloon fully. Now the proximal part of the balloon also expands. The valve gets stretched with splitting up of the commissures (Fig. 17.8).

Step 6: Assessment after Balloon Dilatation

After each dilation of the mitral valve with the balloon, we have to check the LA pressure. For this, remove the stylet, flush the central port of the balloon

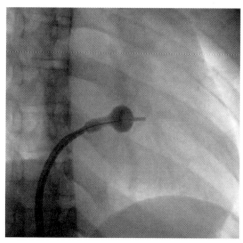

Fig. 17.6: Balloon in the left atrium. It is kept partly inflated to prevent accidental pullback of the balloon into RA. Stylet used for LV entry is also seen through the balloon

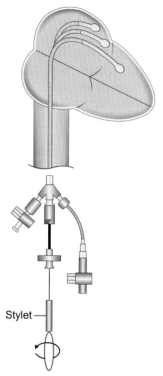

Fig. 17.7: Maneuvering the balloon across the mitral valve into the left ventricle (*Source:* Reproduced with kind permission from Toray Inc.)

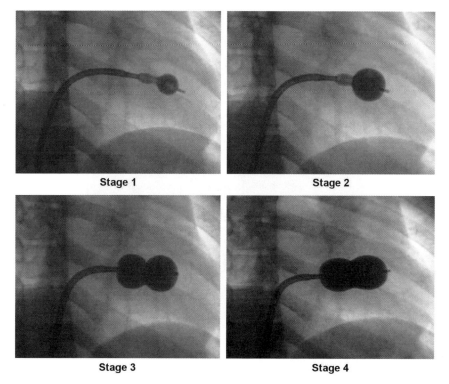

Stage 1   Stage 2

Stage 3   Stage 4

Fig. 17.8: Stages of inflation of the Inoue/Accura balloon

and check the LA pressure. Using the pigtail, we can check the LV end-diastolic pressure and measure the transmitral gradient.

Step 7: Serial Dilatations

If the LA pressure has not fallen or the commissures not given way as assessed by echocardiography, we have to up-size the balloon by increasing the volume of the contrast and do further dilatations. It is always better to note the correct volume of contrast initially in the syringe, as there can be leakage of contrast during the procedure leading to inadequate dilatation.

The assessment of the success of the procedure is done by:

1. Echocardiography showing split of one or more commissures.
2. Decrease in the gradient as assessed by Doppler echocardiography.
3. Decrease in the length or disappearance of diastolic murmur of MS.
4. Checking the left atrial pressure.
5. It is better to check the LV and LA pressure simultaneously as there may be a change in the LVED once the valve is open, either by increased flow across the valve or increase in MR (Fig. 17.9).
6. The "pressure shoot-up sign" (Fig. 17.10) is also considered as an indicator of procedural success.

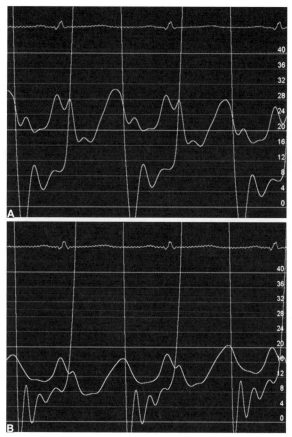

Figs 17.9A and B: Simultaneous pressure tracing of left atrium and left ventricle before (A) and after (B) balloon dilation. See the significant reduction in the left atrial pressure

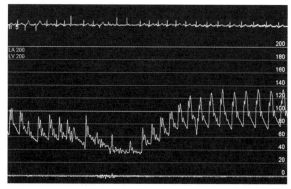

Fig. 17.10: "Pressure shoot-up sign". This is the rise of the aortic pressure over the predilation levels immediately after balloon dilation. This sign indicates that the valve is opened up and there is no significant mitral regurgitation. But the specificity of this sign is questionable

Increase in Mitral Regurgitation

If there is an increase in MR by two grades or the MR has become moderate or more, the PMV procedure has to be stopped. New onset audible MR signifies a significant increase in MR which may warrant stopping the procedure. Assessment of MR by echocardiography may be problematic if the MR jet is eccentric as it may be missed (especially in the cathlab when the echo windows may be poor). An increase in the left atrial V wave, failure of the left atrial mean to drop and the lack of fall in PA pressure, all may be indicators of a significant increase in MR.

MR can be due to excessive split of commissures or due to tear of the valve. Commissural MR up to a moderate degree can be followed up without surgery. But valve tear need to be tackled urgently as the patient could deteriorate anytime (This aspect is detailed in the Chapter on MR– Chapter 55).

Step 8: Removing the Balloon from the Left Atrium

Once the procedure is over, reintroduce the pigtail-shaped wire into the LA and remove the balloon. Never remove the unstraightened balloon through the septum as the bulky balloon can produce a large ASD. Introduce the pigtail wire over the balloon straightener and coil the wire in the LA. Lock the proximal hub of the straightener to the gold hub. Then push the gold and stainless steel tubes together and lock them. The balloon will be in the straightened position. Remove the entire assembly leaving the pigtail wire in the left atrium.

Step 9: Removal of the Left Atrium Wire

To remove the pigtail-shaped LA wire, we have to reintroduce the 7F sheath and the GL/MPA catheter into the LA over the pigtail wire. If the pigtail wire is removed without catheter support, the wire may cut the septum and enlarge the iatrogenic ASD.

Once the pigtail wire is removed, the GL/MPA catheter is used to measure the pulmonary artery pressure and also to obtain blood samples from pulmonary artery, superior and inferior vena cavae. This is to assess the left to right shunt across the ASD and also to measure the cardiac output for calculating the postprocedural mitral valve area by Gorlin's equation.

Once the procedure is over, the venous and arterial sheaths are removed and hemostasis attained.

Postprocedure echocardiogram is performed on the next day and the patient gets discharged.

Chapter 18

Periprocedural Monitoring during PMV

S Venkiteshwaran, Suchith Majumdar

During percutaneous mitral valvotomy (PMV) it is essential to assess the response to balloon dilatation to guide the procedure. Since it is essential to assess hemodynamic responses after each balloon dilatation, we have to rely on a simple, fast and accurate method.

Most reliable method is echocardiography where we can assess three important parameters: (1) the splitting of commissures (which is the most important parameter in assessing the success of a PMV procedure), (2) assessment of 2D mitral valve area and (3) mitral regurgitation (MR). Echocardiographic assessment of MV area is found to correlate well with invasive measurements obtained in the cathlab.[1] It is reported that the periprocedural assessment of pressure half time derived mitral valve area may not be reliable and 2D planimetry derived valve area is more accurate.[2]

But in many cathlabs in the developing world, echocardiography facility may not be available. So we may have to rely on the hemodynamic pressure data obtained in the cathlab. Also Gorlin formula derived valve measurements[4] is reported to be the most heart rate independent indicator of success following valvuloplasty.[3,4] There are few reports that the echo derived valve area may not be reliable especially just following PMV.[5]

Ideally, we should have two pressure transducers measuring left ventricular (LV) and left atrial (LA) pressures simultaneously. Both of them should be zeroed prior to the measurement and be equisensitive. The mitral valve gradient may be directly measured by comparing pressures in the LV and LA (or pulmonary capillary wedge pressure—PCWP). Simultaneous pressures are recorded and the gradients are measured. For best results, the recording speed (100 mm/s) and a recording scale of 0 to 40/50 mm Hg is selected. The gradient across the mitral valve should be measured using an average of five cardiac cycles in patients with normal sinus rhythm and 10 cardiac cycles in patients with atrial fibrillation.

The severity of mitral stenosis can be quantified using measurement of mitral valve area, mitral valve resistance or MV gradient. Mitral valve area (MVA) measurement remains the gold standard in most catheterization laboratories because it includes the three major hemodynamic variables:

transvalvular pressure gradient, cardiac output, and diastolic filling period. By convention, a mitral valve area <1 cm² is considered severe MS. A valve area of 1 to 1.5 cm² is moderate stenosis and a valve area >1.5 cm² is mild stenosis.

The Gorlins formula is the standard for MVA Calculation. It was derived by Dr Richard Gorlin for the calculation of cardiac valvular orifices from flow and pressure gradient data.[4] The Gorlin formula is based on principles of Torricelli's law on round orifices.

$$A = \frac{CO/(DFP \times HR)}{44.3C\sqrt{\Delta P}}$$

C=0.85 (derived by comparing actual and calculated mitral valve areas. Diastolic filling period (DFP) begins at MV opening and continues until end diastole (i.e. LA/LV crossover to peak of R wave in ECG) HR – Heart rate, CO— Cardiac output, $\sqrt{\Delta P}$—square root of transmitral pressure gradient, A—area in cm².

The CO is measured by Fick's principle from saturations of aorta and pulmonary artery (PA) (taken as mixed venous saturation in the absence of shunt). This shall be measured as close in time as possible to the 5 consecutive cardiac cycles which is recorded to measure the gradients taken to calculate MVA. Planimetry of the area between LA and LV pressure tracings of 5 beats are done and divided by the DFP for each beat, giving an average gradient deflection in mm. The mean gradient is calculated as the average gradient deflection in mm multiplied by the scale factor (mm Hg/mm deflection). Next, the average DFP is calculated using the average measured length between initial LA-LV crossover in early diastole and end diastole (peak of R wave by ECG). The average length in mm is divided by paper speed (mm/sec) to give average DFP (Fig. 18.1).

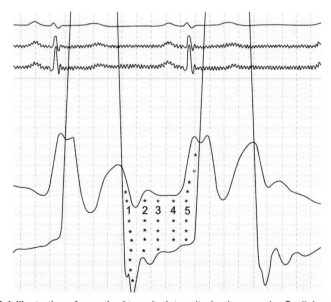

Fig. 18.1: Illustration of a method to calculate mitral valve area by Gorlin's equation

What We do in Our Cathlab in SCTIMST

LA pressure tracing/PCWP—Transducer 1
LV pressure tracing—Transducer 2

We calculate the transmitral mean gradient as follows:

Step I: The simultaneous pressure tracing of LV and LA is recorded with the following settings: (a) the recording speed of 100 mm/s and (b) scale of 0 – 40/50 mm Hg.

Step II: We count the number of small squares of the grid inside the overlapping areas of LA and LV tracings. More than half of a square is counted and less than half ignored. After totaling, we divide this sum by the number of squares on the X-axis covering the overlapped area. We multiply this by scale factor (mm Hg/height of the square in the grid) and get the transmitral gradient (Fig. 18.1).

Step III: DFP calculated from onset of diastole to peak of R wave in ECG. Cardiac output (CO) is obtained by Fick's method.

$$MVA = \frac{CO\,(l/min) \times 1000}{37.7 \times HR \times DFP \times \sqrt{TMG}}$$

$$CO = \frac{VO_2}{1.36 \times Hb\,(gm\%) \times 10 \times (AO\text{-}PA\ saturation)}$$

[VO_2 is calculated from software after entering age, sex, height and weight]

In the example illustrated above, total number of squares is 37, and in X-axis, 5 squares scan the diastolic filling period. So 37/5 = 7.4 is the mean height in "squares" of the pressure gradient on the Y-axis. The height of each square on Y-axis equals 2 mm (Ref. scale factor). Multiplying the mean height of squares by the scale factor, will give the TMG of 14.8 mm Hg.

Pitfalls in Gorlin Equation

1. *Pulmonary capillary wedge pressure (PCWP)*: PCWP can be used in lieu of LA pressure if there is no veno-occlusive disease or cortriatriatum. Proper wedge pressure waveform will resemble the LA pressure waveform with two prominent positive waves, and the mean pressure obtained will be identical to or less than PA diastolic pressure. Blood sample drawn from wedge position should have a saturation close to 100%.
2. *PCWP-LV mismatch*: Phase lag due to late transmission of LA pressure through pulmonary capillary and venous beds can affect the calculation of MVA. Fifty to seventy milliseconds delay is normal and more so if balloon tipped floatation catheter is used. Solution to this issue is to advance PCWP waveform by using a tracing paper by 50 to 70 ms. The peak of the V waves should be adjusted so as to be bisected by the descending limb of

LV pressure tracing. The currently available hemodynamic recorders have the facility to electronically correct the phase lag.

3. *Calibration errors*: This is checked by switching of transducers and verifying the pressure data. Always zero the transducers each time the pressure measurements are done, as zero may shift often.

4. *Early diastasis*: Even when left atrial and LV pressures equalize (diastasis) before the end of diastole, there will be flow through the mitral valve after the point of diastasis. The DFP to be used in valve area calculation should include all of nonisovolemic diastole, not just the period during which gradient is present.

5. *Influence of cardiac output*: Because the square root of the mean gradient is used in the Gorlin formula, the valve area calculation is more strongly influenced by the cardiac output than the pressure gradient. Thus, errors in measuring cardiac output may have profound effects on the calculated valve area, particularly in patients with low cardiac output, in whom the calculated valve area is often of greatest importance.

6. *Influence of mitral regurgitation*: In patients, with mixed mitral stenosis and regurgitation, the use of forward flow as determined by the Fick method or the thermodilution technique overestimates the severity of the valvular stenosis. This overestimation occurs because the Gorlin formula depends on total forward flow across the stenotic valve, not net forward flow. If valvular regurgitation is present, the angiographic cardiac output is the most appropriate measure of flow. If both aortic and mitral regurgitation are present, flow across a single valve cannot be determined and mitral valve area cannot be assessed accurately.

7. *Influence of iatrogenic ASD*: Trans-septal mitral commissurotomy creates an atrial septal defect which may result in significant L→R shunt. For calculating cardiac output by Fick's formula, if PA saturation is taken as mixed venous saturation it may result in fallaciously higher cardiac output, thereby increasing calculated MVA. This can be avoided by computing mixed venous oxygen saturation from superior and inferior vena cava (SVC and IVC) saturations. Levine et al[6-8] occluded the ASD after PMV and found that during septal occlusion, the postvalvotomy cardiac output decreased significantly and the calculated mitral area decreased by 12%.

8. *Problems in estimation of VO_2*: Fick's formula for cardiac output depends on VO_2, which requires pulmonary gas exchange analysis. However, due to practical difficulties it is usually indirectly calculated from normograms. This leads to error in calculation of cardiac output, thereby MVA.

9. If cardiac output is measured by thermodilution technique, presence of tricuspid regurgitation makes cardiac output measurement inaccurate.

10. Failure to calibrate pressure transducers to zero reference point may yield an erroneous gradient. A quick way to check the validity of the gradient is to exchange transducers. If calibrated correctly, it should yield the same gradient.

■ OTHER FORMULAS TO CALCULATE MITRAL VALVE AREA (MVA)

Hakki's Formula

Hakki et al proposed a simplified formula for valve area calculation that does not take into account either heart rate (HR) or left ventricular filling or ejection time. The Hakki's formula[9] can be substituted if the heart rate is within normal range:

$$MVA = \frac{CO\ (l/min)}{\sqrt{Pressure\ gradient\ (mm\ Hg)}}$$

Angel et al[10] suggested a correction factor for Hakki's formula—that an easy correction for heart rate in certain cases, dividing by 1.35 when HR less than 75 beats per min in mitral stenosis, significantly improves the accuracy and validity of Hakki's formula.

Cui's Method

Cui et al from China[11] has proposed a simple formula to obtain the MDLVP. The formula to calculate MVA is MVPG = MLAP – MDLVP = MLAP – LVEDP/2. They noted that the area under the left ventricular pressure during diastole is roughly a triangle with the three corners formed from the intersections of the diastolic filling period (DFP) starting and ending points (mitral valve closure and opening) marking the vertical lines intersecting with the LV pressure line (rising diagonally across diastole, see Fig. 18.2). This triangular area can be estimated from the rectangular area LVEDP × DFP divided by 2.

Thus, the MDLVP is equal to the LVEDP/2. From this key calculation, the mean valve gradient is therefore simplified as the MVG = MLAP – LVEDP/2. Cui et al reported extraordinary strong correlation between the mitral valve areas calculated by the Gorlin and the Hakki formulae.

The MVG obtained by Cui method was not affected by mitral regurgitation, aortic insufficiency, atrial fibrillation, or heart rate unlike that of Hakki. It must be kept in mind that LVEDP is to be measured at the peak of QRS complex.

Cui MVG is very simple, but changes in heart rate will alter the shape of the triangular area under the LV pressure curve, and thus, tachycardia may cause a potential overestimation of valve area.

The advantages of Cui method is that it is very simple and very easy to perform.[12] Secondly, mean mitral pressure gradient calculation by this new method will not necessarily require simultaneously recording left atrial and left ventricular pressures. One can simply pull a catheter back from the left ventricle into the left atrium while recording the pressures after transseptal puncture. This can be easily accomplished, especially with an Inoue balloon catheter during PBMV.[13]

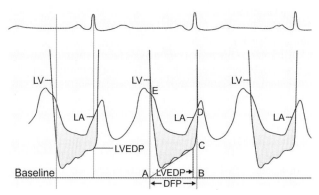

Fig. 18.2: The schematic illustration for calculating mean mitral valve pressure gradient. The area enclosed by left atrial and left ventricular pressure tracings during diastole is used by the standard calculating method, which requires a planimeter. The area of triangle ABC approximates the area under the LV pressure tracing during diastole ($Area_{LVD}$). The LVEDP approximates the height of the triangle ABC. So the mean diastolic LV pressure (MDLVP) can be calculated by dividing the area of triangle ABC by DFP, i.e. MDLVP = (area of triangle ABC)/DFP = (DFP × LVEDP/2)/DFP = LVEDP/2. DFP, diastolic filling period; LA, left atrial pressure tracing; LV, left ventricular pressure tracing; LVEDP, left ventricular end-diastolic pressure (Reprinted with permission from Wiley Inc: Wei Cui, et al. Catheterization and Cardiovascular Interventions 2007;70:754-57)

■ REFERENCES

1. Dev V, Singh LS, Radhakrishnan S, Saxena A, Shrivastava S. Doppler echocardiographic assessment of transmitral gradients and mitral valve area before and after mitral valve balloon dilatation. Clin Cardiol. 1989;12(11):629–33.
2. Krishnamoorthy KM, Radhakrishnan S, Shrivastava S. Simultaneous echocardiographic and catheterisation gradients and mitral valve area during balloon mitral valvuloplasty. Indian Heart J. 1999;51(4):410–3.
3. Harcombe AA, Ludman PF, Wisbey C, Crowley JJ, Sharples L, Shapiro LM. Balloon mitral valvuloplasty: comparison of haemodynamic and echocardiographic assessment of mitral stenosis at different heart rates in the catheterisation laboratory. Int J Cardiol. 1999;68(3):253–9.
4. Gorlin R, Gorlin SG. Hydraulic formula for calculation of the area of the stenotic mitral valve, other cardiac valves, and central circulatory shunts. I. Am Heart J. 1951;41(1):1–29.
5. Nair M, Arora R, Mohan JC, Kalra GS, Sethi KK, Nigam M, et al. Assessment of mitral valvar stenosis by echocardiography: utility of various methods before and after mitral valvotomy. Int J Cardiol. 1991;32(3):389–94.
6. Levin TN, Feldman T, Carroll JD. Effect of atrial septal occlusion on mitral area after Inoue balloon valvotomy. Cathet Cardiovasc Diagn. 1994;33(4):308–14.
7. Kapoor A, Krishnamoorthy KM, Radhakrishnan S, Shrivastava S. Effect of atrial septal defect created during balloon mitral valvuloplasty on calculation of cardiac output and mitral valve area. Indian Heart J. 1996;48(1):37–9.
8. Petrossian GA, Tuzcu EM, Ziskind AA, Block PC, Palacios I. Atrial septal occlusion improves the accuracy of mitral valve area determination following percutaneous mitral balloon valvotomy. Cathet Cardiovasc Diagn. 1991;22(1):21–4.

9. Hakki AH, Iskandrian AS, Bemis CE, Kimbiris D, Mintz GS, Segal BL, et al. A simplified valve formula for the calculation of stenotic cardiac valve areas. Circulation. 1981;63(5):1050–5.

10. Angel J, Soler-Soler J, Anivarro I, Domingo E. Hemodynamic evaluation of stenotic cardiac valves: II. Modification of the simplified valve formula for mitral and aortic valve area calculation. Cathet Cardiovasc Diagn. 1985;11(2):127–38.

11. Cui W, Dai R, Zhang G. A new simplified method for calculating mean mitral pressure gradient. Catheter Cardiovasc Interv Off J Soc Card Angiogr Interv. 2007;70(5):754–7.

12. Kern MJ. The simplified mitral valve gradient calculation by Cui et al. Catheter Cardiovasc Interv Off J Soc Card Angiogr Interv. 2007;70(5):758–9.

13. Abbo KM, Carroll JD. Hemodynamics of mitral stenosis: a review. Cathet Cardiovasc Diagn. 1994;Suppl 2:16–25.

Chapter 19

Anesthetic Management during Percutaneous Mitral Valvuloplasty

Thomas Koshy

Percutaneous mitral valvuloplasty (PMV) has become the procedure of choice in the definitive management of pliable mitral stenosis. The usual medications in the catheterization laboratory for a patient undergoing PMV are sedatives, analgesics and anesthetics.

■ PATIENT EVALUATION PRIOR TO PMV

High-risk patients are identified prior to PMV and the cathlab is set to handle all the possible problems which can arise during PMV. The necessary laboratory studies include a coagulation profile (prothrombin time, platelet count) and hematocrit.[1] ECG and chest X-ray will also be done in all patients.

Patients with significant anemia require additional preparation. Anemia decreases the oxygen carrying capacity of the blood and falsely increases the cardiac output. The pre-existing anemia is made worse by the blood loss associated with the catheterization procedure. Anemia diagnosed weeks before PMV is treated with oral iron supplements. A small percentage of patients may require red cell transfusion before the procedure.[2]

Since, the use of radiographic contrast is very minimal (only during transseptal puncture), renal insufficiency is not a major contraindication for PMV. Prehydration and limiting the volume of contrast (i.e. using echocardiography for assessment of MR thereby avoiding ventriculography) will reduce the risk of worsening renal function.[2] But the surgical team standing-by should be alerted and the patient also should be informed of the possibility of renal dysfunction, if the patient needs a surgical intervention.

Most PMVs are performed using a controlled sedation/analgesia. While general anesthesia (GA) is rarely required for adult patients, it is used in selected patients. Uncooperative or patients on ventilator, hemodynamic instability (before/during catheterization) are the usual indications. Induction of GA shifts the responsibility of the patient's hemodynamic and respiratory stability from the cardiologist to the anesthesiologist.

Since, anesthetics and ventilatory parameters can significantly alter hemodynamics in mitral stenosis (MS), the anesthesiologist should evaluate patient's disease severity and should be familiar with its pathophysiology.

Reduction in mitral valve area limits diastolic filling of left ventricle (LV) and increases left atrial (LA) pressure. High LA pressures in turn results in pulmonary hypertension (PHT) which may ultimately lead to right ventricular (RV) pressure overload. The important cardiovascular management goals in a case of MS are maintenance of LV preload, systemic vascular resistance (SVR) and sinus rhythm if possible and avoidance of tachycardia. Hypoxemia and hypoventilation (which may occur with deep sedation) are poorly tolerated by these patients, as they increase pulmonary vascular resistance. Hypervolemia should also be avoided as it may lead to development of pulmonary edema.[3]

Patients are on multiple medications, which should also be addressed. On the morning of catheterization, cardiac drugs (e.g. β blockers, calcium channel blockers, digoxin, etc.) are routinely continued while diuretic therapy is withheld. Diabetic patients are ideally scheduled in the morning. The protocol for patients on anticoagulants is described elsewhere in this book.

▇ PRECATHETERIZATION PREPARATION

The preparation of the patient begins as soon as the decision is made to perform PMV.

At the very beginning, a general explanation of the procedure and the reason why the procedure is being performed must be told to the patient. The explanation includes the information about precatheterization laboratory tests, access in the groin, length of the procedure, expected stay in the recovery area and the length of the total hospital stay. Patients or the relatives are also informed about the risks of the procedure and consent is to be taken for GA which may be required in a small percentage of patients.

Since, there is a chance of severe mitral regurgitation ending up in MVR, all patients are informed about the need for the surgery under cardiopulmonary bypass (CPB) and the potential complications and also the costs. Blood grouping and cross matching is always done and the availability of blood is confirmed with the blood bank, especially with rare blood groups.

Previous history of contrast exposure and a true contrast reaction if occurred (rash, breathing difficulties, angioedema, etc.) must be recorded. Such patients require premedication with glucocorticoids[2] or de-sensitization. In one large series, Greenberger et al. administered multiple doses of prednisolone (50 mg 3 doses) along with diphenhydramine (50 mg single dose).[4] Though, there was no severe anaphylactic reactions, the incidence of urticarial reactions was 10% in that series.[4] The incidence of allergic reactions may be brought down by the use of nonionic contrast agents in such patients.[5]

▇ PREMEDICATION AND FASTING GUIDELINES

It is better to keep patients (outpatients and inpatients) fasting for 8 hours before the catheterization procedure except for oral medications. Some laboratories allow liquid breakfast up to 3 hours prior to the procedure.

Transesophageal echocardiography is mandatory in every patient to rule out left atrial thrombus. This is usually done on the morning of the day of the procedure. This will also help in assessing mitral regurgitation, aortic regurgitation and the anatomy of the interatrial septum which will aid in transseptal puncture.

Some type of premedication to sedate the patient before the procedure is employed by most laboratories. Premedication can be administered orally or intravenously in the holding area of the catheterization laboratory or at the hospital ward. All patients should receive a secure intravenous line before entering the laboratory for PMV. The usual intravenous medications are midazolam 1–5 mg with fentanyl 25–100 µg.

In our hospital, all patients undergoing PMV are premedicated with 200 mg of hydrocortisone and diphenhydramine (50 mg IV) before the procedure. This is repeated if required. In patients with known contrast allergies undergoing emergency PMV may be given 200 mg of hydrocortisone immediately before the procedure and repeated every 4 hours until the procedure is completed.[6]

PATIENT MONITORING DURING PMV

Standard limb leads are used for ECG monitoring during PMV. Arterial oxygen saturation is routinely monitored in all patients with a pulse oximeter. When PMV is done under GA, invasive hemodynamic monitoring (CVP, femoral/radial artery pressure) allows anesthesiologist to maintain optimal volume status and recognize hemodynamic fluctuations instantaneously. Echocardiographic monitoring in the cathlab is very useful during the procedure, which will aid in the transseptal puncture and also assessing the result of valve dilatation. Echocardiography is most useful in assessing and managing the complications during the procedure.

PATIENT SEDATION

Most PMVs are performed using mild sedation/analgesia along with local anesthetic infiltration at site of vascular puncture. The benzodiazepines/analgesics administered in the holding area (i.e. midazolam with fentanyl) alleviate the patient's anxiety and discomfort during the procedure. These medications also maintain the patient in a very still "steady state" and "cooperative" during the procedure, which is very essential during transseptal puncture. Patient movement during transseptal puncture may lead to major complications during PMV.[7] The other medications used are morphine (0.1 to 0.15 mg/kg body weight) with or without diazepam (0.1 to 0.2 mg/kg body weight). Because sedation induced hypoventilation can result in hypoxia or hypercarbia, patients with PHT, should receive supplemental oxygen and appropriate monitoring using pulse oximetry. Currently use of dexmeditomidine has become more popular for sedation because of its sedative, amnesic, analgesic and anxiolytic effects with minimal respiratory depression.[8] The loading dose of dexmeditomidine ranges from 0.4–1 microgram/kg over 10 minutes followed by a continuous infusion at 0.4–0.7 microgram/kg/hr. The drug can produce modest decreases in blood pressure and heart rate.

▰ GENERAL ANESTHESIA

Though GA is not required for most PMVs, there are patients where it is desirable. GA is indicated in patients on ventilator, significantly symptomatic and not able to maintain a supine position (e.g. presence of orthopnea) and those who develop hemodynamic instability or complications (before/during catheterization). Juvenile mitral stenosis (adolescents) or uncooperative patients may also require GA.

The principles of anesthesia are same as that of a patient undergoing mitral valve surgery for MS. The hemodynamic goals in a case of MS are maintenance of euvolemia and SVR and avoidance of tachycardia. Patients should be premedicated the night before and on the morning of catheterization in such a way to achieve adequate anxiolysis to avoid tachycardia while avoiding over sedation leading to hypoventilation, hypercarbia, hypoxemia thereby avoiding increase of pulmonary artery (PA) pressure. The drugs used for premedication are mentioned above. Medications such as β-blockers, calcium channel blockers or amiodarone taken by the patient preoperatively for control of heart rate should be continued in the perioperative period.

General anesthesia with controlled mechanical ventilation with an endotracheal tube is practiced widely. Radial artery and internal jugular vein may be cannulated for arterial and central venous pressure monitoring. Continuous arterial pressure monitoring facilitates timely management of hemodynamic derangement. Though, a narcotic based anesthetic technique (using morphine or fentanyl) is helpful in avoiding tachycardia, most anesthesiologists frequently use a combination of an inhalational anesthetic (isoflurane or sevoflurane) with a narcotic and a muscle relaxant (preferably vecuronium because of the lack of chronotropic effect). Such a "balanced" anesthetic technique not only achieves the hemodynamic goals but allows early or on-table extubation. The ventilatory adjustments are done to keep the $PaCO_2$ in the normal range but if PHT is present, hemodynamic priority is to decrease PA pressure by inducing mild hypocarbia by way of hyperventilation. Patients are generally extubated at the end of the procedure, if warm and hemodynamically stable. Patients with PHT, RV dysfunction, hemodynamic instability, acute severe MR may require elective postprocedure ventilation.

▰ MANAGEMENT OF COMPLICATIONS

During PMV, patient's hemodynamics can change very suddenly as a result of arrhythmias, high ventricular rate or development of complications like pericardial tamponade, or acute severe MR.[9] Patients can go into atrial Flutter (AF) due to catheter manipulation and may develop hemodynamic instability with high ventricular rate. Cardioversion should not be withheld from such patients. Such patients can be sedated with intravenous anesthetic agent such as etomidate (which has minimal effect on hemodynamics) or titrated doses of propofol.

The procedural mortality ranges from 0 to 3%.[10] The incidence of hemopericardium is reported to be 0.5 to 12%, and embolism 0.5 to 5%.[10]

Though the procedure is successful in 85 to 99% of cases in experienced hands,[2] 2 to 10% of patients may develop severe MR, requiring emergency surgery.[9] Patients who develop significant complications should be mechanically ventilated. Patients who develop acute MR may benefit from vasodilator therapy.

▩ PMV AND THE ANESTHESIOLOGIST

The broad objective of this Chapter has been to provide an overview of the sedation techniques (managed by the cardiologist usually) and the role of the anesthesiologist in a small percentage of patients requiring GA. As success rates of PMV have improved, and complication rates have decreased, and most patients can be managed with sedation, there have been fewer opportunities for the anesthesiologist to manage patients during PMV. The principles of anesthetic management in patients needing GA for PMV, is similar to any patient with MS undergoing mitral valve surgery.

▩ REFERENCES

1. Kozak M, Robertson BJ, Chambers CE. In: Kaplan JA (Ed) Cardiac catheterization laboratory: diagnostic and therapeutic procedures in the adult patient, in Kaplan JA (ed): Kaplan's cardiac anesthesia, 5th edn, Saunders Elsevier, 2006, p 303.
2. Kozak M, Robertson BJ, Chambers CE. Cardiac catheterization laboratory: Diagnositc and therapeutic procedures in the adult patient, Kaplan's cardiac anesthesia, 5th edn, Saunders Elsevier; 2006, p 304.
3. Koshy T, Tambe SP, Sinha PK, Karmarkar V, Bhupali AN, Tempe DK, et al. Case 2--2008 rheumatic mitral stenosis associated with partial anomalous pulmonary venous return. J Cardiothorac Vasc Anesth. 2008;22(2):302–10.
4. Greenberger PA, Patterson R, Tapio CM. Prophylaxis against repeated radiocontrast media reactions in 857 cases. Adverse experience with cimetidine and safety of beta-adrenergic antagonists. Arch Intern Med. 1985;145(12):2197–200.
5. Davidson CJ, Laskey WK, Hermiller JB, Harrison JK, Matthai W Jr, Vlietstra RE, et al. Randomized trial of contrast media utilization in high-risk PTCA: the COURT trial. Circulation. 2000;101(18):2172–7.
6. Greenberger PA, Halwig JM, Patterson R, Wallemark CB. Emergency administration of radiocontrast media in high-risk patients. J Allergy Clin Immunol. 1986;77(4):630–4.
7. Krishnamoorthy KM. Patient movement during transseptal puncture: need for caution. Int J Cardiol. 2003;88(1):113–4.
8. Mitter N, Grogan K, Nyhan D, Berkowitz D. In Kaplan JA, Reich DL, Savino JS (Eds). Pharmacology of Anesthetic Drugs in Kaplan's Cardiac Anesthesia, 6th edn, Saunders Elsevier 2011. p 215.
9. Vahanian A, Palacios IF. Percutaneous approaches to valvular disease. Circulation. 2004;109(13):1572–9.
10. Tempe DK, Gupta B, Banerjee A, Virmani S, Datt V, Marwah C, et al. Surgical interventions in patients undergoing percutaneous balloon mitral valvotomy: a retrospective analysis of anaesthetic considerations. Ann Card Anaesth. 2004;7(2):129-36.

Chapter 20

Intracardiac Echocardiography Imaging in Percutaneous Balloon Mitral Valvuloplasty

Santhosh KG Koshy, Antwon Robinson

■ INTRODUCTION

Real time imaging for accurate and precise delineation of intracardiac structures is important in efficient and safe performance of catheter-based interventional procedures.[1] Rapid technological advancements in ultrasound imaging have been particularly useful for guiding these invasive procedures. Intracardiac echocardiography (ICE), associated with better patient comfort, has emerged as a promising imaging modality to serve as an alternative for the transesophageal echocardiogram (TEE), which is semi-invasive and requires anesthesia for patient comfort during interventional procedures. ICE is a safe procedure and provides both anatomic and physiologic information in real time.

History and Evolution

In the 1960s and 1970s, the use of ultrasound tipped catheters marked the advent of intracardiac ultrasonography.[2-4] The introduction of the intracoronary ultrasound-tipped catheter in the 1980s made clinical intracardiac ultrasonography feasible.[5] These systems provided high-resolution imaging, but because of the high frequency of the transducers (20–40 MHz), tissue penetration was only limited and anatomic intracardiac overviews could not be obtained.[6] The development of the lower frequency transducers with greater imaging depth, made intracardiac imaging with enhanced tissue penetration feasible.[7,8]

Currently, there are six types of ICE catheter systems that are commercially available.[9] First, is a 9 MHz single element transducer incorporated in 9F catheter (Boston Scientific Corp, San Jose, California, USA). Because of poor tissue penetration and far field resolution, imaging of left sided structures is not feasible with this catheter placed in the right heart.[10,11] In addition, the catheter is not steerable; it must be guided by a wire and it lacks Doppler capabilities.

The second catheter available for use is the phased-array catheter. This system uses an 8-10 French single use ultrasound catheter (AcuNav, Biosense Webster, Diamond Bar, CA)[12] which consists of miniaturized 64-element, phased-array transducer. The transducer scans in the longitudinal monoplane, providing a 90° sector image with tissue penetration up to 12 cm for the 10F catheter and 16 cm for the 8F catheter, allowing visualization of left-sided structures from the right heart. The catheter has full Doppler capabilities including color, tissue and spectral Doppler, and four-way articulation of catheter tip provides excellent maneuverability for optimal imaging. Either a femoral or internal jugular approach can be used for introduction of the phased-array catheter.

Clear ICE and EP Med View Flex (St Jude Medical) are 64-element catheters. Clear ICE is derived from the hockey stick catheter, is highly steerable with two sets of electrodes for integration of 3D localization with NavX. Apart from grayscale and tissue Doppler, it also allows for synchronization mapping and 2D speckle tracking. EP Med View Flex uses tissue Doppler at 8-2MHz and allows two-way flex color Doppler and gray scale. Another catheter is SoundStar catheter (Biosense- Webster) which is marketed as a 10F (3.33 mm) device. This device is FDA approved and has integrated ultrasound array (like AcuNav™) but with the Carto magnetic sensor in the tip.[9]

Recently US Food and Drug Administration approved a 3D (volumetric) version of the Siemens AcuNav ICE catheter (Siemens Acuson, Mountain View, CA) for use in clinical setting. The use of this catheter has been found to be safe and useful in guiding percutaneous cardiac structural interventions.[13] This AcuNav V intracardiac ultrasound catheter is a 10-Fr catheter capable of real time reconstruction of volumetric intracardiac images with 3D formatting, and is connected to the Accustom SC2000 console.[50]

Advantages and Limitations

Both transthoracic echocardiography (TTE) and TEE have been used in the past to guide percutaneous interventions in catheterization or electrophysiology laboratories.[13-16] However, there are important limitations for both TTE and TEE during invasive cardiac procedures. TTE does not allow precise visualization of cardiac structures, such as the interatrial septum (IAS) and maintaining sterility of the procedural field is very cumbersome. TEE, while providing excellent intracardiac resolution, requires sedation, is uncomfortable for patients, and may increase the cost of the procedure due to professional and procedural fees.

ICE combines the superior imaging resolution of TEE without exposing patients to the risks of sedation or esophageal intubation. Various studies have reported that images obtained by ICE are either similar,[17,18] or superior to those obtained by TEE.[19] Fluoroscopy time,[20] interventional procedure time, and catheterization laboratory time[21] are also shortened with ICE compared with TEE. ICE also allows direct monitoring of acute procedure-related complications (e.g. thrombus formation, pericardial effusion).

There are several limitations associated with ICE including the large shaft size (10 French), lack of additional catheter features such as ports for guidewires, therapeutic devices, and pressure measurement. Phased-array ICE provides only monoplane image sections, is for single use only and is expensive. While some authors have suggested imaging protocols with ICE,[22] there are still no currently defined standard views for ICE, as are available for TTE and TEE. Finally, even though ICE provides superior image resolution, it is still very difficult to define the exact tip of the catheter due to fact that only two-dimensional imaging is possible with ICE.[17] If visualization of catheter tip is of paramount importance, real-time three-dimensional transesophageal echocardiography may be superior to ICE since the tip of the catheter can be well-defined with real-time 3D TEE. However, the recent introduction of 3D ICE imaging for clinical use addresses this limitation of traditional two-dimensional ICE imaging.[13] Moreover, aortic ICE imaging has been found to be superior to traditional venous ICE imaging to guide transseptal puncture and may prove to be superior to TEE.[24] Possible potential complications that may result from ICE include those associated with right heart catheterization such as pulmonary embolism, pericardial tamponade, and bleeding from the puncture site; however, only vascular complications have been reported in the literature.[19] The need for a separate venous access is also another problem during PMV.

Percutaneous Balloon Mitral Valvuloplasty

Traditionally surgical treatment by open or closed commissurotomy had been the treatment of choice for mitral valve stenosis. However, in selected patients with favorable valve characteristics, a less invasive percutaneous balloon mitral valvuloplasty (PBMV) has emerged as a very popular first line of management for this condition.[23] It was first described by Inoue et al in 1984[24] and the success was later confirmed by Lock et al[25] in children and young adults. This treatment strategy has demonstrated comparable if not better short and intermediate term outcomes[26,27] and equivalent restenosis rates[27] compared to surgical treatment. However, this procedure was and continues to be very dependent on fluoroscopic identification of several anatomical landmarks for its correct completion and efficacy.[23,28] This was especially true for the transseptal puncture as elaborated by Jui-Sung Hung[29] which was noted to be a "vital component of this therapeutic interventional technique". As fluoroscopy is limited regarding the identification of soft tissue structures, other modalities were needed to better elucidate intracardiac structures, define anatomy and reduce and/or quickly identify intraprocedural complications.

Fluoroscopy and Echocardiography

Fluoroscopy has been the primary imaging modality for PMV using the Inoue balloon,[23] and it helps in accurate placement and inflation of the Inoue balloon. Nevertheless, there are several drawbacks to fluoroscopy use.[30] A major limitation is the inadequate resolution of soft tissue structures.[30,31] Also, the exposure of the patient and physician to significant amounts of radiation which is heightened secondary to the complexity of PMV. Additionally, atrial chamber dilatation associated with MS will alter the anatomical orientation of the intracardiac structures, result in suboptimal imaging for procedure guidance. Lastly, the use of iodinated contrast agents, if used, has its inherent potential problems.[30]

Echocardiography (both transthroacic and transesophageal) have been used during the percutaneous treatment of mitral stenosis. Robinson et al[32] noted that TTE was very valuable during the procedure and was helpful in identifying complications from balloon inflation. TTE was also reported to be useful in the actual transseptal catheterization.[33] Similarly, TEE has been cited on multiple occasions as an important adjunct during PBMV.[15,23,34,35] TEE was able to reduce radiation exposure and potential complications.[35,36] However, using TTE or TEE during PBMV has been limited by several factors.[28,30] TTE interferes with the need for a sterile field, and it can be associated with suboptimal visualization of the IAS.[37] Moreover, the risk of radiation exposure to the sonographer with simultaneous echocardiography and fluoroscopy has some concern.[28,37] There are also drawbacks to intraprocedural TEE which include the significant discomfort of prolonged imaging to an awake patient during the procedure.[13] These limitations along with the need for accurate identification of anatomic structures have necessitated the use of a more detailed imaging modality. Hence, ICE has recently emerged as an important imaging tool for guiding PBMV.

Clinical Applicability

A recent review discussed the applications of ICE in a variety of fields.[30] While computed tomography (CT) and magnetic resonance imaging (MRI) can be used to delineate structures within the heart in preparation for a minimally invasive cardiac procedure, these could not be used during the actual procedure. Hence, ultrasound-based imaging allows for better visualization of the intracardiac soft structures regarding transseptal puncture, and specifically ICE could provide superior real-time imaging compared to TTE or TEE and reduce the confines associated with other imaging modalities. Better visualization of the transseptal sheath and dilator apparatus prior to transseptal puncture could be obtained using an ICE based imaging system. Moreover, intracardiac echocardiography has been able to reduce inaccuracy associated with CT imaging prior to a particular procedure.[38,39] Finally, despite the fact that a phase array ICE catheter can cost approximately $2000,[30] it has been shown that the use of ICE is not associated with an increase cost over the use of TEE in the developed world.[40,41] In the developing world, the cost of the catheter is the main limiting factor. Though rotational ICE is limited in its far field view and is not maneuverable, it still can be useful in transseptal puncture. Phase array ICE has a deeper field of depth and steerability, in addition to the opportunity to acquire color flow and Doppler imaging.

Specific Application of ICE in Guiding PBMV

Intracardiac echocardiography (ICE) has been shown to be very beneficial during mitral valvuloplasty (Fig. 20.1) helping to exclude LA appendage thrombus and to provide adequate morphologic characterization of the mitral

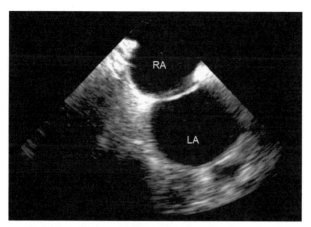

Fig. 20.1: Intracardiac echocardiography view showing longitudinal view
of the atrial septum
Abbreviations: RA, right atrium; LA, left atrium

valve and subvalvular apparatus. There is clinical data supporting the utility
and feasibility of ICE for guiding PBMV. Hung et al[37] studied seven patients
with symptomatic mitral stenosis who were to undergo fluoroscopic guided
PBMV with the addition of a 10 Fr 10 MHz intracardiac echocardiographic
probe. This probe was used without additional discomfort to the patient or
interference with the catheterization procedure. Compared to the conventional
fluoroscopic imaging during PBMV,[29] the use of ICE eliminated the need for
bi-plane fluoroscopy for transseptal puncture as this was done with the frontal
plane view alone. Furthermore, it aids in accurate IAS puncture and helps
to identify postvalvuloplasty mitral regurgitation.[28,42] Since more accurate
intraprocedural assessment of mitral regurgitation is possible, it can also be
useful during mitral valvuloplasty of selected high-risk mitral stenosis patients
with echo scores of more than eight.[43]

Preprocedural Evaluation of the Intracardiac Structures

Delineation of intracardiac structures is important before proceeding with
PBMV. The morphologic details at baseline of the interatrial septum and its
relationship with the other intracardiac structures; the mitral valve including
leaflet mobility and subvalvular thickening; and degree of mitral regurgitation
could be clearly imaged with ICE and is superior to TTE.

Transseptal Puncture

Transseptal puncture, traditionally, has relied on fluoroscopic guidance,[44,45] in
which the important anatomical structures are not displayed directly and the
needle with a sheath were guided entirely by their movement during pullback
from the superior vena cava and by their position within the cardiac silhouette
relative to the catheter in the coronary sinus and/or aortic root.[46] The advent
of ICE allowed the unique opportunity to guide transseptal puncture by direct

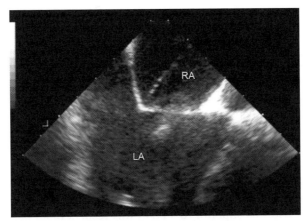

Fig. 20.2: View showing Brockenbrough needle tenting the atrial septum before atrial septal puncture
Abbreviations: LA, left atrium; RA, right atrium

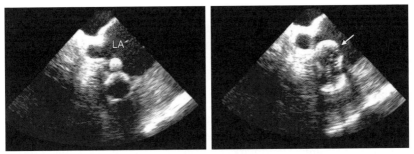

Fig. 20.3: Long axis view of the left ventricle showing different stages of Inoue balloon inflation
Abbreviation: LA, left atrium

imaging of the needle tip within the fossa ovalis region.[47] The right atrial aspect of the fossa shows a clear ridge (the limbus), which is not present on the left atrial side of the septum. The main advantage of ICE is safe navigation in case of anatomical abnormalities such as lipomatous hypertrophy of the septum, atrial septal aneurysm and/or double layer septum. It may also help to reduce the potential complications of transseptal puncture that include aortic puncture, pericardial puncture or tamponade, systemic arterial embolism and perforation of inferior vena caval vein.[48] For optimal visualization, the image is oriented so that the long axis of IAS is perpendicular to the ultrasound beam to maximize echo signal from the structure (Fig. 20.2). During the puncture, a Brockenbrough needle is inserted via a transseptal sheath and dilator system, and directed towards the fossa ovalis. Tenting of the septum at fossa ovalis indicates stable contact of the transseptal dilator at this site (Fig. 20.3). Successful puncture can be confirmed by the appearance of contrast in the LA after contrast injection. The feasibility and utility of intra-aortic ICE imaging guidance for interatrial septal puncture has been tested and is described to be safe in comparison to TEE and venous ICE imaging.[51]

In a case series of 19 patients with mitral stenosis who underwent PBMV with Inoue balloon and ICE guidance, the authors explained in detail the protocol for obtaining images using the intracardiac echocardiography probe.[28] It is noted that although initially both ICE and fluoroscopy were used together to perform IAS puncture and balloon positioning, ICE was used almost exclusively during the former while fluoroscopy was utilized for radiographic documentation of the position of the balloon during inflation. This occurred as the clinical experience of the operators increased. Regarding safety, no patients experienced life-threatening arrhythmias, tamponade, or death as a result of the procedure.

The morphologic details of the mitral valve at baseline including leaflet mobility and subvalvular thickening was achievable with ICE, and it was thought that ICE was superior to TTE in this respect in all patients. It was reported that although the ability to obtain certain views increased with technical experience, some of the views were suboptimal in one patient with an extreme vertical heart axis which was reported as a drawback. Other limitations included incomplete visualization of the LAA and the cost of ICE. Nevertheless, the authors concluded intracardiac echocardiography presented vital structural and valvular information pertinent to the safety and performance of PBMV.

Special Considerations

There are a few special populations that are associated with increased difficulty of transseptal catheterization using fluoroscopy. The amplified risk is because of distorted anatomical landmarks or intracardiac structures which interfere with the accuracy of fluoroscopy. One example of this would be severe left atrial enlargement. A study involving 15 patients (12 with giant left atria, ≥70 mm on M-mode echocardiography) demonstrated the success of transseptal catheterization and subsequent transvenous mitral commissurotomy with ICE.[49] In all 12 patients with giant left atria, the left atrium was noted to have a significant bulge compressing the right atrium, and this interfered with the usual approach of the catheter-needle unit for transseptal puncture. By using ICE, the operators were able to avoid septal dissections with puncture at inappropriate sites.

Furthermore, ICE is also useful in transseptal puncture in the presence of left atrial aneurysm or kyphoscoliosis. Similar to giant left atria, presence of left atrial aneurysm increases the probability of complications during transseptal puncture. Kyphoscoliosis completely distorts the anatomical landmarks and relative cardiac structures on which fluoroscopy are dependent. ICE with its high resolution and depth of imaging is helpful to ensure accurate location of puncture sites and to assist with safe catheterization of left atrium. Currently ICE imaging is being increasingly used for other percutaneous mitral valve procedures like E-repair.[51-53]

CONCLUSION

Intracardiac echo has become a very useful tool in the cardiovascular laboratory. Although it has played a unique role in the electrophysiology laboratory, ICE has made some significant strides in other cardiovascular procedures especially PMV as previously mentioned. ICE has been demonstrated to reduce the amount of fluoroscopy needed during this procedure, and it has overcome some of the limitations of other ultrasound based imaging modalities including the need for sedation (TEE) and interference with sterile fields (TTE). Furthermore, ICE has also improved the ability to overcome anatomic obstacles including left atrial enlargement and kyphoscoliosis. On the other hand, it does have some associated limitations. One limitation is related to the imaging capability of the catheters and second is the cost of the catheters especially in the developing world. The inability of ICE to stand alone as an echocardiographic imaging tool regarding current literature also may be of concern.

REFERENCES

1. Kort S. Intracardiac echocardiography: evolution, recent advances, and current applications. J Am Soc Echocardiogr Off Publ Am Soc Echocardiogr. 2006;19(9):1192–201.
2. Maloney JD, Burnett JM, Dala-Krishna P, Glueck R. New directions in intracardiac echocardiography. J Interv Card Electrophysiol Int J Arrhythm Pacing. 2005;13 Suppl 1:23–9.
3. Glassman E, Kronzon I. Transvenous intracardiac echocardiography. Am J Cardiol. 1981;47(6):1255–9.
4. Bom N, Lancée CT, Van Egmond FC. An ultrasonic intracardiac scanner. Ultrasonics. 1972;10(2):72–6.
5. Pandian NG. Intravascular and intracardiac ultrasound imaging. An old concept, now on the road to reality. Circulation. 1989;80(4):1091–4.
6. Foster GP, Picard MH. Intracardiac echocardiography: current uses and future directions. Echocardiogr Mt Kisco N. 2001;18(1):43–8.
7. Pandian NG, Kumar R, Katz SE, Tutor A, Schwartz SL, Weintraub AR, et al. Real-time, intracardiac, two-dimensional echocardiography: enhanced depth of field with a low-frequency (12.5 mhz) ultrasound catheter. Echocardiogr Mt Kisco N. 1991;8(4):407–22.
8. Seward JB, Khandheria BK, McGregor CG, Locke TJ, Tajik AJ. Transvascular and intracardiac two-dimensional echocardiography. Echocardiogr Mt Kisco N. 1990;7(4):457–64.
9. Hijazi ZM, Shivkumar K, Sahn DJ. Intracardiac echocardiography during interventional and electrophysiological cardiac catheterization. Circulation. 2009;119(4):587–96.
10. Chu E, Fitzpatrick AP, Chin MC, Sudhir K, Yock PG, Lesh MD. Radiofrequency catheter ablation guided by intracardiac echocardiography. Circulation. 1994;89(3):1301–5.
11. Kalman JM, Olgin JE, Karch MR, Lesh MD. Use of intracardiac echocardiography in interventional electrophysiology. Pacing Clin Electrophysiol PACE. 1997;20(9 Pt 1):2248–62.
12. Bartel T, Caspari G, Mueller S, et al. Intracardiac echocardiography–technology and clinical role. J Clin Basic Cardiol. 2002;5:133–7.

13. Schwartz SL, Gillam LD, Weintraub AR, Sanzobrino BW, Hirst JA, Hsu TL, et al. Intracardiac echocardiography in humans using a small-sized (6F), low frequency (12.5 MHz) ultrasound catheter. Methods, imaging planes and clinical experience. J Am Coll Cardiol. 1993;21(1):189-98.

14. Roberts JW, Lima JA. Role of echocardiography in mitral commissurotomy with the Inoue balloon. Cathet Cardiovasc Diagn. 1994;Suppl 2:69-75.

15. Kronzon I, Tunick PA, Schwinger ME, Slater J, Glassman E. Transesophageal echocardiography during percutaneous mitral valvuloplasty. J Am Soc Echocardiogr Off Publ Am Soc Echocardiogr. 1989;2(6):380-5.

16. Levin TN, Feldman T, Bednarz J, Carroll JD, Lang RM. Transesophageal echocardiographic evaluation of mitral valve morphology to predict outcome after balloon mitral valvotomy. Am J Cardiol. 1994;1;73(9):707-10.

17. Hijazi Z, Wang Z, Cao Q, Koenig P, Waight D, Lang R. Transcatheter closure of atrial septal defects and patent foramen ovale under intracardiac echocardiographic guidance: feasibility and comparison with transesophageal echocardiography. Catheter Cardiovasc Interv Off J Soc Card Angiogr Interv. 2001;52(2):194-9.

18. Koenig P, Cao QL. Echocardiographic guidance of transcatheter closure of atrial septal defects: is intracardiac echocardiography better than transesophageal echocardiography? Pediatr Cardiol. 2005;26:135-9.

19. Herrmann HC, Silvestry FE, Glaser R, See V, Kasner S, Bradbury D, et al. Percutaneous patent foramen ovale and atrial septal defect closure in adults: results and device comparison in 100 consecutive implants at a single center. Catheter Cardiovasc Interv Off J Soc Card Angiogr Interv. 2005;64(2):197-203.

20. Bartel T, Konorza T, Arjumand J, Ebradlidze T, Eggebrecht H, Caspari G, et al. Intracardiac echocardiography is superior to conventional monitoring for guiding device closure of interatrial communications. Circulation. 2003;18;107(6):795-7.

21. Boccalandro F, Baptista E, Muench A, Carter C, Smalling RW. Comparison of intracardiac echocardiography versus transesophageal echocardiography guidance for percutaneous transcatheter closure of atrial septal defect. Am J Cardiol. 2004;15;93(4):437-40.

22. Koenig PR, Abdulla R, Cao Q-L, Hijazi ZM. Use of intracardiac echocardiography to guide catheter closure of atrial communications. Echocardiogr Mt Kisco N. 2003;20(8):781-7.

23. Nobuyoshi M, Arita T, Shirai S, Hamasaki N, Yokoi H, Iwabuchi M, et al. Percutaneous balloon mitral valvuloplasty: A review. Circulation. 2009;3;119(8):e211-219.

24. Inoue K, Owaki T, Nakamura T, Kitamura F, Miyamoto N. Clinical application of transvenous mitral commissurotomy by a new balloon catheter. J Thorac Cardiovasc Surg. 1984;87(3):394-402.

25. Lock JE, Khalilullah M, Shrivastava S, Bahl V, Keane JF. Percutaneous catheter commissurotomy in rheumatic mitral stenosis. N Engl J Med. 1985; 12;313(24):1515-8.

26. Turi ZG, Reyes VP, Raju BS, Raju AR, Kumar DN, Rajagopal P, et al. Percutaneous balloon versus surgical closed commissurotomy for mitral stenosis. A prospective, randomized trial. Circulation. 1991;83(4):1179-85.

27. Arora R, Nair M, Kalra GS, Nigam M, Khalilullah M. Immediate and long-term results of balloon and surgical closed mitral valvotomy: a randomized comparative study. Am Heart J. 1993;125(4):1091-4.

28. Green NE, Hansgen AR, Carroll JD. Initial clinical experience with intracardiac echocardiography in guiding balloon mitral valvuloplasty: technique, safety, utility, and limitations. Catheter Cardiovasc Interv Off J Soc Card Angiogr Interv. 2004;63(3):385-94.

29. Hung JS. Atrial septal puncture technique in percutaneous transvenous mitral commissurotomy: mitral valvuloplasty using the Inoue balloon catheter technique. Cathet Cardiovasc Diagn. 1992;26(4):275–84.

30. Kim SS, Hijazi ZM, Lang RM, Knight BP. The use of intracardiac echocardiography and other intracardiac imaging tools to guide noncoronary cardiac interventions. J Am Coll Cardiol. 2009;9;53(23):2117–28.

31. Naqvi TZ. Echocardiography in percutaneous valve therapy. JACC Cardiovasc Imaging. 2009;2(10):1226–37.

32. Robinson NM, Thomas MR, Jewitt DE, Monaghan MJ. The value of transthoracic echocardiography during percutaneous balloon mitral valvuloplasty. J Am Soc Echocardiogr Off Publ Am Soc Echocardiogr. 1995;8(1):79–86.

33. Kronzon I, Glassman E, Cohen M, Winer H. Use of two-dimensional echocardiography during transseptal cardiac catheterization. J Am Coll Cardiol. 1984;4(2):425–8.

34. Goldstein SA, Campbell AN. Mitral stenosis. Evaluation and guidance of valvuloplasty by transesophageal echocardiography. Cardiol Clin. 1993;11(3):409–25.

35. Vilacosta I, Iturralde E, San Román JA, Gómez-Recio M, Romero C, Jiménez J, et al. Transesophageal echocardiographic monitoring of percutaneous mitral balloon valvulotomy. Am J Cardiol. 1992;15;70(11):1040–4.

36. Park SH, Kim MA, Hyon MS. The advantages of On-line transesophageal echocardiography guide during percutaneous balloon mitral valvuloplasty. J Am Soc Echocardiogr Off Publ Am Soc Echocardiogr. 2000;13(1):26–34.

37. Hung JS, Fu M, Yeh KH, Chua S, Wu JJ, Chen YC. Usefulness of intracardiac echocardiography in transseptal puncture during percutaneous transvenous mitral commissurotomy. Am J Cardiol. 1993;1;72(11):853–4.

38. Daccarett M, Segerson N, Gunther J, et al. Blinded correlation study of three-dimensional electro-anatomical image integration and phased array intra-cardiac echocardiography for left atrial mapping. Europace 2007;9:923-6.

39. Zhong H, Lacomis JM, Schwartzman D. On the accuracy of CartoMerge for guiding posterior left atrial ablation in man. Heart Rhythm Off J Heart Rhythm Soc. 2007;4(5):595–602.

40. Alboliras E, Hijazi Z. Comparison of costs of intracardiac echocardiography and transesophageal echocardiography in monitoring percutaneous device closure of atrial septal defect in children and adults. Am J Cardiol. 2004;94: 690-2.

41. Cafri C, de la Guardia B, Barasch E, et al. Transseptal puncture guided by intracardiac echocardiography during percutaneous transvenous mitral commissurotomy in patients with distorted anatomy of the fossa ovalis. Cathet Cardiovasc Intervent 2000;50:463-7.

42. Salem MI, Makaryus AN, Kort S, Chung E, Marchant D, Ong L, et al. Intracardiac echocardiography using the AcuNav ultrasound catheter during percutaneous balloon mitral valvuloplasty. J Am Soc Echocardiogr Off Publ Am Soc Echocardiogr. 2002;15(12):1533-7.

43. Koshy SK, Ahmed S, McMahon W, et al. Utility of intracardiac echocardiography in moderate to high risk percutaneous transvenous mitral balloon commissurotomy [abstr]. Catheter Cardiovasc Interv 2005;65:93.

44. Marcus GM, Ren X, Tseng ZH, Badhwar N, Lee BK, Lee RJ, et al. Repeat transseptal catheterization after ablation for atrial fibrillation. J Cardiovasc Electrophysiol. 2007;18(1):55–9.

45. Bidart C, Vaseghi M, Cesario DA, Mahajan A, Fujimura O, Boyle NG, et al. Radiofrequency current delivery via transseptal needle to facilitate septal puncture. Heart Rhythm Off J Heart Rhythm Soc. 2007;4(12):1573-6.

46. De Ponti R, Zardini M, Storti C, Longobardi M, Salerno-Uriarte JA. Transseptal catheterization for radiofrequency catheter ablation of cardiac arrhythmias. Results and safety of a simplified method. Eur Heart J. 1998;19(6):943–50.

47. Epstein LM, Smith T, TenHoff H. Nonfluoroscopic transseptal catheterization: safety and efficacy of intracardiac echocardiographic guidance. J Cardiovasc Electrophysiol. 1998;9:625-30.

48. B-Lundqvist C, Olsson SB, Varnauskas E. Transseptal left heart catheterization: a review of 278 studies. Clin Cardiol. 1986;9(1):21–6.

49. Hung JS, Fu M, Yeh KH, Wu CJ, Wong P. Usefulness of intracardiac echocardiography in complex transseptal catheterization during percutaneous transvenous mitral commissurotomy. Mayo Clin Proc. 1996;71(2):134–40.

50. Silvestry FE, Kadakia MB, Willhide J, Herrmann HC. Initial experience with a novel real-time three-dimensional intracardiac ultrasound system to guide percutaneous cardiac structural interventions: a phase 1 feasibility study of volume intracardiac echocardiography in the assessment of patients with structural heart disease undergoing percutaneous transcatheter therapy. J Am Soc Echocardiogr. 2014;27(9):978–83.

51. Akkaya E, Vuruskan E, Zorlu A, Sincer I, Kucukosmanoglu M, Ardic I, et al. Aortic intracardiac echocardiography-guided septal puncture during mitral valvuloplasty. Eur Heart J Cardiovasc Imaging. 2014;15(1):70–6.

52. Patzelt J, Seizer P, Zhang YY, Walker T, Schreieck J, Gawaz M, Langer HF. Percutaneous Mitral Valve Edge-to-Edge Repair With Simultaneous Biatrial Intracardiac Echocardiography: First-in-Human Experience. Circulation. 2016;133(15):1517–9.

53. Saji M, Rossi AM, Ailawadi G, Dent J, Ragosta M, Scott Lim D. Adjunctive intra-cardiac echocardiography imaging from the left ventricle to guide percutaneous mitral valve repair with the mitraclip in patients with failed prior surgical rings. Catheter Cardiovasc Interv. 2016;87(2):E75–82.

Section 4

PMV—Techniques and Gadgets

Chapter 21

Different Techniques and Devices for Percutaneous Mitral Valvuloplasty— Introduction

Mohammad A Sherif

■ INTRODUCTION

Rheumatic mitral stenosis (MS) continues to be endemic in developing countries where it is the most frequent valve disease. Although, the prevalence of rheumatic fever has greatly decreased in western countries, it continues to represent an important clinical entity because of immigration from developing countries.[1]

The two major techniques for percutaneous mitral valvuloplasty (PMV) are the double balloon technique (DBT) and the Inoue balloon technique (IBT). The multitrack balloon was introduced as a variant of the DBT that aims at making the procedure easier, as it requires the presence of a single guide wire only.[2]

Cribier et al.[3] introduced the metallic commissurotome (MC), which uses a device similar to the Tubb's dilator used during closed surgical mitral commissurotomy. The results suggest that its efficacy is similar to balloon commissurotomy, but the risk of hemopericardium seems higher because of the device and the presence of a guide wire in the left ventricle (LV). In addition, this technique is more demanding for the operator than the IBT. The potential advantage of metallic commissurotomy is that the dilator is reusable, which reduces the cost of the procedure.

■ HISTORICAL BACKGROUND

The concept of mitral commissurotomy was first proposed by Brunton in 1902 and the first successful surgical mitral commissurotomy was performed in the 1920s. By the late 1940s and 1950s, both transatrial and transventricular closed surgical commissurotomies were considered as accepted clinical procedures. With the development of cardiopulmonary bypass in the 1960s, open surgical mitral commissurotomy and replacement of the mitral valve became the surgical procedures of choice for the treatment of MS.

Kanji Inoue, a cardiovascular surgeon from Japan, began to design and develop a new balloon catheter system in 1976. The balloon was finally perfected in 1980.[4]

The first clinical application of the prototype Inoue balloon catheter was published in 1984.[4] In 1985, Lock et al.[5] used cylindrical polyethylene balloon in 8 children with rheumatic mitral stenosis to perform PMV via transseptal approach. Following Lock's report,[5] Al-Zaibag et al.[6] in 1986 introduced the DBT for treating rheumatic MS.

Palacios et al.[7] in 1987 using a single 25 mm balloon, made the first report of successful PMV in adult patients with calcific MS.

Several modifications of PMV technique have been introduced over the years. The use of transarterial retrograde approach for PMV was reported by Babic et al.[8] Use of bifoil and trifoil balloons were also described. The catheter with a low profile (<14 French) and having a pigtail tip was designed to cross the atrial septum without using a sheath.[9]

A simplified DBT called the multitrack system was developed in Paris by Philip Bonhoeffer and his colleagues, as a valid user-friendly and cost-effective alternative for the treatment of MS.[10]

In 1997, Cribier et al.[11] introduced a new device featuring a metallic valvulotome instead of a balloon for opening the mitral valve. The success of dilatation with the valvulotome was maintained even in patients with high echo scores and in patients with commissural calcification.[12]

TECHNIQUES AVAILABLE FOR PERCUTANEOUS MITRAL VALVOTOMY

There are two major techniques of PMV:
A. Balloon commissurotomy.
B. Metallic (blade) commissurotomy.

Balloon Commissurotomy

Gadgets

1. Cylindrical balloons (over the wire)
   a. Double balloon (two wire, two balloons)
   b. Multitrack system (single wire, two balloons)
   c. Nucleus/JOMIVA balloon (single balloon over the wire)
2. Dumb-bell shaped non-over the wire balloons
   a. Inoue balloon
   b. Accura balloon.

REFERENCES

1. Feldman T, Carroll JD, Herrmann HC, Holmes DR, Bashore TM, Isner JM, et al. Effect of balloon size and stepwise inflation technique on the acute results of Inoue mitral commissurotomy. Inoue Balloon Catheter Investigators. Cathet Cardiovasc Diagn. 1993;28(3):199–205.
2. Bonhoeffer P, Esteves C, Casal U, Tortoledo F, Yonga G, Patel T, et al. Percutaneous mitral valve dilatation with the Multi-Track System. Catheter Cardiovasc Interv Off J Soc Card Angiogr Interv. 1999;48(2):178–83.

3. Cribier A, Eltchaninoff H, Koning R, Rath PC, Arora R, Imam A, et al. Percutaneous mechanical mitral commissurotomy with a newly designed metallic valvulotome: immediate results of the initial experience in 153 patients. Circulation. 1999;99(6):793-9.

4. Inoue K, Owaki T, Nakamura T, Kitamura F, Miyamoto N. Clinical application of transvenous mitral commissurotomy by a new balloon catheter. J Thorac Cardiovasc Surg. 1984;87(3):394-402.

5. Lock JE, Khalilullah M, Shrivastava S, Bahl V, Keane JF. Percutaneous catheter commissurotomy in rheumatic mitral stenosis. N Engl J Med. 1985;313(24):1515-8.

6. Al Zaibag M, Ribeiro PA, Al Kasab S, Al Fagih MR. Percutaneous double-balloon mitral valvotomy for rheumatic mitral-valve stenosis. Lancet. 1986; 1(8484):757-61.

7. Palacios I, Block PC, Brandi S, Blanco P, Casal H, Pulido JI, et al. Percutaneous balloon valvotomy for patients with severe mitral stenosis. Circulation. 1987;75(4):778-84.

8. Babic UU, Vucinic M, Grujicic SM. Percutaneous transarterial balloon valvuloplasty for end-stage mitral valve stenosis. Scand J Thorac Cardiovasc Surg. 1986;20(2):189-91.

9. Berland J, Gerber L, Gamra H, Boussadia H, Cribier A, Letac B. Percutaneous balloon valvuloplasty for mitral stenosis complicated by fatal pericardial tamponade in a patient with extreme pulmonary hypertension. Cathet Cardiovasc Diagn. 1989;17:109-11.

10. Bonhoeffer P, Piéchaud JF, Sidi D, Yonga G, Jowi C, Joshi M, et al. Mitral dilatation with the Multi-Track system: an alternative approach. Cathet Cardiovasc Diagn. 1995;36(2):189-93.

11. Cribier A, Rath PC, Letac B. Percutaneous mitral valvotomy with a metal dilatator. Lancet. 1997;349(9066):1667.

12. Eltchaninoff H, Koning R, Derumeaux G, Cribier A. Percutaneous mitral commissurotomy by metallic dilator. Multicenter experience with 500 patients. Arch Mal Coeur Vaiss. 2000;93(6):685-92.

Chapter 22

The Single Balloon Mitral Valvotomy Catheters

Harikrishnan S, Krishnakumar M, Suji K

The single balloon, non-over the wire devices currently available for PMV are the triple lumen InoueTM balloon catheter and the double lumen AccuraTM balloon catheter (Fig. 22.1). These balloon catheters are manufactured from polyvinyl chloride with a latex balloon attached to the distal end. These single balloon devices are constructed with two layers of latex and a nylon or polyester micromesh "sandwiched" in between. The latex is extremely compliant, whereas the nylon mesh limits the maximum inflated diameter of the balloon and also gives the unique shape and inflation characteristics.

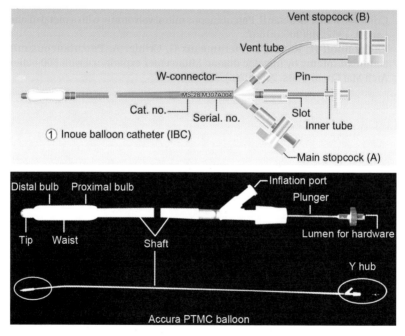

Fig. 22.1: Inoue balloon (top panel) and Accura balloon (lower panel). (Images supplied by Toray Inc. and Vascular Concepts and reproduced with permission)

The different components of the balloon are glued together in most of the areas except in few areas where they are laser welded. This is to be remembered while preparing the balloon and especially when reusing it because it can get detached in vivo during reuse.

Anatomy of Inoue and Accura Balloons

The Inoue balloon has a vent which ends in the balloon lumen. This is to vent the air in the balloon during preparation of the balloon prior to the procedure. The vent extends through the whole length of the balloon shaft from the proximal end of the vent hub and it terminates in the proximal part of the balloon in the balloon lumen. The Accura balloon does not have a vent and this is evident in the proximal part of the balloon shaft (Fig. 22.1).

The Inoue balloon has two small holes on the outer latex layer intended to prevent deflation failure of the balloon. The Accura balloon does not have these holes.

The balloon inflation port opens directly into the shaft of the balloon which is continuous with the balloon lumen. There is a "security thread" which runs from the proximal shaft of the balloon to the balloon (Figs 22.2, 22.4 and 22.5). This is intended to prevent the detachment of the balloon during the procedure.

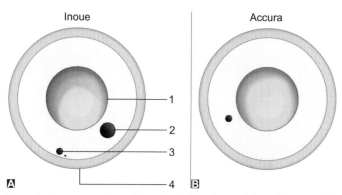

Figs 22.2A and B: Cross-section of the shaft of the Inoue (A) and Accura (B) balloons; 1—Central lumen; 2—Vent tube; 3—Security thread; 4—Shaft. *Note* that the Accura balloon does not have a vent tube

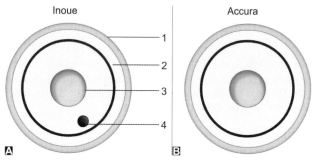

Figs 22.3A and B: Cross-section of the most proximal part of the balloons, 1—Outer latex layer with wire mesh inside, 2—Inner latex layer; 3—Central lumen; 4—End of vent tube. *Note* that the Accura balloon do not have a vent tube

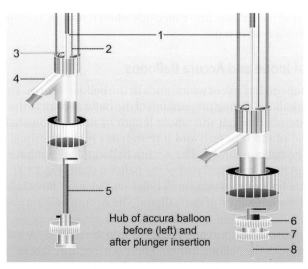

Fig. 22.4: The proximal hub of Accura balloon before (left) and after (right) insertion of the plunger (gold tube). 1—Junction of the gold tube and the central polythene tube; 2—Security thread; 3—Opening on the balloon inflation port; 4—Balloon inflation port; 5—Gold tube (plunger); 6—Proximal part of the gold hub; 7—Proximal hub of silver colored balloon stretching tube; 8—Wire in the central lumen

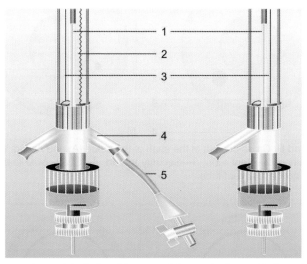

Fig. 22.5: Comparison of the hubs of Inoue and Accura balloons. Both are in the locked position; 1—Central gold hub; 2—Vent tube (only for Inoue); 3—Security thread; 4—Balloon inflation port; 5—Vent port (only for Inoue)

The proximal part of the balloon has a unique design (Figs 22.3A and B). The central lumen of the balloon is formed proximally by the "gold metal tube" which extends 2 cm into the balloon shaft even at the nonstretched (fully pulled back) position (Figs 22.4 and 22.6). The gold metal tube merges with a stiff

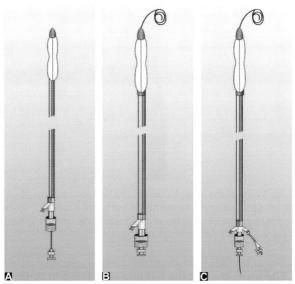

Figs 22.6A to C: (A) Accura balloon, nonstretched;
(B) Accura balloon, stretched; (C) Inoue balloon, stretched

polythene tube which extends through the entire length of the shaft and the balloon till its tip. Only this polythene tube forms the central lumen inside the balloon. That is why it is recommended to push the "gold tube" only with the straightener or the pigtail wire inside, otherwise the slender polythene tube may get kinked (Fig. 36.1–Chapter on trouble shooting).

When the balloon is stretched using the straightener (silver colored), the gold colored tube is pushed inside the shaft of the balloon. The straightener has a lumen which allows the pigtail wire to pass through. The straightener get pushed against the ridge at the tip of the balloon which enabling the stretch of the balloon (Fig. 22.7).

The balloon inflates in three stages. Initially, distal half of the balloon inflates, giving the appearance of a balloon floatation catheter. Secondly, the proximal half of the balloon inflates, creating a dog-bone or dumbbell shape. When positioned across the mitral valve, this facilitates positioning of the balloon device in the valve orifice. Finally, the center position of the balloon inflates, resulting in commissurotomy (Fig. 22.8). The distensibility of the latex material allows each balloon to be inflated over a range of diameter sizes. A single balloon can thus be used to effect sequential dilatation of the valve, by inflating it to serially larger diameters, without removing it from the patient.

Pressure Volume Relationship

Single balloon mitral valvotomy catheters are compliant balloons and are volume driven. The balloon is precalibrated so that inflation with volumes labeled on the inflation syringe result in corresponding inflated diameters of

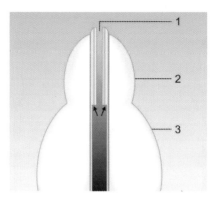

Fig. 22.7: Enlarged view of the tip of Inoue/Accura balloon catheter; 1—Central lumen; 2—Metal hub at the tip; 3—Central lumen inside the balloon made of polythene material. Small arrows indicate the proximal ridge where the balloon stretching metal tube (silver) is going to get placed to allow stretching of the balloon

the balloon. The pressure that the balloon is inflated to is thus different for different inflation volumes. It has a low-pressure zone encompassing the first two-thirds of its range of inflation. The balloon pressure at this point is typically approximately 2 to 3 atmospheres. As the balloon is inflated to its last couple of millimeters of diameter with increasing inflation volumes, the balloon pressure rises towards 4 atmospheres. A smaller size balloon when inflated to its maximal size, such as 26 mm, will generate a higher pressure than a balloon that has larger capacity, such as 30 mm balloon inflated to the same 26 mm (Fig. 22.8). Thus, with similar inflated diameters, smaller balloons will be able to generate more lateral pressure. Higher lateral pressure may be helpful in dilating thick fibrotic valves, but may lead to valve tear and mitral regurgitation.

Inoue and Accura balloons are fundamentally different from conventional balloons, being volume driven and do not have any burst pressure. The size of the balloon reflects the maximum diameter of the middle part of the balloon on full inflation. A 26 mm balloon means, the maximum diameter of the middle part of the fully inflated balloon is 26 mm. Precalibrated volumes will result in corresponding balloon inflated diameters. The intraballoon pressure for initial two-thirds of inflation is 2 to 3 atmospheres and 4 atmospheres during the last couple of millimeters of inflation. The intra balloon pressure transits from the low pressure to the high pressure zone as the balloon is inflated to within 2 mm of the nominal size, e.g. 24 to 26 mm zone in a 26 mm balloon catheter. Each catheter can safely be inflated to maximal diameter of 1 to 2 mm above the nominal size because of the built in safety margin.

Comparison of the pressure volume loop of the Inoue balloon and the Accura balloon (Figs 22.9A and B), illustrates that the Accura balloon can deliver more stable and higher pressures when the balloon is inflated within the stated diameter range. But the proportion of low pressure zone available for balloon dilatation is more with the Inoue balloon.

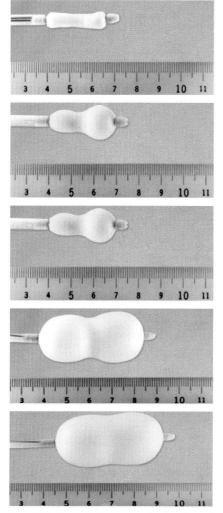

Step 1: Balloon completely deflated.

Step 2: Distal portion partially inflated when a small volume of dilute contrast medium is injected, the distal portion of the balloon inflates first. The balloon may float across the mitral valve, like a thermodilution catheter.

Step 3: Distal portion completely inflated when a larger volume of dilute contrast is injected, the distal portion inflates completely. This aids in seating the balloon on the valve, when it is pulled back from the LV apex to the mitral valve orifice.

Step 4: Hour glass or dumbbell shaped balloon on partial inflation across the mitral valve.

Step 5: Full inflation. Further injection will inflate the balloon to its full extent. The force of this expansion is used to achieve commissurotomy

Fig. 22.8: Inoue balloon showing the five uniquely different inflation stages (*Source*: Toray)

Inoue Balloon PMV System—Description and Specifications

The Inoue balloon catheter is manufactured by Toray (Toray International America Inc. 140 Cypress Station Drive, Suite 210 Houston, Texas 77090). The Inoue balloon catheter is a volume controlled device manufactured of polyvinyl chloride with a balloon attached to the distal end. The balloon has two latex layers between which there is a polyester micromesh. The catheter is 12 F in diameter with a length of 70 cm; the length of each balloon is 2.5 cm (unstretched). Two proximally positioned stopcocks accomplish balloon inflation and catheter venting. A stainless steel tube is used to stretch and slenderize the balloon prior to insertion and a 14 F tapered dilator enlarges the interatrial opening. The stainless steel stylet and guidewire are employed to track the catheter inside the heart and blood vessels. A syringe is used to

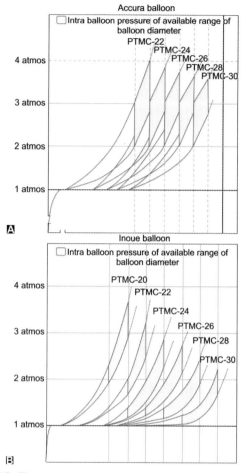

Figs 22.9A and B: The pressure volume relationship of Inoue and Accura balloons (Charts kindly provided by Toray Inc. and Vascular Concepts)

manually inflate the balloon and balloon diameter is measured with a caliper (Ruler) (Fig. 22.10 and Table 22.1).

Name of set item	Purpose
1. Inoue balloon catheter (IBC)	Dilation of valve
2. Balloon stretching tube	Elongation of balloon
3. Dilator	Dilation of the femoral vein puncture site and the interatrial septum
4. Guidewire	Guiding of catheter and dilator
5. Stylet (Spring)	Directing balloon through the valve
6. Syringe	Inflation of balloon
7. Ruler	Measurement of balloon diameter

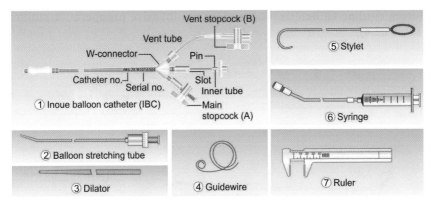

Fig. 22.10: Components of Inoue balloon (*Source:* Toray Inc.)

Table 22.1: Inoue balloon—catheter characteristics and specifications (Toray Inc)

| Catheter No. | Balloon diameter range | Catheter size | | Patient height |
		Fr. Size	Length	
PTMC-30, IMS-30	26 mm–30 mm	12 Fr.	70 cm	>180 cm
PTMC-28, IMS-28	24 mm–28 mm	12 Fr.	70 cm	>160 cm
PTMC-20, IMS-20	22 mm–36 mm	12 Fr.	70 cm	>147 cm
PTMC-30, IMS-30	20 mm–24 mm	12 Fr.	70 cm	≤147 cm
PTMC-22, IMS-22	20 mm–22 mm	12 Fr.	70 cm	≤147 cm
PTMC-20, IMS-20	18 mm–20 mm	12 Fr.	70 cm	≤147 cm

Accura Balloon—Description

The Accura PMV catheter is manufactured from polyvinyl chloride with a balloon attached to the distal end. This is manufactured by Vascular Concepts (Halstead, Essex, United Kingdom, www.vascularconcepts. net). The balloon has also 3 layers, 2 latex layers and 1 micromesh layer. The micromesh layer is sandwiched between the two latex layers. The length of balloon is 2.5 cm (unstretched).

At the proximal end of the balloon, a hub is provided with a stopcock for de-airing the balloon and also to inflate the balloon. A stainless steel metal stretching tube is provided which is inserted into the central lumen to stretch and slenderize the balloon. A 12 French 80 cm tapered medical grade polymer tube called dilator is a provided to enlarge the interatrial septal puncture. A spring guidewire with coiled portion at the distal end is provided to insert the balloon into the LA through the septal puncture (Fig. 22.11 and Tables 22.2 to 22.4).

Balloon Selection

The balloon diameter size is chosen on the basis of the patient's weight, height, and body surface area, as well as the estimated MVA as determined during cardiac catheterization and/or noninvasive preoperative studies (Table 22.4).

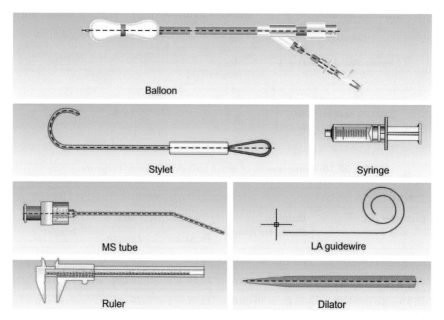

Fig. 22.11: Accura balloon system accessories
(Image supplied by Vascular Concepts)

Table 22.2: Components of the Accura mitral balloon system

1.	Accura balloon	80 cm
2.	Dilator—12 French	80 cm
3.	Stylet—0.38"	80 cm
4.	Metal stretching tube—19 gauge	80 cm
5.	LA guidewire—0.025"	175 cm
6.	Syringe	40 mL
7.	Vernier caliper	0–150 mm

Other factors to be considered in selecting the balloon diameter size include:

Sizing based on Height of the Patient

The reference size (RS) is calculated according to Hung's formula;[1] patient height (in cm) is rounded to the nearest zero and divided by ten, and ten is added to the ratio to yield the RS (in mm), e.g. if the patient height = 166 cm, then RS = 170/10 + 10= 27 mm.[1]

Table 22.3: Accura balloons–specifications and ordering information and the chart showing balloon selection based on patients height

Catalog number	Sizes available	Balloon selection	Patient's height
NM3022	19–22 mm	Max balloon diameter	
NM3024	21–24 mm	29 mm	>180 cm
NM3026	23–26 mm	28 mm	>160 cm
NM3028	25–28 mm	26 mm	>150 cm
NM3029	26–29 mm	24 mm	>150 cm
NM3030	27–30 mm	22 mm	>150

(*Table kindly provided by Vascular Concepts*)

Table 22.4: Selection of Inoue balloon based on patient height, weight and body surface area (*Source*: Toray)

Catheter No.	Available	Maximum range	Patient weight	Patient height	Surface area (m²)
PTMC-30	26–30 mm	30 mm	≥70 kg	≥180 cm	≥1.9
PTMC-28	24–28 mm	28 mm	45–70 kg	160–180 cm	1.6-1.9
PTMC-26	22–26 mm	26 mm	≤45 kg	≤160 cm	≤1.6

Sizing based on the Pathological Condition of the Mitral Valve

In patients with pliable, noncalcified valves as determined by echocardiography, a catheter with a nominal balloon size at least that of the RS (an RS-matched catheter) is used.[1] In contrast, in patients with pre-existing MR, subvalvular disease, and calcified valve, a balloon catheter one size smaller than RS is selected. Therefore in the previous example with an RS of 27 mm, PTMC 28 catheter would be selected for a pliable, noncalcified valve and PTMC-26 catheter would be selected for a calcified valve and/or with severe subvalvular disease.[1]

Sizing based on Age and Expected Physical Activity

For patients with sedentary life style or aged patients, the valve need not be dilated to a size required by active younger patients. If these patients are at high-risk of developing severe MR after PMV, a smaller balloon catheter should be used.[1]

Advantages of the Single Balloon Technique

- A short cycle of positioning-inflation-deflation (5 seconds). Procedure time is only 25–50% of double balloon.[1]
- Left ventricular perforation is also rare as the balloon is engaged into the mitral valve and has a smaller size.
- It does not necessitate a guidewire into the LV.[1]
- It causes minimal hemodynamic disturbance due to rapidity of the procedure. Maximum occlusion time of 2 to 4 seconds only.[1]

- Its strong rubber-nylon micromesh texture resists rupture which is rarely reported. It can stand a pressure of 6 kg/cm^2 (only 2 kg/cm^2 is needed for commissural splitting, i.e. wide margin of safety).[2]
- It is large enough for any mitral valve with only a single balloon needed due to its adjustable sizes.[2,3]
- Less potential for severe MR due to stepwise nature of dilatation and proper positioning across the valve.

COMPARISON BETWEEN INOUE AND ACCURA BALLOONS WITH RESPECT TO SAFETY AND EFFICACY (TABLE 22.5)

816 consecutive patients, who underwent elective BMV in this Institute (SCTIMST) from 1997 to 2003, were included in a retrospective study to assess the safety and efficacy of Accura balloon with respect to the Inoue balloon. The clinical, echocardiographic, and hemodynamic data of 487 patients who underwent BMV with Accura balloon was compared with 329 patients who underwent BMV with Inoue balloon.

Immediate procedural success (93.9% in Inoue group and 91.6% in Accura group p. NS) and complications (6.6% in Inoue group and 5.6% in Accura group p. NS) were comparable between the study groups. The two study population had similar restenosis rate and events at 1 year after BMV. Both balloons could be reused multiple times without compromising on the safety and effectiveness. Accura balloons were less costly than Inoue balloon. The reusability with Accura was slightly more and found to be more cost-effective. Both Accura and Inoue balloon mitral valvotomy balloons are effective in providing relief from hemodynamically significant mitral stenosis in terms of gain in valve area and reduction in transmitral gradient. Both groups have similar procedural success and complication rates, restenosis, and follow-up events at 1 year. Both balloons could be reused multiple times and Accura balloon is found to be more cost effective.[4]

Table 22.5: Comparison between Accura and Inoue balloons

	Inoue	*Accura*
Construction	Triple lumen	Double lumen
Contrast dilution recommended	1:4	1:6–8
Vent holes	Yes	Nil
Blood seepage between layers of balloon	Yes	No
Prevention of deflation failure	Yes	No
Vent holes	Yes – n=2	Nil
Vent tubes	Yes n=1	No
Balloon size attainable (e.g. 26 mm)	+4 mm (e.g. 22-26 mm) +3 mm (e.g. 23-26 mm)	

◾ BLUE ARROW PBMV BALLOON (FIG. 22.12)

Blue Arrow™ PBMV balloon is a balloon manufactured by SYM Shenzen Shineyard Medical Device Company limited, Shenzen, China is currently available. It is also a three port PBMV balloon like the Inoue balloon.

Balloon code	Inflation range	PBMV set code
PBMV-20	16–20 mm	PBMV-20S
PBMV-22	18–22 mm	PBMV-22S
PBMV-24	20–24 mm	PBMV-24S
PBMV-26	22–26 mm	PBMV-26S
PBMV-28	24–28 mm	PBMV-28S
PBMV-30	26–30 mm	PBMV-30S

Item: Catheter	O.D.: 12 F
Catheter length	800 mm
Maximum working pressure	280 KPa
Burst pressure	450 KPa

Item	Purpose	O.D.	Length
Balloon catheter	Dilating mitral valve	12 F	800 mm
Stretching tube	Stretching balloon catheter	1.2 mm	800 mm
Dilator	Dilating puncture site	14 F	700 mm
Guidewire	Guiding balloon catheter	0.025"	1800 mm
Stylet	Directing balloon to mitral valve	0.038"	800 mm

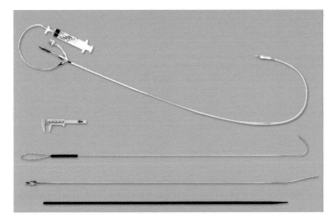

Fig. 22.12: Different components of the Blue Arrow PBMV system.
(*Image Courtesy*: Lifetechmed India)

■ REFERENCES

1. Hung JS, Lau KW. Pitfalls and tips in inoue balloon mitral commissurotomy. Cathet Cardiovasc Diagn. 1996;37(2):188–99.
2. Abdullah M, Halim M, Rajendran V, Sawyer W, al Zaibag M. Comparison between single (Inoue) and double balloon mitral valvuloplasty: immediate and short-term results. Am Heart J. 1992;123(6):1581–8.
3. Chen CR, Cheng TO. Percutaneous balloon mitral valvuloplasty by the Inoue technique: a multicenter study of 4832 patients in China. Am Heart J. 1995;129(6):1197–203.
4. Nair KKM, Pillai HS, Thajudeen A, Tharakan J, Titus T, Valaparambil A, et al. Comparative study on safety, efficacy, and midterm results of balloon mitral valvotomy performed with triple lumen and double lumen mitral valvotomy catheters. Catheter Cardiovasc Interv Off J Soc Card Angiogr Interv. 2012;80(6):978–86.

Chapter 23

Double Balloon Technique

Mohammad A Sherif, Arun Gopalakrishnan

In the early percutaneous valvuloplasty experience, it became apparent that single polyethylene balloons, manufactured in sizes up to 25 mm in diameter, were not sufficiently large to dilate most adult mitral valves.[1] Larger polyethylene balloons (up to 30 mm in diameter) produced adequate results, but resulted in large atrial septal defects when passed across the atrial septum.[2] It was thought that this problem could be overcome by using two smaller balloons, which could be tracked one by one across the interatrial septum. Thus in double balloon antegrade technique, as originally described by Al Zaibag et al[3] and modified by Palacios et al,[4] two balloons (each < 20 mm diameter) are introduced across the mitral valve and simultaneously inflated.[4]

■ DOUBLE BALLOON-TECHNIQUE (DBT)

With the double balloon antegrade technique, the left atrium is accessed through the interatrial septum (antegrade) from the right femoral vein using standard transseptal catheterization equipment.[5] A Mullins sheath is inserted into the left atrium, through which an end-hole balloon tipped catheter can be floated across the mitral valve, avoiding the chordae tendineae. It is then turned in the left ventricular apex using a curved tipped guidewire and advanced out the aortic valve.[6] A long guidewire (260 cm) is then introduced through this catheter from the femoral vein across the atrial septum and the mitral and aortic valves, terminating in the descending aorta. This procedure can be repeated,[3] or a special double lumen catheter used to place a second guidewire adjacent to the first one.[4]

Some operators pass both guidewires through the Mullins sheath without using a second catheter. Two polyethylene balloons are then introduced, one over each guidewire, and simultaneously inflated to dilate the stenotic valve.[1] Advancing the guidewires into the aorta can be technically difficult and time consuming, and some operators prefer to leave them curled in the left ventricle, as with the retrograde aortic technique. This is more likely to cause arrhythmias, provide a less stable position during balloon insertion, and it may increase the risk of left ventricular perforation.[7]

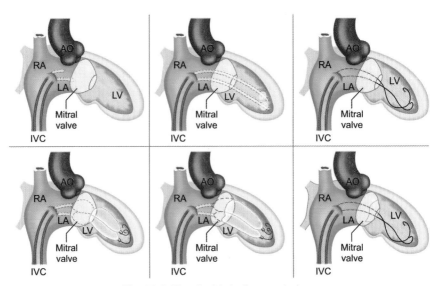

Fig. 23.1: The double balloon technique

When both balloons are introduced through the same septal puncture (Fig. 23.2), the interatrial septum is first dilated with a 6-8 mm diameter balloon to facilitate the passage of the larger balloons. In most adults, two 20 mm diameter balloons give good results.[7,8] In some cases, a combination of smaller balloons may be preferable to avoid over dilating the valve and producing regurgitation.[7,9]

■ BALLOON SIZING

In the early experience, patient's body surface area was used as a reference in choosing the balloon size. Pre-selection of balloon size remains controversial, as the desire for greater improvement must be balanced against the risk of producing severe mitral regurgitation. Usually, balloon sizes are chosen according to the patient's characteristics; body surface area and height or diameter of mitral valve annulus.[10]

Sizing Based on Annulus Diameter

Echocardiography is used to measure the mitral valve annulus diameter in mid-diastole. Reid et al[11] suggested that balloon size is chosen in such a way that the combined diameter of the two balloons were approximately equal to the mitral valve annulus measured by 2D echocardiography. This was thought to decrease the potential of rupture of mitral annulus by over-dilatation.

Chen et al[12] found that the best choice in terms of increase in mitral valve area and prevention of mitral regurgitation is a ratio of (sum of balloon diameters)/(mitral annulus diameter) of 1 to 1.1.

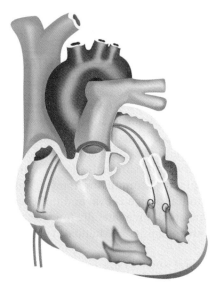

Fig. 23.2: Both balloons are introduced through the same septal puncture and then simultaneously inflated

Reid et al[13] found that MVA immediately after PMV significantly correlated with the effective balloon dilating area (EBDA).

EBDA is calculated as the area of the region formed by two half circles and the trapezoidal region connecting them.[1]

Sizing Based on Body Surface Area

Palacios et al[4] found that the effective balloon dilating diameter normalized to body surface area significantly correlated to the drop in transmitral gradient after PMV. Greater the effective balloon dilating diameter per square meter body surface area, greater will be the drop of transmitral gradient and greater will be the mitral valve area. Single balloon yield was suboptimal compared to double balloon yield.[7,9] Best results were obtained when EBDA/BSA was >3.5/m².

Initial studies by Palacios et al[4] recommended the initial dilatation to be with an EDBA of 4.9 cm² (i.e. 25 mm balloon) to be followed by a bigger combination if the initial results are suboptimal. However, subsequent studies identified that the predictor of moderate to severe mitral regurgitation post double balloon valvotomy was an EBDA/BSA ratio more than 4.0 cm²/m². Hence an EBDA/BSA ratio of 3.5 – 4.0 cm²/m² is considered appropriate for balloon selection by this technique.[14,15]

Several studies have showed that PMV using the DBT is effective and relatively safe.[16-19] The combined analysis of these studies lead to the conclusion that the DBT provides a significant increase in MVA and drop in the transmitral mean pressure gradient associated with significant improvement of the functional status.

The detailed description of studies comparing the effectiveness of DBT with other techniques is given in Chapter 27.

DOUBLE BALLOON TECHNIQUE—ADVANTAGES AND DISADVANTAGES

Double balloon technique is more likely to achieve greater increase in valve area compared to single balloon technique. Several reasons have been postulated. The mechanism of percutaneous balloon mitral valvuloplasty is related to commissural splitting rather than to plastic remodeling of valvular tissue.[20] Thus, the delivery of pressure to the fused commissures is paramount in promoting successful mitral commissurotomy. It has been suggested that because the stenotic mitral orifice is oval and not circular, double balloons selforient and exert maximal force laterally toward the fused commissures, resulting in superior valve opening.[21-23] Multiple in vitro studies have supported the same argument.[24,25]

The acute procedural success are in fact better with double balloon technique than with single balloon valvuloplasty.[26] The post-procedure calculated mitral valve areas were more with double balloon technique as compared with the former. Rihal et al developed a regression equation for final mitral valve area post balloon valvuloplasty: Final mitral valve area = 1.3 × initial mitral valve area + 0.34 × technique + 0.02 where technique = 1 for Inoue balloon and 2 for double balloon (Fig. 23.3).[27]

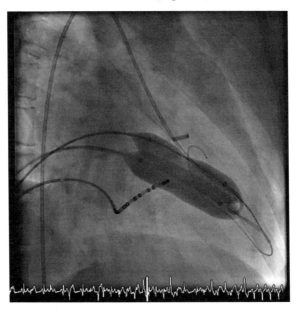

Fig. 23.3: Two 16 mm balloons are introduced through the same septal puncture and the same wire (Boenhoefer system—See Chapter 26 for details) and then simultaneously inflated. Steerable lead in the coronary sinus is also seen. *Figure and Video Courtesy:* Dr PR Stella, Department of Interventional Cardiology, University Medical Center, Utrecht, Netherlands

The ellipsoid balloon dilating surface of the double balloon is technically better suited to the crescent-shaped stenotic mitral valve orifice. Studies have shown that the double balloon produces more longitudinal separation of fused commissures than the Inoue technique.[28] The tension applied to the plane of the mitral commissure is twice the tension applied vertically according to the Laplace's law during simultaneous inflation of the two balloons.[29]

In contrast the dilating forces of the Inoue balloon are radially applied on the fused mitral commissures, potentially contributing to less effective splitting of fused commissures.[26,30]

Double balloon technique is technically more challenging with the need for multiple wire exchanges and difficulty in obtaining stable transmitral balloon positions. Not surprisingly, several workers have documented longer procedure and fluoroscopic times.[30,31] Greater improvement in mitral valve area with this technique also portends a higher incidence of complications. Commissural splitting in double balloon technique occurs preferentially in calcified commissures than in non-calcified commissures.[25] The double balloon technique also requires multiple guidewire exchanges adding to technical complexity. Mitral valve crossing can be difficult, particularly in markedly dilated left atria. The dilating instrument may also add to the complexity in double balloon technique owing to its elliptical shape, unlike the circular one in an Inoue technique.[30] Also there is the difficulty of obtaining a stable position of the balloons across the mitral valve. The incidence of significant procedural complications, such as persistent atrial septal defect and left to right shunt, severe mitral regurgitation, and left ventricular apical perforation was greater in comparison with the Inoue technique in multiple studies.[27,30]

However reported long term event free survival with the double balloon has been comparable with the single balloon technique.[26] This could possibly indicative of limited operator experience with the double balloon technique. It is also notable that there are no randomized trials comparing the two techniques in percutaneous mitral valvotomy. In this regard, the muti-track system offers a more operator friendly procedure incorporating the virtues of the double balloon technique.

■ REFERENCES

1. Herrmann HC, Wilkins GT, Abascal VM, Weyman AE, Block PC, Palacios IF. Percutaneous balloon mitral valvotomy for patients with mitral stenosis. Analysis of factors influencing early results. J Thorac Cardiovasc Surg. 1988;96(1):33–8.
2. Herrmann HC, Kussmaul WG, Hirshfeld JW Jr. Single large-balloon percutaneous mitral valvuloplasty. Cathet Cardiovasc Diagn. 1989;17(1):59–61.
3. Al Zaibag M, Ribeiro PA, Al Kasab S, Al Fagih MR. Percutaneous double-balloon mitral valvotomy for rheumatic mitral-valve stenosis. Lancet. 1986;1(8484):757–61.
4. Palacios I, Block PC, Brandi S, Blanco P, Casal H, Pulido JI, et al. Percutaneous balloon valvotomy for patients with severe mitral stenosis. Circulation. 1987;75(4):778–84.

5. O'Keefe JH Jr, Vlietstra RE, Hanley PC, Seward JB. Revival of the transseptal approach for catheterization of the left atrium and ventricle. Mayo Clin Proc. 1985;60(11):790-5.

6. Lock JE, Khalilullah M, Shrivastava S, Bahl V, Keane JF. Percutaneous catheter commissurotomy in rheumatic mitral stenosis. N Engl J Med. 1985;313(24):1515-8.

7. Herrmann HC, Kleaveland JP, Hill JA, Cowley MJ, Margolis JR, Nocero MA, et al. The M-Heart percutaneous balloon mitral Valvuloplasty Registry: initial results and early follow-up. The M-Heart Group. J Am Coll Cardiol. 1990;15(6):1221-6.

8. Vahanian A, Michel PL, Cormier B, Vitoux B, Michel X, Slama M, et al. Results of percutaneous mitral commissurotomy in 200 patients. Am J Cardiol. 1989;63(12):847-52.

9. Abascal VM, Wilkins GT, O'Shea JP, Choong CY, Palacios IF, Thomas JD, et al. Prediction of successful outcome in 130 patients undergoing percutaneous balloon mitral valvotomy. Circulation. 1990;82(2):448-56.

10. Sancho M, Medina A, Suárez de Lezo J, Hernandez E, Pan M, Coello I, et al. Factors influencing progression of mitral regurgitation after transarterial balloon valvuloplasty for mitral stenosis. Am J Cardiol. 1990;66(7):737-40.

11. Reid CL, McKay CR, Chandraratna PA, Kawanishi DT, Rahimtoola SH. Mechanisms of increase in mitral valve area and influence of anatomic features in double-balloon, catheter balloon valvuloplasty in adults with rheumatic mitral stenosis: a Doppler and two-dimensional echocardiographic study. Circulation. 1987;76(3):628-36.

12. Chen CY, Lin SL, Pan JP, Chang MS. Minimal requirement of effective dilation diameter of balloon(s) in percutaneous transluminal mitral valvotomy. Zhonghua Yi Xue Za Zhi Chin Med J Free China Ed. 1989;44(5):287-92.

13. Reid CL, Chandraratna PA, Kawanishi DT, Kotlewski A, Rahimtoola SH. Influence of mitral valve morphology on double-balloon catheter balloon valvuloplasty in patients with mitral stenosis. Analysis of factors predicting immediate and 3-month results. Circulation. 1989;80(3):515-24.

14. Roth RB, Block PC, Palacios IF. Predictors of increased mitral regurgitation after percutaneous mitral balloon valvotomy. Cathet Cardiovasc Diagn. 1990;20(1):17-21.

15. Palacios IF, Tuzcu ME, Weyman AE, Newell JB, Block PC. Clinical follow-up of patients undergoing percutaneous mitral balloon valvotomy. Circulation. 1995;91(3):671-6.

16. Trevino AJ, Ibarra M, Garcia A, Uribe A, de la Fuente F, Bonfil MA, et al. Immediate and long-term results of balloon mitral commissurotomy for rheumatic mitral stenosis: comparison between Inoue and double-balloon techniques. Am Heart J. 1996;131(3):530-6.

17. Zhang HP, Gamra H, Allen JW, Lau FY, Ruiz CE. Comparison of late outcome between Inoue balloon and double-balloon techniques for percutaneous mitral valvotomy in a matched study. Am Heart J. 1995;130(2):340-4.

18. Park SJ, Kim JJ, Park SW, Song JK, Doo YC, Lee SJ. Immediate and one-year results of percutaneous mitral balloon valvuloplasty using Inoue and double-balloon techniques. Am J Cardiol. 1993;71(11):938-43.

19. Ruiz CE, Zhang HP, Macaya C, Aleman EH, Allen JW, Lau FY. Comparison of Inoue single-balloon versus double-balloon technique for percutaneous mitral valvotomy. Am Heart J. 1992;123(4 Pt 1):942-7.

20. McKay RG, Lock JE, Safian RD, Come PC, Diver DJ, Baim DS, et al. Balloon dilation of mitral stenosis in adult patients: postmortem and percutaneous mitral valvuloplasty studies. J Am Coll Cardiol. 1987;9(4):723-31.

21. Chen CG, Wang YP, Qing D, Lin YS, Lan YF. Percutaneous mitral balloon dilatation by a new sequential single- and double-balloon technique. Am Heart J. 1988;116(5 Pt 1):1161–7.

22. Kasab SA, Ribeiro PA, Zaibag MA, Bitar IA, Idris MT, Shahed M, et al. Comparison of results of percutaneous balloon mitral valvotomy using single and double balloon techniques. Am J Cardiol. 1989;63(1):135–6.

23. Kasab SA, Ribeiro PA, Sawyer W. Comparison of results of percutaneous balloon mitral valvotomy using consecutive single (25 mm) and double (25 mm and 12 mm) balloon techniques. Am J Cardiol. 1989;64(19):1385–7.

24. Reifart N, Nowak B, Baykut D, Satter P, Bussmann WD, Kaltenbach M. Experimental balloon valvuloplasty of fibrotic and calcific mitral valves. Circulation. 1990;81(3):1005–11.

25. Ribeiro PA, al Zaibag M, Rajendran V, Ashmeg A, al Kasab S, al Faraidi Y, et al. Mechanism of mitral valve area increase by in vitro single and double balloon mitral valvotomy. Am J Cardiol. 1988;62(4):264–9.

26. Leon MN, Harrell LC, Simosa HF, Mahdi NA, Pathan AZ, Lopez-Cuellar J, et al. Comparison of immediate and long-term results of mitral balloon valvotomy with the double-balloon versus Inoue techniques. Am J Cardiol. 1999;83(9):1356–63.

27. Rihal CS, Nishimura RA, Reeder GS, Holmes DR. Percutaneous balloon mitral valvuloplasty: comparison of double and single (Inoue) balloon techniques. Cathet Cardiovasc Diagn. 1993;29(3):183–90.

28. Park SJ, Kim JJ, Park SW, Song JK, Doo YC, Lee SJ. Immediate and one-year results of percutaneous mitral balloon valvuloplasty using Inoue and double-balloon techniques. Am J Cardiol. 1993;71(11):938–43.

29. Ruiz CE, Zhang HP, Macaya C, Aleman EH, Allen JW, Lau FY. Comparison of Inoue single-balloon versus double-balloon technique for percutaneous mitral valvotomy. Am Heart J. 1992;123(4 Pt 1):942–7.

30. Bassand JP, Schiele F, Bernard Y, Anguenot T, Payet M, Ba SA, et al. The double-balloon and Inoue techniques in percutaneous mitral valvuloplasty: comparative results in a series of 232 cases. J Am Coll Cardiol. 1991;18(4):982–9.

31. Ramaswamy K, Losordo DW, Rosenfield K, Flynn S, Farley S, Coletta D, et al. Inoue balloon mitral valvuloplasty vs. double balloon technique: procedure duration and radiation exposure. J Am Coll Cardiol. 1991;17(2s1):A253–A253.

Chapter 24

Mitral Valvotomy by Metallic Commissurotome

Mohammad A Sherif, Harikrishnan S

Percutaneous mitral valvotomy (PMV) is the treatment of choice for mitral stenosis, but the cost of the procedure remains a limitation in countries with restricted financial resources, leading to frequent reuse of disposable catheters. To overcome this limitation, a reusable metallic commissurotomy device was developed by Alain Cribier et al. with the goals of both improving the mitral commissurotomy results and decreasing the cost of the procedure.[1]

■ DESCRIPTION OF THE DEVICE

The device consists of a metallic dilator screwed onto the distal end of a disposable catheter. The entire system is made of four components (Fig. 24.1). The catheter has a diameter of 13 F (4.3 mm) and a length of 170 cm.

Its proximal end has a connector for recording distal pressures, and it also allows connection of the activating pliers. Its distal end allows fastening of the dilator. The metallic dilator (Figs 24.2A to C), is made of stainless steel, when closed, is a cylinder 5 cm long and 5 mm wide, with a slightly tapered tip. The distal half of the dilator consists of 2 hemi cylindrical bars 20 mm in length that can be opened out in parallel up to a maximum extent of 40 mm by a lever-arm system. The opening of these 2 bars leads to the separation of the commissures. Furthermore, the dilator contains an internal tube that allows the passage of a traction wire and also the recording of distal pressures.[1]

The metallic head is screwed onto the distal end of the catheter and is detachable. The metallic guidewire is made of stainless steel, with a length of 270 cm and a diameter of 0.035 inch. A metallic bead 2 mm in diameter is soldered at the junction of the stiff core and the 10 cm long floppy distal end. The guidewire is first positioned in the left ventricle; the commissurotome can then be advanced over it until the dilator crosses the mitral valve. Then, the guidewire becomes a traction system that allows the dilator to be opened. For that, the metallic bead is positioned in contact with the distal end of the dilator, and the guidewire is solidly locked into the commissurotome with a threaded fastener located on the activating pliers. Squeezing the arms of the pliers causes a backward traction of the guidewire and the metallic bead that is transmitted

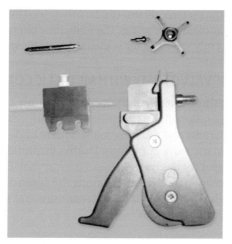

Fig. 24.1: Components of the assembly of the metallic commissurotome

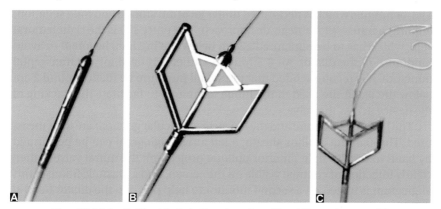

Figs 24.2A to C: The blade in the closed position (A), partly open (B)
and fully open position (C)

to the distal end of the dilator, thus forcing the distal bars to spread apart. The activating pliers are attached to the proximal end of the catheter shaft.

A manual pressure exerted on the arms of the pliers allows the dilator to open according to the mechanism described above, and the release of pressure closes the dilator. The activating pliers comprise several elements:[1]

1. A caliper that allows the degree of opening of the bars to be altered from outside with the help of a cursor. The programmable degrees of opening are 33, 35, 37 and 40 mm.

2. A safety lock that prevents the complete closure of the dilator after the release of pressure exerted on the pilers (it holds the dilator open at 20 mm). To obtain a complete closure of the dilator after withdrawal from the mitral valve, this lock must be activated manually. This security system was designed to avoid any accidental extraction of valvular tissue.

3. A threaded fastener, which is designed to block the metallic guidewire into the commissurotome at the time of opening.

After dilatation, the metallic dilator can be unscrewed from the catheter and can be sterilized by autoclave for reuse. The activating pliers and the guidewire can also be reused. Only the catheter is meant for single use.

◼ MECHANISM OF VALVOTOMY WITH METALLIC COMMISSUROTOME

In clinical practice, this device was shown to act mainly by direct stretching and subsequent separation of the commissures without exerting pressure on the subvalvular apparatus and the valve leaflets there by decreasing the risk of mechanical injury to the valve apparatus. During the initial phase of opening of the bars, the catheter rotates by itself in such a way that the bars are directed where less resistance is encountered, i.e. along the commissural line which is the cause of the high percentage of double commissural splitting, as well as the low rate of mitral regurgitation.[1]

◼ TECHNIQUE

The technique, which is performed under local anesthesia and mild sedation, requires a transseptal antegrade approach. The entry site is the right femoral vein, which has to be punctured ≥2 cm below the inguinal ligament to avoid hindrance to the dilator. An 8 F Mullins catheter is used for the transseptal puncture. It is recommended that the septal puncture be made around 2 cm below the usual site used in the Inoue technique to facilitate the tracking of the device across the valve.

The left atrial pressure and the left atrioventricular gradient are then measured. Through the Mullins sheath, a left atrial angiogram can be performed by hand in the 30° right anterior oblique projection: the mitral valve is then clearly injection of contrast visible on the screen, and a diastolic frame of this angiogram is frozen on a second monitor to help position the dilator head at the time of dilation. Keeping the same projection, a floating balloon catheter is advanced through the sheath and used to cross the mitral valve.

The distal end of the balloon catheter is positioned at the apex of the left ventricle, and the sheath is advanced over it, beyond the mitral valve orifice. The balloon catheter is then removed, and the guidewire of the device is advanced through the sheath in the left ventricle, the metallic bead being positioned at midventricle, i.e. clearly beyond the mitral valve. The Mullins sheath is then removed, and a 14 F polyethylene dilator is advanced over the wire to enlarge the atrial septum puncture site. The same maneuver is then completed by additional dilation with an 18 F dilator, which is also used to enlarge the femoral vein puncture site.[1]

As an alternative technique, a balloon catheter (8 mm in diameter) can be used for enlarging the septum and the femoral puncture site. The commissurotome is then advanced over the wire, and its distal end is placed across the mitral valve. At that time, the guidewire is pulled back until the bead is firmly held against the tip of the valvulotome and then securely fastened by screwing the threaded fastener of the pliers. The dilation can then be performed by squeezing the arms of activating pliers. The desired degree of bar opening is

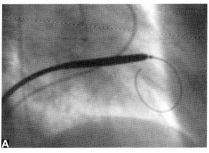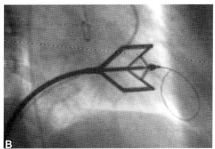

Figs 24.3A and B: Procedure of percutaneous mechanical mitral commissurotomy (PMMC). The device is pushed over guidewire and metallic dilator positioned across mitral valve (A). Then, commissurotomy is performed by opening dilator to its maximum extent (B)

obtained by use of the caliper. After dilation, the device is pulled back into the left atrium, with the guidewire in place in the left ventricle. The transvalvular gradient is assessed, the left atrial pressure being measured with the pressure line of the device (Figs 24.3A and B).

▇ TECHNICAL CONSIDERATIONS[1]

Crossing the Septum and the Mitral Orifice

Despite the length, caliber, and inescapable rigidity of the metallic dilator, the device could easily reach the mitral valve in the vast majority of cases. However, Cribier et.al. reported that 3/153 patients required additional dilatation of the septal puncture site with 8 mm balloon. During the opening phase, the dilator was perfectly stable, and the hemodynamic tolerance was good because of the noninterrupted blood flow.

Positioning the Device Across the Mitral Valve

An optimal positioning of the dilator across the valve before opening can be achieved by several means:[1]

1. A satisfactory position is generally obtained when the distal half of the dilator is located slightly anterior to the aortic orifice in the right anterior oblique (RAO) view which is indicated by the presence of a pigtail catheter placed in the aortic root.
2. When available, the left atrial angiogram obtained after trans-septal catheterization is helpful to locate the free edges of the valve.
3. The transition between the left ventricular and left atrial pressure curves gives an excellent indication of the location of the border of the mitral valve; this can be observed during the withdrawal of the Mullins sheath after the guidewire has been positioned in the left ventricle or by recording these pressures through the pressure lumen of the device.
4. On-line transthoracic two-dimensional echocardiography is frequently used and is an excellent way of optimizing the position of the device.

5. The resistance to the device opening is well-perceived while the arms of activating pliers are squeezed, and this confirms the accurate positioning of the dilator.

Extent of Bar Opening

The extent of bar opening is a significant predictive factor of the immediate percutaneous mechanical mitral commissurotomy (PMMC) results. The device sizing (extent of opening of the bars) is not done according to the measurement of the mitral annulus. In adult patients with a body surface area >1.50 m² and without severe valvular calcification, we can open the device to 40 mm in the beginning itself. In other patients, we can start with 37 mm (or 33 mm in children), with a stepwise increase according to the results.[1] The stepwise approach may be safer also.

The technique of PMMC has several differences from the well-established balloon mitral valvotomy. It requires a lower atrial septal puncture for easy tracking of the catheter, guidewire, and the bulky metal dilator. The PMMC device does not automatically position itself at the mitral orifice, as does the Inoue balloon. Hence, placing the PMMC device at the proper site depends on the experience of the operator and confirmation of successful dilation of the valve with echocardiographic recording after each dilatation.[1]

Despite the resemblance of the instrument used in closed surgical commissurotomy and percutaneous mechanical mitral commissurotomy, some differences do exist, such as the self-positioning of the dilator's bars in the commissures during percutaneous mechanical mitral commissurotomy. A possibility of immediate evaluation of the hemodynamic and echocardiographic results after dilation offers the possibility of subsequent additional dilator openings of a larger size when needed. The main advantage of using the metallic device is, by far, the decrease in procedural cost, because it allows multiple safe reuse after sterilization by autoclaving without any deterioration in the components, thus, favoring countries with limited financial resources that have a high number of cases of mitral stenosis.[2]

Percutaneous mechanical mitral commissurotomy (PMMC) has been used successfully in juvenile mitral stenosis also. Harikrishnan et al.[3] have reported a nonrandomized comparison of 33 juvenile patients (<20 years) who underwent percutaneous transvenous mitral commissurotomy (PTMC) to 33 patients who underwent PTMC with Inoue balloon with similar acute and intermediate term results.

◼ COMPLICATIONS

Although, PMMC is considered as a safe technique for PMV, it carries some risks. The most significant are:
1. Hemopericardium with tamponade resulting from perforation of the left ventricle by the device.
2. Severe mitral regurgitation requiring mitral valve replacement.

■ INITIAL AND LONG-TERM RESULTS

In the initial international experience of PMMC (1995–1998), PMMC was performed at 14 centers in France, India, and Egypt. This clinical experience consisted of 153 patients with broad spectrum of mitral valve deformities. The procedure was successful in 92% of cases and resulted in a significant increase in mitral valve area, from 0.95 ± 0.2 to 2.16 ± 0.4 cm^2. No increase in MR was noted in 80% of cases. Bilateral splitting of the commissures was observed in 87%. Complications reported were severe MR requiring surgery n = 1, pericardial tamponade n = 1, transient cerebrovascular embolic event n = 1. In this series, the maximum number of consecutive patients treated with the same device was 35.[1]

The same group, who published the initial results, later reported a success rate of 93%, in a larger series of 500 patients.[4] Bhat et al[5] published a randomized study comparing PMMC and Inoue balloon commissurotomy (IBMC), and found similar success rates (90.18% Vs 91.8%)(P = NS).

Harikrishnan et al.[6] reported the long-term follow-up results of PMV using metallic commissurotome, in 248 patients by the transseptal technique. They found that the procedure was successful in 230 patients (92.7%). Following PMMC, the transmitral gradient decreased from 14.54 ±5.79 mm Hg to 4.26 ± 2.82 mm Hg (p <0.001). The mitral valve area (MVA) increased from 0.85 ± 0.12 cm^2 to 1.95 ± 0.31 cm^2 (p ≤ 0.001). One patient died due to left ventricular perforation (mortality rate = 0.41%). Another patient who developed a left ventricular tear underwent repair of the tear along with open mitral valvotomy. Four patients developed significant MR from tear of valve leaflets and had to undergo emergency mitral valve replacement. One patient had a transient ischemic attack and 5 patients developed moderate MR caused by excessive split of valve commissures. During the mean follow-up period of 3.34 ± 0.66 years, seven of the 224 patients (3.1%) who were on follow-up, developed mitral restenosis. The clinical improvement following valvotomy persisted in the vast majority of the patients at follow-up of three years indicating the efficacy of the procedure.

■ REFERENCES

1. Cribier A, Eltchaninoff H, Koning R, Rath PC, Arora R, Imam A, et al. Percutaneous mechanical mitral commissurotomy with a newly designed metallic valvulotome: immediate results of the initial experience in 153 patients. Circulation. 1999;99(6):793–9.
2. Bastos MD, Esteves CA, Araújo D, Bastos LA, Eistein M, Santana GP, et al. Percutaneous mechanical mitral commissurotomy performed with a Cribier's metallic valvulotome. Initial results. Arq Bras Cardiol. 2001;77(2):120–31.
3. Harikrishnan S, Nair K, Tharakan JM, Titus T, Kumar VK, Sivasankaran S. Percutaneous transmitral commissurotomy in juvenile mitral stenosis— comparison of long-term results of Inoue balloon technique and metallic commissurotomy. Catheter Cardiovasc Interv. 2006;67:453-9.
4. Eltchaninoff H, Koning R, Derumeaux G, Cribier A. Percutaneous mitral commissurotomy by metallic dilator. Multicenter experience with 500 patients. Arch Mal Coeur Vaiss. 2000;93(6):685–92.

5. Bhat A, Harikrishnan S, Tharakan JM, et al. Comparison of percutaneous transmitral commissurotomy using Inoue balloon technique and metallic commissurotomy—immediate and short-term follow-up results of a randomised study. Am Heart J. 2002;144:1074-80.

6. Harikrishnan S, Bhat A, Tharakan J, Titus T, Kumar A, Sivasankaran S, et al. Percutaneous transvenous mitral commissurotomy using metallic commissurotome: long-term follow-up results. J Invasive Cardiol. 2006;18(2):54–8.

Chapter 25

JOMIVA Balloon

Sajy Kuruttukulam

Joseph et al.[1,2] have developed a simple over-the-wire mitral valvuloplasty balloon catheter (JOMIVA™, Numed, Hopkinton, New York), by modification of a pre-existing balloon-catheter[3,4] (Nucleus™, Numed). This balloon is marketed only in India. The JOMIVA balloon is cylindrical, expands to a fixed size, has two radiopaque markers corresponding to a 4 cm working length, and is made of thin thermoplastic polymer that gives these larger diameter balloons a low crossing profile. The design includes an abrupt distal balloon taper and a short, blunt catheter tip to prevent left ventricular perforation.

The catheter shaft (9 Fr for smaller balloons, 11 Fr for larger balloons) has a coaxial construction that allows for short balloon inflation-deflation times (<6 seconds).

▣ TECHNIQUE

Femoral Approach

The left atrium is accessed through the interatrial septum (antegrade) from the right femoral vein using standard transseptal catheterization equipment. The mitral valve is crossed using a balloon floatation catheter (Fig. 25.1). The J-tip of a 0.035 inch valvuloplasty guidewire (Back-up Meier,™ Boston Scientific, Natick, Massachusetts) is then positioned at the left ventricular apex after manually shaping the stiff shaft just proximal to its soft distal portion into a wide secondary curve (Fig. 25.2). Care is taken during guidewire introduction into the left ventricle to ensure that the tip of the floatation catheter does not abut the ventricular wall, and to ensure that the guidewire tip curled freely as it emerges from the catheter.

Septum is then dilated with 14 French septal dilator which is introduced over the wire (Fig. 25.3). The JOMIVA balloon is then introduced through a 50 cm long, 12 to 14 Fr valved left atrial sheath (Cook, Bloomington, Indiana), and commissurotomy is performed after withdrawing the sheath into the inferior vena cava to allow a more transverse and stable lie of the balloon and the guidewire across the mitral valve (Figs 25.4 and 25. 5).

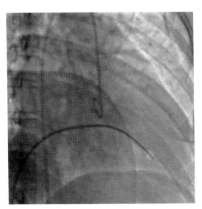

Fig. 25.1: Balloon catheter in LV after septal puncture

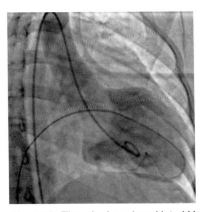

Fig. 25.2: The wire introduced into LV and kept in the optimal position

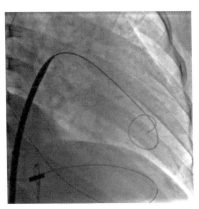

Fig 25.3: Dilatation of the septum with the dilator over the wire kept in LV 📷◀

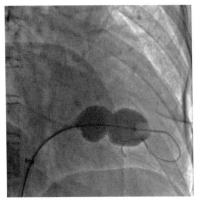

Fig. 25.4: The JOMIVA balloon is tracked over the wire through the left atrial sheath. The waist on the balloon is seen 📷◀

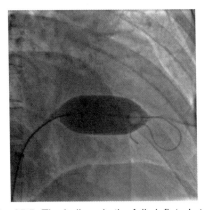

Fig. 25.5: The balloon in the fully inflated state

Jugular Approach

This route is used in patients who have difficulties in IVC access like IVC interruption.[5]

Right internal jugular venous and right radial arterial accesses are obtained, and pulmonary angiography is performed in a 45° right anterior oblique view to acquire a levophase image of the left atrium. Transjugular septal puncture is performed in the same view using an Endrys pediatric transseptal set (Cook™). The atrial septum is punctured the fossa ovalis about 2 cm below the roof of the left atrium, and midway between the aorta and the anterior border of the spine. Bulging of the atrial septum toward the right facilitates obtaining a catch with the needle prior to puncture at the desired location on the septum. A 14 Fr, 20 cm long, J-shaped sheath with a hemostatic valve is inserted into the left atrium, and the mitral valve is crossed using a balloon-floatation catheter. A 0.035 inch Amplatz wire with a large soft J-tip (Cook™) is placed in the left ventricular apex, and valvuloplasty is performed after introducing a JOMIVA balloon through the left atrial sheath.

Reports describing large number of patients who underwent this technique reveals that PMV with JOMIVA balloon is safe and effective and the results are comparable to Inoue balloon technique.[1,2]

◼ REFERENCES

1. Joseph G, Chandy S, George P, George O, John B, Pati P, et al. Evaluation of a simplified transseptal mitral valvuloplasty technique using over-the-wire single balloons and complementary femoral and jugular venous approaches in 1,407 consecutive patients. J Invasive Cardiol. 2005;17:132–8.
2. Routray SN, Mishra TK, Patnaik UK, Behera M. Percutaneous transatrial mitral commissurotomy by modified technique using a JOMIVA balloon catheter: a cost-effective alternative to the Inoue balloon. J Heart Valve Dis. 2004;13(3):430–8.
3. Uruchurtu E, Sánchez A, Solís H, Hernández I, García F, Vázquez A, et al. Immediate results in percutaneous mitral valvuloplasty with the Nucleus balloon. Arch Inst Cardiol México. 2000;70(5):486–91.
4. Angeles-Valdés J, Uruchurtu Chavarin E, Gómez Cruz A. Mitral valvuloplasty: the double balloon technique compared with the "Nucleus" single balloon technique. Arch Cardiol México. 2002;72(4):290–6.
5. Jose J, Kumar V, Joseph G. Transjugular balloon mitral valvotomy in a patient with inferior vena-caval interruption. JACC Cardiovasc Interv. 2012;5(2):243–4.

Chapter 26

Other Gadgets for Percutaneous Mitral Valvotomy

Mohammad A Sherif, Harikrishnan S

In addition to the Inoue balloon, double balloon and metallic commissurotome, there are few other devices available and are in use in different parts of the world. They include the Multi-Track system, Nucleus balloon and its modification, the JOMIVA balloon. The detailed description of JOMIVA balloon is given in the Chapter 25.

■ MULTI-TRACK SYSTEM

The Multi-Track system for PMV was developed by Bonhoeffer et al[1] in France with preliminary results of the first 12 patients published in 1995.

Description of the Device

The Multi-Track system is developed and marketed by NuMED, Inc., Hopkinton, New York, USA. The kit for mitral dilatation is made of 5 components; two balloon catheters, a Multi-Track angiographic catheter, a guidewire and a septal dilator. The guidewire system consists of two separate wires welded at the distal end to form a single wire. The system allows loading two balloon catheters on the same wire. The Multi-Track balloon has a 10 cm nylon plastic shaft and a Multi-Track tip of only 1 cm at the tip [(14, 16, 18 or 20 mm in diameter) × 5 cm in length]. The other balloon catheter is a matched standard monorail balloon catheter.[1]

Selection of the Size of the Balloon Catheters

The sum of the diameters of the two balloons is chosen to be 90–100% of the measured mitral annulus.[2]

Technique

The Multi-Track system is a refinement of the double balloon technique, as it uses a monorail system, but requiring only one guidewire thus easing the procedure compared to the standard double balloon technique (Figs 26.1 and

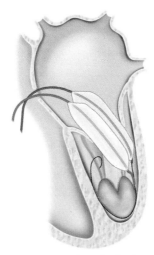

Fig. 26.1: The Multi-Track system across the mitral valve with both balloons inflated (With permission from NuMED, Inc., Hopkinton, New York, USA)

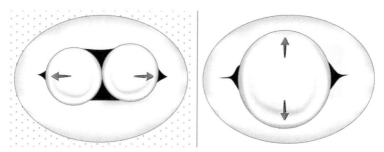

Fig. 26.2: The double balloon system's advantage over the single balloon system. The double balloon will theoretically orient towards the commissures better than the single balloon (With permission from NuMED, Inc., Hopkinton, New York, USA)

26.2). The first steps are almost similar to those done with the Inoue balloon till the step of transseptal puncture. Thereafter a balloon end-hole catheter is introduced into the left atrium through the Mullins sheath. Before passing through the mitral valve, the balloon catheter is inflated in order to avoid its entrapment in the subvalvular apparatus. The mitral valve is then catheterized either directly orienting the catheter slightly anteriorly or by a more indirect approach allowing the catheter to form a large loop in the left atrium. After the balloon catheter is passed through the mitral valve, it is advanced to the apex of the left ventricle and the catheter is then straightened. Then the superstiff preformed 0.035 guidewire is positioned in the left ventricle through the balloon catheter.

The skin and the atrial septum are then dilated with a 14 F long dilator, and then the balloons are loaded onto the guidewire. Initially the first Multi-Track balloon is introduced through the atrial septum and positioned across

Table 26.1: Global results of mitral commissurotomy using the Multi-Track technique between June 1994 and February 2000[3]

	Age (years)	Weight (kg)	score	Area (cm²)		LAP (mm Hg)	
				Pre	Post	Pre	Post
Min.	10	19	3	0.3	1.2	10	2
Max.	86	80	13	1.4	3.1	52	26
Mean	30 ± 12	49 ± 14	8 ± 2	0.75 ± 22	2 ± 0.39	27 ± 8	11 ± 5

the mitral valve. The second balloon is then advanced over the wire and lined up with the first one in the mitral valve. More than half of the balloon length should be positioned in the left ventricle before inflation.[1] Then the balloons are inflated simultaneously under fluoroscopic vision. After deflation the balloons are sequentially removed under fluoroscopic guidance.[1]

In August 2000, Bonhoeffer et al[3] reported the results of 153 patients from 16 centers across all continents (Table 26.1).

Only four patients had a significant increase in mitral regurgitation, two of them needing surgery. In the remaining two patients, there was a progressive clinical improvement.[3] Hemopericardium occurred in four (2.6%) occasions, twice due to trans-septal puncture and twice due to wire perforation of the left ventricular apex. In all cases hemopericardium was successfully drained. Neither thromboembolic nor infectious complications occurred. The technique showed no mortality and demonstrated a low morbidity.[3]

Another advantage of the system is the ability to simultaneously measure the pressure in the left atrium and left ventricle. This can be accomplished by the simultaneous use of two Multi-Track™ catheters, one kept in LV and the other kept in the LA which can be introduced over the Multi-Track wire.

Tariq Ashraf et al. have suggested two modifications to the conventional Multi-Track technique to reduce the complications of MR and LV apical perforation. They hypothesized that the reason for apical perforation was due to the exchange catheter which when inflated the tip of the catheter get erected and caused trauma to left ventricular apex. They have suggested a new algorithm to select the appropriate balloon based on body surface area and also suggested for the placement of wire in the ascending aorta/aortic arch which can prevent the dreadful complication of apical ventricular rupture.[4]

■ NUCLEUS™ BALLOON

This catheter is developed and marketed by NuMED, Hopkinton, New York, USA. The use of this catheter is particularly indicated in stenosis where difficulty is experienced in positioning the balloon across the valve. The NUCLEUS and the new NUCLEUS-X™ balloon valvuloplasty catheter with its coaxial shaft design provides enhanced column strength and pushability combined with a flexible distal tip for optimum steerability (Fig. 26.3). Initial inflation will hold balloon in the desired position, further inflation expands

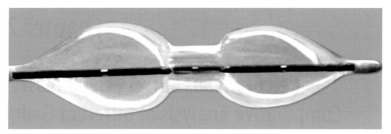

Fig. 26.3: The Nucleus-X balloon
(With permissions from NuMED, Inc., Hopkinton, New York, USA)

the center of the balloon to effect satisfactory dilatation. Platinum marker bands facilitate reliable positioning of the balloon and are located at the 'waist' center and beneath the shoulders of the balloon for clear identification under fluoroscopy.

The Nucleus-X balloon is available in sizes from 18 mm to 30 mm with balloon lengths varying from 4 to 6 centimeters. The shaft size is 9 French, the usable length is 110 cm and the guidewire is 0.035 inches. The introducer sizes vary from 10 to 14 French depending on the size of the balloon.

There are few reports about the use of this balloon from Mexico. The authors report that the Nucleus balloon technique is simpler than double balloon technique and much cheaper than Inoue balloon technique and they claim it is useful in moderately calcified valves.[5] In a comparative study of 15 patients each using the Double balloon technique and Nucleus balloon technique, the Nucleus balloon group performed better.[6]

■ REFERENCES

1. Bonhoeffer P, Piéchaud JF, Sidi D, Yonga G, Jowi C, Joshi M, et al. Mitral dilatation with the Multi-Track system: an alternative approach. Cathet Cardiovasc Diagn. 1995;36(2):189–93.
2. Bonhoeffer P, Esteves C, Casal U, Tortoledo F, Yonga G, Patel T, et al. Percutaneous mitral valve dilatation with the Multi-Track System. Catheter Cardiovasc Interv Off J Soc Card Angiogr Interv. 1999;48(2):178–83.
3. Bonhoeffer P, HA, Yonga G, Yuko-jowi C, Aggoun Y, Saliba Z, Ferreira B, Sidi D, Kachaner J. Technique and results of percutaneous mitral valvuloplasty with the Multi-Track System. Journal of Interventional Cardiology 2000;13:263–8.
4. Asharf T, Memon MA, Rasool SI, Patel N, Panhwar Z, Farooq F, et al. Preventive strategies to fight complications during percutaneous multitrack balloon valvotomy "refining the technique."J Ayub Med Coll Abbottabad JAMC. 2014;26(3):357–60.
5. Uruchurtu E, Sánchez A, Solís H, Hernández I, García F, Vázquez A, et al. [Immediate results in percutaneous mitral valvuloplasty with the Nucleus balloon]. Arch Inst Cardiol México. 2000;70(5):486–91.
6. Angeles-Valdés J, Uruchurtu Chavarin E, Gómez Cruz A. [Mitral valvuloplasty. The double balloon technique compared with the "Nucleus" single balloon technique]. Arch Cardiol México. 2002;72(4):290–6.

Chapter 27

Percutaneous Mitral Valvuloplasty— Comparative Analysis of Different Gadgets

Mohammad A Sherif

Comparison of different gadgets used for PMV should be done by comparing the acute and the long-term results of the procedure. The acute results of PMV in the catheterization laboratory can be assessed using invasive hemodynamics or echocardiography. The following criteria have been proposed for the desired end-point of the procedure: valve area >1 cm^2/m^2 BSA; complete opening of at least one commissure in the absence of more than moderate mitral regurgitation. Post-procedure, the most accurate evaluation of valve area is given by echocardiography using planimetry method. The assessment of mitral regurgitation (MR) is usually done by Doppler color flow.

The only study in the literature that compared all the techniques of PMV was conducted by Sherif et al.[1] In this meta-analysis double balloon technique (DBT), was the commonest gadget used—1148 patients (51%). This was followed by the Inoue balloon technique (IBT) in 914 patients (40.5%), the metallic commissurotome (PMMC) in 142 patients (6%), the Multi-Track system in 33 patients (1.5%), and finally the single balloon technique in 19 patients (1%). The Multi-Track system and the DBT resulted in the largest MVA, the IB and the single balloon resulted in the least increase in MR. The most common complication following PMV was the increase in MR.

El-Sayed et al.[2] reported the first comparative study between IBT, DBT, and PMMC. The three groups were comparable except for the echocardiography score, which was higher in the PMMC group. They found that MVA increased in the three groups, from 0.92 cm^2 to 2.1 ± 0.5 cm^2 with PMMC, from 0.91 ± 0.26 to 1.87 cm^2 with the Inoue balloon, and from 0.94 ± 0.2 to 2.04 with the double balloon (P < 0.0001). The final mitral valve area was significantly larger after PMMC and DBT than after the IBT. Complete split of both commissures were obtained in 60% after PMMC, 50% after double-balloon dilation, and only 20% after Inoue balloon.

There are three large studies comparing the safety and efficacy of different PMV techniques. Arora et al.[3] reported that in their series, DBT was used in 320 patients (6.6%), IBT had the major share being used in 4, 374 patients (90.2%), while the metallic valvulotome was used only in 156 (3.2%) patients. Iung et al.[4]

in their experience of 1024 patients, used Inoue Balloon in 608 patients (59%), the double balloon in 390 patients (38%), and single balloon in 26 patients (2.5%). Chen et al.[5] used only Inoue balloon technique in one of the largest reports of PMV which included 4,832 patients.

In spite of the safety, efficacy and applicability of the IBT, the DBT took the upper hand in the meta-analysis conducted by Sherif et al.,[1] reflecting the importance of economic issues in technique selection. The double balloon set is cheaper, more re-usable and thus much more economic. Although this was intended to be the case for the metallic commissurotome, it represented only 6%, reflecting the fact that this technique is more demanding on the operator than other techniques with a higher incidence of complications.

The IBT differs from the Multi-Track or the double-balloon technique in several important aspects. The dilating shape achieved in the Inoue balloon is circular and different from the elliptic dilating shape achieved in the double-balloons. It is not known whether different dilating shapes produce differences in extent of commissurotomy and whether that might result in different incidences of restenosis and cardiac events.

As regards the increase in mitral valve area (MVA) and the drop in mean trans-mitral pressure gradient (MPG), Sherif et al.[1] found that the Multi-Track system resulted in the largest change in the above mentioned parameters, compared to other techniques. On the other hand, single balloon technique resulted in the smallest change in comparison to all other modalities. Moreover, there were no significant differences among double balloon, Inoue balloon and metallic commissurotome. Regarding increase in MR, it was found that the Multi-Track system resulted in the largest post-PMV increase in the grade of MR. The smallest increase in MR was found with Inoue balloon technique. Moreover, there was no significant difference among double balloon, single balloon and metallic commissurotome regarding the development of significant MR.

▪ INOUE VERSUS DOUBLE BALLOON

Several studies, both randomized and non-randomized, compared IBT to the DBT.[6-9] The analysis of such data leads to the conclusion that the DBT provides a higher final MVA and higher absolute increase of the MVA than the IBT.[10,11] But DBT is a more difficult technique, with a higher complication rate.[10]

Inoue, single and double-balloon techniques have been compared, with the latter demonstrating a larger MVA with a lower incidence of mitral regurgitation. However, the Inoue balloon remains more commonly used because of its ease of use.[8,12]

With double balloons, the dilated mitral valve opening is more oval than the circular shape seen after the use of a single balloon. This may be explained by the fact that the tension applied to the plane of the mitral commissures is twice the tension applied vertically (according to Laplace law) during double-balloon inflation.[9] In contrast, the dilating forces of the Inoue balloon are radially applied to the crescent-shaped mitral orifice, with equal force applied to the free leaflet tissue and the fused commissures, resulting in a less effective splitting of the fused commissures and a greater risk of rupturing the leaflets, the weakest structure of the mitral valve apparatus.[9]

Abdullah et al.[13] compared the results in 60 consecutive patients with severe rheumatic mitral stenosis, who underwent double-balloon PMV by means of a combination of two 20 mm balloon catheters with a similar group of 60 consecutive patients who underwent Inoue balloon mitral commissurotomy. After PMV the hemodynamic measurements showed significant improvement in both groups. There was no significant difference between the groups with regard to clinical or hemodynamic improvement, technical failure rate, inadequacy of dilatation, or complications. However, the DBT was more complex and involved a longer fluoroscopy time.

Trevino et al.[6] compared the immediate results and 2-year follow-up of PMV using the IBT and DBT. The final MVA was 2.0 ± 0.43 cm^2 after IBT and 2.06 ± 0.51 cm^2 after DBT (p = NS). Technical difficulties and complications were more frequent with DBT (16% versus 3.8%; p < 0.001). Severe MR (grade III to IV) occurred in 4.6% of IBT and 4.1% of DBT (p = NS), whereas grade 1 MR was greater with IBT (21% versus 10.2%; p = 0.01). They concluded that there is no significant difference between both techniques with regards to the results and complications.

Bassand et al.[14] compared the immediate hemodynamic results of PMV in two consecutive series of unselected patients from the same institution undergoing valvuloplasty with the double-balloon (161 patients) or the Inoue balloon (71 patients) technique. They found that the magnitude of increase in MVA during percutaneous mitral valvuloplasty did not differ significantly in the Inoue balloon and double-balloon series (1.1 ± 0.2 to 1.95 ± 0.5 and 1.0 ± 0.2 to 1.97 ± 0.5 cm^2 respectively for MVA and 12 ± 3 to 5 ± 2 and 13 ± 4 to 5 ± 2 mm Hg respectively, for mean mitral gradient).

Leon et al.[12] compared the immediate procedural and long-term outcomes of patients undergoing PMV using the IBT und DBT. The DBT resulted in superior immediate outcome, as reflected in a larger post-procedural MVA (1.9 ± 0.7 versus 1.7 ± 0.6 cm^2) and a lower incidence of 3+ MR after PMV (5.4% versus 10.6%). This superior immediate outcome of the DBT was observed only in the group of patients with echocardiographic score ≤8 (post-PMV mitral valve area 2.1 ± 0.7 versus 1.8 ± 0.6). They concluded that, despite the difference in immediate outcome, there were no significant differences in event-free survival at long-term follow-up between the 2 techniques. Compared with the IBT, the DBT resulted in a larger MVA and less degree of severe mitral regurgitation.

Zhang et al.[7] compared the follow-up results of Inoue balloon and double-balloon techniques. They concluded that balloon selection did not appear to influence the clinical outcome at follow-up.

Kang et al.[15] conducted a prospective, randomized trial comparing two procedures in 302 consecutive patients using Inoue or double-balloon technique. They found no significant differences between both techniques in terms of commissural splitting, commissural mitral regurgitation, moderate to severe MR and MVA after PMV. They compared clinical and echocardiographic results of the Inoue balloon and the double-balloon technique for up to eight years, and demonstrated that the Inoue and double-balloon methods resulted in similar long-term outcomes in terms of survival, cardiac events and echocardiographic restenosis. Similar findings were reported by Bugliani et al. also.[16]

■ INOUE BALLOON TECHNIQUE VERSUS PERCUTANEOUS METALLIC COMMISSUROTOMY

Zaki et al.[17] compared the safety, efficacy, and cost of the percutaneous metallic commissurotome with the results of IBT in 80 patients with mitral stenosis (MS). The mean increase in MVA was 0.95 ± 0.19 to 1.7 ± 0.35 cm^2 for metallic commissurotome and 0.97 ± 0.15 to 1.81 ± 0.36 cm^2 for Inoue balloon. They found that bilateral commissural splitting was significantly more common with percutaneous metallic commissurotome than with Inoue balloon (30/39 patients, 76.9%, versus 21/40 patients, 52.5%). Post-procedural severe MR occurred in 1/39 (2.6%) in the percutaneous metallic commissurotome group and in 4/41 (9.8%) in the Inoue balloon group. Because the percutaneous metallic commissurotome device is re-sterilizable, they estimated the cost to be one-fourth the cost of Inoue balloon.

Guerios et al.[18] prospectively randomized 41 patients with rheumatic MS to PMV using the IBT or the PMMC. The success rate was 100 percent in the IBT group and 95 percent in the PMMC group. One patient in the PMMC group developed MR grade 3/4 requiring elective valve replacement. They found that the PMMC provides a significant larger immediate MVA than the IBT, but this difference is no longer significant after a short-term follow- up. Possible explanations include elastic recoil of an initially stretched mitral valve annulus or a more intense inflammatory response. However, PMMC was found superior to IBT in terms of cost-effectiveness.

Left ventricular perforation is very rare with the Inoue balloon catheter because of its low profile and the fact that there is no need for a guidewire in the left ventricle. Furthermore, because of the nature of the Inoue balloon catheter, it always pulls itself away from the apex of the left ventricle towards the mitral valve and maintains its position at the mitral valve orifice during inflation.[19] Therefore, the patient rarely runs the risk of left ventricular perforation by the Inoue balloon catheter. On the other hand, the use of a double balloon catheter or the metallic commissurotome in a patient with a small left ventricle predisposes to left ventricular perforation, especially if the operator was unable to maintain the curled guidewire in the left ventricular apex.[20]

Table 27.1: Immediate and late results reported by Bhat et al.[21]

	IB	*PMMC*	*p value*
MVA pre (cm^2)	0.88+/−0.18	0.89+/−0.19	P = NS
MVA post (cm^2)	1.7+/−0.29	1.86+/−0.34	P = 0.01
MVA (Follow-up) (cm^2)	1.7+/−0.38	1.80+/−0.31	P = NS

Sherif et al.[1] found that the comparison between Inoue balloon technique and PMMC revealed a higher complication rate in PMMC patients (42.5% versus 7%), in contrast to the results of Zaki et al.[17] who found comparable complication rates.

The largest randomized study comparing Inoue balloon and PMMC was reported by Bhat et al. where they randomly performed the procedure in 50 patients each.[21] They found both procedures gave similar procedural success and had similar complication rates.

They also found that PMMC produced larger mitral valve area immediate post-procedure compared to IBT. But at three months, the difference disappeared. The immediate and late results are detailed in Table 27.1.

Guerios et al. has reported similar findings. The mean final MVA was bigger in the PMMC group (2.17 ± 0.13 versus 2.00 ± 0.36 cm^2), but after 6-month and 3-year follow-up, this difference was no longer significant (2.06 ± 0.27 versus 1.98 ± 0.38 cm^2, and 1.86 ± 0.32 versus 1.87 ± 0.34 cm^2 respectively). This finding suggests stretching of the valve is an important mechanism of improvement in valve area with PMMC.

Krishnakumar et al. from India has reported a comparison between the triple lumen Inoue balloon with the double lumen Accura balloon.[22] They have compared the data of 487 patients who underwent PMV with Accura balloon was compared with 329 patients who underwent the procedure with Inoue balloon and found that both are equally effective and safe in terms of immediate and long term outcomes.[22]

From the above data we can conclude that techniques like PMMC and DBT produce better hemodynamic results compared to IBT. But IBT is an easier and a relatively safer procedure compared to other techniques. The learning curve for IBT is also better than others. But when it comes to cost- effectiveness, other techniques scores over IBT. But with the availability of "Inoue like" balloons (e.g. Accura), this technique may become cost- effective also.

■ REFERENCES

1. Sherif MA, Khashaba AA, Gomaa Y, Khaled S, Refaie O, Ramzy A. Pooled analysis of percutaneous mitral valvuloplasty in Egypt. Catheter Cardiovasc Interv Off J Soc Card Angiogr Interv. 2009;73(3):419–25.
2. El Sayed MA, Anwar AM. Comparative study between various methods of percutaneous transvenous mitral commissurotomy; metallic valvulotome, Inoue balloon and, double balloon techniques (VID) study. J Interv Cardiol. 2000;13:357-64.
3. Arora R, Kalra GS, Singh S, Mukhopadhyay S, Kumar A, Mohan JC, et al. Percutaneous transvenous mitral commissurotomy: immediate and long-term follow-up results. Catheter Cardiovasc Interv Off J Soc Card Angiogr Interv. 2002;55(4):450-6.
4. Iung B, Garbarz E, Michaud P, Helou S, Farah B, Berdah P, et al. Late results of percutaneous mitral commissurotomy in a series of 1024 patients. Analysis of late clinical deterioration: frequency, anatomic findings, and predictive factors. Circulation. 1999;99(25):3272-8.

5. Chen CR, Cheng TO. Percutaneous balloon mitral valvuloplasty by the Inoue technique: a multicenter study of 4832 patients in China. Am Heart J. 1995;129(6):1197–203.

6. Trevino AJ, Ibarra M, Garcia A, Uribe A, de la Fuente F, Bonfil MA, et al. Immediate and long-term results of balloon mitral commissurotomy for rheumatic mitral stenosis: comparison between Inoue and double-balloon techniques. Am Heart J. 1996;131(3):530–6.

7. Zhang HP, Gamra H, Allen JW, Lau FY, Ruiz CE. Comparison of late outcome between Inoue balloon and double-balloon techniques for percutaneous mitral valvotomy in a matched study. Am Heart J. 1995;130(2):340–4.

8. Park SJ, Kim JJ, Park SW, Song JK, Doo YC, Lee SJ. Immediate and one-year results of percutaneous mitral balloon valvuloplasty using Inoue and double-balloon techniques. Am J Cardiol. 1993;71(11):938–43.

9. Ruiz CE, Zhang HP, Macaya C, Aleman EH, Allen JW, Lau FY. Comparison of Inoue single-balloon versus double-balloon technique for percutaneous mitral valvotomy. Am Heart J. 1992;123(4 Pt 1):942–7.

10. Rihal CS, Holmes DR Jr. Percutaneous balloon mitral valvuloplasty: issues involved in comparing techniques. Cathet Cardiovasc Diagn. 1994;Suppl 2:35–41.

11. Ribeiro PA, Fawzy ME, Arafat MA, Dunn B, Sriram R, Mercer E, et al. Comparison of mitral valve area results of balloon mitral valvotomy using the Inoue and double balloon techniques. Am J Cardiol. 1991;68(6):687–8.

12. Leon MN, Harrell LC, Simosa HF, Mahdi NA, Pathan AZ, Lopez-Cuellar J, et al. Comparison of immediate and long-term results of mitral balloon valvotomy with the double-balloon versus Inoue techniques. Am J Cardiol. 1999;83(9):1356–63.

13. Abdullah M, Halim M, Rajendran V, Sawyer W, al Zaibag M. Comparison between single (Inoue) and double balloon mitral valvuloplasty: immediate and short-term results. Am Heart J. 1992;123(6):1581–8.

14. Bassand JP, Schiele F, Bernard Y, Anguenot T, Payet M, Ba SA, et al. The double-balloon and Inoue techniques in percutaneous mitral valvuloplasty: comparative results in a series of 232 cases. J Am Coll Cardiol. 1991;18(4):982–9.

15. Kang DH, Park SW, Song JK, Kim HS, Hong MK, Kim JJ, et al. Long-term clinical and echocardiographic outcome of percutaneous mitral valvuloplasty: randomized comparison of Inoue and double-balloon techniques. J Am Coll Cardiol. 2000;35(1):169–75.

16. Bugliani-Pastalka L, Bugliani G, Suter T, Mandinov L, Jenni R, Hess OM. Long-term results after successful mitral valvuloplasty: comparison of Inoue and double balloon technique. Schweiz Med Wochenschr. 2000;130(35):1216–24.

17. Zaki AM, Kasem HH, Bakhoum S, Mokhtar M, El Nagar W, White CJ, El Guindy M. Comparison of early results of percutaneous metallic mitral commissurotome with Inoue balloon technique in patients with high mitral echocardiographic scores. Catheter Cardiovasc Interv. 2002;57:312-7.

18. Guérios EE, Bueno RRL, Nercolini DC, Tarastchuk JCE, Andrade PMP, Pacheco ALA, et al. Randomized comparison between Inoue balloon and metallic commissurotome in the treatment of rheumatic mitral stenosis: immediate results and 6-month and 3-year follow-up. Catheter Cardiovasc Interv Off J Soc Card Angiogr Interv. 2005;64(3):301–11.

19. Cheng TO. Percutaneous balloon mitral valvuloplasty: are Chinese and western experiences comparable? Cathet Cardiovasc Diagn. 1994;31(1):23–8.

20. Ruiz CE, Allen JW, Lau FY. Percutaneous double balloon valvotomy for severe rheumatic mitral stenosis. Am J Cardiol. 1990;65(7):473–7.

21. Bhat A, Harikrishnan S, Tharakan JM, Titles T, Kumar VK, Sivasankaran S, Bimal F, Krishnamoorthy KM. Comparison of percutaneous transmitral commissurotomy with Inoue balloon technique and metallic commissurotomy: immediate and short-term follow-up results of a randomized study Am Heart J 2002;144(6): 1074-80.

22. Nair KKM, Pillai HS, Thajudeen A, Tharakan J, Titus T, Valaparambil A, et al. Comparative study on safety, efficacy, and midterm results of balloon mitral valvotomy performed with triple lumen and double lumen mitral valvotomy catheters. Catheter Cardiovasc Interv Off J Soc Card Angiogr Interv. 2012;80(6):978–86.

Chapter 28

Reuse and Resterilization of PMV Hardware

Suji K, Sethu Parvathy VK

Percutaneous mitral valvotomy (PMV) is established as an effective treatment for mitral stenosis (MS) and is now the procedure of choice. There are different gadgets which are developed and now available for performing percutaneous mitral valvotomy.

However, the cost of the procedure, which results principally from the cost of the balloon catheter used, still remains a limitation to its application in developing countries with limited financial resources, which are, incidentally, those countries with the highest incidence of MS. Consequently, most centers in developing countries reuse these balloon catheters several times, although they are provided as disposable catheters; this introduces potential hazards because of imperfect sterilization and decreasing performance caused by the alteration of the balloon's mechanical properties.

The Inoue balloon has two vent holes that open between the 2 layers of balloon material. The holes are supposed to prevent deflation failure of the balloon. Blood creeps in between these layers during valvotomy, and it is extremely difficult to clear the balloon of this blood, which is a potential hazard for infection. The compliance of the balloon gets altered on repeated usage, leading to decreased efficacy and deflation failure.

Resterilization is practiced widely in the developing world[1-5] and also in the developed world.[6,7] There are several reports of the safe use of resterilized hardware for PMV from developing countries.[8,9] One mitral valvuloplasty balloon can be used safely in six patients after resterilization according to some reports. Devices like metallic commissurotome are intended for re-sterilization and reuse. There are reports of scores of cases done with single metallic commissurotome from different parts of the world.[8,9] There is no mention of device related infection is such reports.

But there are reports of device failure and complications following reuse of balloon catheters and hardware during PMV.[10-13] By careful quality control of resterilized equipment and proper selection of reused hardware, it is possible to safely reuse the hardware multiple times.

In this chapter we will discuss the various aspects of resterilization of PMV hardware.

■ METHODS OF STERILIZATION

The methods of resterilization available for the hardware used for PMV are:
1. Ethylene oxide (EtO) sterilization
2. Glutaraldehyde (CIDEX) sterilization.

Ethylene Oxide

Ethylene oxide (EtO) sterilization is used for products that cannot withstand heat. When the Inoue/Accura balloon catheter was resterilized with EtO, we noticed that the balloon (latex material) and its hub got damaged. Thus, we realized that it is not a good method for resterilizing the balloons.

The most important parameters in the EtO sterilization process are room humidity (RH), temperature and pressure. For EtO use, it is crucial to control RH and temperature within certain limits. Vacuum (pressure) is created to remove air prior to the introduction of EtO, to make sure the EtO gas permeates the product being sterilized.

A typical EtO sterilization cycle involves several stages and usually proceeds as follows:

Pre-conditioning: The product is exposed to a warm, humid environment for at least 12 hours (70% RH, 55°C) to ensure the product is at a uniform temperature and humidity.

Exposure: Vacuum is created and EtO gas is introduced. The product is exposed for 4 to 8 hours usually. During this process the RH is kept at approximately 70% and the temperature at 55°C.

Post-conditioning: The EtO gas is removed by repeatedly creating a vacuum and then introducing air into the sterilization chamber until the EtO gas is cleared out (8 to 12 hours).

It should be noted that generally there is a tremendous variation in exposure times and gas concentration between different hospitals.

The size of the sterilizers can range from small bench-top sterilizers to large sterilizing rooms. Because of problems with toxicity and risk of explosion, many hospitals are choosing to outsource this work rather than perform it themselves. EtO use is therefore becoming a very specialized method of sterilization. A large proportion of all medical devices are sterilized by the EtO method.

In the case of PMV hardware all the components are re-sterilized using EtO except the balloon. In case of Cribier's metallic commissurotome, all the components can be sterilized by using EtO.

Glutaraldehyde Sterilization

The mitral valvuloplasty balloon is resterilized using glutaraldehyde. Active ingredient is 2.45% Glutaraldehyde (Cidex™). The manufacturer's instructions

indicate that a minimum of 10 hours is required for sterilization. Cidex comes in two formulations, Cidex and Cidex-7 (long-life). The shelf-life of activated Cidex is 15 days and of activated Cidex-7 is 28 days. We use glutaraldehyde (Cidex) solution of concentration 2.45% and pH is maintained at 8.2 to 9.2. Maintenance of pH is very important as the efficacy of glutaraldehyde is compromised if there is any change in pH. The pH has to be checked periodically using glutaraldehyde titration method and concentration by Cidex test strips. The method of testing the glutaraldehyde solution is as follows:
- Completely submerge the indicating pads of the strips in the solution
- Hold for one second and remove. Do not shake the strip
- Remove excess solution by holding the strip upright on paper towel
- Read results strictly at 90 seconds
- Pads will be completely purple if it is an effective solution and will be blue if it is ineffective and if so the solution must be discarded.

For checking the pH, usual titration methods performed by chemists should be employed.

▦ RESTERILIZATION PROCESS OF THE PMV HARDWARE

- After the procedure the entire hardware including balloon is cleaned with saline
- All components are wiped and flushed with hydrogen peroxide (H_2O_2) which removes the blood and also kills the microorganisms. Balloon hub has a luer lock (female end) in which blood can stay back. Special care has to be taken here and this blood has to be thoroughly cleansed off
- Balloon contrast port has to be cleaned thoroughly to remove all traces of contrast, otherwise it can get solidified and may interfere with the balloon inflation and deflation mechanisms
- Flush out the residual H_2O_2 with distilled water
- All hardware with the exception of balloon are dried by blowing compressed air through the catheter lumen at a pressure 5.5 to 7 Bars
- Then the components are sealed in window pack, i.e. EtO sterilization pack (Westfield Medical Ltd, Norton). This is a porous pack which will allow the diffusion of EtO through it. Then the packets are send for EtO. (Amsco Steris™, Soma technology, Inc. Bloomfield, USA)
- Accura balloon is resterilized using glutaraldehyde solution.

The balloon is sterilized by immersing the balloon in a large glutaraldehyde tray measuring 100 cm (length) × 12 cm (height) × 15 cm (width) (Fig. 28.1). The balloon catheter is flushed in with cidex and fully immersed and kept in a Cidex tray for a minimum of 24 hours. Cidex solution has to be changed every 14 days. We change the glutaraldehyde solution every 10 days.

▦ STERILIZATION USING HYDROGEN PEROXIDE

Some of the PMV hardware can be sterilized by using H_2O_2. Hydrogen peroxide is strong oxidant and these oxidizing properties allow it to destroy a wide range of pathogens and it is used to sterilize heat or temperature sensitive articles. In medical sterilization hydrogen peroxide is used at higher concentrations, ranging from around 35% up to 90%. The biggest advantage of hydrogen peroxide as a sterilant is the short cycle time. Whereas the cycle time for ethylene oxide (discussed above) may be 10 to 15 hours, the use of very high concentrations of hydrogen peroxide allows much shorter cycle times. Some hydrogen peroxide modern sterilizers, such as the Sterrad NX have a cycle time as short as 28 minutes. Our hospital uses the STERRAD NX Sterilizer which sterilizes medical devices by diffusing hydrogen peroxide vapor into the chamber and then electromagnetically exciting the hydrogen peroxide molecules into a low-temperature plasma state. The combined use of hydrogen peroxide vapor and plasma safely and rapidly sterilizes medical instruments and materials without leaving toxic residues. All stages of the sterilization cycle operate within a dry environment at a low temperature, and thus the cycle is not damaging to compatible instruments sensitive to heat and moisture. The STERRAD NX Sterilizer can be used for both metal and nonmetal devices. Medical devices with materials and dimensions that can be processed in the STERRAD NX Sterilizer Advanced cycle:

- Single-channel stainless steel lumens with an inside diameter of 1 mm or larger and a length of 500 mm or shorter.
- Single-channel PTFE materials with an inside diameter of 1 mm or larger and a length of 850 mm or shorter.

The PMV hardware which can be sterilized with H_2O_2 systems are:

- LV entry stylet
- Balloon straightener
- Left atrial guidewire
- Caliper.

■ RESTERILIZATION OF INOUE BALLOON

Resterilization of Inoue balloon involves more steps since it has two vent holes on the outer latex layer through which blood can enter the space between the latex layers and can get embedded in the nylon mesh between the latex layers. Removal of this blood is pretty difficult and time consuming. This procedure has to be done within minutes after the removal of the balloon from the patient, otherwise cleaning off of the blood will be extremely difficult.

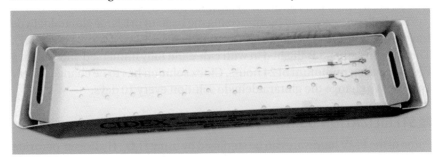

Fig. 28.1: Cidex (Glutaraldehyde) tray in which the Inoue balloons are sterilized

- A mixture of heparinized saline and 30% H_2O_2 is been used for this purpose as the 'cleaning mixture'
- Two technicians are required for this maneuver
- One person has to deflate the inflated balloon to create a negative pressure in the system with 50 mL syringe
- While the negative pressure is applied, the second person has to push the cleaning mixture into the balloon space through the side hole
- Then the other person has to inflate the balloon during which part of solution comes out of the balloon. We have to repeat this process about 20 times to fully evacuate the blood from the system. After this, the mixture of heparinized saline and H_2O_2 has to be removed by the same method with distilled water.

Quality Control

Quality control of the reused hardware is very important. The balloon and the other components of valvotomy system should be thoroughly checked before sending for resterilization. The operator should thoroughly check the balloon and other components for its integrity and effectiveness. The areas which we should carefully inspect are the LA wire at its junction of coiled and straight segment, tip of Brockenbrough needle and the tip of the balloon.

If we carefully inspect each component before reusing, it will definitely reduce the complications related to hardware reuse.

Economic Aspects of Reuse

The economic aspect of reuse of PMV hardware has been reported. In a group of patients with juvenile mitral stenosis, Harikrishnan et al. has compared the economic costs of Inoue balloon catheters (which were reused) to mechanical mitral commissurotomy. They could reuse Inoue balloons six times on an average with significant cost savings. The other components of the valvotomy hardware could also be re-used many times. At 40 months of follow-up, there was no evidence of infection or any problems related to reuse in any of their patients.

■ REFERENCES

1. Reuse of disposables in the catheterization laboratory. Report of the committee appointed by the Cardiological Society of India. Indian Heart J. 1997;49(3):329–31.
2. Unverdorben M, Degenhardt R, Erny D, Scholz M, Wagner E, Köhler H, et al. Clinical and angiographic procedural and mid-term outcome with new versus reused balloon catheters in percutaneous coronary interventions. Indian Heart J. 2005;57(2):114–20.
3. Zubaid M, Thomas CS, Salman H, Al-Rashdan I, Hayat N, Habashi A, et al. A randomized study of the safety and efficacy of reused angioplasty balloon catheters. Indian Heart J. 2001;53(2):167–71.
4. Plante S, Strauss BH, Goulet G, Watson RK, Chisholm RJ. Reuse of balloon catheters for coronary angioplasty: a potential cost-saving strategy? J Am Coll Cardiol. 1994;24(6):1475–81.

5. Mak KH, Eisenberg MJ, Eccleston DS, Brown KJ, Ellis SG, Topol EJ. Cost-efficacy modeling of catheter reuse for percutaneous transluminal coronary angioplasty. J Am Coll Cardiol. 1996;28(1):106–11.

6. Browne KF, Maldonado R, Telatnik M, Vlietstra RE, Brenner AS. Initial experience with reuse of coronary angioplasty catheters in the United States. J Am Coll Cardiol. 1997;30(7):1735–40.

7. Bathina MN, Mickelsen S, Brooks C, Jaramillo J, Hepton T, Kusumoto FM. Safety and efficacy of hydrogen peroxide plasma sterilization for repeated use of electrophysiology catheters. J Am Coll Cardiol. 1998;32(5):1384–8.

8. Harikrishnan S, Nair K, Tharakan JM, Titus T, Kumar VKA, Sivasankaran S. Percutaneous transmitral commissurotomy in juvenile mitral stenosis--comparison of long-term results of Inoue balloon technique and metallic commissurotomy. Catheter Cardiovasc Interv Off J Soc Card Angiogr Interv. 2006;67(3):453–9.

9. Harikrishnan S, Bhat A, Tharakan J, Titus T, Kumar A, Sivasankaran S, et al. Percutaneous transvenous mitral commissurotomy using metallic commissuro-tome: long-term follow-up results. J Invasive Cardiol. 2006;18(2):54–8.

10. Rao PS. Balloon rupture during valvuloplasty. Am Heart J. 1990;119(6):1441–2.

11. Lanjewar CP, Nathani PJ, Kerkar PG. Failure of deflation of an Inoue balloon during percutaneous balloon mitral valvuloplasty. J Intervent Cardiol. 2006;19(3):280–2.

12. Prabhakar D, Thirumalai P, Alagesan R. Valvuloplasty balloon detaching from the stem of a catheter. Indian Heart J. 2001;53(2):206–7.

13. Singla V, Patra S, Patil S, Ramalingam R. Accura balloon rupture during percutaneous trans-septal mitral commissurotomy: a rare and potentially fatal complication. BMJ Case Rep. 2013;2013.

Section 5

Complications Following PMV

Chapter 29

Device-related Complications during Percutaneous Mitral Valvotomy

Harikrishnan S

There are three major complications following PMV: (i) related to septal puncture, (ii) related to the development of mitral regurgitation, and (iii) embolic events. The complications related to these three will be dealt within other chapters.

In this chapter, we are going to deal with other complications related to the balloon devices.

■ BREAKAGE OF COILED LEFT ATRIAL (LA) WIRE

Breakage of the coiled tip of the left atrial stainless steel wire can occur rarely and complicate the PMV procedure. The LA wire has two parts—the distal thin (coiled part) and proximal thick portion. These two parts are welded together. We have seen many times that there is a tendency for the wire to break when the wire is re-used multiple times and the usual point of breakage is this junction. The micro-fractures occurring at this junction of the coiled LA wire may gradually lead to breakage of the wire. The wire may break and get detached and embolise during manipulation. This can be avoided by careful inspection of the junction of the coiled and straight portion of the wire before reuse.

There is another LA wire made of Nitinol (Accura™ PTMC System, Vascular Concepts) (Fig. 29.1), which is a tapering wire, made of a nitinol core extending up to the tip and a nitinol coil wound over the core in the floppy coiled part. The proximal portion of the ribbon is soldered to the main shaft. The soldering is said to be perfect without any bulge, i.e. the soldered portion is practically invisible as it flows along the wire. The use of this wire is thought to reduce this complication of wire breakage, but there are no reports confirming this.

Singh and Panchal have reported a case where the coiled part of the wire broke and remained in the left atrium (Figs 29.2 and 29.3). They tried the Gooseneck™ snare to retrieve the wire, but they were not able to retrieve the broken piece from the left atrium. Since the wire loop was too big, the routinely used snares were not able to catch the broken wire tip. So they had to fashion a snare out of a coronary angioplasty guidewire (.014 inch, 300 cm long) and

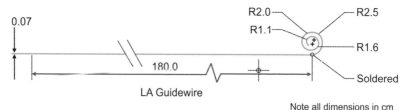

Fig. 29.1: Nitinol left atrial guidewire from vascular concepts

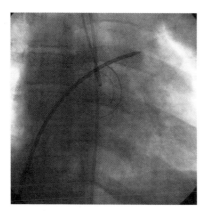

Fig. 29.2: Broken pigtail left atrial guidewire in the left atrium. Pigtail catheter in ascending aorta and Mullins sheath is also seen (*Courtesy:* Dr Parvinder Singh and Dr Falgun Panchal, Baroda Heart Institute and Research Center, India)

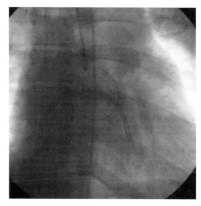

Fig. 29.3: Broken pigtail-shaped left atrial wire in the left atrium. Pigtail catheter in ascending aorta and a large 14 French Mullins sheath is seen (*Courtesy:* Dr Parvinder Singh and Dr Falgun Panchal, Baroda Heart Institute and Research Center, India)

a JR4 diagnostic coronary catheter. The coronary angioplasty guidewire was double looped through the distal end of the catheter to make a snare like loop, while the two working ends were withdrawn through the proximal end of the catheter. Using this snare, the catheter fragment was caught and retrieved and pulled back into a large 14 French sheath (Fig. 29.4). A similar case was reported by Ravindranath et al. who also used a snare fabricated with a coronary angioplasty guidewire.[1]

ENTRAPMENT OF THE PIGTAIL GUIDEWIRE

This is a very rare complication which is reported following PMV. Panneerselvam et al.[2] after successfully completing PMV, was attempting to slenderize the Accura™ mitral valvotomy balloon by passing the pigtail-shaped coiled LA wire. They encountered resistance while passing the balloon stretching tube. They found that the tip of the guidewire got entrapped between the inner balloon lumen and the balloon stretching tube.

But even with force, the slenderizing tube could not be withdrawn as the slenderizing tube was jammed within the lumen of balloon catheter due to friction caused by guidewire entrapment. When the guidewire was advanced further into balloon catheter, the loop kept on increasing (Figs 29.5 and 29.6). When the authors tried to pull out the guidewire or the straightening tube, resistance was encountered. They felt that further forceful withdrawal could potentially fracture the guidewire and hence no further attempt to withdraw the guidewire was made. As the balloon was already slenderized, they decided to pull the entire balloon catheter outside (Fig. 29.7). The problem anticipated was that, withdrawing of the balloon catheter in such a manner could remotely

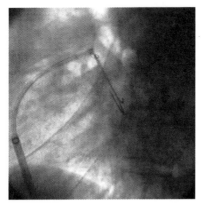

Fig. 29.4: The broken wire caught by the snare going to be pulled back into the large sheath (*Courtesy*: Dr Parvinder Singh and Dr Falgun Panchal, Baroda Heart Institute and Research Center, India)

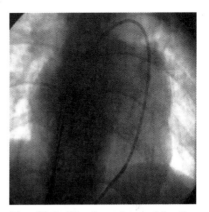

Fig. 29.5: The loop formed by the entrapped 0.025" BMV guidewire can be seen. The balloon catheter resembles a snare unit. The pigtail catheter in pericardium can also be seen (Published with permission, J Clinic Experiment Cardiol. 2011; 2:1)

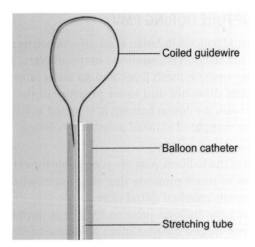

Fig. 29.6: Line diagram illustrating the entrapment of coiled PMV guidewire. The tip of the coiled guidewire can be seen to be stuck between the balloon catheter and balloon stretching tube (Published with permission, J Clinic Experiment Cardiol. 2011; 2:1)

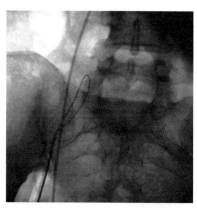

Fig. 29.7: Cine film demonstrating the withdrawal of the balloon catheter along with the looped guidewire from the femoral vein (Published with permission, J Clinic Experiment Cardiol. 2011, 2:1)

result in injury to the interatrial septum and femoral vein. But they succeeded in pulling out the balloon catheter, without manipulating the guidewire. There was no obvious injury to the septum or any other complications.

To prevent such complications, while introducing the guidewire, fluoroscopy should be done compulsorily. This complication can also be prevented by introducing an adequate length of the guidewire into the balloon catheter lumen before advancing the straightening tube. If any resistance is encountered while introducing the balloon stretching tube, further advancement should be avoided and fluoroscopy should be done to assess the cause of resistance. If the guidewire tip is stuck, then the guidewire along with the straightening tube should be withdrawn.

■ BALLOON RUPTURE DURING PMV

Abnormal or unusual balloon inflation is usually caused by a mesh breakage. The Inoue or Accura balloon is composed of three layers. There is an outer latex layer, an intermediate mesh layer, and an inner latex layer. The mesh regulates maximum diameter and inner pressure of the balloon. Due to presence of this mesh, the Inoue balloon is reported to have less incidence of tear and rupture compared to usual polythene balloons.

Mesh breakage may be caused by:
- Over-inflation of the balloon, past the acceptable inner balloon pressure.
- Rapid increase of inner pressure that may occur when the balloon is inflated in a heavily calcified mitral valve.

While preparing the balloon prior to PMV, it is important to note the following: (i) Do not exceed the maximum recommended inflation volume marked on the syringe provided with the balloon catheter, (ii) inject dilute contrast medium slowly to inflate the balloon during test inflations in order to avoid rapid stretching of the mesh layer.

Balloon rupture is a rare occurrence during PMV.[3-7] This happens more frequently in the developing world, where balloon catheters are reused. A deformity of the Inoue balloon catheter (Fig. 29.8) was noted in 4/264 procedures (1.6%) and actual rupture of deformed balloon occurred in one (0.4%) in a series reported by Ho et al.[5] All deformities were found at the distal portion of the Inoue balloon in this series. They have reported that following rupture of the balloon, none of the patients developed neither arterial embolization nor perforation of the cardiac chambers. Ho et al. warns that the deformity of the balloon may portend rupture of the balloon if maximal dilatations are undertaken subsequently.

Schilling et al.[4] reported two cases of balloon tear occurring in the proximal portion of the Inoue balloon. They reported that the rupture was associated with calcific valves.

Two problems which can occur subsequent to rupture of the balloon (Figs 29.9A and B) are: (i) The latex material or the wire mesh can get detached and embolize to the arterial system. Even though it is a possibility, it is not reported so far. (ii) If the contrast mix contains air, which occurs during preparing, it can embolize and produce air embolism in various organs. So when we prepare the balloon, we have to be doubly sure to avoid any air being trapped inside the balloon.

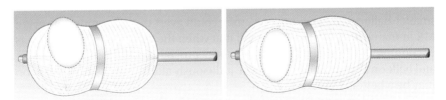

Fig. 29.8: Abnormal balloon dilatation due to mesh stretching
(Figure reproduced with kind permission from Toray Inc.)

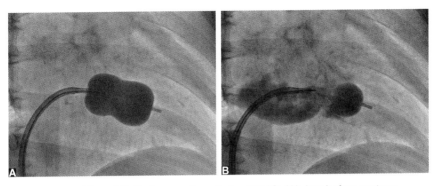

Figs 29.9A and B: Balloon rupture during PTMC: (A) Just before rupture;
(B) Just after rupture

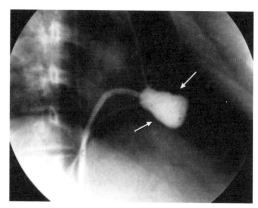

Fig. 29.10: Balloon impasse sign (*Courtesy*: Prof Yoav Turgeman)

BALLOON IMPASSE

In some cases of PMV, the Inoue catheter balloon, although deflated and properly aligned, becomes held up or checked at the mitral valve. This is referred as "balloon impasse" (Fig. 29.10). In a series of 760 patients undergoing the commissurotomy, Lau et al. observed this phenomenon in 13 patients. This is believed to reflect severe obstructive subvalvular disease.

Lau et al.[8] describes that this sign portends severe mitral regurgitation if the usual balloons sizing method is used. When they switched over to smaller balloons in such patients, they could avert the occurrence of severe MR in many. So they recommended that when the "balloon impasse" sign is encountered during the commissurotomy procedure, the catheter selection and balloon sizing method should be judiciously altered and a smaller balloon may be a better choice.

The same phenomenon was also reported by Dugal et al. in a patient who underwent emergency PMV.[9]

REFERENCES

1. Shankarappa RK, Panneerselvam A, Dwarakaprasad R, Nayak MH, Nanjappa MC. Removal of broken balloon mitral valvotomy coiled guidewire from giant left atrium using indigenous snare. Cardiovasc Interv and Ther. 2011;26:60-63.
2. Panneerselvam A, Bhat P, Nanjappa MC. Entrapment of guide wire—A preventable complication of balloon mitral valvotomy. J Clin Exp Cardiol [Internet]. 2011 [cited 2014 Apr 28];02(01). Available from: http://www.omicsonline.org/2155-9880/2155-9880-2-120.digital/2155-9880-2-120.html
3. Chow WH, Chow TC, Cheung KL. Angiographic recognition of a proximal balloon tear during Inoue balloon mitral valvotomy. Cathet Cardiovasc Diagn. 1993;28(3):235-7.
4. Schilling RJ, Francis CM, Shaw TR, Norell MS. Inoue balloon rupture during dilatation of calcified mitral valves. Br Heart J. 1995;73(4):390.
5. Ho YL, Chen WJ, Wu CC, Chao CL, Kao HL, Lee YT. Inoue balloon deformity and rupture during percutaneous balloon valvuloplasty. Cathet Cardiovasc Diagn. 1996;38(4):345-350; discussion 351.

6. Rao PS. Balloon rupture during valvuloplasty. Am Heart J. 1990;119(6):1441–2.
7. Singla V, Patra S, Patil S, Ramalingam R. Accura balloon rupture during percutaneous trans-septal mitral commissurotomy: a rare and potentially fatal complication. BMJ Case Rep. 2013.
8. Lau KW, Hung JS. Balloon impasse: a marker for severe mitral subvalvular disease and a predictor of mitral regurgitation in Inoue-balloon percutaneous transvenous mitral commissurotomy. Cathet Cardiovasc Diagn. 1995;35(4):310-9.
9. Dugal JS, Jetley V, Sabharwal JS, Sofat S, Singh C. Life-saving PTMC for critical calcific mitral stenosis in cardiogenic shock with balloon impasse. Int J Cardiovasc Intervent. 2003;5(3):172–4.

Chapter 30

Complications of Transseptal Puncture and Management

Harikrishnan S, Meera R

One of the important steps in percutaneous mitral valvotomy (PMV) is the transseptal puncture. The main complications of transseptal puncture are hemopericardium and cardiac tamponade. The interventional cardiologist should be able to identify the early signs of cardiac tamponade and act immediately. Otherwise the condition can be fatal.

In the presence of left or right atrial enlargement, the free wall enlarges while the interatrial septum is pushed relatively inferior. Therefore, the likelihood of a high septal puncture is enhanced in the presence of an enlarged left or right atrium. Transesophageal echocardiography or intracardiac echocardiography-guided (TEE or ICE) septal puncture can be helpful in avoiding this complication. The incidence of cardiac perforation has been reported to vary between 1.5% and 4.7% during mitral valvuloplasty.[1,2]

■ SUSPECTED PERICARDIAL TAMPONADE

Hemopericardium and cardiac tamponade are usually recognized during, or immediately after a catheter-based procedure. In a large series of emergency pericardiocentesis following invasive and interventional procedures from Mayo clinic,[3] 57% of patients had significant hemodynamic collapse and 17% needed cardiopulmonary resuscitation (CPR). Rarely, the presentation can be less dramatic, perforation could be inferred by confirmation of a new pericardial effusion by echocardiography.

The finding of a new pericardial effusion in association with acute hemodynamic instability during a catheter-based procedure provides sufficient impetus for rescue pericardiocentesis.

Tempe et al. reported that out of 45 patients who underwent emergency surgery following BMV, 8 were following cardiac tamponade. All of them underwent exploratory thoracotomy, evacuation of clots and repair of the defects which lead to tamponade. Four of them who did not undergo BMV, underwent CMV along with thoracotomy.[4]

It is mandatory to have an echocardiography system available in the cathlab to detect and manage this complication early. It is advisable to have a baseline echocardiographic assessment in the cathlab before the procedure as some patients can have mild pericardial effusion or some artefact like a fatpad which can mimic pericardial collection.

Patients who develop hemopericardium following transseptal puncture may experience chest pain accompanied by hypotension. Any unexplained hypotension following an attempt at transseptal puncture should alert the interventional cardiologist to rule out hemopericardium. When hemopericardium is suspected following septal puncture few points can be used to confirm it.

1. When we inject contrast after the needle puncture, if it spreads beyond the expected limits of the atrium we should suspect entry into the pericardial space.
2. There may be layering of contrast in the pericardial space which can be seen if watched closely by fluoroscopy.
3. Echocardiography is the gold standard to confirm.
4. Loss of cardiac pulsations as evidenced by the immobility of the left heart border and a pericardial halo seen in fluoroscopy are clues to the presence of hemopericardium.

▨ MANAGEMENT

1. When there is only a needle puncture—wait and watch—do not administer heparin. Since the needle prick produces only a small defect, it will close by itself without any sequelae. In such a situation, it is better to defer the valvotomy procedure and postpone it to a later date. If we are proceeding with PMV, we may have to heparinize the patient, which may trigger hemopericardium and even cardiac tamponade.
2. If the effusion is small and not increasing, and the balloon is in the left atrium, it is better to proceed with PMV, as it will reduce the LA pressure and reduce the leak.
3. If we have already dilated the septum using the septal dilator, before the hemopericardium was recognized, the defect already created in the visceral pericardium will be large. Usually such a defect may not close by itself. Also if the hemopericardium is recognized after performing the balloon dilatation, it is advisable to keep the dilator across the suspected defect, which will control the leak to some extent. So reintroduce the pigtail wire, pass the septal dilator and keep it there until the patient reaches the surgical theater.

    If routinely performed a procedure can recognize hemopericardium early. After dilating the septum, before giving heparin, wait for two minutes and perform a screening echocardiography in the PLAX view. This simple and easy step will almost always rule out the presence of hemopericardium and tamponade. A pericardial aspiration set should always be kept ready in the cathlab.
4. If there is significant pericardial collection and hemodynamic compromise, the next thing to do is pericardiocentesis and keep a pigtail catheter inside the pericardial space. After obtaining access to the pericardial space, the

position has to be confirmed. Most of the MS patients have a dilated thin-walled RV, which can be reached accidentally by the pericardial aspiration needle. For confirming the position in the pericardium, we need to pass a long guidewire and see its free movement in the pericardial space beyond the margins of any cardiac chamber. If the wire is in RV, it produces ventricular ectopic beats. Viewing the position of the wire in lateral or LAO view may be important in this regard. Connecting the needle to a pressure transducer is another way to confirm the position inside the pericardium.

Even after we have initiated pericardiocentesis and autotransfusion, the dilator needs to be kept in place till the patient is wheeled to the surgical theater, where the surgical team removes it when the patient is put on cardiopulmonary bypass (CPB). If we remove the dilator, it may result in massive ooze to the pericardium which can be catastrophic.

In the Mayo clinic series,[3] 99% of the patients had relief of tamponade by doing echocardiography guided pericardiocentesis. It is interesting to note that pericardiocentesis was the definitive procedure in 82% of them, though majority of them were electrophysiological (EP) procedures, which cannot be equated to PMV.

In the Mayo clinic series, the ideal entry site selected by 2D echocardiography was located on the chest wall in 62 (67%), while the subcostal position was identified as most suitable in only 22 (24%). Major complications in that series (3%) included pneumothorax (n = 1), right ventricular laceration (n = 1) and intercostal vessel injury with right ventricular laceration (n =1).

REVERSAL OF HEPARIN—PROTAMINE

Once cardiac tamponade is confirmed, it is advisable to reverse the effect of heparin by giving protamine. To calculate the dose required, first calculate the amount of heparin received in the previous 2 hours. The dose of protamine sulfate for reversal of heparin infusion

1. Protamine sulfate 1 mg per 100 units of heparin sodium (received in the previous 2 hours).
2. If the heparin infusion was stopped for more than 30 minutes but less than 2 hours, then use half the dose of protamine sulfate.
3. If the heparin infusion was stopped for greater than 2 hours, then use a quarter of the dose.

The maximum dose of protamine sulfate is 50 mg (single vial of the 50 mg/5 mL).

For reversal of heparin sodium 5000 units given subcutaneously:
- <2 hours: protamine sulfate 25 mg
- >2 hours: protamine sulfate 12.5 mg.

Inject the calculated dose of protamine sulfate into a 100 mL bag of 0.9% NaCl (saline). Run at 10 mL/min until completion of infusion. The patient should be monitored for evidence of hypersensitivity syndrome during and after the infusion. aPTT should be checked periodically to monitor the level of anticoagulation. Obtain blood 15 minutes after the completion of the infusion and check the aPTT to ensure satisfactory reversal. Rebound anticoagulation can occur so it would be prudent to monitor the aPTT every 4–6 hours for the next 24 hours.

■ AUTOTRANSFUSION

Acute cardiac tamponade requires immediate paracentesis pericardii and drainage. Direct retransfusion of the pericardial blood via the femoral venous sheath helps maintain blood pressure. In case of PMV, it is better to get another venous access as we will be using the venous access at the groin to keep the dilator across the pericardial rent. If we are not able to get another venous access, then the aspirated blood can be infused into the arterial line. But retransfusion of a large volume of pericardial blood may be associated with complications, such as air embolism, hemolysis or thromboembolism.

The salvaged blood can be collected, filtered with the autotransfusion apparatus and then antologously retransfused to the patient, which is called autotransfusion.[5] Autotransfusion is usually not associated with adverse events like cerebrovascular events, infection, hemolysis or fat embolism.

Although autotransfusion would decrease or eliminate the need for allogeneic transfusion during pericardiocentesis, it is not proven that autologous transfusion would decrease the need for surgical intervention.

Autotransfusion can be accomplished by specialized instruments—the aspirated blood can be transferred to the Cell Saver (Hemonetics, MA, USA) or the autotransfusion apparatus (Hemonetics, MA, USA) where the blood undergoes a washing process before resuspension in saline and is transferred to a sterile collection bag as packed RBCs at a hematocrit of 50–60%. The blood is then returned to the patient via a peripheral route.

The volumes of aspirated and autotransfused blood should be recorded to maintain adequate volume status in patients with mitral valve disease.

Some patients develop cardiac tamponade due to stitch phenomenon.[4] In patients with enlarged left atrium, there is no atrial septum in the region beyond or near the right lateral and inferior borders of the LA. The overlapping walls of RA and LA form this region. If this region is punctured, the catheter/needle may perforate the right atrial wall and then re-enter the LA (the so-called "stitching phenomenon") through the pericardial space (Fig. 30.1).[6] This is a dangerous situation as the blood enters the pericardial space both from LA and RA. So this complication needs to be tackled without delay by surgery.

The surgical management of the other complications arising out of PMV is detailed in Chapter 35.

■ THROMBUS FORMATION IN THE SEPTAL PUNCTURE SITE

Thrombus formation at the puncture site following PMV has been reported. Raman et al. have reported one case where they found a large thrombus attached to the IAS at the puncture site[7] (Fig. 30.2). The patient was managed with intensification of anticoagulation and the clot disappeared. We also had one case where we found a large clot the next day following BMV (Fig. 30.3).

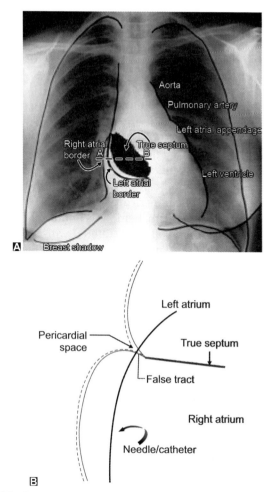

Figs 30.1A and B: Schematic diagram in frontal projection shows absence of true atrial septum near the lateral and inferior aspects of left atrial border. (B) Schematic diagram at plane AB; (A) Shows the path traversed by the catheter/needle from right atrium across pericardial space to left atrium (Published with permission from Vijay Trehan, et al. Novel nonsurgical method of managing cardiac perforation during percutaneous transvenous mitral commissurotomy. Indian Heart J. 2004;56:328-32)

She was offered surgery to remove the clot, but she refused. This patient was continued on heparin and the clot disappeared after 4 days without any complications. There is another case reported in the Turkish literature on a similar complication, but that patient had pericardial effusion in addition.[8]

The management of such patients is not clear. Since all the cases had the clot detected following a successful procedure, the surgery was only to remove the clot. But the danger of leaving a large intracardiac clot needs to be considered in making decisions in managing such patients.

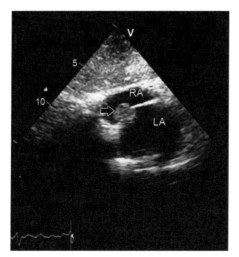

Fig. 30.2: Shows clot in the IAS following PMV.
Abbreviations: LA, left atrium; RA, right arium
(*Image Courtesy:* Padmakumar R, Professor of Cardiology, KMC, Manipal)

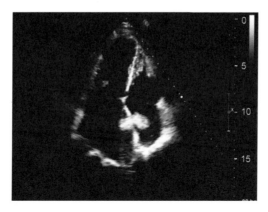

Fig. 30.3: Show clot at the septal puncture site visualized next day following BMV. Patient refused surgery, clot disappeared on heparinization without any sequelae

■ REFERENCES

1. Friedrich SP, Berman AD, Baim DS, Diver DJ. Myocardial perforation in the cardiac catheterization laboratory: incidence, presentation, diagnosis, and management. Cathet Cardiovasc Diagn. 1994;32:99-107.
2. Isner JM. Acute catastrophic complications of balloon aortic valvuloplasty. The Mansfield Scientific Aortic Valvuloplasty Registry Investigators. J Am Coll Cardiol. 1991;17:1436-44.
3. Teresa S M Tsang, William K Freeman, Marion E Barnes Ms, Guy S Reeder, Douglas L Packer, James B Seward. Rescue echocardiographically guided pericardiocentesis for cardiac perforation complicating catheter-based procedures-The Mayo Clinic Experience. JACC. 1998;32(5):1345-50.

4. Tempe DK, Gupta B, Banerjee A, Virmani S, Datt V, Marwah C, et al. Surgical interventions in patients undergoing percutaneous balloon mitral valvotomy: a retrospective analysis of anaesthetic considerations. Ann Card Anaesth. 2004;7(2):129–36.

5. Gao Ling-yun, Tang Ri-bo, Dong Jian-zheng, Liu Xing-peng, Long De-yong, Yu Rong-hui, et al. Autotransfusion in the management of cardiac tamponade occurring during catheter ablation of atrial fibrillation. Chinese Medical Journal 2010;123(7):961-3.

6. Trehan V, Mukhopadhyay S, Yaduvanshi A, Mehta V, Roy TNS, Nigam A, et al. Novel non-surgical method of managing cardiac perforation during percutaneous transvenous mitral commissurotomy. Indian Heart J. 2004;56(4):328–32.

7. Raman VG, Ramachandran P, Kansal N. An unusual complication of cardiac catheterisation during BMV. BMJ Case Rep. 2011.

8. Yüksel İÖ, Küçükseymen S, Çağırcı G, Arslan Ş. [A case of percutaneous mitral balloon valvuloplasty complicated by pericardial effusion and thrombus formation on the interatrial septum]. Türk Kardiyol Derneği Arş Türk Kardiyol Derneğinin Yayın Organıdır. 2014;42(8):747-50.

Chapter 31

Neurological Complications Related to Percutaneous Mitral Valvotomy

Sajith Sukumaran

Extensive experience has accumulated over several decades concerning the association of systemic embolism and rheumatic heart disease. According to pioneering observations,[1] a minimum of 20% of patients with rheumatic heart disease experience a thromboembolic complication at some time, and 40% of these arterial emboli involve the brain. Embolic events are the cause of death in 16–35% of adults dying of rheumatic heart disease. Embolism is most likely to occur when the dominant valvular lesion is that of mitral stenosis either alone or in combination with aortic valve disease or mitral insufficiency. Isolated aortic valve disease is rarely associated with embolic events.

Neurological complications are common consequences of invasive cardiac procedures including mitral valve surgery and catheter-based interventions and can limit the benefits of such procedures. These post-procedural complications are mainly in the form of stroke or hypoxic ischemic encephalopathy. Many more patients develop subtle, but permanent cognitive sequelae, which are most often left clinically under-recognized. Adverse cerebral outcomes significantly increase duration of hospital stay including intensive care. This is in addition to the subsequent morbidity and need for prolonged care and rehabilitation. Therefore, prevention of periprocedural neurological complications is of utmost importance.

▥ SYSTEMIC EMBOLISM IN PATIENTS WITH MITRAL STENOSIS

Mitral stenosis, the most common rheumatic valvular disease associated with embolic complications, is the valvular lesion most often treated by catheter-based interventions. Though early interventions help to prevent systemic embolism, the procedure has been associated with a small but significant risk of periprocedural embolic complications including embolic stroke. The risk of periprocedural stroke has been found to be 1.1–5.4% in different series.[2]

■ FACTORS ASSOCIATED WITH SYSTEMIC EMBOLIZATION

There are many important predictors of systemic embolism in patients with mitral stenosis with or without atrial fibrillation. Many studies have revealed that for patients in sinus rhythm, embolization was related to age, mitral valve area and left atrial dimensions. Coexistence of significant aortic regurgitation or left atrial thrombi predict high-risk of thromboembolism even in the absence of atrial fibrillation.[3]

For patients in atrial fibrillation, previous embolism is the most important predictor for subsequent events. Atrial fibrillation, age[4-6] and previous embolism[7] correlate with increased incidence of systemic embolism. Age, on its own merit, is closely related to the prevalence of atrial fibrillation[8] and to a history of embolization.[4-6] The risk conferred by left atrial smoky echoes [left atrial spontaneous echo contrast (LASEC)] by transesophageal echocardiography (TEE) has been controversial in different studies, irrespective of the presence of atrial fibrillation.[3,9] Cardiac catheterization in presence of an intracardiac thrombus seemingly increases the risk, however, data in this regard is largely lacking. Rarely, embolization of material from the mitral valve has been reported, which was confirmed by histopathology.[1]

▌ PERCUTANEOUS BALLOON MITRAL COMMISSUROTOMY AND SYSTEMIC EMBOLISM

Since its introduction in 1984 by Inoue et al., Percutaneous mitral balloon valvuloplasty (PMBV) has been accepted as an effective procedure for the treatment of severe mitral stenosis with immediate and short-term results comparable to those of surgical commissurotomy. Over the past years, several large series of patients undergoing PMV have demonstrated low rates of significant complications, such as perforation, tamponade, severe mitral regurgitation (MR), embolic strokes and death.[10-12]

Presently, percutaneous balloon mitral commissurotomy (PBMC) has become one of the standard, and often first-line treatment for patients with mitral stenosis.[13-17] It has been found to be a negative predictor of systemic embolism in patients with mitral stenosis in atrial fibrillation for the rest of their life.[3,18] The identification of PBMC as an independent negative predictor of systemic embolism favors the early use of this procedure in patients with mitral stenosis who are in atrial fibrillation. Because the procedure seemed to be an independent negative predictor, it would help patients, regardless of their anticoagulation status. Furthermore, earlier intervention may also be beneficial in patients in sinus rhythm as it delays or prevent the development of atrial fibrillation and systemic embolism. However, as mentioned before, the risk of periprocedural embolic stroke can be significant (in up to 1.1–5.4 %).

▌ PREVENTION OF CARDIOEMBOLIC STROKE IN RHEUMATIC MITRAL STENOSIS DURING PERCUTANEOUS MITRAL INTERVENTIONS

Anticoagulation reduces the incidence of systemic embolism in patients with mitral stenosis and atrial fibrillation. Anticoagulation may be prudent not only in patients in atrial fibrillation and patients with a previous systemic embolism but also in patients in sinus rhythm showing left atrial thrombi on echocardiography. Therefore, echocardiography should be carefully performed to look for any evidence of left atrial thrombus.

Early percutaneous balloon mitral commissurotomy may be another effective measure (regardless of anticoagulation status) to help prevent systemic embolism in patients with mitral stenosis. The incidence of embolic events can be favorably influenced by routine preprocedure transesophageal echocardiography (TEE), avoiding intervention in patients with left atrial thrombi.[2]

■ PERIPROCEDURAL STROKE AND TREATMENT OPTIONS

Timely detection of periprocedural stroke is probably the most important factor which determines the treatment outcome. Early detection, while the arterial sheath is still in situ, allows rapid access for intra-arterial thrombolysis. Presence of a cardiac in situ clot and its fragmentation and subsequent embolization has long been remained as a concern in the past, especially with intravenous thrombolysis. The embolic potential of cardiac thrombus may be directly related to duration of its formation, as recently formed poorly adherent thrombus is more likely to dislodge. The morphology of thrombus can also help to predict subsequent embolization. Thrombus protrusion and mobility are associated with an increased embolic risk.[19] It should, however, be emphasized that patients should not be denied the benefits of thrombolytic therapy and potential reduction in morbidity and mortality that can be achieved with this treatment, unless the associated risks are appreciable (Fig. 31.1).

There are reports where patients with cardiac thrombus were treated with intravenous thrombolytic therapy using tissue plasminogen activator (tPA) for acute ischemic stroke without further systemic embolic complications.[20] Patients who develop cerebral embolism as a result of dislodgement of embolic material from the aortic arch due to intra-arterial catheter manipulation or those who develop fresh intracardiac or catheter-related thrombus formation and subsequent cerebral embolism can be subjected to thrombolytic procedure without concern of thrombus fragmentation and systemic embolization. This complication can be further alleviated by the use of intra-arterial (mechanical rather than pharmacological) thrombolysis.

For patients fully heparinized for cardiac intervention, though intra-arterial mechanical thrombolysis (IAT - Mechanical) is a logical and effective treatment option, intracranial bleeding complications are always a concern. Achievement of recanalization without complication, to a great extend is related to the technique as well as the skill of the interventionist.

By eliminating the need for thrombolytics, mechanical thrombectomy has made endovascular treatment feasible in many circumstances in which intra-arterial thrombolysis (IAT) has been previously judged unsafe. In patients with in situ cardiac thrombus also, mechanical thrombectomy may prove to be a safe and effective option. The major disadvantages of endovascular recanalization techniques include relative complexity of the procedure, the

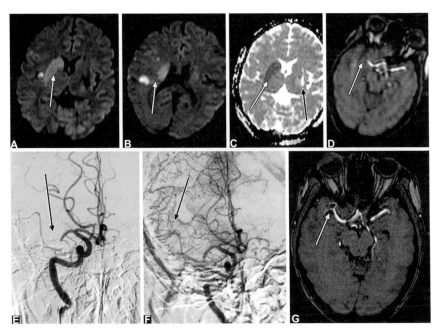

Figs 31.1A to G: (A and B) Axial diffusion-weighted imaging showing an acute infarct involving the right gangliocapsular region and insular cortex (white arrow); (C) Axial apparent diffusion coefficient map showing previous infarction in the lateral putamen and external capsule region (black arrow); (D) Axial time-of-flight source images of the circle of Willis angiogram showing total occlusion of the M1 segment of the right middle cerebral artery (white arrow) with poor visualization of the right middle cerebral artery branches; (E) Pre-thrombolytic digital subtraction angiogram of the right internal carotid artery showing total occlusion of the right M1 segment of the middle cerebral artery (black arrow); (F) Post-thrombolytic digital subtraction angiogram showing flow in the branches of the right middle cerebral artery (black arrow); (G) Axial time-of-flight source images of the circle of Willis angiogram showing recanalization of the M1 segment of the right middle cerebral artery (white arrow) and opening of right middle cerebral artery branches. Reproduced with permission from Elsevier, Meenakshi-Sundaram, et al. Complete recovery following intra-arterial tenecteplase administration in a woman with acute ischemic stroke. Journal of Clinical Neuroscience. 2013;20(12);1786-8.

level of technical expertize, relatively low availability, excessive trauma to the vasculature leading to vasospasm, dissection or rupture, and fragmented thrombus causing distal embolization into previously unaffected territories.[21] Nevertheless, the advantages of mechanical therapy appear to significantly outweigh its disadvantages and risks, as reflected in the results of recent multicenter trials.[22-24] Moreover improvement in technique and devices (e.g. solitaire device) in the recent past has demonstrated better and faster revascularization and improved clinical outcome.[25]

There is a report of use of embolic protection devices in both carotids by Blake et al.[26] in an old lady with severe MS and mobile LA clot. They deployed

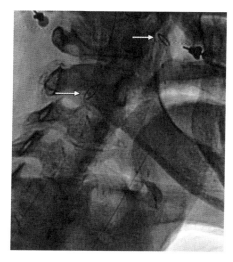

Fig. 31.2: Right anterior oblique image of neck demonstrating bilateral internal carotid artery filters (arrows). (Reprinted with permission from Wiley Sons, Blake JW, Hanzel GS, and O'Neill WW Neuroembolic protection during percutaneous balloon mitral valvuloplasty. Catheterization and Cardiovascular Interventions. 2007; 69(1):52-5.)

EZ-FilterWire devices (Boston Scientific, Natick, Massachusetts) in both the right and left internal carotid arteries using 6 French JR4 guide catheters (Fig. 31.2). Adequate apposition of the FilterWire nitinol loops were confirmed angiographically. Then PMV was performed with Inoue balloon with good result. No neurological or systemic embolic events occurred during the procedure.

In situations where thrombectomy devices or expertize are not available, use of smaller doses of intra-arterial tPA can be considered. However, safety of this treatment option in fully heparinized patients is largely unknown. Though cardioembolic strokes generally have increased propensity for hemorrhagic transformation, early detection and intervention can help to reduce the risk of this serious complication.

To summarize, the incidence of embolic cerebrovascular events during percutaneous mitral interventions can be reduced significantly by routine preprocedure transesophageal echocardiographic (TEE) screening. Early detection and treatment are the most important factors which determine the neurological outcome after embolic stroke. Therefore, the importance of looking for neurological deficits in the periprocedural period cannot be overemphasized. In those patients who develop periprocedural stroke, an emergent cerebral angiography followed by intra-arterial mechanical thrombolysis is the most appropriate treatment option. Angiographically negative (no demonstrable intracranial arterial occlusions) patients may be treated conservatively and such patients generally have a presumable good outcome.

Since, there are no clear-cut guidelines and there are concerns regarding complications, the treatment option has to be decided on a case-to-case basis, based on careful clinical evaluation and neurovascular imaging.

■ REFERENCES

1. Abernathy WS, Willis PW. Thromboembolic complications of rheumatic heart disease. Cardiovasclin. 1973;5:131-75.
2. Harrison JK, Wilson JS, Hearne SE, Bashore TM. Complications related to percutaneous transvenous mitral commissurotomy. Cathet Cardiovasc Diagn. 1994;(Suppl 2):52-60.
3. Chiang CW, Lo SK, Ko YS, Cheng NJ, Lin PJ, Chang CH. Predictors of systemic embolism in patients with mitral stenosis: A prospective study. Ann Intern Med.1998;128(11):885-9.
4. Casella L, Abelmann WH, Ellis LB. Patients with mitral stenosis and systemic emboli: hemodynamic and clinical observations. Arch Intern Med. 1964; 114: 773-81.
5. Coulshed N, Epstein EJ, McKendrick CS, Galloway RW, Walker E. Systemic embolism in mitral valve disease. Br Heart J. 1970;32:26-34.
6. Chiang CW, Lo SK, Kuo CT, Cheng NJ, Hsu TS. Noninvasive predictors of systemic embolism in mitral stenosis. An echocardiographic and clinical study of 500 patients. Chest. 1994;106:396-9.
7. Easton JD, Sherman DG. Management of cerebral embolism of cardiac origin. Stroke. 1980;11:433-42.
8. Benjamin EJ, Levy D, Vaziri SM, D'Agostino RB, Belanger AJ, Wolf PA. Independent risk factors for atrial fibrillation in a population-based cohort. The Framingham Heart Study. JAMA. 1994;271:840-4.
9. Rittoo D, Sutherland GR, Currie P, Starkey IR, Shaw TR. A prospective study of left atrial spontaneous echo contrast and thrombus in 100 consecutive patients referred for balloon dilation of the mitral valve. J Am Soc Echocardiogr. 1994;7(5):516-27.
10. The National Heart, Lung and Blood Institute Balloon Valvuloplasty Registry: Complications and mortality of percutaneous balloon mitral commissurotomy. Circulation. 1992;85:2014-24.
11. Farhat MB, Ayari M, Maatouk F, et al. Percutaneous balloon versus surgical closed and open mitral commissurotomy: Seven-year follow-up results of a randomized trial. Circulation. 1998;97:245-50.
12. Nobuyoshi M, Hamasaki N, Kimura T, et al. Indications, complications and short-term clinical outcome of percutaneous transvenous mitral commissurotomy. Circulation. 1989;80:782-92.
13. Inoue K, Owaki T, Nakamura T, Miyamoto N. Clinical application of transvenous mitral commissurotomy by a new balloon catheter. J Thorac Cardiovasc Surg. 1984; 87:394-402.
14. Vahanian A, Michel PL, Cormier B, Vitoux B, Michel X, Slama M, et al. Results of percutaneous mitral commissurotomy in 200 patients. Am J Cardiol. 1989; 63: 847-52.
15. Ruiz CE, Allen JW, Lau FY. Percutaneous double balloon valvotomy for severe rheumatic mitral stenosis. Am J Cardiol. 1990;65:473-7.
16. Hung JS, Chern MS, Wu JJ, Fu M, Yeh KH, Wu YC, et al. Short- and long-term results of catheter balloon percutaneous transvenous mitral commissurotomy. Am J Cardiol. 1991;67:854-62.
17. Chiang CW, Hsu LA, Chu PH, Ko YS, Ko YL, Cheng NJ, et al. On-line multiplane transesophageal echocardiography for balloon mitral commissurotomy. Am J Cardiol. 1998;81:515-8.

18. Liu TJ, Lai HC, Lee WL, Wang KY et al. Percutaneous balloon commissurotomy reduces incidence of ischemic cerebral stroke in patients with symptomatic rheumatic mitral stenosis. Int J Cardiol. 2008;123(2):189-90.
19. Stratton JR, Nemanich JW, Johannessen KA, Resnick AD. Fate of left ventricular thrombi in patients with remote myocardial infarction or idiopathic cardiomyopathy. Circulation. 1988;78:1388-93.
20. Segura T, Herrera M, Garcia-Muñozguren S, Zorita MD. Thrombolytic treatment in stroke in patients with intracardiac thrombus: Presentation of one case. Neurologia. 2005;20:149-52.
21. Nogueira RG, Schwamm LH, Hirsch JA. Endovascular approaches to acute stroke, part 1: Drugs, devices, and data. Am J Neuroradiol. 2009;30:649-61.
22. Gobin YP, Starkman S, Duckwiler GR, Grobelny T, et al. MERCI 1: A phase 1 study of Mechanical Embolus Removal in Cerebral Ischemia. Stroke. 2004;35(12):2848-54.
23. Smith WS, Sung G, Saver J, Budzik R, et al. and Multi-MERCI Investigators, Mechanical thrombectomy for acute ischemic stroke: final results of the Multi MERCI trial. Stroke. 2008;39(4):1205-12.
24. Shi ZS, Loh Y, Walker G, Duckwiler GR. MERCI and Multi-MERCI Investigators. Clinical outcomes in middle cerebral artery trunk occlusions versus secondary division occlusions after mechanical thrombectomy: pooled analysis of the Mechanical Embolus Removal in Cerebral Ischemia (MERCI) and Multi MERCI trials. Stroke. 2010;41(5):953-60.
25. Nguyen TN, Malisch T, Castonguay AC, Gupta R et al. Balloon guide catheter improves revascularisation and clinical outcomes with the solitaire device: Analysis of the North American solitaire acute stroke registry. Stroke. 2014; 45(1): 141-5.
26. Blake JW, Hanzel GS, O'Neill WW. Neuroembolic protection during percutaneous balloon mitral valvuloplasty. Catheterization and Cardiovascular Interventions. 2007;69(1):52-5.

Chapter 32

Thromboembolic Complications during Balloon Mitral Valvotomy

Dash PK

■ INTRODUCTION

Embolic phenomena is a potential and severe complication of percutaneous balloon mitral valvuloplasty (BMV) and can be devastating, since the rheumatic process itself is quite prevalent in the younger population (the average age of a person undergoing BMV in our institution is 27.9 years). The incidence of systemic embolism during BMV has been reported to be less than 5% and only 0.6% with the Inoue technique. This is less than that reported in closed commissurotomy series and about the same as in open commissurotomy.

Incidence and Etiology

The exact incidence of embolic phenomena during is difficult to estimate due to the ubiquitous nature and variability in presentation. Since these phenomena may be transient without lasting effects of any physical nature, they may be overlooked in some cases unless meticulously sought. Various factors linked to the occurrence of these features include—underlying rhythm during BMV, LA dilation and remodelling due to long standing rheumatic disease process, presence of spontaneous echo contrast (SEC) in the left atrial appendage (LAA), inadequate anticoagulation and inherent tendency to increased coagulability seen in patients with rheumatic MS.

Risk Factors for Systemic Embolism during BMV

Atrial fibrillation (AF) is a definite risk factor due to predilection to form thrombi in the left atrium and left atrial appendage LAA due to low velocity blood transit in these chambers and especially the stagnation of blood in the LAA. In fact most reports of embolic phenomena reported in literature have reported them in patients in AF. In our experience, all 7 cases of definite embolism with clinical manifestations where transient ischemic attack (TIA) occurred or residual defects persisted, happened to be in patients in AF. In other large-scale analyses of complications of balloon mitral valvotomy, embolic complications have been reported to be to the tune of 1.5%,[1] with most reported complications occurring before the routine use of TEE for ruling out clots in LA and LAA.

For patients in sinus rhythm, age [relative risk (RR), 1.12 (95% CI, 1.04 to 1.21)], the presence of a left atrial thrombus [RR, 37.1 (CI, 2.82 to 487.8)], mitral valve area [RR, 16.9 (CI, 1.53 to 187.0)], and the presence of significant aortic regurgitation [RR, 22.4 (CI, 2.72 to 184.8)] were positively associated with embolism. For patients in AF, previous embolism [RR, 3.11 (CI, 1.66 to 5.85)] was positively associated with embolism; percutaneous balloon mitral commissurotomy [RR, 0.37 (CI, 0.18 to 0.79)] was a negative predictor.[2] Notably, the most important factor for new embolic event in BMV patients was history of previous embolism.

Similarly, other studies[2,3] concluded that percutaneous balloon commissurotomy reduces incidence of ischemic cerebral stroke in patients with symptomatic rheumatic mitral stenosis, furthering the proof that early mitral commissurotomy is beneficial.

Predictors of Systemic Embolism in Patients Undergoing BMV

Few predictors of systemic embolism in patients with mitral stenosis have been identified by noninvasive methods. However, consistently researchers have found that markers of inflammation are increased in patients of mitral stenosis, and these may have a potential role in promoting hypercoagulability. Markers of platelet activity (P-selectin), fibrinolysis (d-dimer), thrombin activity [prothrombin fragments 1, 2 (PF1,2) and thrombin–antithrombin III complex (TAT)], and inflammation [interleukin 1β (IL-1β)] have been found to be significantly higher than the control patients and significantly decreased after BMV. P-selectin change correlated with the changes in left atrial diameter (LAD), pulmonary artery systolic pressure (PASP), and IL-1β. d-Dimer change had similar correlations, LAD, PASP, and IL-1β. The PF1,2 change correlated with the change in IL-1β. The TAT change correlated with the changes in LAD. The IL-1β change correlated with the changes in PASP. MS is associated with increased inflammatory, platelet, thrombin, and fibrinolytic activities that decrease after BMV. Altered hemodynamics and reduced inflammatory activity may have a potential role in these changes.

Spontaneous echo contrast (SEC) due to slow moving blood in LAA and LA are an indicator and predisposing factor for development of clots in these areas and a harbinger of embolic events. The SEC can be graded by Fatkin's classification[4] and there is a linear predilection between denser SEC (higher blood echogenicity) and the predilection for clot formation in LA and LAA, hence the need to repeat the TEE prior to the BMV procedure cannot be overstressed.

In a prospective study of left atrial spontaneous echo contrast and thrombus by Ritto et al.[5] in 100 consecutive patients undergoing BMV lower peak systolic pulmonary vein flow velocity (SVm) (24 ± 12 versus 45 ± 11 cm/sec; $p < 0.001$), and correspondingly lower systolic velocity-time integral (4.0 ± 2.6 vs 7.9 ± 2.9 cm; $p < 0.001$) were seen in patients with SEC than had patients without SEC.

There were no significant associations between SEC and either mitral valve area or anticoagulant therapy. SVm and AF were found to be independent predictors of SEC. In patients in sinus rhythm, SVm was the only independent predictor of SEC.

Neurological Embolism and its Management

Neurological embolism may range from cognitive dysfunction from multiple small emboli to the cortex and subcortical regions, to transient ischemic attacks to a full blown stroke in some cases. An MRI-assisted imaging study of the brain done at our Institute (SSIHMS Whitefield)[6] in patients undergoing BMV was conducted in 35 consecutive MS patients <30 years between July 2005 and September 2006. 17 were in AF and 18 in SR and pre- and post-BMV MRI brain were done to look at microinfarcts. It revealed that none of the patients in SR had microembolic infarcts whereas 1 patient in AF had microembolic infarct. Thus, we concluded that TEE may be obviated in MS patients in SR patients, if below 30 years age, though larger studies are required to corroborate the same.

It is ostensibly unclear how to treat patients who have systemic embolism during BMV because giving systemic intravenous thrombolytics across the board runs the risk of dislodging further emboli to the brain. However, if the thrombus has formed due to hardware manipulation or from the aortic arch during catheter manipulation, this option is still worth a try, though it would be unlikely or practical to expect any RCT to prove or disprove the same.

Blake et al.[7] have even reported BMV by using bilateral carotid Filter Wire EZ filters in an old patient with mobile LA clot.

Role of TEE in Preventing Thromboembolic Episodes during BMV

In a study of almost 9,000 patients presented at National CSI 2010, from SSIHMS Whitefield Bangalore,[8] we studied risk factors for thromboembolic events among age group <30 years. We concluded that those who did not have high risk features for clot formation [AF, past thromboembolism, RV failure, Severe SEC (Fatkins grade III)], did not suffer any thromboembolic event. Thus, in this patient subset, routine pre-BMV TEE could be safely avoided.

Experiences from Our Institutes

Since, the occurrence of embolic complications is itself a rare phenomenon with only case reports and anecdotal experiences across world literature, we thought, it prudent to share illustrative experiences over the last 25 years from our institutions where BMV is commonly done.

Among the patients who have sustained thromboembolic events at our Institutes over the past 25 years with almost 35,000 BMV procedures done, are the following:

Case 1: A 35-year-old lady from Nepal complained of inability to move the left side of her body and facial deviation 2 hours after PTMC. She was maintaining adequate INR before the planned BMV and was in AF and had also undergone a preprocedural TEE, which was normal. An urgent MRI study of the brain revealed parietal and temporal lobe infarcts with multiple areas of embolization ("shower of emboli"), most probably from manipulation during the procedure. She was treated with oral antiplatelet and anticoagulant therapy, along with physiotherapy and recovered almost completely over the next 6 months.

Case 2: A 28-year-old laborer from Odisha complained of inability to see from the left eye less than an hour after BMV. CT of the brain and orbit was unremarkable (MRI was not available). He recovered in less than 24 hours (i.e. IA) with full return of vision to normal. He was discharged on oral anti-coagulants and aspirin. Another similar case was encountered in a 36-year-old lady where the loss of vision in one eye improved in less than 2 hours post-procedure without any residual deficits.

Case 3: In the days before preprocedural TEE was mandated by protocol, a devastating case of post BMV embolism occurred in a 14-year-old girl in AF. She had undergone a preprocedural TEE, two days prior to the BMV which was reportedly normal. After septal puncture, the arterial BP plummeted to near zero level. Urgent TTE revealed no pericardial fluid or tamponade, however, the rapidity of the decline in BP arose suspicion of thrombus dislodgement across the mitral valve orifice or into the LVOT. Indeed an intraprocedural TEE done after intubating the patient showed a LA roof thrombus, adjacent to the pulmonary vein ostia which had probably fragmented with the daughter emboli obstructing the mitral valve. Despite an emergent attempt at sending the patient for surgery, she succumbed to the event. This event also highlights the need for detailed "nook-and corner" evaluation of LA for clots in LAA/LA/LA roof/PV ostia.

Case 4: Another devastating case of embolism during BMV occurred in a 46-year-old lady in AF in 2013. The procedure went off smoothly with the mitral valve area increasing 1.8 sq cm after the BMV and only trivial mitral regurgitation. 30 minutes after shifting to the step-down CCU, the patient began hypotensive and complained of chest pain. She was rushed back to the cathlab by which time she had begun unresponsive. Despite cardiac massage and high inotrope dosage, systolic BP hovered in the sixties only. Echo revealed no pericardial collection, but severely hypocontractile LV with 20% ejection fraction. ECG revealed ST elevation in aVR with global ST segment depression. An urgent coronary angiogram confirmed left main artery ostial occlusion. Despite a successful attempt at LMCA stenting with IABP support, the acute injury was too much to sustain life and the patient succumbed in 2 hours. We believe in retrospect that the thrombus probably originated from the pigtail that was kept in the aortic cusps to serve as a landmark during septal puncture. A point to mention is that this event had occurred despite heparinization at 100 U/kg body wt (Figs 32.1 to 32.3).

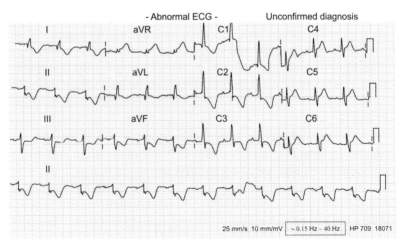

Fig. 32.1: Thirty minutes after the PTMC procedure patient developed hypotension (SBP 70 mm Hg) and ECG showed ST segment elevation in aVR and V4-6 and ST depression in Leads I, II, III, aVF and V1-3. Echo showed a globally hypokinetic LV with LVEF 30%, No pericardial effusion. We suspected LMCA/LAD occlusion

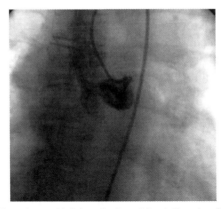

Fig. 32.2: LCA injection showed total occlusion of the left main with thrombus. PCI was done to LMCA, LAD and LCX with 7Fr XB guide. Thrombus aspiration was done which achieved TIMI 3 flow in LAD. Intracoronary Gp IIb/IIIa inhibitor and adenosine was given. Persistent thrombus in LCX with TIMI 0 flow seen. LCX was wired and thrombus aspiration and balloon dilation were done. Intracoronary STK was given. TIMI 2 flow was achieved in LCX. After restoration of flow, hemodynamics stabilized

Case 5: A case of peripheral embolization occurred in one of our patients almost 2 hours after the balloon mitral procedure. The patient presented with sudden onset paraparesis and bilateral lower limb pain 1 hour after the BMV. Clinical examination revealed cold lower limbs with loss of pulses bilaterally. An urgent peripheral angiogram revealed saddle embolus at aortoiliac bifurcation. Catheter directed thrombolysis was given for 24 hours after which the thrombus resolved significantly, and the patient underwent a successful aortobiiliac angioplasty the next day.

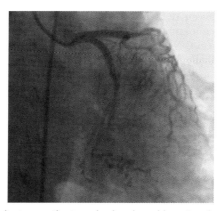

Fig. 32.3: After 10 minutes, patient again developed hypotension; IABP was inserted through the left femoral artery. Patient developed gross pulmonary edema and was intubated and ventilated, following which was treated with diuretics. Balloon atrial septostomy was done. Metabolic acidosis was corrected. Despite high inotrope support, patient remained in refractory hypotension, followed by electromechanical dissociation. Cardiac massage was continued. Despite all measures patient could not be salvaged due to severe ischemic LV dysfunction, contributed by diabetes mellitus, distal coronary embolization and global microvascular dysfunction

CONCLUSION

Patients with mitral stenosis have a predilection for clot formation due to the presence and contributive effects of various markers of inflammation present in increased amounts. Thromboembolic complications during BMV are generally uncommon, though a majority of them occur with underlying factors, such as AF and dense LA SEC (spontaneous echo contrast). Preprocedural TEE is very helpful in determining LA/LAA clots and it is imperative to repeat it on the morning of the planned procedure even if done earlier.

REFERENCES

1. Hung JS, Lau KW, Lo PH, Chern MS, Wu JJ. Complications of Inoue balloon mitral commissurotomy: impact of operator experience and evolving technique. Am Heart J. 1999;138(1 Pt 1):114–21.
2. Chiang CW, Lo SK, Ko YS, Cheng NJ, Lin PJ, Chang CH. Predictors of systemic embolism in patients with mitral stenosis. A prospective study. Ann Intern Med. 1998;128(11):885–9.
3. Hasan-Ali H, Mosad E. Changes in platelet, coagulation, and fibrinolytic activities in mitral stenosis after percutaneous mitral valvotomy: role of hemodynamic changes and systemic inflammation. Clin Appl Thromb Hemost. 2015;21(4):339–47.
4. Fatkin D, Loupas T, Jacobs N, Feneley MP. Quantification of blood echogenicity: evaluation of a semiquantitative method of grading spontaneous echo contrast. Ultrasound Med Biol. 1995;21(9):1191–8.
5. Rittoo D, Sutherland GR, Currie P, Starkey IR, Shaw TR. A prospective study of left atrial spontaneous echo contrast and thrombus in 100 consecutive patients referred for balloon dilation of the mitral valve. J Am Soc Echocardiogr Off Publ Am Soc Echocardiogr. 1994;7(5):516–27.

6. Chaudappa S, Praveen AV, Dash PK. MRI brain before and after PTMC in patients high risk for systemic embolisation. Indian Heart J. 2007;58:427.
7. Blake JW, Hanzel GS, O'Neill WW. Neuro-embolic protection during percutaneous balloon mitral valvuloplasty. Catheter Cardiovasc Interv. 2007;69(1):52–5.
8. Dash PK. Outcome of BMV in 4000 patients. SSIHMS experience. Indian Heart J. 2010.

Chapter 33

Arrhythmias and Its Management during Percutaneous Mitral Valvotomy

Shomu R Bohora

■ INTRODUCTION

Rheumatic heart disease is a disease predominantly affecting the valves. Arrhythmia is secondary to the structural abnormalities, especially atrial enlargement and fibrosis caused by hemodynamic changes, though inflammation may also contribute to the genesis of arrhythmia.

Atrial flutter and atrial fibrillation (AF) are the most common arrhythmias associated with rheumatic heart disease and mitral stenosis (MS). Valvular heart disease comprise 8 to 25% of the cause of atrial fibrillation depending on the geographic location and sex of the patient.[1,2] Patients with mitral stenosis frequently worsen symptomatically due to onset of atrial arrhythmia, which is due to loss of atrial contribution to cardiac output and due to irregular and fast heart rates decreasing the diastolic filling time. Once atrial tachycardia sets in, generally there is a rapid progression of symptoms and heart failure, and unlike in patients with structurally normal heart, chances of spontaneous termination of tachycardia are remote.

Arrhythmias during percutaneous mitral valvotomy (PMV) and management of atrial arrhythmias pre- and post-PMV is discussed in brief.

■ ARRHYTHMIAS DURING PMV

Hardware manipulation within the atrium and the ventricles during PMV can cause procedure-related transient arrhythmias and they are not uncommon. In patients who are in sinus rhythm, atrial ectopics (Fig. 33.1A), transient atrial tachycardia (Figs 33.2A and B), and atrial flutter (Fig. 33.3) are commonly seen during septal puncture, catheter manipulation in right atrium and manipulation of balloon in the left atrium. Ventricular ectopics (Fig. 33.1B) or short runs of ventricular tachycardia may be seen during catheter manipulation in the right ventricle or during balloon or pigtail catheter entry into the left ventricle. Gentle manipulation of hardware would reduce the chances of such arrhythmias and withdrawal of catheter immediately upon recognition of arrhythmia should stop the

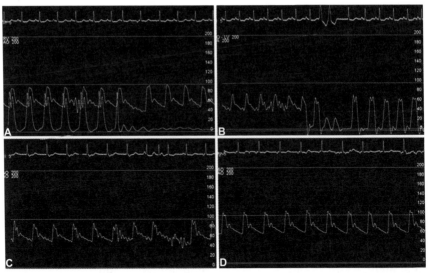

Figs 33.1A to D: Recordings during PMV showing arrhythmia during hardware manipulation: (A) Atrial ectopic during catheter withdrawal form right ventricle to right atrium; (B) Ventricular ectopics during catheter withdrawal from pulmonary artery to right ventricle; (C) Junctional rhythm followed by atrial ectopies during septal puncture; (D) Low atrial rhythm during septal dilatation

same. In an occasional patient, atrial tachycardia may persist even after the procedure is completed and should be treated by either chemical or electrical cardioversion on completion of the procedure.

Septal puncture, septal dilatation, balloon dilatation and pain during the procedure can induce vagal activation and reflex bradycardia and occasionally result in slow junctional rhythm (Figs 33.1C and 33.4) or slow ectopic atrial rhythm (Fig. 33.1D). Transient right bundle branch block due to catheter manipulation is not uncommon. Complete heart block occurring during PMV is rare (Fig. 33.5) and if irreversible may require pacemaker implantation.[3,4] Left bifascicular block may be seen during balloon inflation.[5] Unexplained inappropriate sinus tachycardia or bradycardia with hypotension should raise the suspicion of tamponade and should immediately be ruled out by doing transthoracic echocardiography.

Control of heart rate during the procedure in patients having AF or even sinus rhythm is important. Patient should be on adequate rate control drugs preprocedure and if required intravenous drugs can be given for rate control during the procedure. Success of PMV is important in maintaining sinus rhythm. Better the result of PMV, more the chance that the patient would remain in sinus rhythm on follow-up.[6] Serum potassium should be monitored especially in patients taking diuretics and correction should be done prior to PMV to avoid arrhythmias during the procedure. Digoxin dose should be adjusted to avoid toxicity.

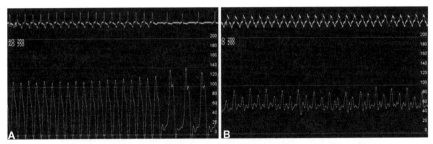

Figs 33.2A and B: Atrial tachycardia during PMV: (A) Atrial tachycardia with spontaneous termination; (B) Atrial tachycardia with bundle branch block

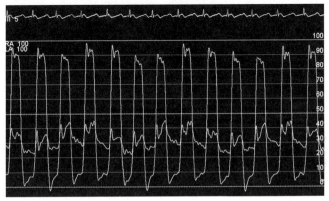

Fig. 33.3: Atrial flutter during PMV. Both left atrial and left ventricular pressure tracings are seen

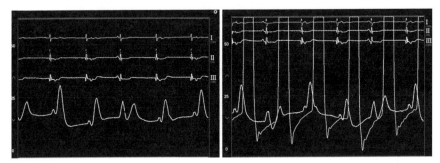

Fig. 33.4: Junctional rhythm during PMV. Sinus rhythm and junctional rhythm with retrograde p wave and the effect of p waves in the left atrial pressure tracing is seen

■ PREPROCEDURE MANAGEMENT OF ATRIAL FIBRILLATION

Atrial tachyarrhythmias can be observed in 18% patients who undergo PMV for the first time.[7] Increasing risk of developing AF in rheumatic mitral stenosis occurs with increasing age, longer duration of disease, greater mitral valve score, larger size of the left atrium (LA) and significant disease of

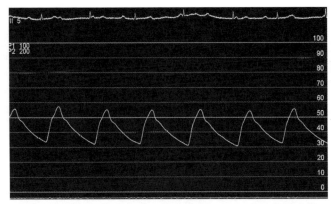

Fig. 33.5: Complete heart block with narrow QRS escape occurring during catheter manipulation for transseptal puncture. The patient made an uneventful recovery and had a successful procedure

other valves, which supports the opinion that AF is a marker of widespread rheumatic damage.[8,9] Coarse AF as defined by fibrillatory wave amplitude of >1 mm in lead V1, is a marker of advanced disease and associated with higher thromboembolic complications as compared to fine AF.[10] Presence of AF in an asymptomatic patient in presence of moderate to severe MS is an indication to consider PMV (Class II a).[11]

All patients with rheumatic mitral stenosis and AF should be on oral anticoagulation for at least 3 weeks prior to procedure, unless there is an emergency, as the risk of clot formation and subsequent thromboembolism is high.[12] Even after adequate anticoagulation, transesophageal echocardiography (TEE) is advisable to exclude LA and LA appendage clots prior to PMV. Patients who are on warfarin should be switched over to heparin when warfarin therapy is discontinued prior to PMV to normalize INR. This is essential to avoid thromboembolic complications.

Rate control in patients with AF and MS is an acceptable strategy till the time PMV is planned, unless there is a necessity of achieving sinus rhythm due to severe symptoms or due to hemodynamic compromise. High heart rates can precipitate pulmonary edema in patients with critical MS. Adequate heart rate control by using appropriate oral or intravenous beta-blockers, calcium channel blockers, digoxin and rarely amiodarone, alone or in combination, is required preprocedure.[12] Preprocedure anxiety related tachycardia can be avoided and treated by beta-blockers and sedation. Antiarrhythmic drugs should be initiated in patients who are planned for elective cardioversion post-PMV to improve the success of conversion and maintenance of sinus rhythm.

Other arrhythmias like atrioventricular nodal reentrant tachycardia, atrioventricular reentrant tachycardia, and ventricular arrhythmia may coexist independently and needs to be treated on their own merit. However, valvular disease may cause difficulties in treatment of these arrhythmias due to abnormal valvular as well as chamber morphology.

POSTPROCEDURE MANAGEMENT OF ATRIAL FIBRILLATION

In patients with chronic AF, measures should be undertaken to restore sinus rhythm immediately following PMV.[13] Atrial arrhythmias which started during the procedure should be addressed immediately post-procedure. The chances of thromboembolism when converting to sinus rhythm are minimal as patient would have been properly anticoagulated and LA or LA appendage clot already excluded prior to the procedure. The hemodynamic improvement after a successful PMV makes maintaining sinus rhythm easier.

The optimal strategy to treat AF after PMV should be individualized. Patients with rheumatic heart disease and AF benefit from achieving and maintaining sinus rhythm.[14] With AF duration ≤12 months and post-PMV LA size ≤45 mm, sinus rhythm is easier and safer to achieve and maintain.[15,16] Moreover, patients benefit from restoration and maintenance of sinus rhythm in terms of improved AF-related symptoms, 6 minute walk test and Quality of life (QOL). Rhythm control should, therefore be considered as the preferred initial therapy for this group of patients.[15,16] Additionally, patients who have intractable symptoms due to atrial fibrillation but the duration of AF is longer or the LA size is larger may also be considered for cardioversion though the success may be less.

Chemical or electrical cardioversion can be planned immediately post-PMV or at 6 weeks or 12 weeks of PMV.[13,15,17] Chemical cardioversion may be effective in 39% of patients,[15] while others require electrical (DC) cardioversion in addition to drugs. Overall success rates in achieving sinus rhythm is 85 to 90%[13-15] (Figs 33.6A and B). The most frequent drug used for chemical cardioversion is amiodarone which can be loaded orally or intravenously depending on the timing of cardioversion.[13,15,17] All patients who are planned for DC cardioversion should have been adequately loaded with amiodarone (10 grams given over a period of days in divided doses). Ibutilide, dofetilide, propafenone and flecainide may also be effective though have not been specifically studied for efficacy in the rheumatic population.[12]

At one year around 50% patients maintain sinus rhythm on medications.[13,14,17,18] Maintaining sinus rhythm correlates with younger age group, absence of concomitant aortic valve disease and a smaller LA size.[15,17,18]

Long-term maintenance of sinus rhythm again depends on duration of preceding AF. The chances of maintaining sinus rhythm in patients who were in AF for less than 2 years is 95% as compared to 64% if the duration of AF was more than 2 years.[15] Successful maintenance of sinus rhythm with amiodarone can be predicted by the degree to which LA size is reduced and mitral valve area is increased.[19] Amiodarone should be continued long-term if possible for maintaining sinus rhythm in a dose of 100–400 mg/day as the chances of maintaining sinus rhythm are higher.[12,14,15] Sotalol and dronedarone can also be used for maintaining sinus rhythm but have not been studied in rheumatic mitral stenosis.[12]

Maze procedure done either surgically[20] or using a cool-tipped catheter[21] is effective in patients being operated for rheumatic mitral disease to convert

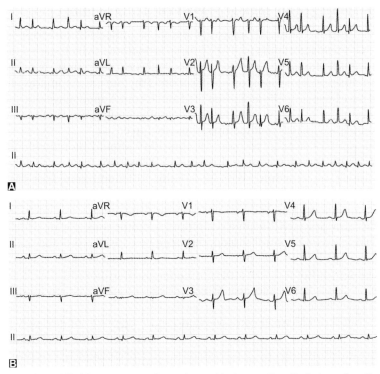

Figs 33.6A and B: Management of a patient with rheumatic mitral stenosis with atrial fibrillation: (A) Basal ECG showing AF; (B) Post DC cardioversion ECG showing successful conversion to sinus rhythm

and maintain sinus rhythm. Similarly, hybrid therapy using radiofrequency catheter ablation along with PMV is safe and feasible and significantly improves the AF free survival rate compared to drug therapy alone.[22-24] In a study of 20 patients by Machino et al. at a mean follow-up period of 4.0 +/– 2.7 years, 8 patients (80%) in the radiofrequency catheter ablation group maintained SR, as compared to 1 (10%) in the cardioversion and drug therapy group.[24] However, rheumatic atrial fibrillation may require ablation around the coronary sinus ostium and the atrial septum in addition to the standard treatment protocol.[25]

ATRIAL FLUTTER

There is practically no difference in approach to a patient with rheumatic mitral stenosis and atrial flutter as compared to atrial fibrillation.[12] An isthmus line by radiofrequency ablation may not be effective as flutter may arise from LA or the coronary sinus.[25]

CONCLUSION

Arrhythmias are commonly seen in patients undergoing PMV. Gentle hardware manipulation and alertness on the part of the operator will prevent any sustained arrhythmia during the procedure in patients who are in sinus rhythm.

Atrial fibrillation is the predominant arrhythmia encountered during PMV and the optimal strategy to manage this arrhythmia should be individualized for either rate or rhythm control. The postprocedure management of atrial fibrillation like conversion to and maintenance of sinus rhythm should be planned along with PMV.

■ REFERENCES

1. Ntep-Gweth M, Zimmermann M, Meiltz A, Kingue S, Ndobo P, Urban P, et al. Atrial fibrillation in Africa: clinical characteristics, prognosis, and adherence to guidelines in Cameroon. Europace. 2010;12(4):482-7.
2. Lévy S, Maarek M, Coumel P, Guize L, Lekieffre J, Medvedowsky JL, et al. Characterization of different subsets of atrial fibrillation in general practice in France: the ALFA study. The College of French Cardiologists. Circulation. 1999;99(23):3028-35.
3. Maté I, Sobrino JA, Calvo L, Rico J, Oliver JM, Sobrino N, et al. Atrioventricular block at the nodal level and block of an accessory pathway during percutaneous mitral valvuloplasty. Rev Esp Cardiol. 1990;43(1):56-8.
4. Evora PR, Finzi LP, Haddad J, Secches AL, Ribeiro PJ, Vicente WV. Complete heart block after percutaneous mitral valvotomy with Inoue balloon. Arq Bras Cardiol. 1996;66(3):149-52.
5. Fernandez F, Soria R, Rocha P. Left bifascicular block and percutaneous mitral valvuloplasty. Ann Cardiol Angéiologie. 1991;40(8):469-73.
6. Abe S, Matsubara T, Hori T, Nakagawa I, Imai S, Ozaki K, et al. Effect of percutaneous transvenous mitral commissurotomy for the preservation of sinus rhythm in patients with mitral stenosis. J Cardiol. 2001;38(1):29-34.
7. Peixoto EC, de Oliveira PS, Netto MS, Villella RA, Labrunie P, Borges IP, et al. Percutaneous balloon mitral valvoplasty. Immediate results, complications and hospital outcome. Arq Bras Cardiol. 1995;64(2):109-16.
8. Srimahachota S, Boonyaratavej S, Wannakrairoj M, Udayachalerm W, Sangwattanaroj S, Ngarmukos P, et al. Percutaneous transvenous mitral commissurotomy: hemodynamic and initial outcome differences between atrial fibrillation and sinus rhythm in rheumatic mitral stenosis patients. J Med Assoc Thail 2001;84(5):674-80.
9. Kabukçu M, Arslantas E, Ates I, Demircioglu F, Ersel F. Clinical, echocardiographic, and hemodynamic characteristics of rheumatic mitral valve stenosis and atrial fibrillation. Angiology. 2005;56(2):159-63.
10. Mutlu B, Karabulut M, Eroglu E, Tigen K, Bayrak F, Fotbolcu H, et al. Fibrillatory wave amplitude as a marker of left atrial and left atrial appendage function, and a predictor of thromboembolic risk in patients with rheumatic mitral stenosis. Int J Cardiol. 2003;91(2-3):179-86.
11. Vahanian A, Baumgartner H, Bax J, Butchart E, Dion R, Filippatos G, et al. Guidelines on the management of valvular heart disease: The Task Force on the Management of Valvular Heart Disease of the European Society of Cardiology. Eur Heart J. 2007;28(2):230-68.
12. Fuster V, Ryden LE, Cannom DS, Crijns HJ, Curtis AB, Ellenbogen KA, et al. ACC/AHA/ESC 2006 guidelines for the management of patients with atrial fibrillation: full text: A report of the American College of Cardiology/American Heart Association Task Force on practice guidelines and the European Society of Cardiology Committee for Practice Guidelines (Writing Committee to Revise the 2001 Guidelines for the Management of Patients With Atrial Fibrillation)

Developed in collaboration with the European Heart Rhythm Association and the Heart Rhythm Society. Europace. 2006;8(9):651–745.

13. Langerveld J, Hemel NM, Kelder JC, Ernst JMPG, Plokker HWM, Jaarsma W. Long-term follow-up of cardiac rhythm after percutaneous mitral balloon valvotomy. Does atrial fibrillation persist? Europace. 2003;5(1):47–53.

14. Vora A, Karnad D, Goyal V, Naik A, Gupta A, Lokhandwala Y, et al. Control of rate versus rhythm in rheumatic atrial fibrillation: a randomized study. Indian Heart J. 2004;56(2):110-6.

15. Kapoor A, Kumar S, Singh RK, Pandey CM, Sinha N. Management of persistent atrial fibrillation following balloon mitral valvotomy: safety and efficacy of low-dose amiodarone. J Heart Valve Dis. 2002;11(6):802–9.

16. Hu CL, Jiang H, Tang QZ, Zhang QH, Chen JB, Huang CX, et al. Comparison of rate control and rhythm control in patients with atrial fibrillation after percutaneous mitral balloon valvotomy: a randomised controlled study. Heart. 2006;92(8): 1096–101.

17. Kavthale SS, Fulwani MC, Vajifdar BU, Vora AM, Lokhandwala YY. Atrial fibrillation: how effectively can sinus rhythm be restored and maintained after balloon mitral valvotomy? Indian Heart J. 2000;52(5):568–73.

18. Krittayaphong R, Chotinaiwatarakul C, Phankingthongkum R, Panchavinnin P, Tresukosol D, Jakrapanichakul D, et al. One-year outcome of cardioversion of atrial fibrillation in patients with mitral stenosis after percutaneous balloon mitral valvuloplasty. Am J Cardiol. 2006;97(7):1045–50.

19. Guo GB-F, Hang C-L, Chang H-W, Wu C-J, Fang C-Y, Chen C-J. Prognostic predictors of sinus rhythm control by amiodarone and electrical cardioversion in patients undergoing percutaneous transluminal mitral valvuloplasty for rheumatic atrial fibrillation. Circ J. 2007;71(7):1115–9.

20. Sternik L, Luria D, Glikson M, Malachy A, First M, Raanani E. Efficacy of surgical ablation of atrial fibrillation in patients with rheumatic heart disease. Ann Thorac Surg. 2010;89(5):1437–42.

21. Abreu Filho CAC, Lisboa LAF, Dallan LAO, Spina GS, Grinberg M, Scanavacca M, et al. Effectiveness of the maze procedure using cooled-tip radiofrequency ablation in patients with permanent atrial fibrillation and rheumatic mitral valve disease. Circulation. 2005;112(9 Suppl):I20–25.

22. Miyaji K, Tada H, Ito S, Naito S, Yamada M, Hashimoto T, et al. Percutaneous transvenous mitral commissurotomy and radiofrequency catheter ablation in patients with mitral stenosis. Circ J. 2005;69(9):1074–8.

23. Adragão P, Machado FP, Aguiar C, Parreira L, Cavaco D, Ribeiras R, et al. Ablation of atrial fibrillation in mitral valve disease patients: five year follow-up after percutaneous pulmonary vein isolation and mitral balloon valvuloplasty. Rev Port Cardiol. 2003;22(9):1025–36.

24. Machino T, Tada H, Sekiguchi Y, Tanaka Y, Naito S, Yamasaki H, et al. Hybrid therapy of radiofrequency catheter ablation and percutaneous transvenous mitral commissurotomy in patients with atrial fibrillation and mitral stenosis. J Cardiovasc Electrophysiol. 2010;21(3):284–9.

25. Nair M, Shah P, Batra R, Kumar M, Mohan J, Kaul U, et al. Chronic atrial fibrillation in patients with rheumatic heart disease: mapping and radiofrequency ablation of flutter circuits seen at initiation after cardioversion. Circulation. 2001;104(7): 802–9.

Chapter 34

Deflation Failure of Mitral Valvuloplasty Balloon

Pranav Bansal, Mamtesh Gupta, Jagdish Dureja

One of the dreaded nightmares in cardiac catheterization lab is failure of deflation of valvuloplasty balloon whilst the assembly is in situ. Even though percutaneous balloon valvuloplasty has established its reputation over decades for being a safe procedure, occasional complications still do occur, especially when the standard safety protocols and guidelines are bypassed. Rare complications include moderate to severe valvular regurgitation in 2–3%, systemic embolization in 1–3% and even death in 0.1–1% of cases.[1,2]

Presently, the technique for valvuloplasty employs use of percutaneous latex made, Inoue or Accura balloon. Balloon assembly malfunction is a rare phenomenon, but almost always reported on repeated use of the balloon. The commonly reported assembly related complications include tear, rupture or deflation failure of the balloon.[3-6] The problem with deflation failure in-vivo is that the bulky inflated balloon cannot be withdrawn from the heart, while its prolonged presence can incite arrhythmias, thromboembolism, compromise left atrial filling and cardiac output, leading to increased morbidity and mortality.[7] Even if a partially deflated balloon is forcibly pulled back across the interatrial septum (IAS), it will increase the size of the iatrogenic ASD leading to a significant LR shunt.[5]

The first case of complete deflation failure of a mitral valvuloplasty balloon was reported in 1996 by Patel et al. while using a bifoil balloon.[8] Of the innumerable BMV's performed worldwide, currently fewer than ten cases of deflation failure of various valvuloplasty balloons have been reported in literature, the last being reported in 2012.[6-8] Reports reveal that balloon malfunction is higher (20%) with reused balloons as compared to newly used assemblies (<0.1%), though this data is highly misleading owing to frequent under-reporting in developing or third world countries.[9]

Possible Mechanisms of Deflation Failure of Inoue Balloon Assembly

1. Repeated sterilization and usage damages the latex of the balloon, leading to herniation of its walls, externally or internally (Fig. 34.1). Contrast can enter between the two layers of balloon which can produce one-way valve like mechanism which may lead to deflation failure (Fig. 34.2).[6]

2. Forceful insertion of balloon catheter through skin can produce kink in the shaft, commonly at the junction of distal end of the shaft assembly and proximal end of the balloon, thus occluding the lumen of inflation tube.[7]

3. Forceful and rapid inflation of balloon whilst within mitral valvular apparatus can lead to rupture, dissection or herniation of walls of the inner lumen of the inflation tube. This also produces ball-valve type obstruction, i.e. fluid can be pushed into the balloon on injection but fails to retrieve on aspiration, due to luminal collapse.[6]

4. If the dilution of contrast used for inflating the balloon is not optimal (1:4 or 1:3), high viscosity of the solution may lead to sticking and clogging of inner walls of inflation tube.[9]

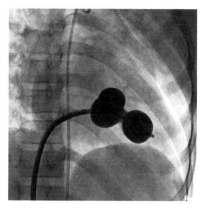

Fig. 34.1: Bulging wall of damaged balloon as seen on fluoroscopy in vivo [*Courtesy:* Dr Charan P Lanjewar, with permission, Journal of Interventional Cardiology 2006;19(3):280–2]

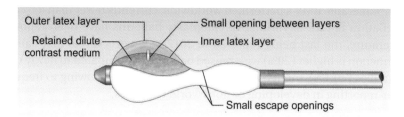

Fig. 34.2: One-way valve mechanism leading to collection of contrast between 2 layers of PMV balloon [*Courtesy:* Dr Charan Lanjewar, with permission, Journal of Interventional Cardiology. 2006;19(3):280-2]

5. On repeated exposure, the possibility of chemical reaction between the latex walls of balloon and ethylene trioxide (ETO) gas during sterilization process cannot be ruled out. Changes in the wall color or texture can serve as a warning sign of increasing stiffness and likely malfunction of balloon assembly.

Methods to Prevent Deflation Failure of PMV Balloon

Though, recommended for single use only, the Inoue or Accura Balloon are used multiple times in developing countries, owing to the high cost of the balloon assembly.[9] We believe that after using 3–4 times, the balloon assembly should be best avoided, as it can malfunction in vivo. The following steps can minimize the incidence of unexpected balloon assembly malfunction:

1. Check for proper functioning of balloon assembly (inflation ports, connections, balloon inflation and deflation, etc) ex vivo, prior to the procedure. Remove any residual air bubbles in the balloon.
2. During balloon insertion through femoral route avoid excessive strain on the catheter. Vertical puncture and vertical entry should be avoided.
3. Perform only gradual and serial dilatation of mitral valve apparatus, as forcible and rapid dilatation can damage the balloon and cause its wall to herniate internally or externally (Fig. 34.3).
4. Residual contrast between the walls can solidify and interfere with the proper inflation or deflation of the balloon. So after each use, the balloon should be thoroughly cleansed for removal of any residual contrast.

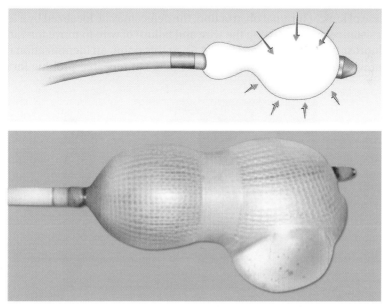

Fig. 34.3: Bulging weak and thin wall of damaged PMV balloon demonstrated ex vivo and in sketch (arrows)

Management Options in Case of Deflation Failure of Balloon Assembly

Failure to deflate the Inoue balloon, is an emergent situation. The key to management lies in exploring the possible cause of deflation failure and working on the best option to deal it. Based on previous successful attempts, a few management strategies are discussed below.

Dos

- Try to identify the possible cause of deflation failure.
- Consider sedation if patient is anxious.
- Check for the uniform shape of PMV balloon on fluoroscopy and rule out external herniation of balloon wall.
- Perform repeated aspirations using 20 mL syringe and check for any dye retrieval for at least 10 minutes. If the dye comes out in small volumes, occlusion may be partial and repeated aspirations may deflate the balloon. Minute volumes of warm saline injection and aspiration may also help in restoring luminal patency by decreasing stickiness of walls, if inappropriately concentrated contrast had been used.
- Using a larger syringe (50 mL) may generate a higher negative pressure during aspiration and facilitate retrieval of the dye.
- Pass a J-shaped stylet through the central lumen of balloon catheter. Free passage will rule out kink in the shaft of catheter while occlusion will locate the affected site on fluoroscopy.
- Try passing a coronary angioplasty guidewire [e.g. Balance middle weight (BMW) wire of 0.014 inch 2 gauge] through inflation port in the lumen with gentle rotations and try to restore the patency of lumen (Fig. 34.4).[9] In case of kink or luminal obstruction, the defect may be localized by a feel of resistance on negotiating the wire and failure of wire to move forward on fluoroscopic visualization (Fig. 34.5). At this point, an identification mark on wire may be made with a marker pen. On repeated probing forward

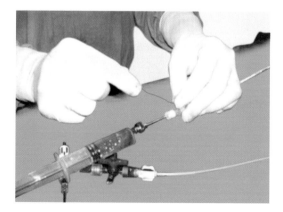

Fig. 34.4: Coronary angioplasty guidewire (0.014 inch) is being introduced through the balloon inflation port

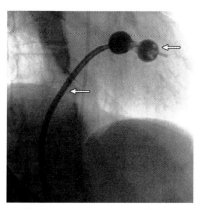

Fig. 34.5: Partially deflated PMV balloon stuck inside the left atrium with some retained air (upper arrow) inside. Coronary guidewire in the shaft of the balloon is seen (lower arrow)

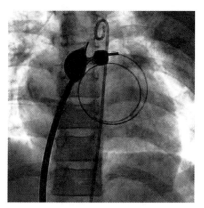

Fig. 34.6: Balloon puncture via spring needle (*Courtesy:* Dr Charan P Lanjewar, with permission, Journal of Interventional Cardiology. 2006;19(3):280–2)

passage of guidewire through this resistance can be well identified with the help of these markings. After removal of guidewire gentle and sustained aspiration will retrieve the dye in most of the cases.

- Another successful method of balloon deflation was reported by Charan Lanjewar et al.[6] A spring guidewire was passed through inflation tube to rupture the balloon internally, using the pointed end of wire under fluoroscopic guidance (Fig. 34.6). In a recent report, similar technique was employed by using reverse end of 0.025" spring coil LA to perforate the balloon (Fig. 34.7).[7]

During these maneuvers, PBMV balloon should be stationed near the septum to avoid undesirable motions in the vigorously contracting left atrium. Maneuvering of wire should be done with a gentle, steady and guarded hand movement, because even the slightest needle overshoot can lead to more serious complications like cardiac perforation and tamponade. Prior to the rupture, PBMV balloon should be free of air bubbles as sudden release of air in left atrium can lead to arrhythmias, fall in cardiac output or

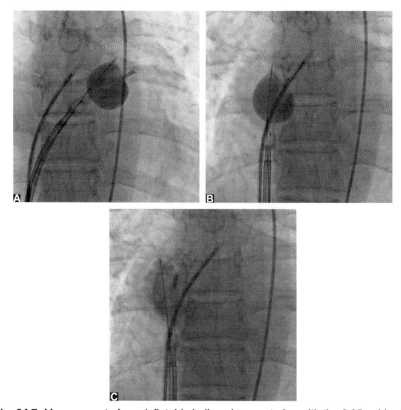

Fig. 34.7: Management of nondeflatable balloon by puncturing with the 0.25 guidewire proximal tip. (A) Tenting of balloon by reverse end of 0.025" spring coil LA wire (B). Prior to rupture balloon (C). Rupture of the balloon by 0.025" spring coil LA wire [Reproduced with permission from Hore et al. Journal of the Indian College of Cardiology. 2012 (2) 135–9][1]

embolism. Though, the severity of complications which can be produced by release of 5–10 mL of air in atrial cavity is a topic of debate.

- Yet another reported method of deflation includes puncturing the balloon using a transseptal puncture needle (Figure 34.8). Patel et al.[8] introduced a Mullins catheter via femoral vein to the left atrium and placed a Brockenbrough needle inside the catheter. After pulling the balloon catheter back gently against the interatrial septum, the proximal end of inflated balloon was repeatedly punctured and deflation of balloon was achieved.

- In one report, nondeflation of balloon catheter occurred in an infant with transposition of the great arteries (D-TGA) undergoing a Rashkind (atrial) septostomy. Deflation in that case was achieved with a fine-gauge needle introduced percutaneously via a transhepatic approach.[10]

- If all measures fail, removal of balloon assembly will require surgery to exteriorize the left atrium. Puncturing the balloon via a wide bore needle or incision via a scalpel will easily facilitate the removal of the balloon

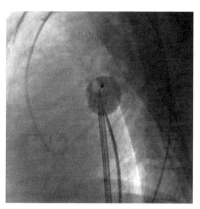

Fig. 34.8: Attempting puncturing the balloon from outside by transseptal puncture needle. [Reproduced with permission from Hore et al. Journal of the Indian College of Cardiology. 2012;(2):135–9]

assembly, thereafter. Morbidity and mortality are high following emergency open heart surgery as deaths have been reported due to hemorrhagic myocardial infarction after removal of inflated balloon.[11]

After successful deflation is achieved, try to identify the cause of deflation failure ex vivo.

Don'ts

- Avoid introducing air into the balloon while checking or restoring patency. If puncturing of balloon is opted as the last report, this air can embolize to cerebral, cardiac or end arterial circulation and cause devastating complications.
- Do not over inflate the balloon in a myth that over inflation might lead to rupture of the balloon. This is because PMV balloons can sustain 2.5–3 times the recommended volumes and it is unlikely that we will be able to rupture the balloon in this manner. This technique has shown failure in previous reports[8] though, on the contrary, has been successfully used to deflate Foley's catheter in urinary bladder.[12]
- Avoid excessive negative aspiration as it can collapse the luminal walls in case of luminal dissection or promote sticking of the walls with viscous dye (both ionic and nonionic).

■ CONCLUSION

Failure to deflate the valvuloplasy balloon is a rare complication of where identification of the cause is crucial for a successful deflation. In face of such complication, attempt all possible maneuvers [i.e. negative aspiration, dilution of contrast, recanalization of lumen by balanced middle weight (BMW) 0.014" or stiff coronary guidewire, perforate the balloon by reverse end of 0.025" spring coil wire or transseptal needle].

Considering the cost of equipments, reuse of hardware for PMV is a reality in the developing world. There are few reports of safe reuse of PMV hardware in the literature.[13] If proper care is taken and a thorough inspection of the balloon and other hardware is done before the procedure we can avoid many of these complications.

■ REFERENCES

1. Jeffery J Popma, Donald S Baim, Frederic S Resnic. Percutaneous coronary and valvular intervention; Braunwald's heart disease (8th edition); Philadelphia: Saunders; 2008:pp1646-55.
2. Hung Jui-Sung, Lau Kean-Wah, Lo Ping-Han Chern Ming-Shyan, Wu Jong- Jen. Complications of Inoue balloon mitral commissurotomy: Impact of operator experience and evolving technique. American Heart Journal. 1999;138(1):114–21.
3. Dev V, Shrivastava S. Balloon rupture during valvuloplasty. Am Heart J. 1990; 119:1441–2.
4. Kerkar PG, Dalvi BV. Unusual tear in Inoue balloon during PTMV in a patient with calcific mitral stenosis. Cathet Cardiovasc Diagn. 1994;31:127-9.
5. Ishikura F, Nagata S, Yasuda S, Yamashita N, Miyatake K. Residual atrial septal perforation after percutaneous transvenous mitral commissurotomy with Inoue balloon catheter. Am Heart J. 1990;120:873–78.
6. Charan P Lanjewar, Pratap J Nathani, Praffula G Kerkar. Failure of deflation of an Inoue balloon during percutaneous balloon mitral valvuloplasty. Journal of Interventional Cardiology. 2006;19(3): 280-2.
7. Hore DR, Rambhau D, Tiwari N. Failure to deflate balloon-A rare complication after successful percutaneous balloon mitral valvuloplasty. Journal of Indian College of Cardiology. 2012; (2):135-9.
8. Patel MT, Dani S. Unsuccessful deflation of a bifoil balloon during percutaneous balloon mitral valvuloplasty. Cathet Cardiovasc Diagn. 1996;37: 290-2.
9. Bansal P, Gupta M, Yadave R, Agarwal D. Deflation failure of Accura balloon in left atrium during balloon mitral valvuloplasty. The Internet Journal of Cardiology, 2010.
10. Nigel J Wilson, JA Gordon Culham, George GS Sandor. Successful treatment of a nondeflatable balloon atrial septostomy catheter. Pediatric Cardiology. 1990;11(3): 150-2.
11. Park SJ, Park SW, Kim JJ, Lim CM, Kim SW, Lee JK. A Case of Deflation Failure of Inoue Balloon. Korean Circ J. 1990;20(2):256-9.
12. Ta-Chong Lin, Hueh Long Shieh, Mao Sheng Lin, Chow Tse Chen, Chi Shiang Wu, Yi Ching Lin. An Alternative Technique for Deflation of a Nondeflating Balloon in a Small Caliber F8 Foley Catheter in Women. JTUA. 2009;20:32-3.
13. Harikrishnan S, Nair K, Tharakan JM, Titus T, Kumar VKA, Sivasankaran S. Percutaneous transmitral commissurotomy in juvenile mitral stenosis-comparison of long term results of Inoue balloon technique and metallic commissurotomy. Catheter Cardiovasc Interv. 2006;67(3):453–9.

Chapter 35

Emergency Surgery after Percutaneous Mitral Valvotomy

Praveen Reddy Bayya, Praveen Kumar Neema, Praveen Kerala Varma

▓ INTRODUCTION

Inoue and colleagues[1] in 1984 described percutaneous transmitral commissurotomy as an effective alternative to closed mitral valvuloplasty (CMV) for mitral stenosis (MS). Reported complications of PMV include mitral regurgitation (MR), cardiac tamponade, complete heart block, thromboembolism, and left-to-right shunt across the septal puncture.

Emergency surgery is rarely needed for the complications resulting from PMV. It may be required, however, for massive hemopericardium resulting from left ventricular or atrial perforation unresponsive to pericardiocentesis or, for severe MR leading to hemodynamic collapse or refractory pulmonary edema.[2]

Incidence

During PMV, the appearance of a new or the increase of a previously mild MR is frequent[2,3] but the development of severe MR is about 4%.[2-5] Cardiac perforation and tamponade occur in 0.5 to 12%[4,5] of patients, though recent reports show much lower incidence.[6] Tamponade and/or perforation are the most common indication for emergency cardiac surgery and the most common cause of death in the catheterization laboratory.[4] Emergency surgery is rarely required (<1%).[4]

Hemopericardium and Cardiac Tamponade

Patients who develop hemopericardium following transseptal puncture may experience chest pain accompanied by hypotension. Any unexplained hypotension following an attempt at transseptal puncture should alert the interventional cardiologist to rule out hemopericardium. Mild pericardial effusion following the introduction of only the transseptal needle may settle by itself and may not need pericardiocentesis. Hemopericardium recognized after the septal dilator has dilated the interatrial septum will need pericardiocentesis. When it is recognized, it is recommended to keep the septal dilator across the tear with the tip in the LA, which will prevent ooze to the pericardium to some extent. The next thing to do is pericardiocentesis and to keep a pigtail catheter inside the pericardial space. Even after the initiation of pericardiocentesis and autotransfusion, the dilator needs to be kept in place till the patient is wheeled to the surgical theater, where the surgical team removes it while the patient is put on cardiopulmonary bypass. Removing the dilator can result in massive bleeding into the pericardium, which can be catastrophic. The presentation of hemopericardium occurring after a left ventricular tear will be more dramatic as the left ventricular pressure is much higher. The hemodynamic compromise will be sudden and needs immediate pericardiocentesis, autotransfusion and surgery.

Mechanism of Hemopericardium

Pericardial hemorrhage may be related to transseptal catheterization or perforation of the left ventricular apex. The interatrial septal puncture is the critical step in performing PMV. In the presence of left or right atrial enlargement, the free wall enlarges while the inter-atrial septum is pushed relatively inferior. Therefore, the likelihood of a high septal puncture is enhanced in the presence of an enlarged left or right atrium (Fig. 35.1). TEE-guided septal puncture can be helpful in avoiding this complication.[6]

Exaggerated movements of the guidewires or the balloon/devices can lead to perforation of the left ventricular apex.[5] In our series, cardiac tamponade occurred in eight cases: before dilatation in seven patients and during dilatation in one patient. The causes of cardiac tamponade included left atrial roof puncture in four cases, left atrial appendage tear in two cases, left ventricular tear in one case, and right atrial roof tear in one case.[6]

Some patients develop cardiac tamponade due to stitch phenomenon. In patients with enlarged left atrium, there is no atrial septum in the region beyond or near the right lateral and inferior borders of the LA. The overlapping walls of RA and LA form this region. If this region is punctured, the catheter/needle may perforate the right atrial wall and then re-enter the LA (the so-called "stitch phenomenon") through the pericardial space. This is a dangerous situation as the blood enters the pericardial space both from LA and RA. So, it has to be tackled without delay by surgery (Fig. 35.1).

Management of Hemopericardium and Cardiac Tamponade

When hemopericardium is suspected it has to be confirmed by echocardiography. Loss of cardiac pulsations as evidenced by the immobility of the left heart border and a pericardial halo seen in fluoroscopy are clues to the presence of hemopericardium.

Tamponade events secondary to a puncture during transseptal catheterization are of variable gravity, but can be well-tolerated.[7]

Echocardiography will confirm the existence of pericardial fluid that had been absent before PMV.[8] Pericardiocentesis in the catheterization laboratory usually allows stabilization of the patient's condition and secondary transfer for cardiac surgery.[5] In these circumstances, it is logical to simultaneously treat the hemopericardium as well as the mitral valve pathology.[8]

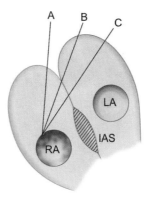

Fig. 35.1: Various mechanisms of CT in our series. In presence of enlarged right atrium (RA) or left atrium (LA), interatrial septum (IAS) is displaced inferiorly, leading to high puncture. A and B lead to roof puncture, whereas C leads to LAA perforation (Published with permission from Varma PK, et al. J Thorac Cardiovasc Surg 2005;130:772-6.)

Hemopericardium secondary to perforation of the LV necessitates immediate control of the ventricular tear. Patients need to undergo emergent cardiopulmonary bypass and suturing of left ventricular perforation.

It is mandatory to inspect the visceral surface of the pericardium as there is a possibility that there may be multiple leaks. There is a chance of the needle entering the right ventricle while attempting pericardiocentesis. This rent also needs to be inspected and closed. There are reports of injury to the coronary artery (left anterior descending coronary artery) while attempting pericardiocentesis, this also needs to be checked perioperatively.

■ ACUTE MITRAL REGURGITATION

Presentation

Clinical tolerance to acutely produced severe MR is variable, while some patients require emergency surgery, others do not need it,[3] and even a few may have a decrease in the severity of MR over time.[8] The onset of chest pain[7] and massive pulmonary edema associated with serious hemodynamic instability refractory to medical therapy frequently signifies severe trauma to the mitral apparatus. Despite a reduction in diastolic mitral gradient the mean left atrial pressure fails to drop because of a significant increase[3] (even more than 100 mm Hg) in the left atrial V wave[2] accompanied by an increase in left ventricular end diastolic pressure and a significant drop in cardiac output.[2]

The acute rise in left atrial pressure lead to acute rise in pulmonary pressure and right ventricular afterload, decreased coronary perfusion, ischemia and right ventricular failure. Associated septal shift and falling left ventricular preload leads to a vicious cycle of myocardial ischemia and hemodynamic collapse and needs to be addressed emergently before the onset of end organ damage.

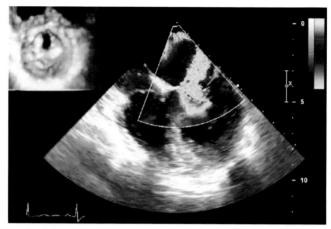

Fig. 35.2: The preoperative TEE picture of a patient who developed severe MR following PMV. Inset – 3D picture showing tear in the AML

Pande et al. has reported that patients undergoing MBV with an RVSP >76 mm Hg and the presence of noncommissural calcium on the mitral valve leaflet, or those who develop an RVSP of 77 mmHg following the procedure will very likely require emergency MVR.

Transthoracic echocardiography allows precise identification of the lesion (Fig. 35.2).[8] and allows quantification of MR. Large central MR jet (area >40% of LA area), a wall impinging jet of any size, swirling into LA and Doppler vena contracta width >0.7 cm all denote severe MR9. Hypotension and hypoxia are the common manifestations. Orthopnea and pulmonary edema are documented less frequently.[9]

Mechanism of Mitral Insufficiency

Post-PMV MR most commonly occurs at the site of successful commissural split.[2,5] Commissural MR, and the less frequently occurring anterior mitral leaflet prolapse, is usually mild and of no clinical consequence.[2]

In contrast, severe MR following PMV is an unpredictable event[2] and is almost always due to noncommissural tearing of the anterior or posterior mitral leaflet with disruption of the valve mechanism, and less frequently due to damage to the subvalvular apparatus, mainly chordal rupture.[3]

The influence of mitral anatomy in the production of MR is still controversial and studies have failed to identify patients who subsequently developed severe MR.[3,10,11]

Nevertheless, surgically excised mitral valves of patients with severe MR often show certain anatomical characteristics, which, alone or together, may have contributed to an undesirable transmission of balloon pressure forces with the result of valve disruption instead of the expected commissural cleavage. These are: uneven mitral leaflets, with thick areas coexisting with more normal or even thin areas; severe and extensive fusion, thickening and foreshortening of subvalvular structures; and calcium in one or both commissures.[3] Commissural and paracommissural fibrocalcific dystrophy represent sites of greater resistance that hinder commissural splitting, leading to delivery of the balloon pressure to the relatively thin AML and causing the tear.[6] However, in the presence of rigid, unyielding commissures, areas with lesser resistance can "give way." The posterior leaflet is often rolled up and thickened, whereas a more pliable anterior leaflet becomes vulnerable. In the case of severely thickened and foreshortened subvalvular structures, an excessive tension might be transmitted at the insertion site of the chordae in the leaflet, which produces a leaflet tear extending from the insertion point to the mitral annulus.[3] The "string-plucking effect" leading to chordal rupture and severe MR has also been reported.[12]

Other mechanisms noted are paracommissural tears,[8,9] rupture of the papillary muscle,[5,8] or excessive commissural splitting.[5] The thickening and shortening of subvalvular structures is often underestimated by echocardiography.[3]

In our experience, only tear of the leaflet caused acute, severe MR necessitating emergency surgery. The leaflet tear led to severe elevation of left atrial pressure, and in the presence of unrelieved MS, the clinical picture of pulmonary edema ensued. Most of our patients had pulmonary arterial hypertension before PMV (mean pulmonary artery pressure 68.6 +/–26.2 mm Hg).[6] Acute MR in the presence of severe pulmonary arterial hypertension leads to hemodynamic compromise.[11] Three of our patients with acute MR had previous CMV. The mitral valve was distorted after previous commissurotomy. More often, the valve was heavily fibrosed and thickened, with severe subvalvular pathology.

Even though excellent results have been reported from one large series,[10] the natural progression of rheumatic disease with the fibrocicatricial changes of commissurotomy could make the mitral valve anatomy heavily deformed, leading to transmission of balloon pressure in an unpredictable way that would cause valve damage.[6]

Management of Mitral Insufficiency

Acute severe MR most often require surgery. Mortality is significantly high when time interval to surgery is more than 24 hours, cause being multiorgan dysfunction secondary to low cardiac output. Hence, it is extremely important that patients are taken up for surgery at the earliest, before the vicious cycle and consequences of low output manifest.[9] In most cases of acute severe MR, following PMV, mitral valve replacement becomes necessary because of the severity of the underlying valve disease.[5] Valve commissures are often severely fibrotic, with severe subvalvular pathology and paracommissural calcium making the valve unsuitable for repair.[6] Conservative surgery combining suture of the tear and commissurotomy, has been performed successfully in patients with less severe valve deformity.[5] Though the need for valve replacement is more closely related to the extent of valve disease than to the tear itself,[5,8] leaflet tears can often be irregular and extending to and involving the mitral annulus, deterring attempts at valve repair.[6]

Mortality and Morbidity

The cost and time constraints of having an operating room and the surgical and anesthetic team on standby have led many centers to relax this practice; however, this has also proved costly at times.[8] Emergency surgery after PMV is associated with significant mortality and morbidity in the postoperative period.[6] Sudden elevation of right ventricular systolic pressure as a result of MR and hypotension could lead to right ventricular subendocardial ischemia, which may manifest as low cardiac output in the postoperative period. Early ventilation and surgery, with the capacity for an on-site circulatory support system could decrease adverse outcomes.[6,8,12] Death as a complication of cardiac perforation is usually a result of LV perforation and not usually a complication of transseptal catheterization.[4]

■ REFERENCES

1. Inoue K, Owaki T, Nakamura T, Kitamura F, Miyamoto N. Clinical application of transvenous mitral commissurotomy by a new balloon catheter. J Thorac Cardiovasc Surg. 1984;87(3):394–402.
2. Essop MR, Wisenbaugh T, Skoularigis J, Middlemost S, Sareli P. Mitral regurgitation following mitral balloon valvotomy. Differing mechanisms for severe versus mild-to-moderate lesions. Circulation. 1991;84(4):1669–79.
3. Hernandez R, Macaya C, Bañuelos C, Alfonso F, Goicolea J, Iñiguez A, et al. Predictors, mechanisms and outcome of severe mitral regurgitation complicating percutaneous mitral valvotomy with the Inoue balloon. Am J Cardiol. 1992; 70(13):1169–74.
4. Complications and mortality of percutaneous balloon mitral commissurotomy. A report from the National Heart, Lung, and Blood Institute Balloon Valvuloplasty Registry. Circulation. 1992;85(6):2014–24.
5. Vahanian A, Iung B, Cormier B. Mitral valvuloplasty. In: Topol EL, Editor. Textbook of interventional cardiology. 4th edn. Philadelphia: WB Saunders; 2003.p.921-40.
6. Varma PK, Theodore S, Neema PK, Ramachandran P, Sivadasanpillai H, Nair KK, et al. Emergency surgery after percutaneous transmitral commissurotomy: operative versus echocardiographic findings, mechanisms of complications, and outcomes. J Thorac Cardiovasc Surg. 2005;130(3):772–6.
7. Acar C, Deloche A, Tibi PR, Jebara V, Chachques JC, Fabiani JN, et al. Operative findings after percutaneous mitral dilation. Ann Thorac Surg. 1990;49(6):959–63.
8. O'Shea JP, Abascal VM, Wilkins GT, Marshall JE, Brandi S, Acquatella H, et al. Unusual sequelae after percutaneous mitral valvuloplasty: a Doppler echocardiographic study. J Am Coll Cardiol. 1992;19(1):186–91.
9. Nanjappa M, Ananthakrishna R, Setty SKH, Bhat P, Shankarappa RK, Panneerselvam A, et al. Acute severe mitral regurgitation following balloon mitral valvotomy: echocardiographic features, operative findings, and outcome in 50 surgical cases. Catheterization and Cardiovascular Interventions. 2013; 81:603–8.
10 Sharma S, Loya YS, Desai DM, Pinto RJ. Balloon valvotomy for mitral restenosis after open or closed surgical commissurotomy. Int J Cardiol. 1993;39(2):103–8.
11. Tempe DK, Mehta N, Mohan JC, Tandon MS, Nigam M. Early hemodynamic changes following emergency mitral valve replacement for traumatic mitral insufficiency following balloon mitral valvotomy: Report of six cases. Anesthesiology 1998;89:1583.
12. Chern M-S, Chang H-J, Lin F-C, Wu D. String-plucking as a mechanism of chordal rupture during balloon mitral valvuloplasty using Inoue balloon catheter. Catheter Cardiovasc Interv. 1999;47(2):213–7.

Chapter 36

Troubleshooting of Single Balloon Catheters— Inoue and Accura Balloons

Harikrishnan S

■ INTRODUCTION

Inoue or Accura balloons are gadgets which can be used usually without any major issues once the operator is well-trained. The operator should have adequate knowledge about the structure of the balloon before using it. Improper usage of the balloon results in damage to the balloon and can also harm the patient by increasing the procedure time and radiation exposure.

Few issues faced while using the balloon are the following—kinking, twisting of the inner balloon lumen and tear in the balloon. These issues are being dealt with in this Chapter. Other issues like nondeflation of the balloon and detachment of the balloon from the shaft are described elsewhere in this book.

Kinking of the Balloon

Kinking of the balloon is one of the most common problems which happens during PMV using Inoue or Accura balloon. This happens because of the unique construction of the balloon.

One should realize that the central lumen inside the balloon per se is made of a polythene tube which does not have adequate strength to keep the balloon stretched by itself. So, it requires the support of the balloon stretching tube or the LA guidewire to keep the balloon stretched.

Kinking while Inserting the Balloon

If the gold hub tube is pushed into the balloon without the support of the balloon stretching tube it results in kinking of the balloon (Figs 36.1 and 36.2).

Kinking while Removing the Balloon

If the operator is not careful, kinking can also happen while removing the balloon. The fact to be kept in mind is that the innermost polythene tube does not have the strength to keep the balloon stretched without the support of the balloon stretching tube (Fig. 36.3). So, while withdrawing the balloon

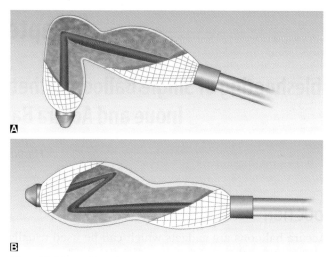

Figs 36.1A and B: Kinking of the balloon: (A) An acute angle; (B) A zig-zag which is difficult to be noticed externally. (With kind permission from Toray Inc.)

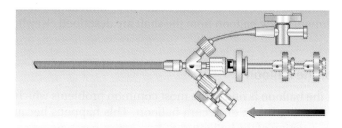

Fig. 36.2: Cause of kinking—when the gold hub is pushed forwards without the support of the balloon stretching tube (With kind permission from Toray Inc.)

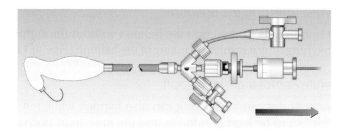

Fig. 36.3: Cause of kinking—if the balloon stretching tube is pulled back without pulling back the gold hub and without guidewire support it can result in kinking (With kind permission from Toray Inc.)

from the left atrium, the gold hub and the balloon stretching tube should be withdrawn only together unless the guidewire is in place and fully protruded from the balloon tip and coiled in the LA. This caution disregarded, the catheter could bend at an acute angle resulting in damage to the device or difficulty in carrying out the procedure. Never use a kinked balloon.

Troubleshooting When the Balloon is Kinked
(Adapted from Toray Inc.[1])

Solutions to Kinking: Follow Steps 1 to 6

Step 1: Unlock the inner tube from the W-connector and pull it out until resistance is felt (do not attempt to reconnect the hub of the balloon stretching tube to the inner tube while the inner tube is still locked into the W-connector).

Step 2: Inflate the balloon completely, then deflate immediately.

Step 3: Insert the guidewire.*

Step 4: Insert the balloon stretching tube* into the inner tube and secure the hubs with the luer lock.

Step 5: Advance the inner tube (with the balloon stretching tube locked) into the W-connector. Place the pin of the inner tube into the slot on the W-connector and secure the lock. This way the balloon will be stretched normally.

Step 6: Withdraw the catheter from the patient and discard it. Use a new Inoue balloon catheter.

Loss of Balloon Volume

We prepare the balloon and keep the desired volume of diluted contrast in the syringe. It is always recommended to do a pretesting with the volume in the syringe and check the actual inflation volume. In the developing world where the syringes are obtained from different vendors, there may be a chance of having wrong volume in the syringe. This can lead to under dilation or over dilation of the balloon, both of which can be problematic.

But if the proximal hub of the balloon is loosened (in an attempt to pull back the gold hub in case there is resistance) there is a chance of contrast leakage. This may result in inadvertent under-dilatation of the valve if not recognized on time.

---

* If the guidewire or balloon stretching tube cannot be inserted correctly into the inner tube following the above procedure, the balloon cannot be stretched and this may result in difficulty when removing the kinked balloon through the interatrial septum and/or the femoral vein puncture site. In this case, the kinked balloon should be carefully removed using the best clinical judgment.

To prevent this complication always note the balloon volume before each dilatation. If loss of volume is found, replenish the volume before the balloon dilatation.

Twisting of the Inner Tube of the Balloon

Twisting of the inner tube lumen occurs when there is a rotation of the inner tube at its attachment to the W-connector end of the Inoue balloon (Fig. 36.4). It is very important to hold the W-connector and not the inner tube during catheter manipulation, this will avoid twisting of the inner tube. It is equally important to hold the W-connector and not the inner tube during manipulation of the stylet to direct the balloon through the mitral valve (Fig. 36.5).

If the inner tube is found to be twisted, gently try to rotate it in the opposite direction and confirm untwisting by passing a guidewire or the stylet very gently.

If balloon kinking or twisting of the inner tube occurs, there is a possibility that the guidewire may get stuck in the balloon catheter and the balloon may not get stretched. Never insert/advance the balloon stretching tube under these conditions. If the balloon stretching tube is inserted under these conditions, it may also get stuck. In the event of a balloon kink or twisted tube, there is a possibility of the stylet also getting stuck. Withdrawing the guidewire or stylet by force may cause damage to the tip of the guidewire or stylet, leading to even separation of the tip.

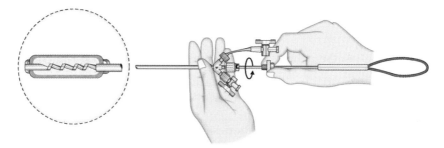

Fig. 36.4: Cause of twisting of the inner tube of the balloon due to manipulation of the gold hub (With kind permission from Toray Inc.)

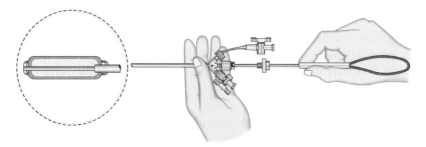

Fig. 36.5: Correct way to manipulate the balloon holding the W-connector and the stylet (With kind permission from Toray Inc.)

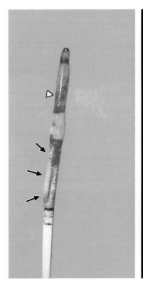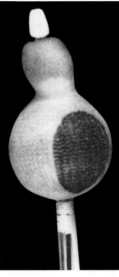

Fig. 36.6: Tear in the proximal balloon exposing the mesh (arrows). The distal part of the balloon with the normal smooth glistening appearance of latex is seen (arrowhead). The right panel shows the in vitro appearance of the balloon in a case reported by Kerkar et al. [Published with permission from Wiley Inc. Cathet Cardiovasc Diagn. 1994;31(2):127-9]

Tear in the Balloon

The Inoue balloon has different compliance characteristics. The distal segment being the most compliant inflates first, followed by the proximal and finally the middle segment (Fig. 36.6).

But when there is a tear in the outer layer of the proximal segment of the balloon, this unique inflation mechanism may fail, making the proximal segment most compliant and therefore getting inflated first. When the proximal segment inflates before the distal (i.e. reverse of the normal), a possibility of balloon rupture should be anticipated. However, a similar rent in the outer layer of the distal segment would not change the order of inflation and would therefore remain unrecognized.

Tear in the balloon can lead to rupture with its incident complications.[2-5] The detailed description of balloon rupture is given in the chapter on "Device related complications"—Chapter 29.

Troubleshooting in the Event of a Tear

Though, it is advisable to remove the balloon from the system and use a new balloon, in the event of a suspected tear, there are other methods to tackle the problem. Patel et al. have described a method to circumvent the problem of the reverse sequence of balloon inflation in the event of a tear. The sequence of balloon inflation has been described as follows: When there is a tear, the deflation sequence is also reversed. The proximal portion deflates first followed by the distal portion. So, Patel et al. hitched the balloon against the mitral valve as soon as the proximal segment of the balloon is deflated. Then the balloon is rapidly inflated opening the valve (Figs 36.7A to D).

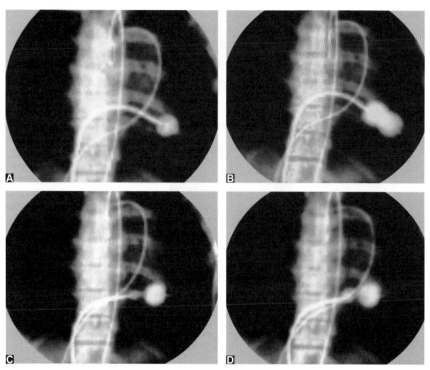

Figs 36.7A to D: Steps of the modified Inoue technique to troubleshoot a large proximal segment tear during percutaneous balloon mitral valvuloplasty: (A) Inflation of the proximal segment; (B) Inflation of the distal segment followed by the middle segment. Leading to a completely inflated Inoue balloon; (C) Hitching of the inflated distal segment across the mitral valve following deflation of the middle and proximal segments; (D) Inflation of the proximal and middle segments, leading to removal of the waist [Published with permission from Patel et al. Indian Heart J. 2003;55(2):178-9][4]

Since, a tear in the distal balloon will not alter the inflation-deflation sequence, there is no need for modification of the technique in case of a distal tear.

■ REFERENCES

1. http://www.torayusa.com/medical/ibpd.htm.
2. Kerkar PG, Vora AM, Sethi JP, Kale PA, Dalvi BV. Unusual tear in Inoue balloon during percutaneous balloon mitral valvuloplasty in a patient with calcific mitral stenosis. Cathet Cardiovasc Diagn. 1994;31(2):127-9.
3. Chow WH, Chow TC, Cheung KL. Angiographic recognition of a proximal balloon tear during Inoue balloon mitral valvotomy. Cathet Cardiovasc Diagn. 1993;28(3):235-7.
4. Patel T, Shah SC, Ranjan A. The modified Inoue technique: a simple troubleshooting approach to a proximal segment tear of an Inoue balloon. Indian Heart J. 2003;55(2):178-9.
5. Hung JS, Lau KW. Pitfalls and tips in inoue balloon mitral commissurotomy. Cathet Cardiovasc Diagn. 1996;37(2):188-99.

Section 6

PMV in Special Situations

Chapter 37

Percutaneous Mitral Valvotomy in Pregnancy

Shyam Sundar Reddy

MITRAL STENOSIS AND PREGNANCY

Although rheumatic heart disease has become a rare entity in affluent societies, it is still prevalent in the developing world. In the third world, cardiac disease remains an important cause of maternal mortality. Rheumatic heart disease remains the most common type of heart disease in pregnant women in developing countries, and up to 75% of these patients have mitral stenosis (MS).[1-6]

Pregnancy is a hyperdynamic state characterized by an increase in cardiac output, heart rate and oxygen consumption. The hemodynamic changes associated with pregnancy may be viewed as normal adaptation to the 15-20% increase in oxygen consumption required by the fetus. During the first trimester, blood volume increases up to 60% above the values in the nonpregnant state. Cardiac output begins to rise during the first 10 weeks, reaching a peak 30–45% above the resting nonpregnant state by around 20th week. The increase in cardiac output is associated with a fall in systemic vascular resistance, which results in either a fall or no change in blood pressure, and a widened pulse pressure. Mean heart rate rises, average 10–20 beats/minute at term; most of this increase occurring by the eighth week. These changes are most significant between the 24th and 26th week of gestation and can be explained by an increase in blood volume, the presence of a placental arteriovenous fistula and the hormones produced by the fetus and the placenta.[7,8]

The normal mitral valve has no pressure gradient across, and the increased cardiac output of pregnancy is well tolerated. However, in MS a gradient exists between the left atrium (LA) and ventricle, the magnitude of which depends on the severity of the stenosis and blood flow. Thus, at a given severity of MS the gradient depends on flow. This flow is equivalent to cardiac output and is determined by heart rate and diastolic filling period. Thus, as cardiac output increases during pregnancy, mitral valve flow increases resulting in an increased gradient across the valve. The resultant increase in left atrial pressure causes pulmonary venous hypertension and an increased risk of pulmonary edema. The pulmonary arterial and right ventricular pressures are elevated and right ventricular failure eventually may ensue. The presence of MS in pregnancy leads not only to low systemic perfusion, but also to pulmonary congestion in as many as 25% of patients.[7-11]

During labor and delivery, extra demands are placed on the cardiovascular system. The cardiac response to pain during contractions and the increased amount of blood returning to the heart from the contracting uterus represents an additional 20% rise in cardiac output. The largest fluid shifts occur after delivery when the normal pregnant patient (due to shift of blood from placenta) experiences an increase in cardiac output of up to 65% during the immediate postpartum period. In addition, tachycardia resulting from pain, stress of labor, inappropriate vasodilatation or prostaglandin-agonist therapy can precipitate pulmonary edema in women with MS.[10] This occurs as tachycardia is accompanied by a disproportionate reduction of diastolic filling period across the mitral valve and results in elevated left atrial pressures with consequent increased risk of pulmonary edema.[7-11]

Concomitant aortic valve disease, anemia and cardiac arrhythmias may further aggravate the abnormal hemodynamics of mitral stenosis. Atrial irritability may be increased during pregnancy and atrial fibrillation can lead to catastrophic pulmonary edema during late pregnancy as well as thrombus formation and additional risk of cerebrovascular embolization.[7-11]

It is, therefore, not surprising that MS in pregnancy, if not treated appropriately, is associated with a high maternal and perinatal mortality. The rate of maternal death rate is nearly 1% and varies directly with NYHA class (0.4% in class I or II, 6.8% for class III or IV). The highest risk is during the intrapartum and postpartum period. In the presence of atrial fibrillation (AF) maternal mortality is further increased to 14–17%. Similarly, perinatal mortality rates are low in class I-II but increase to 12–31% in patients in NYHA Class III-IV.[2-6]

Ideally, if severe symptomatic MS is diagnosed in a nonpregnant woman desiring pregnancy, it should be treated by percutaneous mitral valvotomy or surgical intervention before the patient conceives. However, for several reasons, this is not always possible. Many of the patients will be detected to have MS for the first time during pregnancy.

■ MEDICAL THERAPY

During pregnancy patients with severe MS present a challenging problem because of a high rate of fetal and maternal complications. Although medical treatment is always recommended as first-line therapy, the medications have their own limitations. One must also consider the untoward effects of some drugs in this particular setting. Diuretics are known to decrease placental perfusion. The tachycardia is of sinus origin and is unresponsive to digoxin because the increased sympathetic tone in pregnancy overrides the vagal effect of digoxin.[12,13]

Beta-blocker is often effective in slowing the exertional tachycardia and may allow pregnancy to continue without the need of intervention.

However, some patients may not be able to tolerate the dose of beta-blockers sufficient to prevent tachycardia. Beta-blocker therapy in pregnancy has been reported in largely uncontrolled retrospective studies to be associated with fetal growth restriction, bradycardia or hypoglycemia in the newborn infant. However, some studies using beta-blockers, such as atenolol, indicate that growth restriction is not significant if exposure is minimal and confined to the latter part of pregnancy.[14,15]

INTERVENTIONS IN MITRAL STENOSIS IN PREGNANCY

Relief of mitral valve obstruction is needed when symptoms persist despite medical therapy. Surgical mitral valvotomy, closed (CMV) or open (OMV) has a significant risk of fetal death. With open surgical commissurotomy performed under general anesthesia and extracorporeal circulation, fetal mortality is between 15% and 33%. Closed commissurotomy carries a lower risk to the fetus, although a 5% to 15% of fetal loss has been associated with this technique as well.[16-19] Zitnik et al. have reported a 5% rate of maternal mortality and a 33% of fetal mortality in 22 pregnant women undergoing closed mitral commissurotomy.[18] Becker et al. described one death and 20% of fetal loss in 68 patients after surgical mitral commissurotomy.[19] However, the closed procedure is thought to be less effective than the open commissurotomy and may be more difficult in cases of severe stenosis, calcification, thrombi, or regurgitation. In addition, surgical experience with closed commissurotomy has declined over the last few decades because the technique has been largely replaced by open commissurotomy or percutaneous techniques in most centers.

Jain et al. reported a comparison of 48 patients with mitral stenosis who had intervention before delivery and those who had no intervention and found that the incidence of preterm labor in the test group (1/18) was lower than that in the control group (10/30) (P = 0.035). The groups did not differ in mode of delivery, mean birth weight, or neonatal complications.[20]

PERCUTANEOUS MITRAL VALVOTOMY (PMV) IN PREGNANCY

Percutaneous mitral valvotomy is an effective alternative for the management of patients with mitral stenosis during pregnancy. It was first performed by Inoue et al. in 1984[21] and has proved to be a safe procedure for the mother and child, with outstanding short-term results. The Inoue technique seems to be particularly attractive as fluoroscopy time is short in this method. A comparison of PMV with CMV has shown equivalent efficacy.[22] The hazards of PMV are related to hemodynamic changes during the procedure, radiation hazards and complications like MR and pericardial tamponade. The hemodynamic risks during PMV are due to hypotension from compression of the inferior vena cava when the mother is in the supine position for a prolonged period and/or due to the prolonged inflation and deflation of the balloon during dilatation of the mitral valve. This may cause fetal distress, leading to an increased likelihood of delivery by cesarean section.[23]

Depending upon the dose level, radiation during pregnancy may result in intrauterine growth restriction, microcephaly, leukemia or other malignancies later in life. Avoidance of PMV during organogenesis, the use of an abdominal shield, and avoidance of left ventricular angiography have significantly reduced the hazard of radiation to the mother and the fetus. The average estimated radiation dose received by the fetus during PMV procedure is 0.2 rad, which is much below the allowed safe dose of 5 rad. Therapeutic abortion is recommended when the fetus is exposed to 10 rad or more.[24,25] Farhat et al. reported no clinical abnormalities in 44 children whose mothers had been submitted to a PMV after a follow-up of 28 months.[26]

In pregnant women, some technical problems may be encountered during the PMV procedure. The hypercoagulable state in pregnancy necessitates a quick transseptal puncture, after which heparin needs to be administered. The gravid uterus may compress and distort the inferior vena cava, making passage of catheters difficult. The elevated diaphragm near term may alter the usual lie of the interatrial septum, making it more horizontal. Thus, it is crucial to assess the interatrial septum in detail before performing the transseptal puncture. The high cardiac output state of pregnancy produces higher gradients across the MV, which should be kept in mind while assessing the result of PMV.[27]

Percutaneous mitral valvotomy can be performed whenever possible, starting from the 12th week of gestation, to avoid the inherent risks of radiation (organogenesis). However, in the presence of unstable clinical conditions, PMV can be performed irrespective of the gestational age. Successful PMV during pregnancy should improve the patient's clinical condition, permitting a pregnant woman to return to NYHA functional class I or II as a consequence of improved hemodynamics and MVA. PMV should permit gestation to reach full-term, offering the fetus good conditions for adequate intrauterine development and better clinical conditions to the mother until delivery.[27-30]

◼ PMV IN PREGNANCY—PROCEDURAL DETAILS

Since PMV in pregnancy is technically a demanding procedure, it should be undertaken by operators who are well-experienced in PMV procedures. PMV is performed in the fasting state in the catheterization laboratory.

Preferably, it should be done in the morning hours as the patient is fasting overnight. Surgical and gynecology back-up is usually arranged and kept ready.

To limit fetal radiation exposure, all patients will have their abdomen shielded with lead sheets from the diaphragm to pubic symphysis. There are lead shields available for this purpose.[31] We attach two lead shield sheets together using a adhesive tape and that is used to cover the anterior abdomen. The posterior body is protected by a lead sheet on the cathlab table on which the patient will be lying on (Figs 37.1 and 37.2). The lead shields used for covering the anterior abdomen should be light weight, so that it will not compress the gravid uterus.

Limiting fluoroscopy should be one of the primary aims while performing PMV in pregnancy. Fluoroscopy time should be monitored during the

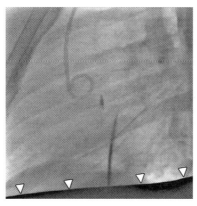

Fig. 37.1: Fluoroscopic view of performing septal puncture in a pregnant patient for severe MS. Note the lead shield protecting the fetus (arrowheads)

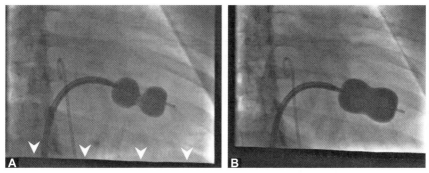

Figs 37.2A and B: Fluoroscopic view of successful balloon dilatation in a pregnant patient during PMV. Note the lead shield protecting the fetus (arrowheads)

procedure and fluoroscopy used only when absolutely necessary. Left ventriculography and right heart catheterization are usually avoided to reduce the fluoroscopy time.

All PMV procedures are usually performed under local anesthesia with the Inoue (or similar balloon) technique using the transseptal, anterograde left-sided cardiac approach. Maximum balloon size possible is determined according to the patients' height (height in centimeters/10 + 10).

Right femoral artery and venous access is obtained. Initially, a Goodale Lubin (GL) or Multipurpose catheter is introduced into the innominate vein using an exchange length 0.35" guidewire. This is then exchanged for a Mullins sheath or dilator. It is always better to obtain a blood sample to assess the SVC saturation which will give an idea about the hemodynamic status of the patient.

Then the Brockenbrough septal puncture needle is introduced into the Mullins sheath and simultaneously the assistant puts the pigtail catheter in the noncoronary sinus of the aortic root. Septal puncture is done usually in lateral view and LA is entered and the pressure is recorded. Then the pigtail-shaped LA wire is introduced into the LA, septum is dilated and Heparin 100 IU/kg is given intravenously. Subsequently, the balloon is introduced and MV dilatation is done.

Stepwise dilatations of 0.5 mm should be done until a successful result is obtained or there is any evidence of increasing mitral regurgitation. A successful optimal outcome is defined as a final post-PMV mitral valve area (MVA) of >1.3 cm^2 or an increase in MVA of 25% compared to the preprocedural MVA, in the absence of severe MR. It is advisable to be conservative in pregnant patients as our aim is to avoid MR and mitral valve replacement at any cost as it can be catastrophic to the mother and the fetus.

SHORT- AND LONG-TERM OUTCOMES FOLLOWING PMV IN PREGNANCY

Gupta et al. in a series of 40 patients who underwent PMV in pregnancy demonstrated a procedural success of 97.5% (39/40). 11 patients, in whom PMV was performed before 20 weeks of pregnancy, subsequently underwent medical termination of pregnancy uneventfully. 18 patients had a normal delivery, three underwent cesarean section for fetal distress, one had a preterm delivery, and there was one stillbirth. Full-term delivery data were available in 23 babies—all were healthy without any complications.[32] Nercolini et al. in a series of 44 consecutive PMV in pregnant patients showed a procedural success in 95% with no major complications. Data available from 37 patients showed that 30 patients (81%) reached term and delivered normal infants. Seven patients (18.9%) delivered prematurely, resulting in two fetal deaths; one patient delivered a stillborn. Both studies proved the efficacy and safety of PMV in pregnant patients.[33]

Mangione et al. followed up 23 patients for 5.33 ± 6 3.12 years, 91% of them were in FC I and II. Two patients (9%) who remained in FC III underwent a repeat successful PMV; no further intervention was required. There were no embolic events or death related to the procedure. Echocardiography showed an initial increase in mitral valve area from 1.14 ± 0.22 cm^2 to 2.01 ± 0.21 cm^2 ($P < 0.0001$). During long-term follow-up, the MVA decreased to a mean of 1.75 ± 0.24 cm^2 ($P < 0.0001$). Initial transmitral valve gradient decreased from 17.73 ± 4.56 mm Hg to 5.91 ± 1.80 mm Hg ($P < 0.0001$) and increased to 8.95 ± 3.58 ($P - 0.002$) during long-term follow-up. Twenty one children (96%), aged 4.91 ± 2.8 years, showed normal growth and development, and no clinical abnormalities were observed.[34] The report by Mishra et al. also showed a very good outcome in pregnant patients who underwent PMV.[35]

Routray et al. in study of PMV in 40 pregnant women showed that mitral valve area increased from 0.82 ± 0.34 to 1.9 ± 0.4 cm^2 (P-0.001). One patient had pericardial tamponade. Mean fluoroscopy time was 5.5 ± 3.8 minute. There was one stillbirth, no maternal death/abortion/intrauterine growth restriction. All 39 babies were normal at birth. One baby died at 7 months due to pneumonia. On follow-up for 36 ± 15 months, all 38 babies maintained normal growth and development without any thyroid disease or malignancy.[36]

Esteves et al.[37] in their study of 71 consecutive pregnant women who underwent PMV—reported procedural success of 100% with a significant increase in mitral valve area from 0.9 ± 0.2 to 2.0 ± 0.3 cm^2 (p < 0.001). At the end of pregnancy, 8% of the patients were in New York Heart Association functional class I or II. At a mean follow-up of 44 ± 31 months, the total event-free survival rate was 54%. The mean gestational age at delivery time was 38 ± 1 week. Preterm deliveries occurred in 9 patients (13%), including 2 twin pregnancies. The remaining 66 of 75 newborns (88%) had normal weight (mean 2.8 ± 0.6 kg) at delivery. At long-term follow-up of 44 ± 31 months after birth, the 66 children exhibited normal growth and development and did not show any clinical abnormalities.

Harikrishnan et al.[38] reported the data of 36 patients, with a procedural success rate of 97.2% (35/36) and no maternal mortality. All patients symptomatically improved and had uneventful deliveries. The children had normal growth and development at a follow-up of 2.8 ± 3.3 years.

Gulraze et al. has reported the 17 years outcome following mitral balloon valvuloplasty in pregnancy. They reported that PMV is a safe and useful procedure during pregnancy, with no short-or long-term adverse effects on the mothers and their obstetric future. The children born of subsequent pregnancies exhibited normal physical and mental development.[39] All these data shows that PMV can be safely performed in pregnancy with good short-term results. These patients had excellent outcomes following the procedure and majority had normal deliveries. The babies also had normal growth and development.

Manjunath et al. reported 15 years of PTMC experience.[40] Out of 12,555 patients who underwent BMV, 605 were pregnant. Majority were in NYHA class III and IV. 47 patients were in acute pulmonary edema. Single balloon (Inoue or Acura) was used in all the patients. Average fluoroscopy time was 5.1 + 2.5 minutes. Procedure was successful in 95.2% of patients. Mean left atrial pressure dropped from 32 + 16 to 14 + 5 mm Hg and mitral valve orifice area increased from 0.8 + 0.4 to 1.85 + .03 cm^2. Mild to moderate MR was seen in 10.5% of patients and 1.6% had severe MR. Serious complications like tamponade occurred in 1.8%, CVA in 0.4% and mortality in 0.7% of patients.

Krishna et al., who analyzed the Feto-maternal outcomes in 40 patients of RHD.[41] 14 patients (35%) underwent PTMC (10 patients prior to pregnancy and 4 patients during pregnancy). Obstetric outcome were good with no maternal mortality noted. Maternal morbidity in terms of CCF was associated with severity of disease. Surgical correction of lesion prior to pregnancy was associated with better pregnancy outcome. 30% preterm births were noted in those who underwent balloon mitral valvuloplasty (BMV) prior to pregnancy compared to 50% preterm births for those who underwent during pregnancy. One perinatal mortality was seen in patients who underwent BMV in present pregnancy.

In a study by Seyfollah Abdi et al., in which they analyzed 33 consecutive patients undergoing PTMC during pregnancy.[42] Mitral valve area increased from $0.83 \pm 0.13 \text{ cm}^2$ to $1.38 \pm 0.29 \text{ cm}^2$ (P = 0.007). Mean gradient of mitral valve decreased from 15.5 ± 7.4 mm Hg to 2.3 ± 2.3 mm Hg (P = 0.001). Pulmonary artery pressure decreased from 65.24 ± 17.9 to 50.45 ± 15.33. No maternal death, abortion, intrauterine growth restriction was observed and only one stillbirth occurred.

In another unreported study from our institution, wherein we compared the outcomes between PTMC and pregnant and nonpregnant women and also the maternal, fetal morbidity and mortality. Sixty two consecutive pregnant women were included in the study and were compared with 121 age matched nonpregnant females who underwent PTMC during the same period. There was no significant difference between the baseline clinical and demographic data of the two groups. MS mean gradient was higher in pregnant patients and more patients had PAH; other parameters were similar in both the groups. The mean fluoro time was 4.5 ± 3.6 minutes and the gestational age at BMV was 27.9 ± 4.1 weeks. Success was attained in >90% in both the groups, and the results were comparable. One patient in the pregnant group, who had to undergo emergency BMV, subsequently died due to sepsis in spite of successful BMV. On follow-up for 4.2 ± 2.7 years the incidence of AF, restenosis, event-free survival and functional class was similar in both the groups. Event free survival at last follow-up was comparable in both groups [56 (88.9%) vs 110 (90.9%)]. Follow-up data regarding delivery details was available in 51 patients (82.25%) only. Out of which successful outcomes were seen in 48 (84.1%) patients. Among the patients with successful outcomes 30 patients (58.8%) had a normal vaginal delivery, 17 (33.3%) underwent elective cesarean and 1(1.96%) had to undergo emergency cesarean (for obstetric reason). Three patients had a preterm delivery. Low birth weight was seen in 19 (39.6%) children and very low birth weight in 1 (2.1%) child. On follow-up for mean duration of 4.8 ± 2.9 years, 33 children (68.8%) had no evidence of any malnutrition. The predictors of low birth weight were low MVA, PAH and high LA (m) on multivariate analysis. On follow-up for 4.82 ± 2.97 years, all children had normal growth and development with no major congenital abnormalities.

KEY POINTS

- Pregnancy imposes significant hemodynamic stress to patients with severe mitral stenosis
- PMV is the procedure of choice in patients who need an intervention for mitral stenosis in pregnancy
- PMV can be safely performed in pregnancy with good short-term results
- These patients have excellent outcomes following the procedure and majority will have normal uneventful deliveries
- The babies born out of this pregnancy usually have normal growth and development.

REFERENCES

1. Szekely P, Snaith L. Maternal mortality in rheumatic heart disease. In: Szekely P, Snaith L (Eds). Heart and Pregnancy. Edinburgh: Churchill Livingstone; 1974. pp. 129–33.
2. McFaul PB, Dornan JC, Lamki H, Boyle D. Pregnancy complicated by maternal heart disease. A review of 519 women. Br J Obstet Gynaecol. 1988;95(9):861–7.
3. Vijaykumar M, Narula J, Reddy KS, Kaplan EL. Incidence of rheumatic fever and prevalence of rheumatic heart disease in India. Int J Cardiol. 1994;43(3):221–8.
4. Visser AA, Coetzee EJ, Grolier CJF, Cronje HS. Cardiac disease. In: Cronje HS, Grolier CJF, Visser AA (Eds). Obstetrics in Southern Africa. Pretoria: JL Van Schaik; 1996. p. 229.
5. Desai DK, Adanlawo M, Naidoo DP, Moodley J, Kleinschmidt I. Mitral stenosis in pregnancy: a four-year experience at King Edward VIII Hospital, Durban, South Africa. BJOG Int J Obstet Gynaecol. 2000;107(8):953–8.
6. Hameed A, Karaalp IS, Tummala PP, Wani OR, Canetti M, Akhter MW, et al. The effect of valvular heart disease on maternal and fetal outcome of pregnancy. J Am Coll Cardiol. 2001;37(3):893–9.
7. McAnulty JH, Morton MJ, Ueland K. The heart and pregnancy. Curr Probl Cardiol. 1988;13(9):589–665.
8. Walters WA, MacGregor WG, Hills M. Cardiac output at rest during pregnancy and the puerperium. Clin Sci. 1966;30(1):1–11.
9. Bhagwat AR, Engel PJ. Heart disease and pregnancy. Cardiol Clin. 1995;13(2):163–78.
10. Clark SL, Phelan JP, Greenspoon J, Aldahl D, Horenstein J. Labor and delivery in the presence of mitral stenosis: central hemodynamic observations. Am J Obstet Gynecol. 1985;152(8):984–8.
11. Ducey JP, Ellsworth SM. The hemodynamic effects of severe mitral stenosis and pulmonary hypertension during labor and delivery. Intensive Care Med. 1989;15(3):192–5.
12. Sullivan JM, Ramanathan KB. Management of medical problems in pregnancy--severe cardiac disease. N Engl J Med. 1985;313(5):304–9.
13. Szekely P, Snaith L. Obstetric care and the fetus in rheumatic heart disease. In: Szekely P, Snaith L (Eds). Heart Disease and Pregnancy. Edinburgh: Churchill Livingstone; 1974.p.137.
14. Wichman K, Rydén G, Karlberg BE. A placebo controlled trial of metoprolol in the treatment of hypertension in pregnancy. Scand J Clin Lab Investig Suppl. 1984;169:90–5.
15. Butters L, Kennedy S, Rubin PC. Atenolol in essential hypertension during pregnancy. BMJ. 1990;301(6752):587–9.
16. Pavankumar P, Venugopal P, Kaul U, Iyer KS, Das B, Sampathkumar A, et al. Closed mitral valvotomy during pregnancy. A 20-year experience. Scand J Thorac Cardiovasc Surg. 1988;22(1):11–5.
17. Goon MS, Raman S, Sinnathuray TA. Closed mitral valvotomy in pregnancy—a Malaysian experience. Aust N Z J Obstet Gynaecol. 1987;27(3):173–7.
18. Zitnik RS, Brandenburg RO, Sheldon R, Wallace RB. Pregnancy and open-heart surgery. Circulation. 1969;39(5 Suppl 1):I257–62.
19. Becker RM. Intracardiac surgery in pregnant women. Ann Thorac Surg. 1983;36(4):453–8.
20. Jain S, Maiti TK, Jain M. Fetomaternal outcome among women with mitral stenosis after balloon mitral valvotomy. Int J Gynaecol Obstet Off Organ Int Fed Gynaecol Obstet. 2013;121(2):119–22.

21. Inoue K, Owaki T, Nakamura T, Kitamura F, Miyamoto N. Clinical application of transvenous mitral commissurotomy by a new balloon catheter. J Thorac Cardiovasc Surg. 1984;87(3):394–402.

22. De Souza JA, Martinez EE Jr, Ambrose JA, Alves CM, Born D, Buffolo E, et al. Percutaneous balloon mitral valvuloplasty in comparison with open mitral valve commissurotomy for mitral stenosis during pregnancy. J Am Coll Cardiol. 2001;37(3):900–3.

23. Sananes S, Iung B, Vahanian A, Acar J, Salat-Baroux J, Uzan S. Fetal and obstetrical impact of percutaneous balloon mitral commissurotomy during pregnancy. Fetal Diagn Ther. 1994;9(4):218–25.

24. Brent RL. The effect of embryonic and fetal exposure to X-ray, microwaves, and ultrasound: counseling the pregnant and nonpregnant patients about these risks. Semin Oncol. 1989;16(5):347–68.

25. Gray JE. The radiation hazard—let's put it in perspective. Mayo Clin Proc. 1979;54(12):809–13.

26. Ben Farhat M, Gamra H, Betbout F, Maatouk F, Jarrar M, Addad F, et al. Percutaneous balloon mitral commissurotomy during pregnancy. Heart Br Card Soc. 1997;77(6):564–7.

27. Kalra GS, Arora R, Khan JA, Nigam M, Khalilullah M. Percutaneous mitral valvotomy during pregnancy. Cathet Cardiovasc Diagn. 1994;33:28-30.

28. Martínez-Reding J, Cordero A, Kuri J, Martínez-Ríos MA, Salazar E. Treatment of severe mitral stenosis with percutaneous balloon valvotomy in pregnant patients. Clin Cardiol. 1998;21(9):659–63.

29. Cheng TO. Percutaneous Inoue balloon valvuloplasty is the procedure of choice for symptomatic mitral stenosis in pregnant women. Catheter Cardiovasc Interv Off J Soc Card Angiogr Interv. 2000;50(4):418.

30. Fawzy ME, Kinsara AJ, Stefadouros M, Hegazy H, Kattan H, Chaudhary A, et al. Long-term outcome of mitral balloon valvotomy in pregnant women. J Heart Valve Dis. 2001;10(2):153–7.

31. Sivadasanpillai H, Ganapathi S, Tharakan J. Letter by Sivadasanpillai et al. Regarding article, "management of severe mitral stenosis during pregnancy."Circulation. 2012;126(1):e15; author reply e16.

32. Gupta A, Lokhandwala YY, Satoskar PR, Salvi VS. Balloon mitral valvotomy in pregnancy: maternal and fetal outcomes. J Am Coll Surg. 1998;187(4):409–15.

33. Nercolini DC, da Rocha Loures Bueno R, Eduardo Guerios E, Tarastchuk JC, Pacheco AL, Pia de Andrade PM, et al. Percutaneous mitral balloon valvuloplasty in pregnant women with mitral stenosis. Cathet Cardiovasc Interventions 2002;57:318-22.

34. Mangione JA, Lourenco RM, Dos Santos ES, Shigueyuki A, Mauro MF, Cristovao SA, et al. Long-term follow-up of pregnant women after percutaneous mitral valvuloplasty. Cathet Cardiovasc Interventions. 2000;50:413-7.

35. Mishra S, Narang R, Sharma M, Chopra A, Seth S, Ramamurthy S, et al. Percutaneous transseptal mitral commissurotomy in pregnant women with critical mitral stenosis. Indian Heart J. 2001;53(2):192–6.

36. Routray SN, Mishra TK, Swain S, Patnaik UK, Behera M. Balloon mitral valvuloplasty during pregnancy. Int J Gynaecol Obstet Off Organ Int Fed Gynaecol Obstet. 2004;85(1):18–23.

37. Esteves CA, Munoz JS, Braga S, Andrade J, Meneghelo Z, Gomes N, et al. Immediate and long-term follow-up of percutaneous balloon mitral valvuloplasty in pregnant patients with rheumatic mitral stenosis. Am J Cardiol. 2006;98(6):812–6.

38. Sivadasanpillai H, Srinivasan A, Sivasubramoniam S, Mahadevan KK, Kumar A, Titus T, et al. Long-term outcome of patients undergoing balloon mitral valvotomy in pregnancy. Am J Cardiol. 2005;95(12):1504–6.

39. Gulraze A, Kurdi W, Niaz F, Fawzy M. Mitral balloon valvuloplasty during pregnancy: The long-term up to 17 years obstetric outcome and childhood development. Pak J Med Sci. 2014;30(1):86–90.

40. CN Manjunath, Prabhavathi. Mitral valve disease : Advances in catheter interventions. Medicine Update 2010; 20: 368-74.

41. Gurav SR, Algotar KM. Foetomaternal outcome in rheumatic mitral valve. Bombay Hosp J [Internet]. 2012 [cited 2015 Apr 7];54(2). Available from: http://www.bhj.org.in/journal/2012-5402-april/download/253-258.pdf.

42. Abdi S, Salehi N, Ghodsi B, Basiri HA, Momtahen M, Firouzi A, et al. Immediate results of percutaneous trans-luminal mitral commissurotomy in pregnant women with severe mitral stenosis. Clin Med Insights Cardiol. 2012;6:35–9.

Chapter 38

Percutaneous Mitral Valvotomy in Juvenile Mitral Stenosis

Randeep Singla

Percutaneous mitral valvotomy (PMV) has become the treatment of choice for rheumatic mitral stenosis (MS). PMV yield results similar to open surgical commissurotomy and better results than closed commissurotomy.[1,2] However, juvenile MS was not adequately represented in these studies. Juvenile MS has been defined as symptomatic MS in age less than 20 years.[3] However, many subsequent studies showed similar immediate, mid-term and long-term results of PMV in juvenile MS as well.[4-6] The incidence of juvenile mitral stenosis ranged from 16% to 27% in these series of PMV.[4,5,7] Even in children less than 12 years of age, PMV has been shown to be safe and effective.[8]

◼ INDICATION FOR PMV IN JUVENILE MITRAL STENOSIS

The current guidelines don't give any age specific difference in the therapeutic management of MS and hence the standard criteria for timing and type of intervention are also applicable in juvenile group.[9] Juvenile MS is frequently associated with severe symptoms, high transmitral gradients and severe pulmonary hypertension and hence require early therapeutic intervention.

◼ VALVE MORPHOLOGY

Mitral valve structure as assessed using Wilkins score is most important predictor of successful PMV and restenosis.[10] Juvenile patients tend to have pliable valves with minimal calcification, lesser subvalvular pathology and hence, a lower MV score as compared to adults.[11] In a study by Gamra et al. an echo scores >8 was found in 15% juveniles as compared to 37% in adults. The mean mitral echo score was significantly lower in juveniles compared to adults.[4]

◼ PMV PROCEDURE IN JUVENILE MITRAL STENOSIS

Small children may require general anesthesia for the procedure. Since, the inadvertent movements of the patients during the procedure can be catastrophic, it is better to have the procedure under sedation especially in small children.

■ VASCULAR ACCESS

Since the patients have a smaller body frame compared to adults, it is better to obtain the arterial and venous access little spaced to avoid AV fistula. It is advised to have the arterial access with a 4F or 5F sheath to avoid arterial access problems.

■ BALLOON SELECTION AND DILATATION

Good procedural outcomes had been demonstrated using double balloon technique, Inoue technique[4] and metallic commissurotome[10] in juvenile MS.[4,5,12] The size of the balloon is selected based on the height based formula. However, in children less than 12 years, a balloon size smaller than that derived from height has been shown to be equally effective and safer with lesser incidence of acute MR.[13]

In cases of Cribier's metallic commissurotomy, extent of bar opening is based on the body surface area and the mitral valve morphology. The initial bar opening is set at 37 mm if the patients had a BSA of 1.5 m^2 or more and if they have no significant calcium in the mitral valve. Patients with smaller body frames have the bar opening set to 33 mm or 35 mm and increased to 35, 37 or 40 mm according to the result after initial dilatations.

Grossly enlarged left and right atria, thickened and calcified interatrial septum, severely diseased and distorted valves—factors that makes transseptal puncture and balloon passage more difficult in adults are rarely encountered in juvenile patients. This makes the procedure easier, smoother and shorter in these young patients.

Immediate Hemodynamic Results

Juvenile patients show significant improvement in hemodynamic parameters after PMV. The immediate hemodynamic results in children have been shown to be similar to adults with significant improvement in MV area and fall in LA mean and PA pressures.[6] In a study by Gamra et al., juvenile patients when compared to adults had lesser incidence of residual stenosis, but with no significant difference in invasively determined mean left atrial pressure, systolic pulmonary arterial pressure, or pulmonary vascular resistance both before and immediately after valvotomy.[4] In a multivariate analysis, absence of prior surgical commissurotomy and younger age had been shown to be significant predictors of the gain in mitral valve area.[14]

■ COMPLICATIONS

As compared to adults, PMV in juveniles is associated with a low complication rates. No procedure related major complications (severe MR, tamponade or systemic embolism) was reported among 110 juveniles undergoing PMV compared to 8.4% in adult group).[4] In a series 107 juvenile patients[5] undergoing PMV, only one patient each had cardiac tamponade and severe MR requiring emergency mitral valve replacement.[6] No procedure related mortality was reported in three large juvenile PMV series.[4-6]

Low complication rates in this group are attributed to the more favorable valve anatomy in the young as demonstrated by a lower echocardiographic score. Similarly, low-risk of embolic episodes has been attributed to smaller LA size and low incidence of AF in these patients. LA or LAA thrombus is only rarely seen in patients in the juvenile age group.

Long-term Outcome

One study which reported 10 years follow-up among patients who underwent BMV for Juvenile MS[3] revealed a low event rate and no mortality. The probability of event-free survival was 90% at 5 years and 74% at 10 years in juvenile patients.[4] In comparison, the event-free survival rate was 80% at 1 year, 71% at 2 years, 66% at 3 years and 60% at 4 years in a large adult registry.[15] In a study by Fawzy et al. there was no significant difference between juveniles and adults in the incidence of restenosis or event-free survival rate after a mean follow-up of 5 years.[5]

Although, juveniles tend to have severe pulmonary arterial hypertension before PMV, they exhibit rapid resolution of pulmonary hypertension with no significant difference in pulmonary artery pressure between juveniles and adults on follow-up.[5]

Restenosis

It has been hypothesized that children and adolescent patients may be more prone to restenosis because of the higher likelihood of smoldering rheumatic activity or recurrence of rheumatic fever in this age group. However, both mid-term and long-term studies had consistently shown similar or lower restenosis rates in juveniles as compared to adults.[4-6] Restenosis rate of 1.8% on mid-term follow-up and 12% to 16% on long-term follow were observed in juvenile mitral stenosis.[4-6] MV echocardiographic score has been shown to be the only significant predictor of mitral valve restenosis and the lower scores seen in the juvenile group likely contributes to lower restenosis rates in them.[16]

Repeat PMV in Juvenile MS

Most juvenile patients with mitral valve restenosis have pliable mitral valve apparatus suitable for a repeat procedure.[4,5] In a study by Gamra et al. all juvenile patients with restenosis underwent successful PMV. In the same study only 40.2% adult patients had valves suitable for repeat balloon mitral commissurotomy. Repeat PMV for juvenile MS give good outcomes.[4]

PMV in very Young Children

In a small subset of juvenile patients (~10%), the disease process and hemodynamic impairment develop unusually rapidly and became symptomatic before 12 years of age.[17] The safety and efficacy of PMV in these young children has been reported in few small case series and case reports[13,17-19] Some of these patients were found to have thick fibrotic valves and severe subvalvar pathology.[17] Two technical aspects need special consideration in these patients during PMV. Firstly, due to small body frames, procedural success is better defined by MV index (MVA indexed to body surface area) rather than MVA. Postprocedural MV index >1 cm^2/m^2 body surface area or the achievement of more than a 50% increase in MVA from basal area without major complications is considered to be an adequate hemodynamic result.[17] Secondly, the choice of balloon size in this group need special mention. The risk of MR and valve damage in this group can be reduced by performing serial dilations starting with balloon diameters that are 2 to 4 mm smaller than the maximum balloon size derived from height-based formula.[17]

▦ REFERENCES

1. Ben Farhat M, Ayari M, Maatouk F, Betbout F, Gamra H, Jarra M, et al. Percutaneous balloon versus surgical closed and open mitral commissurotomy: seven-year follow-up results of a randomized trial. Circulation. 1998;97(3):245–50.
2. Reyes VP, Raju BS, Wynne J, Stephenson LW, Raju R, Fromm BS, et al. Percutaneous balloon valvuloplasty compared with open surgical commissurotomy for mitral stenosis. N Engl J Med. 1994;331(15):961–7.
3. Roy S. Juvenile mitral stenosis in India. The Lancet. 1963;282:1193–6.
4. Gamra H, Betbout F, Ben Hamda K, Addad F, Maatouk F, Dridi Z, et al. Balloon mitral commissurotomy in juvenile rheumatic mitral stenosis: a ten-year clinical and echocardiographic actuarial results. Eur Heart J. 2003;24(14):1349.
5. Fawzy ME. Long-term clinical and echocardiographic results of mitral balloon valvotomy in children and adolescents. Heart. 2005;91:743–8.
6. Joseph PK, Bhat A, Francis B, Sivasankaran S, Kumar A, Pillai VR, et al. Percutaneous transvenous mitral commissurotomy using an Inoue balloon in children with rheumatic mitral stenosis. Int J Cardiol. 1997;62(1):19–22.
7. Bahl VK, Chandra S, Kothari SS, Talwar KK, Sharma S, Kaul U, et al. Percutaneous transvenous mitral commissurotomy using Inoue catheter in juvenile rheumatic mitral stenosis. Cathet Cardiovasc Diagn. 1994;Suppl 2:82–6.
8. Kothari SS, Ramakrishnan S, Kumar CK, Juneja R, Yadav R. Intermediate-term results of percutaneous transvenous mitral commissurotomy in children less than 12 years of age. Catheter Cardiovasc Interv. 2005;64(4):487–90.
9. Bonow RO, Carabello BA, Chatterjee K, de Leon AC, Faxon DP, Freed MD, et al. 2008 Focused update incorporated into the ACC/AHA 2006 guidelines for the management of patients with valvular heart disease: a report of the American College of Cardiology/American Heart Association Task Force on Practice Guidelines (Writing Committee to Develop Guidelines for the Management of Patients With Valvular Heart Disease). Circulation. 2008;118(15):e523–e661.
10. Wilkins GT, Weyman AE, Abascal VM, Block PC, Palacios IF. Percutaneous balloon dilatation of the mitral valve: an analysis of echocardiographic variables related to outcome and the mechanism of dilatation. Br Heart J. 1988;60(4):299–308.
11. Bhayana JN, Khanna SK, Gupta BK, Sharma SR, Gupta MP, Padmavati S. Mitral stenosis in the young in developing countries. J Thorac Cardiovasc Surg. 1974;68(1):126–30.

12. Harikrishnan S, Nair K, Tharakan JM, Titus T, Kumar VKA, Sivasankaran S. Percutaneous transmitral commissurotomy in juvenile mitral stenosis--comparison of long term results of Inoue balloon technique and metallic commissurotomy. Catheter Cardiovasc Interv. 2006;67(3):453–9.

13. Kothari SS, Kamath P, Juneja R, Bahl VK, Airan B. Percutaneous transvenous mitral commissurotomy using Inoue balloon in children less than 12 years. Cathet Cardiovasc Diagn. 1998;43(4):408–11.

14. Herrmann HC, Ramaswamy K, Isner JM, Feldman TE, Carroll JD, Pichard AD, et al. Factors influencing immediate results, complications, and short-term follow-up status after Inoue balloon mitral valvotomy: a North American multicenter study. Am Heart J. 1992;124(1):160–6.

15. Dean LS, Mickel M, Bonan R, Holmes DR Jr, O'Neill WW, Palacios IF, et al. Four-year follow-up of patients undergoing percutaneous balloon mitral commissurotomy: a report from the National Heart, Lung, and Blood Institute Balloon Valvuloplasty Registry. J Am Coll Cardiol. 1996;28(6):1452–7.

16. Ben-Farhat M, Betbout F, Gamra H, Maatouk F, Ben-Hamda K, Abdellaoui M, et al. Predictors of long-term event-free survival and of freedom from restenosis after percutaneous balloon mitral commissurotomy. Am Heart J. 2001;142(6):1072-9.

17. Kapoor A, Moorthy N, Kumar S. Inoue balloon mitral valvotomy in a 4-year-old boy: to treat fulminant rheumatic mitral stenosis. Tex Heart Inst J. 2012;39(1):108-11.

18. Krishnamoorthy KM, Tharakan JA. Balloon mitral valvulotomy in children aged < or = 12 years. J Heart Valve Dis. 2003;12(4):461–8.

19. Essop MR, Govendrageloo K, Du Plessis J, van Dyk M, Sareli P. Balloon mitral valvotomy for rheumatic mitral stenosis in children aged < or = 12 years. Am J Cardiol. 1993;72(11):850–1.

Chapter 39

Transjugular Percutaneous Mitral Valvotomy

Boonjong Saejueng, Sudaratana Tansuphaswadikul

Since, the introduction of Inoue balloon in 1984, it has been extensively used worldwide in percutaneous mitral commissurotomy (PTMC) because of its efficacy, low-risk of complications and, especially, ease of the procedure with a short learning curve. Under the hands of experienced operators, the rate of technical success defined as completion of transseptal access and mitral valve dilatation with Inoue technique is approaching 99% using traditional transfemoral access.[1,2] As a result, most valvular interventionists are not familiar with transjugular PTMC.

Till the present time, limited number of patients with mitral stenosis have been treated with transjugular approach.[3-7] Advantage of transjugular venous access is clearly demonstrated among mitral stenosis patients who have venous abnormalities caused either by congenital (Figs 39.1 and 39.2) or acquired

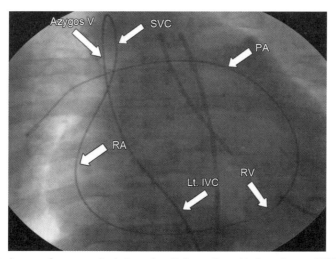

Fig. 39.1: A case of severe mitral stenosis with impediment to transfemoral PTMC from abnormal venous drainage: A guidewire coursing from the left inferior vena cava, the azygos vein, the superior vena cava, the right atrium, the right ventricular, the main pulmonary artery to the right pulmonary artery: The pigtail catheter coursing from the aorta to the left ventricle is also seen

Abbreviations: Azygos V, azygos vein; SVC, superior vena cava; RA, right atrium; PA, pulmonary artery; Lt IVC, left inferior vena cava; RV, right ventricle

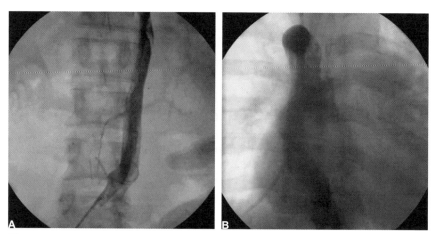

Figs 39.2A and B: (A) Venogram showing the left inferior vena cava at the lumbar level; (B) The left inferior vena cava continues as the azygos vein that drains into the superior vena cava

disorders that preclude transfemoral PTMC. A group of transfemoral technical failure due to cardiac anatomic distortion may earn benefit from transjugular approach instead of referring the patients for valve surgery.

■ TRANSJUGULAR INTERATRIAL SEPTAL PUNCTURE

Landmark for Optimal Puncture

Landmark for septal puncture derived from Inoue's angiographic method in frontal view is suitable for traditional transfemoral approach.[8,9] In order to use transjugular approach, it is recommended to use different puncture point from fluoroscopy in 45-degree right anterior oblique (RAO) projection.[3] This projection allows the septum to be viewed enface and maximizes separation of the anterior aorta and posterior cardiac borders. A stop-frame of levophase left atrial image from pulmonary angiography is kept as a reference.[6] The appropriate site of puncture is 2 cm (a vertebral body height) below the roof of the left atrium and midway between imaginary vertical lines passing through the pigtail catheter tip located at the aortic valve and the anterior border of thoracic spine (Fig. 39.3). This puncture point is above fossa ovalis and is classified as a high atrial septal puncture. High atrial septal access facilitates balloon crossing into the left ventricle in transjugular approach. However, very high puncture (less than 1 or 2 cm from atrial roof) should be avoided because it is associated with high incidence of cardiac tamponade. If interatrial septum is punctured at fossa ovalis or low atrial septum, the over-the-wire technique is helpful in delivering the balloon through mitral valve orifice.

■ PROCEDURE OF SEPTAL PUNCTURE

After left internal jugular vein is cannulated with 8 French sheath, a J-shaped 0.032-inch guidewire is advanced into inferior vena cava. The Mullins catheter

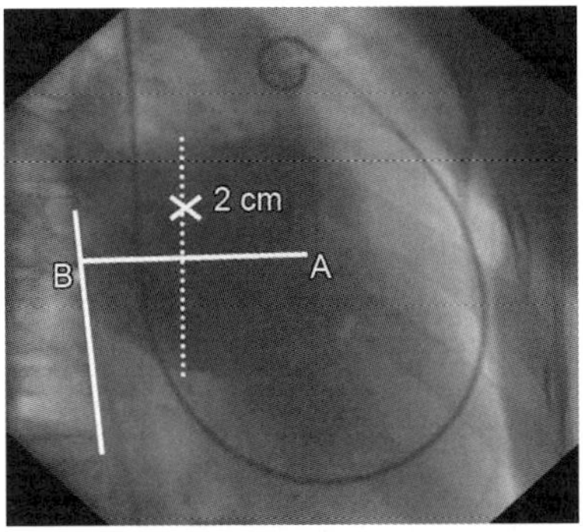

Fig. 39.3: Pulmonary angiogram showing levoplase of the left atrium in 45° RAO view as a reference in septal puncture: A recommended puncture site at 2 cm below the roof of the left atrium at vertical line passing through midway of horizontal line from the tip of a pigtail catheter at the aortic cusps and the anterior border of thoracic spine

(dilator) is inserted over the guidewire, the guidewire is removed and the Brockenbrough needle is delivered into the catheter to a point 2–3 mm from the catheter tip. Shankarappa et al. has used the pediatric septal puncture needle (Medtronic Inc.).[6]

Increased curvature of transseptal needle used in transjugular PTMC is recommended to avoid septal dissection caused by oblique passage of the needle through the septum. The external needle index is generally kept pointing between 7 and 8 o'clock (view from the head end of the patient) and the needle-fitted transseptal catheter is slowly withdrawn cranially. When the tip of the catheter is at the target, the catheter with the concealed needle is pushed slightly and the catheter tip is fixed against the atrial septum. The needle is pushed forward while fixing the catheter. After confirming needle entry in the left atrium using contrast media injection or pressure monitoring, the needle indicator is directed toward 9 o'clock and both the needle and the catheter are simultaneously advanced 2 cm into the left atrial cavity. Then, only the catheter is introduced 2 cm further with the needle held fixed. Finally, the needle is withdrawn and a curved 0.025 wire is inserted into left atrium followed by immediate heparinization. The skin and septum are dilated by a 14 French long dilator.

Although, it is inconvenient to perform on-table transesophageal echocardiography (TEE), TEE guidance (Fig. 39.4) is useful for visualizing the appropriate puncture site and preventing serious complications.[10] The equipment for puncture used in daily clinical practice is too long and unwieldy for transjugular access. Pediatric transseptal set, if available, will make the procedure easier while reducing the working field considerably.

MITRAL VALVE DILATATION PROCEDURE

Method of advancing the Inoue balloon catheter into the left atrial cavity is as mentioned traditionally. However, neither conventional direct nor loop method is chosen for crossing the mitral valve orifice. When compared to the femoral venous approach, the jugular approach provides a more direct route to the mitral valve without having a balloon catheter bent over backward to cross the mitral valve. A right anterior oblique projection is selected for mitral

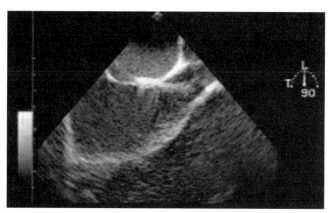

Fig. 39.4: Transesophageal echocardiography guidance confirming the tip of the needle in the left atrium: The shaft of the needle placing in the superior vena cava

valve crossing. If septum is punctured high enough, it is possible to use a stylet in directing the balloon catheter into the left ventricle. Reshaping the usual "U"-shaped to "S"-shaped stylet is helpful. The balloon catheter with the stylet inside is retracted and rotated clockwise to be aligned with the apex-mitral valve axis. When the balloon catheter is positioned close to the mitral valve orifice signaled by to-and-fro movement, advancement of the catheter and stylet as a unit is performed during diastole.

In case of low puncture (below the level of aortic valve) or failure to cross with the stylet, over-the-wire technique using a 0.025-inch guidewire is preferable to guide the Inoue balloon across the mitral valve. With the Mullins sheath directed towards the mitral valve, a 0.025 inch coiled guidewire is directly introduced into the left ventricle and manipulated to obtain optimal coiling of the guidewire in LV. The balloon catheter is advanced into the LV over the same coiled guidewire (Fig. 39.5A). Balloon was positioned across the MV and inflated (Figs 39.5B to D). Stepwise dilatation process is recommended to prevent severe mitral regurgitation.

Other single balloon technique may be applied for mitral valve dilatation as an alternative choice or a complement to Inoue balloon technique. With this technique, a 14 French J-shaped sheath with hemostatic valve is placed into the left atrium. A balloon floating catheter inserted into the sheath is advanced from the left atrium to the left ventricle. The J-shaped sheath is manipulated through the line of a balloon catheter until the tip of the sheath positioning closed to mitral valve orifice. A 0.035 wire with a large, soft J-tip is introduced through the sheath into the left ventricle. Finally, the balloon is thread over the wire across the mitral valve and is inflated. If diameter of single balloon is large enough (up to 30 mm), the mitral valve area after procedure is expected to be acceptable. In case of failure to cross the mitral valve with the Inoue balloon, predilatation with single balloon (Figs 39.6A and B) eases the second attempt of Inoue balloon crossing and complete the Inoue technique.

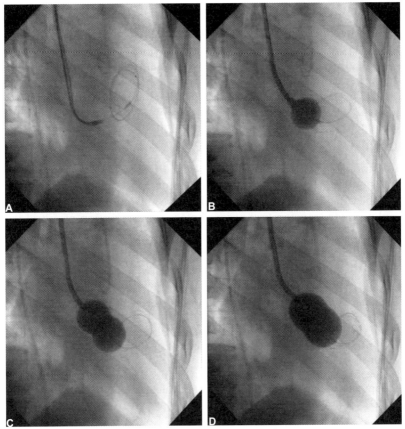

Figs 39.5A to D: Dilation of mitral valve with Inoue balloon: (A) The balloon catheter threaded along curved 0.025 guidewire into the left ventricle; (B) Inflation of distal balloon; (C) Inflation of proximal balloon with the mid-portion of the balloon located at the mitral valve orifice; (D) Full expansion of the balloon 📷◀

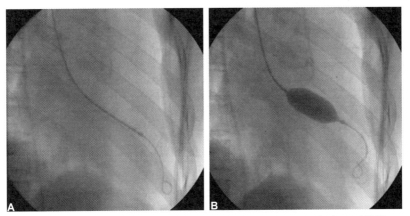

Figs 39.6A and B: Mitral valve dilatation using single balloon technique: (A) Mansfield balloon (20 mm) positioned at mitral orifice; (B) Full dilatation of the balloon

■ COMPLICATIONS

Procedure-related complications including cardiac tamponade, emergency surgery, severe mitral regurgitation and embolization have been reported and are assumed to be similar to transfemoral approach. Very high puncture resulting in cardiac tamponade should be avoided. Another concern is greater radiation exposure to operators in work field compared to transfemoral approach.

■ CONCLUSION

Transfemoral PTMC still remains the standard intervention in patients with mitral stenosis. However, transjugular venous is a challenging access and should be considered in candidates who have any impediment to successful completion via transfemoral access before the last option of mitral valve surgery.

■ REFERENCES

1. Hung JS, Lau KW, Lo PH, Chern MS, Wu JJ. Complications of Inoue balloon mitral commissurotomy: impact of operator experience and evolving technique. Am Heart J. 1999;138(1 Pt 1):114-21.
2. Iung B, Nicoud-Houel A, Fondard O, Hafid Akoudad, Haghighat T, Brochet E, et al. Temporal trends in percutaneous mitral commissurotomy over a 15-year period. Eur Heart J. 2004;25(8):701-7.
3. Joseph G, Baruah DK, Kuruttukulam SV, Chandy ST, Krishnaswami S. Transjugular approach to transseptal balloon mitral valvuloplasty. Cathet Cardiovasc Diagn. 1997;42(2):219-26.
4. Joseph G, George OK, Mandalay A, Sathe S. Transjugular approach to balloon mitral valvuloplasty helps overcome impediments caused by anatomical alterations. Catheter Cardiovasc Interv. 2002;57(3):353-62.
5. Saejueng B, Tansuphaswadikul S, Kanoksin A, Hengrussamee K, Assavahanrit J, Chantadansuwan T. Transjugular approach as a challenging access in PTMC: case report. J Med Assoc Thail Chotmaihet Thangphaet. 2005;88(7):997-1002.
6. Shankarappa RK, Math RS, Chikkaswamy SB, Rai MK, Karur S, Dwarakprasad R, et al. Transjugular percutaneous transvenous mitral commissurotomy (PTMC) using conventional PTMC equipment in rheumatic mitral stenosis with interruption of inferior vena cava. J Invasive Cardiol. 2012;24(12):675-8.
7. Jose J, Kumar V, Joseph G. Transjugular balloon mitral valvotomy in a patient with inferior vena-caval interruption. JACC Cardiovasc Interv. 2012;5(2):243-4.
8. Hung JS. Atrial septal puncture technique in percutaneous transvenous mitral commissurotomy: mitral valvuloplasty using the Inoue balloon catheter technique. Cathet Cardiovasc Diagn. 1992;26(4):275-84.
9. Inoue K, Lau KW, Hung JS. Percutaneous Transvenous Mitral Commissurotomy: Grech ED, Ram DR (Eds), Practical Interventional Cardiology (Martin Dunitz: China, 2002;373-87.
10. Hengrussamee K, Tansuphaswadikul S, Kehasukcharoen W. The Advantages of Intraprocedural Transesophageal Echocardiography in Percutaneous Transseptal Mitral Commissurotomy. Asian Heart Journal. 1999;7:8-15.

Chapter 40

Percutaneous Prosthetic Mitral Balloon Valvotomy

Col. Subroto Kumar Datta

"Medicine is a science of uncertainty and an art of probability."

William Osler

■ INTRODUCTION

Structural valve deterioration begins in prosthetic valves by five years of implantation.[1]

Stented bioprosthetic valves are derived from glutaraldehyde preserved aortic porcine valves. Degeneration is seen in the form of gradual breakdown of collagen matrix and focal calcification. The calcification starts in basal attachments of the leaflets and closure lines of commissures. The importance of dynamic stress is suggested by predisposition of commissural involvement.

Less than 5% show noninfected thrombus which may calcify or produce stenosis. Cuspal loosening, tears, perforation, infective endocarditis are other causes of degeneration. The tears occur along commissures, centrally or along calcific deposits.[2]

In vitro balloon dilation of excised stented porcine valves from aortic and mitral valves position has been studied by Waller et al. (Fig. 40.1). Balloon dilatation resulted in commissural splitting (18/20), cuspal fractures (9/20), strut fracture (3/20) and embolization of material (6/20). There was no annular rent seen in any case.[3]

Idiopathic inflammatory deposition of fibroconnective tissue as early as one year of bioprosthetic mitral implant has been reported in the absence of adverse risk factors like young age <40 years, smoking, chronic renal disease, hemodialysis, hyperlipidemia.[4]

■ CASE SELECTION/INDICATION

Balloon dilatation of stented bioprosthetic valves is justified as a bailout procedure where the risk of conventional open heart valve replacement is considered to be unacceptably high due to poor cardiac condition and presence of serious comorbidities which adversely impact the clinical outcome of valve replacement.

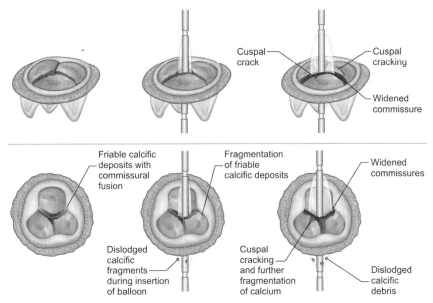

Fig. 40.1: Results and mechanisms of catheter balloon valvuloplasty in degenerative stenotic porcine bioprosthetic valves[2]

Isolated case reports have shown the feasibility of a safe but often suboptimal relief of obstruction.[5] It is possible for an experienced operator to perform the procedure safely by suitable preprocedural screening as a bridging procedure in a back to the wall situation.

◼ EVALUATION

A detailed clinical profile, echocardiographic and fluoroscopic evaluation can be used to confirm the presence of degenerative obstructive valve disease, rule out valve instability, endocarditis, regurgitation and thrombus.

◼ ECHO

Transthoracic and transesophageal echo defines the left ventricular function, chamber dimensions, associated valvular lesions of aortic tricuspid, pulmonary valves, pulmonary hypertension and their severity. The presence of thrombus in the left ventricle, left atrium, atrial appendage, prosthetic valve is carefully ruled out.

The prosthetic valve is carefully defined. Leaflets of bioprosthetic leaflets are thickened, show reduced excursion. Presence of paravalvular leaks, calcification, thrombus, vegetation is carefully assessed. The valve function is determined by Doppler transvalvular gradient, valve area by pressure half time. Any valvular regurgitation is likely to worsen with ballooning.

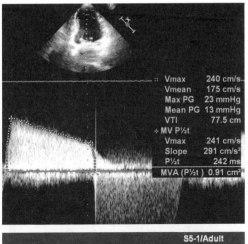

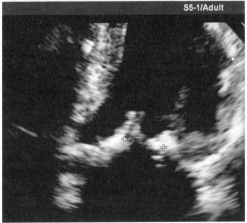

Fig. 40.2: The four chamber view allows optimal visualization of the valve, leaflets and estimation of valve area, transmitral gradients

SELECTION AND SIZING OF BALLOON

The self-centering Inoue balloon has been used by us successfully in performing the procedure in two cases. The size of balloon was 1.0–1.1 times the maximum diameter measured in any view in transthoracic or transesophageal echo. The four chamber view is generally appropriate to profile the inner lumen of the stented valve in mitral position (Fig. 40.2).

PROCEDURE

The conventional fluoroscopy-guided transseptal approach for antegrade balloon dilatation is used for both transeptal puncture and entry into the left ventricle across the bioprosthetic valve. The patient is appropriately heparinized. The distal balloon is inflated in the left ventricular cavity. It is

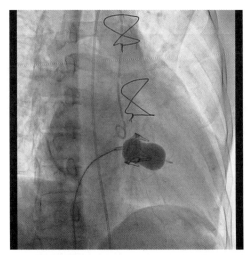

Fig. 40.3: Right anterior oblique image of balloon dilatation
of bioprosthetic valve in mitral position

then pulled back till the waist engages the leaflets and the proximal end of
the balloon is across the valve suture ring in the right anterior oblique view.
Fluoroscopic inflation of the balloon was accepted by us as the end point of the
procedure (Fig. 40.3). No effort was made to eliminate transvalvular gradient.
After inflation of the balloon it is withdrawn into the left atrium.

Left atrial and ventricular pressures were recorded pre- and postprocedure.
Echocardiographic evaluation for residual gradient, regurgitation is done
postprocedure and repeated after 24 hours.

■ FOLLOW-UP

Both our cases have maintained improvement in valve area and symptom
relief at one year postprocedure (Fig. 40.4). Both have not required redo valve
replacement.

■ DISCUSSION

Percutaneous options for relief of bioprosthetic restenosis in mitral position is
still second to surgical valve replacement. Successful transapical valve in valve
(VIV) implantation has been described in small series of high risk patients
with multiple comorbidities.[6] The procedure is best performed in hybrid labs
and understandably has a significant mortality. This option is not available in
India. It is not likely to be affordable to majority of recipients of bioprosthetic
valves. The VIV in mitral position is an "off-label" indication of the Sapiens valve
often performed for clinical compulsions. The migration of the percutaneous
implanted valve has been reported.[7]

The manufacturer and echo determined inner diameters of the valve do
not match. The echo dimensions are consistent with fluoroscopic sizing and
easy to obtain predictably.

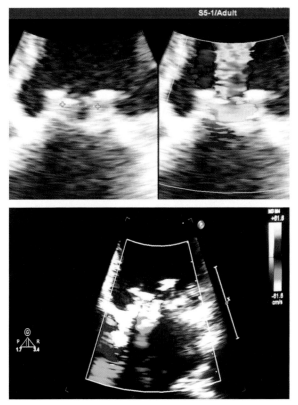

Fig. 40.4: Pre- and postdilatation echo of stented bioprosthetic mitral valve at one year follow-up. *Note* the appearance of mitral regurgitation

Repeat inflations may potentially predispose to embolization. They were avoided.

The reporting of few successful procedures maybe misleading. There is a very real probability that procedures with adverse outcomes may not be reported. Regional or national registry data can be of great value to overcome this problem.

REFERENCES

1. Rahimtoola SH. Choice of prosthetic valve in adults: an update. JACC. 2010; 55(22):2413-16.
2. Waller B, Mckay C, Vantassel J, Allen M. Catheter balloon valvoplasty of stenotic porcine bioprosthetic valves; part I: Anatomic considerations. Clin Cardiol. 1991; 14:686-91.
3. Waller B, Mckay C, Vantassel J, AllenM. Catheter balloon valvoplasty of stenotic porcine bioprosthetic valves; part II: Mechanisms, Complications, and recommendations for clinical use. Clin Cardiol. 1991;14:764–72.
4. Bajaj M, Abuissa H, Main ML. Rapid bioprosthetic valve degeneration resulting in severe mitral stenosis. J Am Soc Echocardiogs. 2008;21(1):90.e1.

5. Bekeredjian R, Katus HA, Rottbauer W. Valvuloplasty of a stenosed mitral bioprothesis. J Invasive Cardiol. 2010;22:E97–E98.

6. Seiffert M, Conradi L, Baldus S, Schirmer J, Knap M. Transcatheter mitral valve-in valve implantation in patients with degenerated bioprosthesis. J Am Coll Cardiol Intv. 2012;5:341–9.

7. Bapat VN, Khaliel F, Ihlberg L. Delayed migration of Sapien valve following a transcatheter mitral valve-in–valve implantation. Catheterization and Cardiovascular Interventions. 2014; 83:E150-E154.

Chapter 41

Tackling Subvalvular Disease during Balloon Mitral Valvotomy

CN Manjunath, Prabhavathi, BC Srinivas

▇ INTRODUCTION

Subvalvular apparatus (SVA) includes chordae tendinae, two papillary muscles and adjacent left ventricular free wall. In rheumatic mitral stenosis (MS), subvalvular disease was noted in 40% of autopsy specimens and two-thirds of patients undergoing open mitral commissurotomy.[1,2]

Subvalvular disease results from two closely related mechanisms: (1) a late manifestation of healed inflammation following acute rheumatic valvulitis, (2) superimposed turbulence that induces fibrosis.[3]

Rheumatic process results in fusion (agglutination), thickening, retraction, shortening, and calcification of the chordae. The free interchordal space diminishes and the "leaflet – chordae tendinae tunnel" available for diastolic flow is limited.

Assessment of the Subvalvular Apparatus

Echocardiography is the main tool for assessing the subvalvular disease. One can visualize the chordae plastered to the papillary muscles resulting in severe shortening (Fig. 41.1, Video-1). Marked color turbulence and multiple jets in subvalvular region suggest significant disease (Fig. 41.2, Video-2).

We can also measure the submitral orifice in the short axis view (Figs 41.3A and 41.3B, Video 3A and 3B). However, echocardiography underestimates subvalvular pathology when compared to intraoperative assessment.

During balloon mitral valvotomy (BMV), significant subvalvular disease is suspected when:

1. Left atrial (LA) pressure is high despite less than severe MS at commissural level (with normal heart rate)
2. Disproportionate pulmonary arterial hypertension (PAH)
3. Difficulty in balloon reaching left ventricular (LV) apex
4. Frequent slipping of balloon during initial inflations
5. The balloon Impasse sign (Figs 41.4A and 4B, Video-4A and 4B)

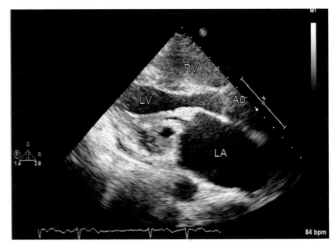

Fig. 41.1: Transthoracic echocardiography showing severe subvalvular thickening (Video-1) [Reproduced with permission from Nanda NC, Textbook of echocardiography. India: Jaypee publications; 2013]
Abbreviations: RV, right ventricle; LV, left ventricle; LA, left atrial; AO, aorta

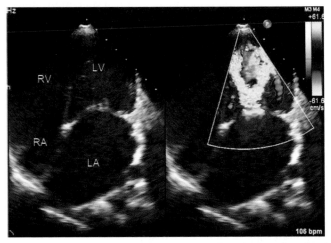

Fig. 41.2: Transthoracic echocardiography with color Doppler imaging showing severe subvalvular thickening producing multiple inflow jets simulating "sun-rays" (Video-2) [Reproduced with permission from Nanda NC, Textbook of echocardiography. India: Jaypee publications; 2013]
Abbreviations: RV, right ventricle; LV, left ventricle; RA, right atrium; LA, left atrium

6. The "balloon compression" sign is a result of the distorted inflated balloon configuration at the subvalvular level (Fig. 41.5A, Video-5A), instead of having the typical "hourglass" appearance (Fig. 41.5B, Video-5B)

Balloon mitral valvotomy (BMV) in presence of severe submitral disease is challenging and pose several obstacles. In severe submitral stenosis, balloon entry into LV can be difficult. In such cases, predilating and releasing submitral stenosis with peripheral angioplasty balloon facilitates subsequent entry of

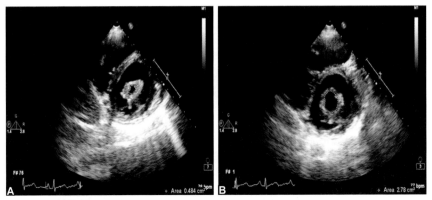

Figs 41.3A and B: Impact of measuring MVA at proper plane: Cross-sectional area measured at chordal level in a patient with severe subvalvular level shows MVA of 0.0484 cm² (A) whereas in same patient at the level of commisures MVA is 2.78 cm². (B) Video-3A and 3B [Reproduced with permission from Nanda NC, Textbook of echocardiography. India: Jaypee publications 2013]

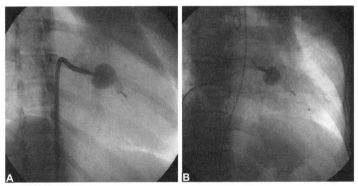

Figs 41.4A and B: Fluroscopic image showing resistance in reaching LV apex secondary to severe subvalvular obstruction resulting in distorted shape of Inoue balloon "Impasse sign" (Video-4A and 4B)

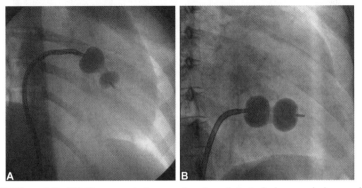

Figs 41.5A and B: (A) Fluroscopic image showing distorted abnormal shape of distal balloon"balloon compressions" sign due to severe subvalvular obstruction (Video-5A). (B) Normal shape of Inoue balloon during inflation in patient without significant subvalvular stenosis (Video-5B)

balloon catheter. This can be achieved either through antegrade approach or retrograde approach.

Submitral Release from Antegrade Approach[4]

A 45-year-old female presented with severe symptomatic mitral stenosis with mitral valve orifice area of 1.0 cm² at cuspal level and 0.4 cm² at chordal level. The submitral apparatus was extensively diseased with thickening and fusion (Figs 41.6A and B, and Video- 6A). BMV was attempted with conventional method. However, the balloon catheter failed to enter LV despite several attempts.

Hence, over the wire technique[5] of LV entry was tried. In this technique, 0.025" coiled guidewire is directly placed in the LV through the Mullin's sheath and then the balloon is passed over this wire. But there was resistance to the entry of balloon catheter and the entire assembly backed out into the LA due to severe submitral disease (Fig. 41.7A, Video-7A). Submitral orifice diameter (6 mm) was smaller than the diameter of the unstretched balloon (8 mm).

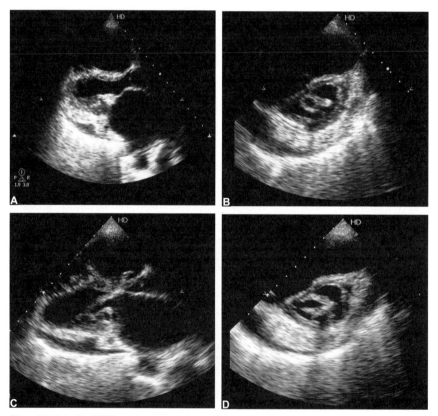

Figs 41.6A to D: (A) Transthoracic echocardiography showing severe submitral stenosis; (B) Transthoracic echocardiography in short axis at mitral valvular level showing severe mitral stenosis (MVOA:1.0 cm²); (C) Post-BMV transthoracic echocardiography showing wide opening of mitral valve and opened submitral stenosis; (D) Post-BMV transthoracic echocardiography showing posteromedial commissural split with MVOA:2.0 cm²

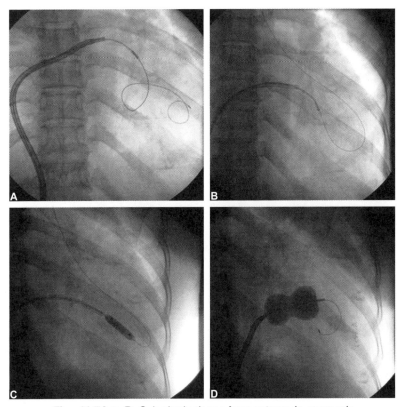

Figs 41.7A to D: Submitral release from antegrade approach

Then we planned to dilate the submitral apparatus with a peripheral balloon. A 0.035" Terumo wire was introduced into the LV with support of right Judkin's catheter (Fig. 41.7B, Video-7B). The distal end of the Terumo wire was parked in the right subclavian artery. An 8 × 20 mm OPTA® ProPeripheral angioplasty balloon (Cordis Corporation) was passed over the Terumo wire and the submitral apparatus was serially dilated (Fig. 41.7C, Video-7C). The Terumo wire was then exchanged for a coiled guidewire. Now, the BMV balloon catheter entered the LV cavity easily and the procedure was completed (Fig. 41.7D, Video-7D). Final result was good with mitral valve orifice area of 2.0 cm². Medial commissure was split and the submitral fusion was released (Fig. 41.6C, 6D, Video-6C). There was no chordal tear or mitral regurgitation which may complicate dilatation of the submitral structures.

Submitral Release from Retrograde Approach

A 50-year-old female presented with severe mitral restenosis (post-BMV 10 years) and NYHA class III dyspnea. Echocardiography revealed severe noncalcific mitral stenosis (MVOA 0.9 cm²), severe submitral fusion and severe PAH (PASP 80 mm Hg). A small atrial septal defect (ASD) with left to right shunt (10 mm) was also noted.

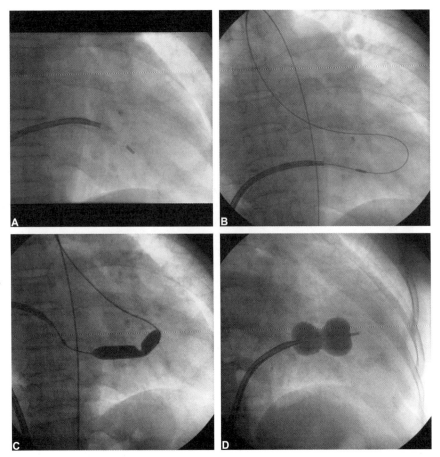

Figs 41.8A to D: Submitral release from retrograde approach

Conventional antegrade BMV was attempted using 26 mm Accura balloon. However, the balloon catheter could not reach the LV apex despite several attempts (Fig. 41.8A, Video-8A). To enhance the support for proper balloon passage, a 0.035″ exchange length (260 cm) Terumo guidewire was introduced into aorta. Still, the Balloon catheter did not pass through. We realized that it was due to severe submitral disease and we planned to tackle submitral first from retrograde approach.

The Terumo wire was advanced into right femoral artery and was snared from the arterial end creating a venoarterial loop (Fig. 41.8B, Video-8B). An 8 × 40 mm OPTA® Properipheral angioplasty balloon was introduced from the arterial end, towards the submitral apparatus. The submitral apparatus was serially dilated with the balloon introduced from the arterial end (Fig. 41.8C, Video-8C). Now, the Accura balloon could be introduced antegradely into LV easily and the BMV was completed successfully (Fig. 41.8D, Video-8D).

Balloon dilatation of subvalvular stenosis: In patients with predominant submitral stenosis, in spite of commissural split the gradient across mitral

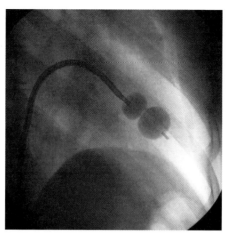

Fig. 41.9: Balloon dilatation of subvalvular stenosis using Inoue balloon (Video-9)

valve may remain high and mitral valve may not open satisfactorily. In such situations, controlled, graded and careful dilation of submitral stenosis using same Accura/Inoue balloon (Fig. 41.9, Video-9) may yield optimal result. However, risk of chordal rupture, papillary muscle rupture/avulsion resulting in severe MR should be considered.

■ CONCLUSION

In severe submitral disease, balloon entry into the LV can be challenging. Releasing submitral stenosis with peripheral angioplasty balloon, followed by valve dilatation with BMV balloon catheter achieves higher success rate with minimal risk of mitral regurgitation. Both antegrade and retrograde techniques are effective.

■ REFERENCES

1. Rusted IE, Scheifley CH, Edwards JE. Studies of the mitral valve, II: certain anatomic features of the mitral valve and associated structures in mitral stenosis. Circulation. 1956;14:398–406.
2. Mullin MJ, Engleman RM, Isom OW, Boyd AD, Glassman E, Spencer FC. Experience with open mitral commissurotomy in 100 consecutive patients. Surg. 1974;76(6):974–82.
3. Olson LJ, Subramanian R, Ackermann DM, et al. Surgical pathology of the mitral valve: a study of 712 cases spanning 21 years. Mayo Clin Proc. 1987;62:22–34.
4. Nanjappa MC, Bhat P, Panneerselvam A. Modified technique of BMV for severe submitral stenosis. J Invasive Cardiol. 2011;23(9):387–8.
5. Manjunath CN, Srinivasa KH, Patil CB, Venkatesh HV, Bhoopal TS, Dhanalakshmi C. Balloon mitral valvuloplasty: our experience with a modified technique of crossing the mitral valve in difficult cases. Cathet Cardiovasc Diagn. 1998;44:23–6.

Chapter 42

Over-the-Wire Techniques during PMV

KS Ravindranath, Ravi S Math, CN Manjunath

Traditionally, four methods have been described for the entry of the percutaneous mitral valvuloplasty (PMV) balloon from the left atrium (LA) into the left ventricle (LV)[1]: (1) the direct method, (2) vertical method, (3) horizontal (sliding method), and (4) loop method. Many a times, these methods fail and recourse may have to be taken to more advanced techniques like the over-the-wire (OTW) technique. This Chapter deals with OTW techniques related to Inoue/Accura balloons (together called as PTMC balloons henceforth).

The OTW technique relies on the placement of a stiff wire directly into the LV and then threading the PTMC balloon over the stiff wire. The method was first proposed by Meier.[2] His technique involved the following steps: (a) placement of a 0.020-inch back-up J-tip wire in the left ventricle over a diagnostic right Judkin's catheter positioned in the left atrium (LA), (b) advancement of the diagnostic right Judkin's catheter into the LV, (c) positioning of the pre-shaped 0.025-inch pigtail Inoue wire in the left ventricle, and (d) introduction of the Inoue balloon over the wire.

The second method advocated by Mehan and Meier[3] involved: (a) crossing the mitral valve with a balloon floatation catheter (Swan-Ganz), (b) maneuvering the balloon catheter into the aorta, (c) positioning of a 0.021-inch long 'back-up' valvuloplasty guidewire through this catheter in the descending aorta, and (d) introduction of the Inoue balloon over the wire.

Manjunath et al. have modified Meir's technique and simplified the steps.[4] The steps involved are: (1) placing the 0.025" coiltip guidewire in the LA; (2) the Mullin sheath is reintroduced into the LA over the coiltip guidewire, and the coiled portion of the guidewire is withdrawn into the sheath; (3) positioning of the Mullin's sheath near the mitral orifice (Fig. 42.1A) and placement of the coiltip guidewire directly into the LV (Fig. 42.1B, Video–1). This step may initially appear to be difficult because of the pigtail tip. However, with some perseverance and practice it can be easily achieved; (4) This is followed by further advancement of the Mullin sheath into the LV cavity (Fig. 42.1C) for obtaining optimal coiling of the coiltip guidewire (atleast 2-3 coils) (Fig. 42.1D, Video–2) (if not previously done, septal dilatation with the 14 Fr dilator may be done over the coiltip guidewire); (5) Introducing the Inoue balloon catheter over the wire into the LV cavity (Video-3). The PTMC balloon should not be deslenderized until atleast 2/3rd of the balloon has crossed the IAS (Fig. 42.1E, F, Video-4) keeping a sustained forward push on the coiltip guidewire. After crossing the mitral valve, the balloon is positioned across the valve and the dilation performed in the usual way (Fig. 42.1G, H, Video-5). While removing the coiltip guidewire from the LV, it is essential that the wire is withdrawn with the PTMC balloon still placed in the LV to avoid slicing of the submitral apparatus. Only when the wire is inside the balloon, should the entire assembly be withdrawn into LA (Fig. 42.1I). No additional accessories like

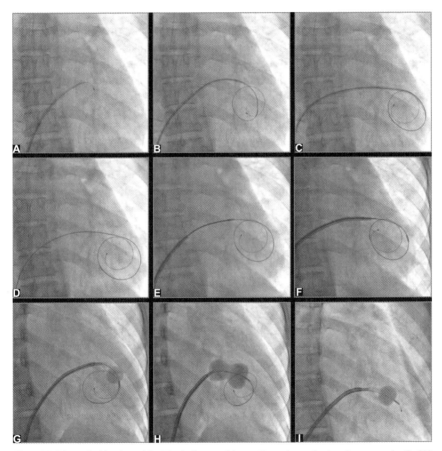

Figs 42.1A to I: Manjunath's Technique of 'over-the-wire mitral valve crossing": (A) Positioning of the Mullin's sheath near the mitral orifice; (B), placement of the coiltip guidewire directly into the LV; (C) Further advancement of the Mullin sheath into the LV cavity; (D) Optimal coiling of the coiltip guidewire (atleast 2-3 coils); (E) introducing the PTMC balloon catheter over the wire into the LV cavity. The PTMC balloon should not be de-slenderised until at least 2/3rd of the balloon has crossed the IAS; (F) De-slenderised PTMC balloon advanced into LV cavity; (G) Distal half of PTMC balloon inflated; (H) PTMC balloon withdrawn up to the mitral valve and proximal half inflated; (I) PTMC balloon in LV. Coiltip guidewire withdrawn into balloon before withdrawing entire assembly

back up guidewires, right Judkins catheter or floatation catheters are required, thus preventing additional expenses. As the coiltip guidewire is directly introduced into the LV, multiple exchanges involved in other conventional OTW techniques are avoided, resulting in lesser fluoroscopic, procedural time and high success rate. Since, the technique is associated with frequent ventricular ectopics and nonsustained ventricular tachycardia; it has been felt that this may make the patient hemodynamically unstable. An analogy may be drawn to balloon aortic valvuloplasty where during the placement of the extrastiff-wire into the LV, similar ectopy is noted. However, once the wire has a stable position the rhythm stabilizes. Similar findings are noted in the OTW technique. During the wire insertion, ectopy is near-universal. Once optimum coiling of the coiltip guidewire is obtained, the ectopy disappears. Another concern has been that the 0.025″ coiltip guidewire provides inadequate support with resultant prolapse of the balloon into LA. The trick here is that the PTMC balloon should not be deslenderized until atleast 2/3rd of the balloon has crossed the IAS. Lastly, Abhaichand et al.[5] have expressed a concern that the guidewire may get inserted between the chordate tendinae which may get damaged during balloon inflation leading to severe mitral regurgitation. In our experience, we have not found this to be a concern over the past 15 years. When 2–3 optimal coils of the coiltip guidewire are made in the LV, the possibility of entering the subvalvular apparatus is precluded due to the large diameter of the coils. Identifying the "balloon impasse" or "balloon compression" signs will prevent inadvertent inflation of the balloon in the subvalvular apparatus.[6]

We have found the above technique to be useful in a number of situations, such as giant LA, low puncture, thick IAS, LA/LAA (left atrial appendage) clot, critical MS, dextrocardia/malposed cardia, jugular PTMC, etc. This technique is especially useful in the presence of LA/LAA clot. The presence of a LA thrombus is a contraindication for PMV due to the risk of systemic embolization. Manjunath et al.[7] classified LA thrombus based on their location, extension, and mobility as assessed by TTE/TEE (Figure 53.4, Chapter 53). Patients were considered for PTMC if they had type Ia, type Ib and type IIa LA clots. Patients were anticoagulated (INR 2.0–3.0) for 8–12 weeks. A deliberate low IAS puncture was performed. The modified OTW as described earlier was used. By adopting this technique, the LA is virtually excluded from the track of the septal dilator and balloon catheter exchanges and hence the possibility of disturbing the thrombus is negligible. In a prospective study, 108 patients with LA/LAA thrombus successfully underwent PMV. There were no thromboembolic episodes during the procedure (Table 42.1, Fig. 42.2). There was one case of transient ischemic attack which occurred 6 hours after a successful balloon mitral valvuloplasty (BMV). There was significant and comparable improvement in the mitral valve area, mitral valve gradient, LA mean and pulmonary artery systolic pressure following the procedure. All these procedures performed by experienced operators who had performed more than 500 BMVs. More recently, Ravindranath et al.[8] reported the use of the OTW technique in transjugular PTMC. In the event of a low puncture, LV entry was difficult in one of the four cases of transjugular PTMC. The OTW

Table 42.1: PTMC results in 108 patients with LA/LAA clot

	Study group (n = 108)	*Control group (n = 2,622)*
Age (years)	27 ± 8	26 ± 9
MV score >8	46 (42.6%)	943 (36%)
MVO area by ECHO (cm²)		
Pre-BMV	0.8 ± 0.2	0.9 ± 0.2
Post-BMV	1.8 ± 0.2	1.9 ± 0.2
CVA—Stroke	0	5 (0.19%)
CVA—TIAs	1 (0.92%)	8 (0.31%)
Peripheral embolic episodes	0	3 (0.11%)
Moderate to severe MR	2 (1.85%)	32 (1.22%)
MR requiring emergency MVR	1 (0.92%)	20 (0.76 %)
Cardiac tamponade	1 (0.92%)	40 (1.52%)
In hospital death	0	5 (0.19%)
Suboptimal results	2 (1.85%)	49 (1.87%)

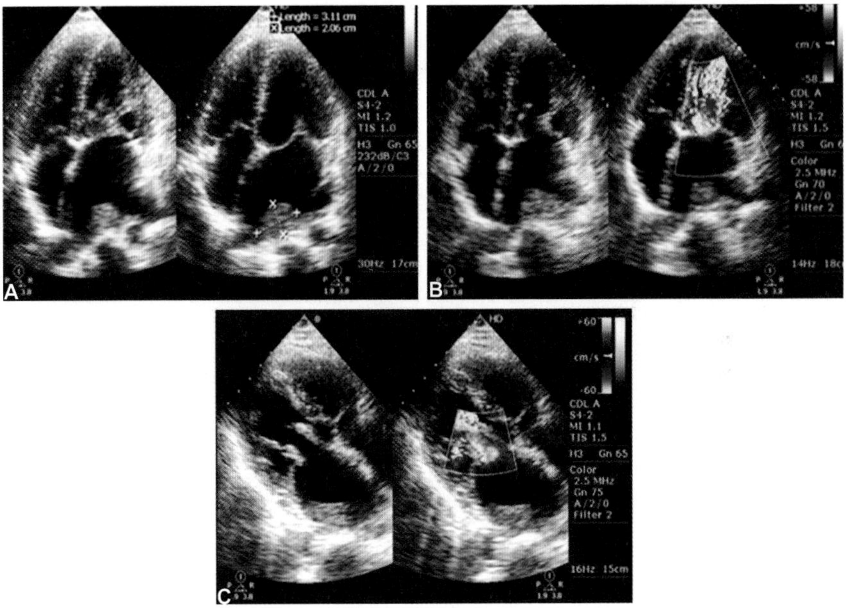

Figs 42.2A to C: TTE still frames of a patient before PTMC (A) and after PTMC (B and C) showing intact LA roof clot

technique was successfully used to enter the LV and the PTMC was successfully performed (Figs 42.3A to F). Deora et al.[9] used a 0.035″, hydrophilic, 260-cm long glidewire over a 4 Fr AR-1 diagnostic coronary catheter to enter the LV. The hydrophilic wire was then exchanged with a 0.035″ Amplatz super-stiff

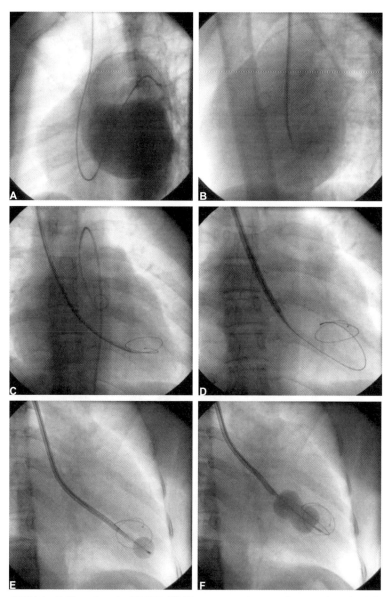

Figs 42.3A to F: Transjugular PTMC: (A) Pumonary artery angiogram done to delineate the left atrium and the interatrial septum in the levophase; (B) Septal puncture done in the left anterior oblique (LAO) cranial view midway between the pigtail and the spine; (C) A 0.025" coil wire maneuvered into the left ventricle over the Mullins sheath; (D) Septal dilatation was done with a 14 F dilator; (E) Accura balloon entering the left ventricle over the coil wire; (F) Balloon dilatation done

guidewire, which was coiled in vitro to make extra loops of its floppy portion. The Inoue PTMC catheter was slenderized directly over this super-stiff wire without its metal stylet and gradually negotiated to park across the stenotic mitral valve orifice. Tandar et al.[10] used an arteriovenous loop to track the Inoue balloon. They advanced a 260 cm 0.032" wire over the Mullins sheath into the LV from where the wire was snared using a gooseneck snare inserted through the femoral artery over a 5 Fr multipurpose-1 catheter. The 0.032" wire was withdrawn to the abdominal aorta while advancing the 0.32 wire from the venous system. The Inoue balloon was then tracked over the arteriovenous loop. Since, the 0.032" wire is unsheathed within the LV, traction during the establishment of the AV loop can transect the MV apparatus leading to mitral regurgitation. A safer alternative would have been to advance the 0.032" wire over a balloon floatation catheter into the LV and then further into the aorta from where it could be snared.

For all OTW techniques, with wire positioned in the LV, direct measurement of LA pressure is not possible (except if the PTMC balloon is exchanged for a multitrack catheter). The success (or otherwise) of the PMV procedure has to be monitored with transthoracic echocardiogram. Mitral regurgitation may be over-estimated due to the wire interfering with leaflet coaptation.

The OTW technique forms an important armamentarium in the cases of difficult LV entry and in the presence of LA/LAA clot.

▓ REFERENCES

1. Hung JS, Lau KW. Pitfalls and tips in Inoue balloon mitral commissurotomy. Cathet Cardiovasc Diagn. 1996;37:188–99.
2. Meier B. Modified Inoue technique for difficult mitral balloon commissurotomy. Cathet Cardiovasc Diagn. 1992;26:316-18.
3. Mehan VK, Meier B. Impossibility to cross a stenotic mitral valve Bwith the Inoue balloon: success with a modified technique. Indian Heart J. 1994;46:51–2.
4. Manjunath CN, Srinivasa KH, Patil CB, Venkatesh HV, Bhoopal TS, Dhanalakshmi C. Balloon mitral valvuloplasty: our experience with a modified technique of crossing the mitral valve in difficult cases. Cathet Cardiovasc Diagn. 1998;44:23–6.
5. Abhaichand RK, Joseph G. Letter to the editor: Re Manjunath et al., Catheterization and Cardiovascular Interventions. 1999;46:117.
6. Manjunath CN, Srinivasa KH. Reply to the letter to the editor by Abhaichand and Joseph. Catheterization and Cardiovascular Interventions. 1999; 46:117–18.
7. Manjunath CN, Srinivasa KH, Ravindranath KS, Manohar JS, Prabhavathi B, Dattatreya PV. Balloon mitral valvotomy in patients with mitral stenosis and left atrial thrombus. Catheter Cardiovasc Interv. 2009; 74(4):653-61.
8. Shankarappa RK, Math RS, Chikkaswamy SB, Rai MK, Karur S, Dwarakprasad R, et al. Transjugular percutaneous transvenous mitral commissurotomy (PTMC) using conventional PTMC equipment in rheumatic mitral stenosis with interruption of inferior vena cava. J Invasive Cardiol. 2012;24(12):675-8.
9. Deora S, Vyas C, Shah S. Percutaneous transvenous mitral commissurotomy: a modified over-the-wire technique for difficult left ventricle entry. J Invasive Cardiol. 2013;25:471-3.
10. Tandar A, Badger R, Whisenant BK. Mitral valvuloplasty with the Inoue balloon tracked over an arteriovenous wire. Catheter Cardiovasc Interv. 2012;80:987-90.

Chapter 43

PMV Performed with other Percutaneous Interventions

Dinesh Choudhary, Harikrishnan S

Mitral stenosis can be associated with lesions of other valves or these patients have other unrelated diseases like coronary artery disease or even congenital heart disease. Occasionally, we need to perform percutaneous interventions in these patients along with percutaneous mitral valvuloplasty (PMV). In this chapter, we will discuss about some situations where we need to perform other interventions along with PMV.

PMV AND PERCUTANEOUS VALVOTOMY OF OTHER VALVES

Several previous small series and case reports about combined percutaneous mitral and tricuspid valvuloplasty have demonstrated feasibility, safety and efficacy of the procedure with excellent immediate outcome and the benefit being maintained on the intermediate term.[1-6] Case reports of combined aortic/mitral and combined aortic/tricuspid have also shown feasibility and safety.[7,8] A few cases of combined triple valvuloplasty (mitral, aortic and tricuspid) are reported in the literature to date.[9,10] Recently, Rifaie et al. has reported a series of 11 patients who underwent valvotomy of another valve along with PMV.[11]

WHICH VALVE TO TACKLE FIRST?

When we are planning intervention in multiple valves, the distal valve has to be tackled first. This is because if we are relieving the obstruction in proximal stenosis, e.g. tricuspid valve in case of BMV or BMV in case of BAV, this will lead onto sudden flooding of blood into LA or LV (respectively) and can lead to sudden hemodynamic and clinical deterioration leading to pulmonary edema. Krishnan et al.[12] did BMV before tackling the aortic valve, but none of their patients had any clinical deterioration.

However, in patients with advanced aortic valve obstruction with left ventricular dysfunction, the risk may be genuine. In such cases, it may be advisable to do retrograde aortic dilatation first, followed by transvenous mitral valvotomy. Sharma, et al.[3] also dilated the aortic valve before the MV in all their patients; however, the transseptal puncture was performed before the aortic balloon valvotomy.

Rifaie et al. did PMV before PAV.[11] Since, PAV requires heparin anticoagulation, and PMV requires transseptal puncture (with an inherent risk of hemopericardium, especially on anticoagulation), they preferred to do PMV before PAV. PTV was also done after PMV, as they thought that the hemodynamic parameters will change once the pulmonary artery pressure comes down following a PMV. In case when the patient required procedure of all three valves, they performed PMV and PAV together in one setting and PTV was done in another setting to avoid patient as well as operator fatigue.[11]

◼ PMV AND PERCUTANEOUS AORTIC VALVOTOMY

Bicuspid artic valve (BAV) for degenerative aortic valve disease has lost its popularity, with only cases where it is performed only as a palliative procedure or as a bridge to surgery. The newly developed percutaneous aortic valve replacement is replacing the role of BAV even in those previously mentioned situations. But the scenario of rheumatic aortic valve stenosis is different.

Rheumatic aortic stenosis is characterized by commissural fusion which—in the absence of calcification or with minimal calcification—would easily yield under balloon dilatation, a mechanism exactly similar to PMV.

Sharma et al.[3] has reported the 2-year outcome of 10 patients who underwent BAV and BMV for combined rheumatic aortic and mitral valve disease. The transaortic gradient decreased from 93.56 ± 17.7 mm Hg to 28.56 ± 7.8 mm Hg ($p < 0.0005$) and the valve area increased from 0.37 ± 0.05 cm^2 to 1.03 ± 0.25 cm^2 ($p < 0.005$). Symptomatic and hemodynamic results were sustained at 23.5 ± 9.1 months.

Rifaie et al.[11] has reported the long-term outcome of 10 patients with rheumatic aortic stenosis who underwent BAV along with PMV. They reported a good immediate outcome with the peak systolic gradient coming down from 69 mm Hg to 28 mm Hg. Only one patient developed increase in AR of one grade following BAV. At long-term follow-up of mean 24 months, the peak gradient remained at a mean value of 29 mm Hg and the mean aortic valve area was 2.1 ± 0.2 cm^2, and the peak systolic pressure gradient across the valve was 29.8 ± 8.1 mm Hg, none of the patients developed restenosis of the aortic valve.

Sayed M Abdou et al.[13] recently published their experience in percutaneous valvuloplasty using the Inoue balloon in 14 patients with combined rheumatic mitral and aortic stenosis (AS) in a single stage procedure via antegrade transseptal approach. The study group was characterized by relatively young age (mean 37.5 +/- 9.6 years). Aortic followed by mitral valvuloplasty via antegrade approach resulted in a fall of transaortic peak pressure gradient (PG) from 59 mm Hg to 25 mm Hg (P 0.012) and mean from 49 mm Hg to 16 mm Hg (P 0.043), mean transmitral gradient decreased from 14 mm Hg to 5.3 mm Hg. Aortic valve area increased significantly from 0.7 cm^2 to 1.4 cm^2 (P 0.042) and mitral valve areas from 1.08 cm^2 to 1.92 cm^2. The procedures were well-tolerated without development of significant valvular regurgitation or thromboembolism. During follow-up, 2 patients died due to lung cancer and sudden death at months 48 and 100. Five patients received delayed surgery after mean duration of 73.4 +/- 39.7 months. The study results suggest that balloon aortic valvuloplasty can be more durable in younger patients with rheumatic AS than in elderly patients with degenerative AS. Concurrent antegrade, transseptal Inoue balloon aortic and mitral valvuloplasty, is feasible and safe, and provides excellent immediate results as one-stage procedure.

In view of the results of the above three studies, which are the largest studies percutaneous valvotomy of rheumatic aortic valves, we would suggest that patients with rheumatic severe aortic stenosis and minimal calcification should be given a chance for PAV, particularly in young females with childbearing potential, in order to defer the need for valve replacement by the surgical route. We also have to note that these patients almost always have mitral valve disease associated with them as isolated rheumatic aortic stenosis is extremely rare to find. These patients will end up in double valve replacement with its intending surgical risks, costs, availability and long-term follow-up including anticoagulation.

BAV ALONG WITH PMV—TECHNIQUES

Retrograde Technique

It is the most commonly employed technique. The series by Sharma et al.[3] used Mansfield balloons for the procedure. Rifaie et al.[11] used the retrograde approach in 8 out of 9 patients. The advantage of the procedure is that it is easy, if the valve can be crossed. There is no need to use the railroad technique by snaring the wire, etc. The disadvantage is the requirement of a large sheath through the arterial side which will lead to access site complications. The Mansfield™ or Tyshak™ balloons can be used for this procedure. The balloon chosen is usually 90–100% of the size of the annulus. Sharma et al. reported that balloon size selected for aortic valve was equal to or 1–2 mm smaller than the aortic annulus as measured on aortography.

Antegrade Technique

Krishnan et al.[12] and Bahl et al.[14] have reported few patients whom they did BMV and BAV together using the antegrade technique. Antegrade or transseptal approach for balloon aortic valvotomy (BAV) is an attractive alternative to retrograde route; it has the advantage of crossing the valve along the jet of flow besides avoiding complications at the arterial access site. After balloon mitral valvotomy (BMV), Mullins sheath is introduced into the LV across the mitral valve. The Mullins sheath is gently advanced to the LV apex and a loop is made with the help of a J-tip exchange length guidewire. The wire is negotiated into the left ventricular outflow and then across the aortic valve. This wire is tracked into the descending aorta. Then this wire is exchanged for an extra-stiff wire which will allow the tracking of the balloon across the aortic valve. Then the appropriate sized balloon is tracked from the venous side and through the IAS, LV and aortic valve. Bahl et al.[14] and Krishnan[12] et al. (Figs 43.1 and 43.2) have used Inoue balloon for doing BAV.

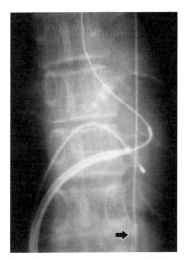

Fig. 43.1: Snare (arrow) stabilizing the guide wire while Inoue catheter attempts to cross aortic valve (With permission from Elsevier, MN Krishnan et al., International Journal of Cardiology 2007;114:e9–e11)

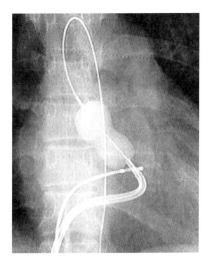

Fig. 43.2: Inoue balloon inflated across the aortic valve (With permission from Elsevier, Krishnan MN, et al. International Journal of Cardiology 2007;114:e9–e11)

To avoid the problem of wire dislodgement and losing the position of the balloon, people have reported to snare the distal end of the wire in the descending aorta and holding it to maintain stability of the system (Fig. 43.3). To prevent squeezing out of the balloon by the high LV pressure, it is advisable to pace the right ventricle at 200–240 bpm which will produce a state of near asystole (Figs 43.4 to 43.6).

There are three advantages of this approach when this is combined with a BMV. One is that we are already having a left atrial access which will make the procedure easier. Next is the obvious merit of avoiding insertion of large calibre arterial sheath, the third advantage is that this approach may make crossing the tightly stenotic valve easier. Sakata et al.[15] and Eisenhauer et al.[16] reported that compared to retrograde approach, transseptal cases produced a better hemodynamic result. Sakata et al. found that antegrade group had 20% additional increase of aortic valve area and 20% greater reduction of transaortic valve gradient compared to the retrograde approach along with technical advantages as described above. Eisenhauer et al. showed that increase in aortic valve area was significantly greater ($P = 0.039$) along with delayed total follow-up mortality in antegrade approach.

Both found that the conventional cylindrical or isodiametric balloons may not be able to achieve optimal stretching and compression of the aortic leaflets because of constraints produced by the aortic annulus or the ascending aorta. The largest Inoue balloon (30 mm) does provide a larger dilating diameter than the biggest available conventional balloon (25 mm). Optimal dilatation is achieved by overstretching the leaflets back into the sinuses of Valsalva along

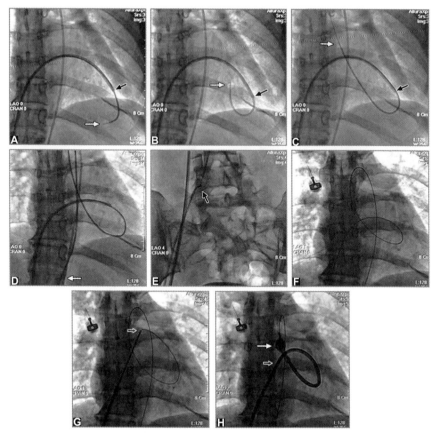

Figs 43.3 A to H: Technical sequence in antegrade transseptal Inoue balloon aortic valvuloplasty. (A) Balloon wedge catheter (white arrow) is advanced to left ventricle through Mullins sheath (black arrow); (B) With slight deeper seating of Mullins sheath in left ventricle, balloon catheter is advanced to form a wide up-ticking loop in left ventricle; (C) With counterclockwise rotation of catheter, its tip balloon is directed towards outflow tract and then to ascending aorta across aortic valve; (D) Guided by a 260 cm 0.0245 inches PTFE-coated wire, balloon catheter is advanced to abdominal aorta alongside preexisting pigtail catheter; (E) Wire is exteriorized with a snare (black arrow) for anchoring outside arterial sheath; (F) Balloon catheter and Mullins sheath are removed, leaving guidewire with a wide loop in left ventricle; (G) Stretched Inoue-balloon catheter is advanced over guidewire to left atrium (open white arrow); (H) Inoue-balloon catheter is destretched and stretch metal tube is withdrawn to leave its tip (open white arrow) about 2 cm into the left atrium beyond atrial septum. Thereafter, catheter manipulation is supported by guide wire, anchored at both distal and proximal ends, as well as by stretch metal tube fixed across atrial septum (open white arrow). Catheter balloon is advanced to ascending aorta to initiate valve dilatation, following slight inflation of balloon (white arrow) (Abdou SM. Catheter Cardiovasc Interv. 2013;82:E712–17) (Published with permission from Wiley Inc.)

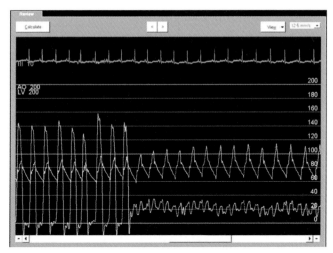

Fig. 43.4: Hemodynamic tracing in the cathlab in a patient with rheumatic mitral and aortic stenosis. The tracing in white is the pullback from left ventricle to left atrium. Simultaneous pressure in the ascending aorta is seen. *Note* the elevated LA pressure and also the gradient across the aortic valve

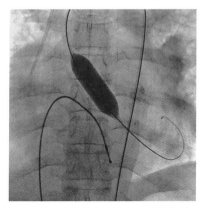

Fig. 43.5: Balloon aortic valvotomy being performed initially prior to PMV. *Note* the temporary pacing wire in the right ventricle. The RV is paced at 200–240 bpm to prevent squeezing out of the balloon by the high LV pressure

with annular stretching with a dumbbell-shaped balloon like Inoue. The short term benefits results due to annular dilatation and fractures of nodular calcium. In patients with commissural fusion and preserved leaflet architecture, aggressive dilatation may lead to long-term benefits with separation of the commissures. The fit of the distal bulbous end of the Inoue balloon into the sinuses of Valsalva during approximation of annulus by waist of the balloon usually help to achieve a more complete dilatation, commissural separation and/or fracture. This self-positioning dumbbell configuration, coupled with size adjustability, can generate improved initial hemodynamic benefit.

PMV and Balloon Pulmonary Valvotomy

Rheumatic involvement of pulmonary valve is rare. Quadrivalvar involvement in RHD is very rare with few case reports. [17-21] Successful surgical management of rheumatic quadrivalvular disease is reported.[21] Percutaneous intervention for rheumatic trivalvular disease (mitral, aortic and tricuspid valves) is also reported.[22,23]

There is a possibility that rheumatic pulmonary stenosis may be missed in cases of rheumatic mitral stenosis and pulmonary hypertension. The high RV systolic pressure may be attributed to pulmonary arterial hypertension and pulmonary stenosis may be missed if careful Doppler interrogation of pulmonary valve is not done.

We have reported two cases of balloon pulmonary valvotomy along with PMV (in the same sitting), done presumably for rheumatic pulmonary stenosis[22] (Figs 43.7 and 43.8). Both patients were males, 47 and 23 years old. Echocardiographic evaluation showed severe valvular pulmonary stenosis (Fig. 43.8), severe mitral stenosis with mild mitral regurgitation (MR), mild aortic stenosis (AS) and moderate organic tricuspid regurgitation. Since, both patients were noted to have normal pulmonary valve 10–17 years prior, it was presumed that the pulmonary involvement was also rheumatic in origin. Since, the mitral valve was pliable and suitable for percutaneous mitral valvotomy, both cases were planned for balloon mitral valvotomy (BMV) and balloon pulmonary valvotomy (BPV) in the same sitting.

Balloon mitral valvuloplasty BMV was successfully done by the anterograde transseptal approach using 24 mm Inoue balloon. The pulmonary annulus measured by echocardiography was 22 mm. So, the same Inoue balloon was used to dilate the pulmonary valve. BPV was done with the same (24 mm) Inoue balloon (Fig. 43.7). It was difficult to track the pigtail-shaped wire (usually used along with Inoue balloon) into the pulmonary artery. So, a 300 cm long, 0.025 extra support (Cook Inc.) guidewire was used and the wire tip parked in the distal RPA. The Inoue balloon was tracked over the wire and BPV was done successfully with the gradient across the pulmonary valve decreasing from 80 mm Hg to 10 mm Hg.

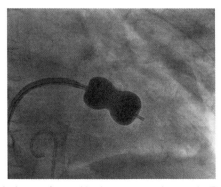

Fig. 43.6: PMV being performed in the same patient as in Figure 43.5, Inoue balloon across mitral valve during concurrent PMV and BAV

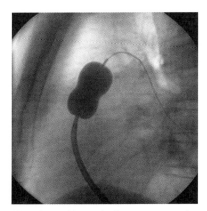

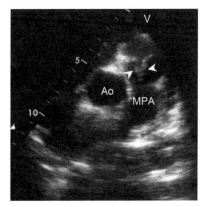

Fig. 43.7: Inoue balloon across the pulmonary valve during pulmonary valvotomy. *Note* the extra support wire in the pulmonary artery 📷◀

Fig. 43.8: Echocardiographic picture showing the thickened and doming pulmonary valve due to rheumatic origin. This was dilated and yielded on ballooning producing good hemodynamic benefit *Abbreviations*: AO, aorta; MPA, main pulmonary artery

The second case was done with two Inoue balloons of two sizes. BMV was done by 26 mm Inoue balloon and BPV was done by 22 mm Inoue balloon with good hemodynamic result. In this case, we could park the pigtail wire in the left pulmonary artery which allowed tracking of the Inoue balloon across the pulmonary annulus.

These cases are already reported. This is the only report describing percutaneous pulmonary valvotomy and mitral valvotomy in rheumatic heart disease. In both these cases, both procedures were done with the Inoue balloon. BMV using Inoue balloon has become the standard technique. Use of Inoue balloon in pulmonary valvotomy is also described.[23]

The problem with usage of Inoue balloon in BPV is the difficulty in tracking and parking the pigtail wire in the pulmonary artery. We had difficulty in tracking the pigtail in one case and we had to use a 0.025 extra support (Cook Inc.) 300 cm guidewire to track the Inoue balloon.

▦ PMV AND BALLOON TRICUSPID VALVOTOMY

Rheumatic mitral and tricuspid stenosis is also a common association. Double-valve balloon valvotomy is feasible and safe and provides excellent immediate and intermediate-term follow-up results in selected patients with multivalve disease. Sharma et al.[3] did mitral and tricuspid balloon valvotomy as a single staged procedure in 10 patients. The mitral valve area increased from 0.78 ± 0.21 cm^2 to 2.05 ± 0.56 cm^2 ($p < 0.0005$) and tricuspid valve area increased from 1.11 ± 0.41 cm^2 to 2.52 ± 0.69 cm^2 ($p < 0.0005$). The excellent symptomatic and hemodynamic results were sustained at 30.3 ± 9.8 months of follow-up. Rifaie et al.[11] also published 2 cases of combined PMV and BTV and concluded that combined percutaneous balloon dilatation of rheumatic mitral and tricuspid stenosis is feasible with fairly adequate immediate and long-term outcomes.

TRIPLE VALVE INTERVENTION

Percutaneous intervention for all the three valves has been reported, though extremely rare.[24] Goel et al.[10] reported the case of a 26-year-old male, who underwent valvotomy of all the three valves. The mitral and tricuspid valves were dilated using the same Inoue balloon, whereas the aortic stenosis was dilated using the pigtail-tipped balloon. Sobrino et al.[9] reported two patients with combined rheumatic mitral, aortic and tricuspid stenosis in which triple percutaneous valvuloplasty was performed in a single sitting. Here also the sequence of dilatation is worth discussing. Ideally, it should be tricuspid, mitral and aortic in that order.

PERCUTANEOUS CORONARY INTERVENTION AND PMV

In the developing world, since CAD is rising in prevalence, interventionalists may come across more and more cases where CAD and RHD may coexist. Occasionally, we come across cases where we need to perform both percutaneous coronary intervention (PCI) and percutaneous mitral valvotomy in the same patient.

There are four reports in the literature describing combined coronary angioplasty and PMV.[25-28] We have reported one case from our center.[28] In two of the above-mentioned reports,[25,26] PCI was done first, while we performed PMV as the first procedure.[28] Since, there is a chance of significant mitral regurgitation (MR) leading to mitral valve replacement (MVR) in a small percentage of patients, we thought of doing PMV as the first procedure. If the patient develops MR, he can have mitral valve replacement (MVR) and a bypass graft to the coronaries. Since PCI of a simple Type A lesion in LAD coronary artery (like that was in our patient) is almost completely safe, we opted to do it after PMV. One of the reported cases who had PMV and PCI together, had PCI to the LAD and the other one had PCI to the right coronary artery.

Percutaneous coronary intervention requires anticoagulation with heparin. For PMV, the patient is anticoagulated only after septal puncture and the subsequent septal dilatation for fear of cardiac tamponade. Anticoagulation after LA entry and subsequently performing PCI is the technique described in the two cases reported[1,2] but keeping a pigtail wire in the LA for a long time in the thrombogenic milieu of mitral stenosis is dangerous, and if by any chance LA access is lost, repuncturing the septum is dangerous in view of the anticoagulation.

These are the two arguments we put forward for performing PMV as the initial procedure. Otherwise the technique of both procedures are not in any way different from any other case, except the fact that we have to be very careful in performing the PCI, to prevent any complication which will end-up in surgery, when we had already dilated the mitral valve successfully.

■ REFERENCES

1. Ashraf T, Pathan A, Kundi A. Percutaneous balloon valvuloplasty of coexisting mitral and tricuspid stenosis: single-wire, double-balloon technique. J Invasive Cardio. 2008;20 (4):E126-8.
2. Sancaktar O, Kumbasar SD, Semiz E, Yalcinkaya S. Late results of combined percutaneous balloon valvuloplasty of mitral and tricuspid valves. Cathet Cardiovasc Diagn. 1998;45:246-50.
3. Sharma S, Loya YS, Desai DM, Pinto RJ. Percutaneous double valve balloon valvotomy for multivalve stenosis: immediate results and intermediate-term follow-up. Am Heart J. 1997;133:64-70.
4. Shrivastava S, Radhakrishnan S, Dev V. Concurrent balloon dilatation of tricuspid and calcific mitral valve in a patient of rheumatic heart disease. Int. J Cardio. 1988;20:133-7.
5. Sharma S, Loya YS, Daxini BV, Sundaram U. Concurrent double balloon valvotomy for combined rheumatic mitral and tricuspid stenosis. Cathet Cardiovasc Diagn. 1991;23:42-6.
6. Bahl VK, Chandra S, Sharma S. Combined dilatation of rheumatic mitral and tricuspid stenosis with Inoue balloon catheter. Int J Cardiol. 1993;42:178-81.
7. Mechmeche R, Cherif A, Elmnouchi R. Percutaneous balloon valvotomy for combined rheumatic mitral and aortic stenosis. Tunis Med. 2008;86:598-9.
8. Shrivastava S, Goswami KC, Dev V. Concurrent percutaneous balloon valvotomy for combined rheumatic tricuspid and aortic stenosis. Int J Cardio. 1993;38(2):183-6.
9. Sobrina N, Calvo Orbe L, Merino JL, Peinado R, Mate I, Rico J, et al. Percutaneous balloon valvuloplasty for concurrent mitral, aortic and tricuspid rheumatic stenosis. Eur Heart J. 1995;16(5):711-3.
10. Goel Sl, Desai OM, Shah LS. Concurrent balloon dilatation of rheumatic trivalvular stenosis. Cathet Cardiovasc Diagn. 1995;36(5):283-6.
11. Rifaie O, El-Itriby A, Zaki T, Abdeldayem TM, Nammas W. Immediate and long-term outcome of multiple percutaneous interventions in patients with rheumatic valvular stenosis. EuroIntervention. 2010;6(2):227-32.
12. Krishnan MN, Syamkumar MD, Sajeev CG, Venugopal K, Johnson F, Vinaykumar D, et al. Snare-assisted anterograde balloon mitral and aortic valvotomy using Inoue balloon catheter. Int J Cardiol. 2007;114(1):e9-11.
13. Abdou SM, Chen YL, Wu CJ, Lau KW, Hung JS. Concurrent antegrade transseptal inoue-balloon mitral and aortic valvuloplasty. Catheter Cardiovasc Interv. 2013;82:E712–17.
14. Bahl VK, Chandra S, Goswami KC, Manchanda SC. Balloon aortic valvuloplasty in young adults by antegrade, transseptal approach using Inoue balloon. Cathet Cardiovasc Diagn. 1998;44(3):297–301.
15. Sakata Y, Syed Z, Salinger MH, Feldman T. Percutaneous balloon aortic valvuloplasty: antegrade transseptal vs. conventional retrograde transarterial approach. Catheter Cardiovasc Interv. 2005;64(3):314–21.
16. Eisenhauer AC, Hadjipetrou P, Piemonte TC. Balloon aortic valvotomy revisited: the role of the Inoue balloon and transseptal antegrade approach. Catheter Cardiovasc Interv. 2000;50(4):484–91.
17. Talwar S, Jayanthkumar HV, Sharma G, Kumar AS. Quadrivalvular rheumatic heart disease. Int J Cardiol. 2006;106(1):117-8.
18. Kumar AS, Iyer KS, Chopra P. Quadrivalvular heart disease. Int J Cardiol. 1985;7(1):66-9.

19. Krishnamoorthy KM. Images in cardiovascular medicine. Rheumatic stenosis of all four valves. Tex Heart Inst J. 2002;29(3):224-5.
20. Jai Shankar K, Jaiswal PK, Cherian KM. Rheumatic involvement of all four cardiac valves. Heart. 2005;91(6):e50.
21. Kumar N, Rasheed K, Gallo R, Al-Halees Z, Duran CM. Rheumatic involvement of all four heart valves: preoperative echocardiographic diagnosis and successful surgical management. Eur J Cardiothorac Surg. 1995;9(12):713-4.
22. Harikrishnan S, Bijulal S, Krishnakumar N, Ajithkumar VK. Combined mitral and pulmonary valvotomy with Inoue balloon in rheumatic quadrivalvular disease. J Heart Valve Dis. 2011;20(1):112-3.
23. Lau KW, Hung JS. Controversies in percutaneous balloon pulmonary valvuloplasty: timing, patient selection and technique. J Heart Valve Dis. 1993;2(3):321-5.
24. Konugres GS, Lau FY, Ruiz CE. Successive percutaneous double-balloon mitral, aortic, and tricuspid valvotomy in rheumatic trivalvular stenoses. Am Heart J. 1990;119(3 Pt 1):663-6.
25. Chow WH, Yip AS, Chow TC. Concurrent balloon dilation in a patient with mitral stenosis and coronary artery disease. A case report. Angiology 1994;45:489–92.
26. Rothlisenberger C, Kaufmann U, Meier B.Combined percutaneous balloon mitral valvotomy and coronary angioplasty with stent implantation. Cathet Cardiovasc Diagn. 1995;36:183–5.
27. Ramondo A, Chioin R, Rigatelli G. Simultaneous coronary angioplasty and percutaneous mitral valvuloplasty: a case report (Italian with English abstract). Ital Heart J Suppl. 2000;1 (2):266-9.
28. Harikrishnan S, Bhat A, Tharakan J. Percutaneous balloon mitral valvotomy and coronary stenting in the same sitting. Heart Vessels. 2003;18:150–2.

Chapter 44

Balloon Tricuspid Valvotomy along with PMV

Harikrishnan S, Amit Kumar Chaurasia

Rheumatic tricuspid stenosis (TS) can also be successfully dilated by means of balloon valvotomy (Fig. 44.1).[1,2] Isolated TS without TR is rare in MS. But when TS is seen it is almost always associated with MS. When MS and TS exist together, concurrent percutaneous balloon valvuloplasty can be performed in suitable cases.[3-9]

Initially, double balloon technique was used for balloon tricustid valvotomy (BTV),[1,4] but now most of the cases are performed with Inoue balloon.[3,6,8]

When mitral and tricuspid stenoses coexist in a patient, the sequence of balloon dilation is first the mitral valve, then the tricuspid. This sequence is important, because of the concern that concomitant mitral stenosis may lead to worsening pulmonary congestion should the obstruction at the tricuspid valve is relieved initially. On the other hand, in the presence of mitral stenosis with marked elevation of left atrial pressure, a prompt decrease of left atrial pressure following successful balloon mitral valvuloplasty through the transseptal approach may bring about an abrupt right-to-left shunting across the atrial septum, thereby inducing serious systemic hypoxemia. So a fast BTV is recommended by some people.[10]

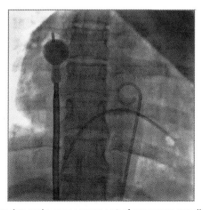

Fig. 44.1: Invasive hemodynamic measurement of pressure gradient across the tricuspid valve. Note the balloon flotation catheter in the RV and the Inoue balloon in the RA. The pigtail in the descending aorta is also seen

Technique

Balloon selection: Sharma et al. decided the size of the balloon for BTV on the basis of the measurement of the tricuspid annulus on right ventriculography (Figs 44.2 to 44.4). They have used either the same-sized Inoue balloon or balloons with size 1–2 mm smaller than the measured annulus. Most labs report that they used the same balloon which was used for PMV as it is cost-effective. The same balloon can be used at least as the initial balloon for BTV. Tricuspid annulus measured by echocardiography in the apical 4 chamber view can also be used for this purpose.[4]

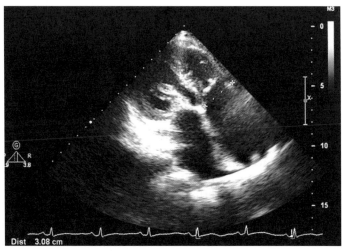

Fig. 44.2: Apical 4 chamber view which is used to measure the tricuspid annulus

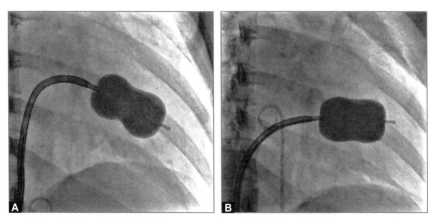

Figs 44.3A and B: (A) Balloon across the mitral valve; (B) Balloon across the tricuspid valve. Both images are acquired in the RAO 30° view

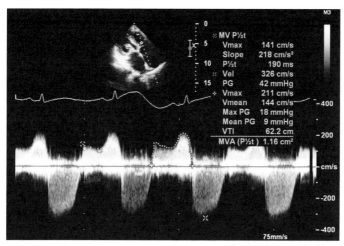

Fig. 44.4: Doppler flow evaluation of tricuspid valve flow indicating severe TS with a mean gradient of 9 mm Hg. PHT valve area is 1.16 cm². TR flow velocity is also seen

Inoue Balloon Technique

The Inoue balloon after PMV is slenderized and withdrawn into the right atrium across the transseptal access. The coiled stainless steel pigtail-shaped guidewire is taken out so as to render the Inoue balloon catheter flexible. The J-shaped balloon introducer stylet is used to direct and float the Inoue balloon across the tricuspid valve into the right ventricle.

Instead of the counter clockwise rotation employed in case of mitral valve, Patel et al. recommends clockwise rotation of the stylet to introduce the balloon across the tricuspid valve. The partially inflated distal portion of the balloon is withdrawn until it straddled against the tricuspid valve and the balloon is fully inflated to the capacity depending on the size of the annulus of the tricuspid valve till the waist disappears. Here also serial dilations are recommended.

Bhargava et al. has proposed an algorithm for using the Inoue balloon in BTV.[11] They suggest that the Inoue balloon catheter usually found to float swiftly into the right ventricle (RV) without using the J-stylet. But in some cases it may be difficult to negotiate the tricuspid valve by "floatation technique" especially in those with distorted right atrial anatomy and severely stenosed tricuspid valve.

Bhargava Algorithm for BTV Using Inoue Balloon

Step 1: Simply float the Inoue balloon into the RV like the Swan-Ganz catheter.
Step 2: If step 1 fails, use the J-stylet with clockwise rotation.
Step 3: If step 2 fails, use the J-stylet and utilize the Swan-Ganz property of the Inoue balloon to enter the RV.
Step 4: If step 3 fails, use the "over-the-wire" technique, particularly in severely stenosed valves and distorted right atrial anatomy.

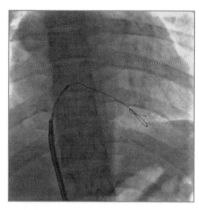

Fig. 44.5: Over-the-wire entry of Inoue balloon across tricuspid valve

Over-the-Wire Technique

Balloon tricuspid valvotomy (BTV) may pose technical challenges in situations like a severely stenosed valve with significantly dilated right atrium. If there is difficulty in crossing the tricuspid valve, the over-the-wire technique can be employed. The wire is usually kept in the RV (Fig. 44.5), till the balloon dilation is completed.[12,13] If the wire in the RV is inducing ectopics and ventricular tachycardia, the wire can be kept in the pulmonary artery also.

Positioning of the Inoue balloon over-the-wire across the stenosed valve may at times be difficult due to inadequate support from the right atrium and the relative stiffness of the shaft of the catheter. In the double balloon technique, proper placement of both the balloons may sometimes be difficult because the balloons slide over each other during inflation.[11]

Complications Related to BTV

Possible complications include damage to the tricuspid apparatus leading to significant tricuspid regurgitation. The technique using Inoue balloon is reported to be safer than using the double balloon. The over-the-wire techniques will have the wire related complications also to be accounted for.

■ REFERENCES

1. Al Zaibag M, Ribeiro P, Al Kasab S. Percutaneous balloon valvotomy in tricuspid stenosis. Br Heart J. 1987;57(1):51–3.
2. Cemin R, Mautone A, Donazzan L, Oberhollenzer R. Inoue balloon valvuloplasty for rheumatic tricuspid valve stenosis: an excellent technique with some intrinsic difficulties. J Cardiovasc Med Hagerstown Md. 2014;15(3):263–5.
3. Bahl VK, Chandra S, Mishra S. Concurrent balloon dilatation of mitral and tricuspid stenosis during pregnancy using an Inoue balloon. Int J Cardiol. 1997;59(2):199–202.
4. Sharma S, Loya YS, Daxini BV, Sundaram U. Concurrent double balloon valvotomy for combined rheumatic mitral and tricuspid stenosis. Cathet Cardiovasc Diagn. 1991;23(1):42–6.

5. Sobrino N, Calvo Orbe L, Merino JL, Peinado R, Mate I, Rico J, et al. Percutaneous balloon valvuloplasty for concurrent mitral, aortic and tricuspid rheumatic stenosis. Eur Heart J. 1995;16(5):711–3.
6. Bahl VK, Chandra S, Sharma S. Combined dilatation of rheumatic mitral and tricuspid stenosis with Inoue balloon catheter. Int J Cardiol. 1993;42(2):178–81.
7. Shrivastava S, Radhakrishnan S, Dev V. Concurrent balloon dilatation of tricuspid and calcific mitral valve in a patient of rheumatic heart disease. Int J Cardiol. 1988;20(1):133–7.
8. Bahl VK, Chandra S, Goel A, Goswami KC, Wasir HS. Versatility of Inoue balloon catheter. Int J Cardiol. 1997;59(1):75–83.
9. Bethencourt A, Medina A, Hernandez E, Coello I, Goicolea J, Laraudogoitia E, et al. Combined percutaneous balloon valvuloplasty of mitral and tricuspid valves. Am Heart J. 1990;119(2 Pt 1):416–8.
10. Cheng TO. Concurrent balloon valvuloplasty for combined mitral and tricuspid stenoses. Int J Cardiol. 1997;61(2):197.
11. Bhargava B, Mathur A, Chandra S, Bahl VK. Tricuspid balloon valvuloplasty: can the balloon be floated into the right ventricle? Cathet Cardiovasc Diagn. 1996;38(3):333–4.
12. Patel TM, Dani SI, Shah SC, Patel TK. Tricuspid balloon valvuloplasty: a more simplified approach using inoue balloon. Cathet Cardiovasc Diagn. 1996; 37(1):86–8.
13. Shaw TR. The Inoue balloon for dilatation of the tricuspid valve: a modified over-the-wire approach. Br Heart J. 1992;67(3):263–5.

Chapter 45

PMV in Patients with Atrial Fibrillation

Krishnakumar M

The development of atrial fibrillation (AF) is a common sequelae in patients with long-standing mitral stenosis, and it is associated with hemodynamic and clinical decompensation. Leon et al. have pointed out that the presence of AF is associated with inferior immediate and long-term outcome after PMV.[1] This chapter discusses the mechanism of AF, its effect on PMV and then the long-term outcome following PMV in patients with AF.

■ MECHANISM OF ATRIAL FIBRILLATION IN MITRAL STENOSIS

Atrial fibrillation (AF) can occur in clinically normal individuals[2] and as a complication of virtually every known form of cardiac disease. It does, however, have a preferential tendency to develop in certain specific cardiac conditions, of which mitral valve disease is the most noteworthy. The incidence of AF in mitral stenosis has been estimated at 40%.[3]

Earlier studies dealing with possible factors in the development of AF in patients with mitral stenosis (MS) have not shown consistent results. Fraser and Turner[4] concluded from a study of 269 patients with mitral valve disease that AF bears no direct relationship to severity of mitral disease. Atrial enlargement, on the other hand, has been found with greater frequency in patients with AF than in those in sinus rhythm. This relationship has been established by estimation of atrial size by left atrial volumetric determinations.[5] Although Loogen[6] suspected some correlation between severity of MS and left atrial size, Pech and Munster[7] could not reach similar conclusions on the basis of atrial volume determinations. Other investigators[8-10] have also been unable to find a consistent relationship between atrial size and various hemodynamic parameters in MS.

The mechanical consequences of MS, although not expressed by any single hemodynamic measurement, may be assumed to traumatize the left atrium, providing prerequisites for the electrophysiologic in homogeneity of atrial conduction times and refractory periods that are demonstrable in experimental AF.[11-13] Once present, AF leads to a further increase in the degree of left atrial enlargement that was initially the result of obstruction at the mitral valve. The

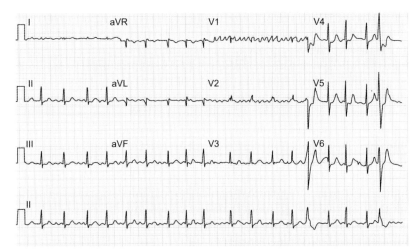

Fig. 45.1: Patient with AF and severe MS. The coarse fibrillation waves are seen in lead V1. Sometimes, it will be difficult to differentiate between flutter and fibrillation

arrhythmia is self-sustaining, and the vicious cycle is further perpetuated by the advancing age of the patient. The relationship between severity of MS and incidence of AF will tend to be obliterated by considering together both older individuals who have MS in a mild, nonprogressive form[14] who, because of their age, are more prone to develop AF, and younger patients in whom the hemodynamic effect of mitral stenosis may be sufficient to initiate the arrhythmia. Patients with MS who remain in sinus rhythm may be presumed to have noncompliant, hypertrophied atria which usually resist significant dilatation. Whether or not a given patient remains in sinus rhythm or develops AF must depend, at least in part, on the individual properties of cardiac muscle, as well as possibly, the rapidity of the development of the mitral valve lesion.

Established AF (Fig. 45.1) is associated with structural alterations in the atrium consisting of fibrosis, loss of muscle mass, and disruption of normal architecture.[15] These morphologic changes lead to atrial enlargement. There is a suggestion that such anatomic abnormalities are related to rheumatic activity. But many facts can be cited against this proposition—(1) AF is exceedingly rare in the early stages of rheumatic fever, when rheumatic activity is highest and when microscopic changes in the myocardium are demonstrated, (2) non-rheumatic diseases associated with overload of atrium, such as nonrheumatic mitral regurgitation and atrial septal defect are associated with as high an incidence of AF, (3) isolated rheumatic aortic valve disease shows only a very low incidence of AF.[15]

Problems

When AF supervenes, blood flow in the atrial appendage and in the body of the atrium becomes even more disorganized, with low velocity, multidirectional flow patterns, blood flow stasis and development of atrial thrombi. This swirling pattern of low velocity flow is often evident as spontaneous contrast on echocardiography, particularly when using a high-frequency transducer from a transesophageal approach. Approximately 17% of patients undergoing surgery for MS have left atrial thrombus, and in approximately one-third of these patients the thrombus is restricted to the atrial appendage.[16]

The prevalence of AF in patients with MS increases with age, severity of MS and lower cardiac output.[21] AF was present in 17% of patients aged 21–30 years, 45% of those aged 31–40 years, 60% of those older than age 51 years in one series.[17] The association of AF with age appears to be partly independent of the effect of disease severity since another series of patients undergoing valvuloplasty have a prevalence of AF ranging from 4% in younger patients[18] in India to 45% in an older North American population.[19] In a series of patients older than 65 years of age undergoing valvuloplasty, the prevalence of AF was 74%.[20] A high prevalence of AF (60%) was noted in MS patients who had associated pulmonary hypertension.[20]

The association between AF and left atrial thrombus formation is well known. Most atrial thrombi occur in the atrial appendage, possibly related to the larger size of the left atrial appendage and less effective emptying in MS compared to patients who have other reasons for AF.[21] In patients with MS, AF is associated with a higher prevalence of embolic events, compared to sinus rhythm.[22] In a series of 737 patients, in patients older than 35 years of age the incidence of systemic embolism was 32% in those with AF versus 11% in those in sinus rhythm.[23]

The higher risk for embolic events in AF in MS, compared to patients without mitral valve disease, is also well documented.[24] The Framingham study estimated a 17 fold increase in the risk of stroke in patients with AF and MS compared to a 5-fold increased risk for AF in the absence of mitral valve disease.[24] An European series estimated the risk of embolic events in MS with AF as 3.6 cases per 1000 patient-years in those with moderate stenosis and 5.7 cases per 1000 patient-years in those with severe MS.[25] A study of 500 MS patients identified AF and spontaneous left atrial contrast as risk factors for systemic embolism.[26] In addition, MS with AF is associated with excess mortality; Gajewski et al. reported a 5 years survival for mitral stenosis patients with AF of only 64% compared to 85% in patients with AF but no mitral valve disease.[27] The onset of AF with loss of atrial contraction often leads to hemodynamic/clinical decompensation (decrease in cardiac output and increase in left atrial pressure). This seems to be primarily due to the effect of diastolic filling time of the accelerated ventricular rate, rather than to the loss of atrial booster function. The shortened diastole further compromises the reservoir function, the major mechanism of left ventricular filling.

Medical Management

Embolic events are best prevented by interventions to relieve mitral valve obstruction prior to the development of excessive left atrial enlargement and AF. When AF does occur, efforts should be directed toward restoration of sinus rhythm through mechanical intervention to increase mitral valve area if appropriate, or through electrical cardioversion in conjunction with pharmacological therapy.[28] Both short-term cardioversion and pharmacologic therapy followed by valvuloplasty or surgery may be needed for maintenance of sinus rhythm. If efforts to achieve and maintain sinus rhythm are unsuccessful, attention should be directed to pharmacological rate control and long-term anticoagulation. Rapid ventricular rates are poorly tolerated in MS due to impaired ventricular filling. Rate control, usually by pharmacological depression of conduction in the atrioventricular node, allows an adequate time interval for diastolic filling of the left ventricle across the stenotic mitral valve. Standard approaches to rate control are appropriate in patients with MS, including treatment with a beta-blocker, a calcium channel blocker, or a combination of agents, depending on the specific clinical circumstances for each patient.[28]

With persistent AF, anticoagulation to achieve a therapeutic international normalized ratios (INR) of 2 to 3 is particularly important in patients with MS given the high-risk of embolic events.[28] Although transesophageal echocardiographic evaluation for left atrial thrombus has been proposed to allow earlier cardioversion in patients with AF, the risk of left atrial thrombus is so high among patients with mitral stenosis that it is prudent to consider therapeutic anticoagulation for at least 4 weeks prior to cardioversion.[29] Similarly, all patients with MS being considered for balloon mitral valvotomy should undergo transesophageal echocardiography shortly before the procedure given the high-risk of embolic complications if a left atrial thrombus is present.[30] In patients undergoing surgical intervention for MS, another proposed approach to restoration of sinus rhythm is the Cox-Maze procedure. This procedure aims to surgically create a single electrical pathway from the sinus node to the AV node, while isolating the abnormal electrical activity of the left and right atrial tissues. An alternative procedure is electrophysiological mapping with isolation of the pulmonary vein orifice.[31]

Technical Difficulties in PMV

Hemodynamic assessment of the severity of MS from cardiac catheterization data is time consuming, particularly for patients in AF. The most accurate method use a hydraulic formula, such as that of Gorlin and Gorlin, which requires measurement of the cardiac output and the mean mitral valve gradient over 10 consecutive cardiac cycles (by planimetry or from digitized signals). The dependence of the end diastolic mitral valve gradient on heart rate has long been appreciated.[32-35] It may be particularly difficult to interpret the end diastolic gradient at extremes of heart rate and in patients in AF. Transmitral gradient depends on interactions between the length of preceding cardiac cycles and hemodynamic factors including left atrial filling and the inotropic and lusitropic state of the left ventricle, which may be particularly complex in AF.[36]

Noninvasive assessment of the severity of MS by conventional or Doppler echocardiography (Figs 45.1 and 45.2) or both is convenient and reliable. Care

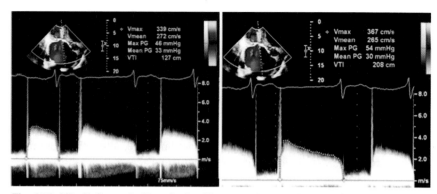

Fig. 45.2: Mitral inflow velocities obtained from a patient who is in AF. See the differences in the MV gradients obtained from a short (46/33 mm Hg) and a long (54/30 mm Hg) diastole

is needed in interpretation because these methods may be inaccurate at fast heart rates and at high flows.[37]

Long-term Outcome

We have done a retrospective study to examine the effect of AF on the immediate and long-term outcome of patients undergoing balloon mitral valvotomy (BMV). 818 consecutive patients, who underwent elective BMV in SCTIMST from 1997 to 2003, were included in the study. Of them, 95 were in AF. The clinical, echocardiographic and hemodynamic data of these patients were compared with those of 723 patients in normal sinus rhythm (NSR). Immediate procedural results and long-term events were compared between the two study groups. Patients with AF were older (29.4 ± 10.1 vs. 39.9 ± 9.9 years; $p < 0.001$) and presented more frequently with New York Heart Association (NYHA) class III-IV (32.9% vs. 53.7%; $p < 0.001$), echocardiographic score >8 (24.9% vs. 47.4%; $p < 0.001$) and with history of previous surgical commissurotomy (11.5% vs. 33.7%; $p < 0.001$). Patients in the AF group had higher pulmonary artery pressure (36.1 ± 15 vs. 33.6 ± 10.9 mm Hg) and transmitral gradients (15.7 ± 5.9 vs. 13.6 ± 5.4 mm Hg; $p = 0.041$). In patients with AF, BMV resulted in inferior immediate and long-term outcomes, as reflected in a lesser post-BMV mitral valve area (1.6 ± 0.4 vs. 1.3 ± 0.4 cm²; $p = 0.032$) and a lower event-free survival (freedom of death, reintervention, mitral valve replacement surgery, stroke and death) at a mean follow-up time of 6 years (93.6% vs. 86.3%; $p = 0.016$). In the group of patients in AF, Wilkin's echocardiographic score >8 ($p = 0.004$) was identified as the sole independent predictor of combined events at follow-up. Thus, AF was found as a marker for clinical and morphologic features associated with inferior results after BMV.

▌ RESTORATION AND MAINTENANCE OF SINUS RHYTHM IN ▌ MITRAL STENOSIS

This aspect is described in detail in the Chapter 33 on Arrhythmias and PMV.

Arguably, the most important proximate cause of AF in MS is LA stretch caused by raised LA pressure. In addition to reducing LA pressure, percutaneous transvenous mitral commissurotomy (PMV) has been shown to favorably alter atrial refractoriness[38] and conceivably set the stage for reversion to SR (Figs 45.3 and 45.4). However, most patients in chronic AF before PMV fail to revert to SR in the absence of an aggressive antiarrhythmic strategy.[39,40] Furthermore, only a few of the patients who do revert remain in SR at follow-up (Fig. 45.5).[39]

Therefore, combining PMV with an aggressive antiarrhythmic strategy offers the best prospect of rhythm control. This has previously been attempted in nonrandomized studies, with favorable results. Duration of AF, LA size and age are the principal determinants of successful cardioversion and maintenance of

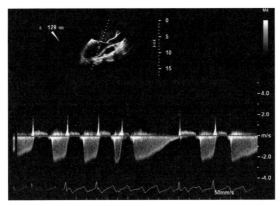

Fig. 45.3: Doppler tracing obtained by TEE across the mitral valve in a patient with atrial flutter. The ECG showing atrial flutter and the beat-to-beat variation in the pressure gradient is shown clearly. Here we have average five beats to estimate the gradients across the mitral valve

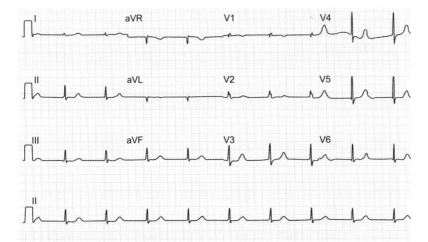

Fig. 45.4: The same patient in Figure 45.3 underwent electrical cardioversion, went into slow junctional rhythm which reverted in 12 hours to sinus rhythm as seen in Figure 45.4

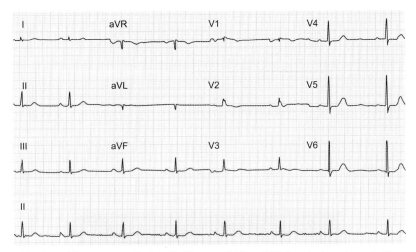

Fig. 45.5: The same patient as in Figures 45.3 and 45.4 restoring sinus rhythm following cardioversion

SR.[40,41] Hu and colleagues reported the results of the first randomized controlled trial of a rate versus rhythm control strategy immediately following PMV.[42] The authors reported remarkable success with a rhythm control strategy (96% of the patients were in SR at one year) with concomitant improvements in symptom status, exercise capacity, and quality of life.

REFERENCES

1. Leon MN, Harrell LC, Simosa HF, Mahdi NA, Pathan A, Lopez-Cuellar J, et al. Mitral balloon valvotomy for patients with mitral stenosis in atrial fibrillation: immediate and long-term results. J Am Coll Cardiol. 1999;34(4):1145–52.
2. Orgain ES, Wolff L, White PD. Uncomplicated auricular fibrillation and auricular flutter. Arch Intern Med. 1936;57:493.
3. Wood P. Diseases of the heart and circulation. Philadelphia: JB Lippincott Company;1968. p. 625.
4. Fraser HR, turner RW. Auricular fibrillation; with special reference to rheumatic heart disease. Br Med J. 1955 Dec 10;2(4953):1414–8.
5. Arvidsson H. Angiocardiographic observations in mitral disease with special reference to volume variations in the left atrium. Acta Radiol Suppl. 1958; 158:1–124.
6. Loogen F, Panayotopoulos SN. Vorhofflimmern and Mitralfehler. Dsch Med Wochenschr 1963;88:19.
7. Pech HJ, Münster W. [Volume determination of the left atrium by means of angiocardiography]. Cardiologia. 1968;53(3):129–38.
8. Melhem RE, Dunbar JD, Booth RW. The "B" lines of Kerley and left atrial size in mitral valve disease. Their correlation with the mean left atrial pressure as measured by left atrial puncture. Radiology. 1961;76:65–9.
9. Chen JT, Behar VS, Morris JJ Jr, McIntosh HD, Lester RG. Correlation of Roentgen findings with hemodynamic data in pure mitral stenosis. Am J Roentgenol Radium Ther Nucl Med. 1968;102(2):280–92.

10. Simon G. The value of radiology in critical mitral stenosis. Clin Radiol. 1964;15: 99–105.
11. Hudson RE. The human pacemaker and its pathology. Br Heart J. 1960;22:153–67.
12. Trautwein W, Kassebaum DG, Nelson RM, Hechth. Electrophysiological study of human heart muscle. Circ Res. 1962;10:306–12.
13. Singer DH, Harris PD, Molin JR, Hoffman BF. Electrophysiological basis of chronic atrial fibrillation. (abstr) Circulation. 1967;35 (suppl II): II-239.
14. Selzer A, Cohn KE. Natural history of mitral stenosis: a review. Circulation. 1972;45(4):878–90.
15. Bailey GW, Braniff BA, Hancock EW, Cohn KE. Relation of left atrial pathology to atrial fibrillation in mitral valvular disease. Ann Intern Med. 1968;69(1):13–20.
16. Waller BF. Etiology of mitral stenosis and pure mitral regurgitation. In: Waller BF (Eds). Pathology of the Heart and Great Vessels. New York: Churchill Livingstone;1988:pp.101-48.
17. Deverall PB, Olley PM, Smith DR, Watson DA, Whitaker W. Incidence of systemic embolism before and after mitral valvotomy. Thorax. 1968;23(5):530–6.
18. Arora R, Kalra GS, Murty GS, Trehan V, Jolly N, Mohan JC, et al. Percutaneous transatrial mitral commissurotomy: immediate and intermediate results. J Am Coll Cardiol. 1994;23(6):1327–32.
19. Multicenter experience with balloon mitral commissurotomy. NHLBI Balloon Valvuloplasty Registry Report on immediate and 30-day follow-up results. The National Heart, Lung, and Blood Institute Balloon Valvuloplasty Registry Participants. Circulation. 1992;85(2):448–61.
20. Tuzcu EM, Block PC, Griffin BP, Newell JB, Palacios IF. Immediate and long-term outcome of percutaneous mitral valvotomy in patients 65 years and older. Circulation. 1992;85(3):963–71.
21. Hwang JJ, Li YH, Lin JM, Wang TL, Shyu KG, Ko YL, et al. Left atrial appendage function determined by transesophageal echocardiography in patients with rheumatic mitral valve disease. Cardiology. 1994;85(2):121–8.
22. Chiang CW, Lo SK, Ko YS, Cheng NJ, Lin PJ, Chang CH. Predictors of systemic embolism in patients with mitral stenosis. A prospective study. Ann Intern Med. 1998;128(11):885–9.
23. Coulshed N, Epstein EJ, McKendrick CS, Galloway RW, Walker E. Systemic embolism in mitral valve disease. Br Heart J. 1970;32(1):26–34.
24. Wolf PA, Dawber TR, Thomas HE Jr, Kannel WB. Epidemiologic assessment of chronic atrial fibrillation and risk of stroke: the Framingham study. Neurology. 1978;28(10):973–7.
25. Horstkotte D, Niehues R, Strauer BE. Pathomorphological aspects, aetiology and natural history of acquired mitral valve stenosis. Eur Heart J. 1991;12 Suppl B:55–60.
26. Chiang CW, Lo SK, Kuo CT, Cheng NJ, Hsu TS. Noninvasive predictors of systemic embolism in mitral stenosis. An echocardiographic and clinical study of 500 patients. Chest. 1994;106(2):396–9.
27. Gajewski J, Singer RB. Mortality in an insured population with atrial fibrillation. JAMA J Am Med Assoc. 1981;245(15):1540–4.
28. Prystowsky EN, Benson DW Jr, Fuster V, Hart RG, Kay GN, Myerburg RJ, et al. Management of patients with atrial fibrillation. A Statement for Healthcare Professionals. From the Subcommittee on Electrocardiography and Electrophysiology, American Heart Association. Circulation. 1996;93(6):1262–77.
29. Stoddard MF, Dawkins PR, Prince CR, Longaker RA. Transesophageal echocardiographic guidance of cardioversion in patients with atrial fibrillation. Am Heart J. 1995;129(6):1204–15.

30. Rittoo D, Sutherland GR, Currie P, Starkey IR, Shaw TR. A prospective study of left atrial spontaneous echo contrast and thrombus in 100 consecutive patients referred for balloon dilation of the mitral valve. J Am Soc Echocardiogr Off Publ Am Soc Echocardiogr. 1994;7(5):516–27.
31. Sueda T, Imai K, Ishii O, Orihashi K, Watari M, Okada K. Efficacy of pulmonary vein isolation for the elimination of chronic atrial fibrillation in cardiac valvular surgery. Ann Thorac Surg. 2001;71(4):1189–93.
32. Wood P. An appreciation of mitral stenosis: II. Investigations and results. Br Med J. 1954;1(4871):1113–24.
33. Nakhjavan FK, Katz M, Shedrilovzky H, et al. Hemodynamic effects of exercise, catecholamine stimulation and tachycardia in mitral stenosis and sinus rhythm at comparable heart rates. Am J Cardiol. 1969;23:659-66.
34. Manchanda SC, Ramesh L, Roy SB. Haemodynamic effects of atrial pacing in rheumatic mitral stenosis. Br Heart J. 1974;36(7):636–40.
35. Grossman W, McLaurin LP. Dynamic and isometric exercise during cardiac catheterisation. In: Grossman W, (eds.) Cardiac catheterization and angiography. Philadelphia: Lea and Febiger; 1980. pp.215-22.
36. Keren G, Meisner JS, Sherez J, Yellin EL, Laniado S. Interrelationship of mid-diastolic mitral valve motion, pulmonary venous flow, and transmitral flow. Circulation. 1986;74(1):36–44.
37. Sagar KB, Wann LS, Paulson WJ, Lewis S. Role of exercise Doppler echocardiography in isolated mitral stenosis. Chest. 1987;92(1):27–30.
38. Soylu M, Demir AD, Ozdemir O, Topaloğlu S, Aras D, Duru E, et al. Evaluation of atrial refractoriness immediately after percutaneous mitral balloon commissurotomy in patients with mitral stenosis and sinus rhythm. Am Heart J. 2004;147(4):741–5.
39. Langerveld J, van Hemel NM, Kelder JC, Ernst JMPG, Plokker HWM, Jaarsma W. Long-term follow-up of cardiac rhythm after percutaneous mitral balloon valvotomy. Does atrial fibrillation persist? Eur Eur Pacing Arrhythm Card Electrophysiol J Work Groups Card Pacing Arrhythm Card Cell Electrophysiol Eur Soc Cardiol. 2003;5(1):47–53.
40. Kapoor A, Kumar S, Singh RK, Pandey CM, Sinha N. Management of persistent atrial fibrillation following balloon mitral valvotomy: safety and efficacy of low-dose amiodarone. J Heart Valve Dis. 2002;11(6):802–9.
41. Kavthale SS, Fulwani MC, Vajifdar BU, Vora AM, Lokhandwala YY. Atrial fibrillation: how effectively can sinus rhythm be restored and maintained after balloon mitral valvotomy? Indian Heart J. 2000;52(5):568–73.
42. Hu CL, Jiang H, Tang QZ, Zhang QH, Chen JB, Huang CX, et al. Comparison of rate control and rhythm control in patients with atrial fibrillation after percutaneous mitral balloon valvotomy: a randomized controlled study. Heart. 2006;92(8):1096-101.

Chapter 46

Percutaneous Mitral Valvotomy in Dextrocardia

Harikrishnan S, Krishnakumar Nair

Distorted cardiac anatomy of dextrocardia produces technical difficulties during percutaneous mitral valvotomy. During PMV, there may be difficulties experienced in interatrial septal puncture and left ventricular entry. There are only a few reports of PMV in dextrocardia.[1-8] This may be due to the fact that many of these patients undergo surgical commissurotomy due to the technical difficulties involved in the percutaneous procedure.[9,10]

Many modifications are proposed to tackle the anatomical variations in this situation. The newer version of cathlab equipments are able to provide image inversion in the left-right orientation. This will take care of most of the problems of PMV in dextrocardia. The radiographic images can be acquired in the inverted position and can be used as fluoroscopic guidance for the septal puncture, as described by Nallet et al.[4] and Namboodiri et al.[11] The inverted fluoroscopic settings, which will simulate normal anatomy (pseudo-views), facilitate easy manipulation of the transseptal needle and balloon in the LA. We get a pseudo-AP view when the C-arm is in the AP position with the image inverted left-right and a pseudo-right anterior oblique (RAO) 30° view when the C-arm was in the left anterior oblique (LAO) 30° view (Figs 46.1 to 46.4).

Transseptal catheterization is usually performed from the left groin to reduce the puncture needle angulation at the confluence of the iliac veins to the left-sided inferior vena cava. The descent of the needle assembly is recommended in the mirror-image position, i.e. the 7 to 9 o'clock position of the external indicator of the needle instead of the usual 4–6 o'clock position. The reference position is the ceiling as 12 o'clock (Fig. 46.4).

The delineation of the IAS is the most important and difficult step in transseptal puncture in such difficult anatomies. Verma et al. used levophase pulmonary angiography for IAS delineation in a patient with isolated dextrocardia and normal atrial situs. We utilized this technique in one of our cases, and we found it was considerably helpful in delineating the IAS fluoroscopically (Figs 46.3A and B). The catheter placed in the noncoronary aortic sinus marked the anterosuperior limit of the IAS (Fig. 46.5).

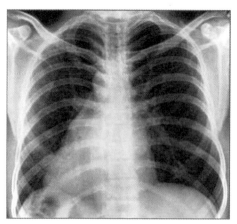

Fig. 46.1: Chest X-ray in posteroanterior view suggesting situs inversus, dextrocardia and pulmonary venous hypertension

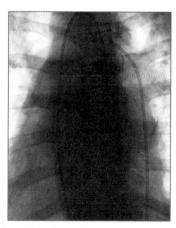

Fig. 46.2: Frontal view of the cardiac silhoutte with the pigtail catheter in the aortic root and MPA catheter in the superior vena cava, consistent with mirror-image dextrocardia

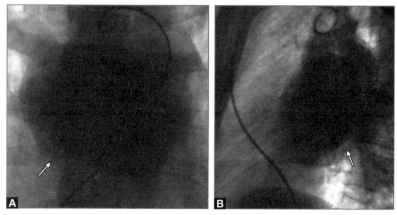

Figs 46.3A and B: Levophase pulmonary angiography in pseudo-AP and left lateral views delineating the interatrial septum (white arrows)

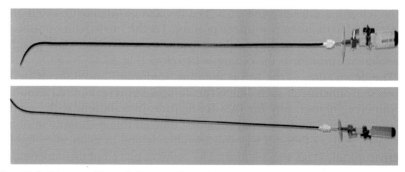

Fig. 46.4: The position of the needle pointer in case of transseptal puncture in dextrocardia. Note that compared to the usual needle orientation of 3–4 o'clock, in dextrocardia, we have to go to 7–8 o'clock position

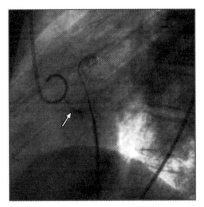

Fig. 46.5: Transseptal puncture in a left lateral view. Contrast is being injected into the cavity of the left atrium through the needle across the interatrial septum. Contrast staining of the interatrial septum is marked with a white arrow. A pigtail catheter is placed in the noncoronary aortic sinus

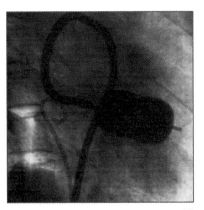

Fig. 46.6: Fully-expanded Accura™ balloon across the mitral valve, with the reverse loop in the left atrium 🎥

When there are other problems like IAS aneurysm it can compound the difficulties arising out of the difficult anatomy. In the presence of the septal aneurysm, contrast injection into the atria to delineate the IAS will be very useful. In situations like dextrocardia, there can be difficulties in crossing the mitral valve and dilating it. Crossing the mitral valve and balloon dilatation is done in pseudo RAO-view, that is LAO 30 view. Sometimes it may be necessary to resort to other techniques like reverse loop entry to cross and dilate the mitral valve (Fig. 46.6).

■ REFERENCES

1. Raju R, Singh S, Kumar P, Rao S, Kapoor S, Raju BS. Percutaneous balloon valvuloplasty in mirror-image dextrocardia and rheumatic mitral stenosis. Cathet Cardiovasc Diagn. 1993;30(2):138–40.
2. Patel, Dani, Thakore, Chaq, Shah, Shah, et al. Balloon mitral and aortic valvuloplasty in mirror-image dextrocardia. J Invasive Cardiol. 1996;8(3):164–8.
3. Chow WH, Fan K, Chow TC. Balloon mitral commissurotomy in a patient with situs inversus and dextrocardia. J Heart Valve Dis. 1996;5(3):307–8.
4. Nallet O, Lung B, Cormier B, Porte JM, Garbarz E, Michel PL, et al. Specifics of technique in percutaneous mitral commissurotomy in a case of dextrocardia and situs inversus with mitral stenosis. Cathet Cardiovasc Diagn. 1996;39(1):85–8.
5. Joseph G, George OK, Mandalay A, Sathe S. Transjugular approach to balloon mitral valvuloplasty helps overcome impediments caused by anatomical alterations. Catheter Cardiovasc Interv Off J Soc Card Angiogr Interv. 2002;57(3):353–62.
6. Verma PK, Bali HK, Suresh PV, Varma JS. Balloon mitral valvotomy using Inoue technique in a patient of isolated dextrocardia with rheumatic mitral stenosis. Indian Heart J. 1999;51(3):315–7.

7. Tavassoli A, Pourmoghaddas M, Emami M, Mousavizadeh M, Emami Meybodi T. Percutaneous transvenous mitral commissurotomy in a patient with situs inversus and dextrocardia: a case report. ARYA Atheroscler. 2011;7(1):47–50.

8. Kulkarni P, Halkati P, Patted S, Ambar S, Yavagal S. Percutaneous mitral balloon valvotomy in a case of situs inversus dextrocardia with severe rheumatic mitral stenosis. Cardiovasc Revasc Med. 2012;13(4):246–8.

9. Said SA, Veerbeek A, van der Wieken LR. Dextrocardia, situs inversus and severe mitral stenosis in a pregnant woman: successful closed commissurotomy. Eur Heart J. 1991;12(7):825–8.

10. Ramasamy D, Zambahari R, Fu M, Yeh KH, Hung JS. Percutaneous transvenous mitral commissurotomy in patients with severe kyphoscoliosis. Cathet Cardiovasc Diagn. 1993;30(1):40–4.

11. Namboodiri N, Harikrishnan SP, Ajitkumar V, Tharakan JA. Percutaneous mitral commissurotomy in a case of mirror-image dextrocardia and rheumatic mitral stenosis. J Invasive Cardiol. 2008;20(1):E33–35.

Chapter 47

Balloon Mitral Valvotomy—Left Femoral Vein Approach and in Venous Anomalies

Rajesh Muralidharan

Transseptal puncture and percutaneous balloon valvotomy has traditionally been performed through right femoral vein. This is a less tortuous route and provides the greatest ease in transseptal puncture and balloon mitral valvotomy. For a variety of reasons, percutaneous access from right femoral vein (RFV) is not always possible and another site must be used. A frequent alternative percutaneous access site is the left common femoral vein.

There are very few reports of PMV through LFV in the literature.[1-3]

The main concerns are the problems faced during septal puncture and tracking of the balloon-dilator assembly through the acute angulation in the left femoral vein-inferior vena cava (LFV-IVC) route which can produce significant traction on IVC. Rarely this acute angulation can lead to perforation of the Mullins sheath system.[4,5] There can also be difficulties in engaging the Brockenbrough needle into the fossa ovalis, which is more parallel than perpendicular, leading to dissection of atrial septum on attempts to advance the catheter and the needle.

Tejas Patel et al.[2] have reported a case where they performed PMV using the Inoue balloon through the left femoral route. Their patient was a 45-year-old Indian female with narrow build and narrow pelvis causing less acute angulation of left iliac vein combined with dilated inferior vena cava (IVC) attributable to severe TR. We have done one case through the left femoral vein and this patient was also of a small frame.

The difficulties of the left femoral vein approach can be minimized by two techniques: (1) Bending the trunk of the patient to the right in order to straighten the course of the catheter and the needle (Figs 47.1 and 47.2). (2) Increasing the distal curvature of the needle to approx 40 degrees also facilitates in achieving a more favorable catheter position (Fig. 47.3). (3) Pre-shaping the Brockenbrough needle, with a gentle curve about 15 cm proximal to its tip in the same direction. The group of Tejas Patel reported the use of all the three techniques (modification of the angle of the needle at the tip and 15 cm proximally) and bending the patient.

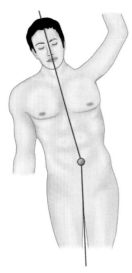

Fig. 47.1: Bending of the thorax to the right straightens the course of the catheter and the needle thereby decreasing the traction on the inferior vena cava and patient discomfort

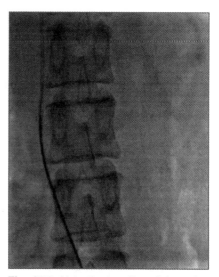

Fig. 47.2: Note the bending of the spine to the right to facilitate smooth passage of the catheter and the needle 📷◀

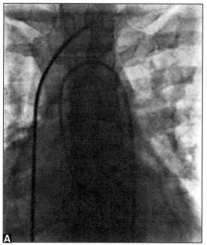

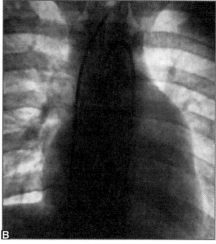

Figs 47.3A and B: Note the modified angle of transseptal needle in transseptal puncture from the left femoral vein access (A) compared to the usual angle in transseptal puncture from the right femoral vein access (B)

Vyas et al. encountered significant resistance at the junction of the inferior vena cava (IVC) and left iliac vein. The acute angle at the junction prevented the entry of the stiff Brockenbrough needle, the septal dilator and the Inoue Balloon into the IVC. At this point, the authors used what they described as

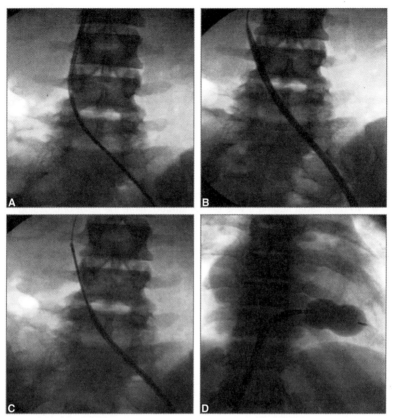

Figs 47.4A to D: (A) Negotiation of a Mullins dilator through left femoral vein approach (LFVA); (B) Septal dilator could be traversed across the acute venous angle, using the "telescoping" technique; (C) Slenderized Inoue percutaneous transvenous mitral commissurotomy catheter was advance using the same technique; (D) PTMC was performed successfully using the LFVA

a "telescoping" technique, i.e. simultaneous gentle push of the needle while pulling the Mullins dilator. (Figs 47.4A to D). This maneuver allowed smooth entry of the needle into the IVC and then SVC by minimizing the friction at the venous angulation.

In a series of 6 patients reported by Rawal et al. all patients underwent successful balloon mitral valvotomy through the left femoral venous approach. Patients had mild to moderate pain during the procedure. In variance with our technique, Rawal et al.[1] relied only on altering the curvature of the transseptal needle to achieve a successful transseptal catheterization and not on positioning the patient. There is another report of PMV through the left femoral vein in a pregnant patient, where there was a congenital anomaly of the venous system (Figs 47.5A and B).[6]

In conclusion, right femoral vein remains the preferred access for percutaneous balloon mitral valvotomy. Left femoral vein approach may be resorted to as an alternative. Bending the thorax to the right and re-shaping

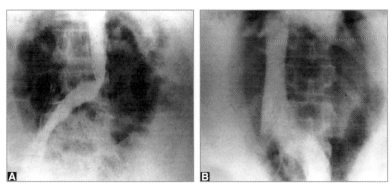

Figs 47.5A and B: Inferior vena cava angiogram showing the major abdominal venous system. No right canal segment was demonstrated. *Note* the point of crossing of the inferior vena cava to the right at the renal vein level (Reprinted with permission from Aggarwala, et al. Asian Cardiovasc Thorac Ann. 1998;6:227-8).

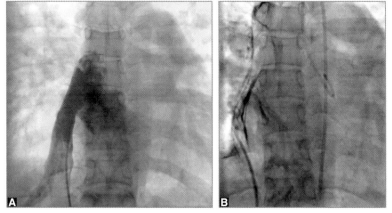

Figs 47.6A and B: (A) The venous angiogram showing the drainage of IVC into mid RA; (B) Dissection of the septum extending to IVC and SVC (AP view)

the needle facilitates septal puncture with minimal discomfort to the patient although patients may have mild lower abdominal or back pain at the time of needle manipulation in the pelvis. Jugular approach is another method if there is a problem with right femoral access, but it requires expertize and different set of hardware (See chapter 39).

■ BMV IN OTHER VENOUS ANOMALIES

Other types of venous anomalies can give rise to problems during BMV. Two cases which we came across are illustrated below.

Case I

26-year-old female was detected to have mitral stenosis when evaluated for a medical check up prior to emigration. She was referred to us after an attempt of PMV elsewhere, when the procedure was abandoned because she developed

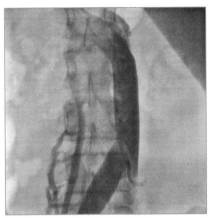

Fig. 47.7: IVC angiogram showing the IVC crossing from the right side to the left side and then back to the right side. This patient successfully underwent BMV through this anomalous vein

pericardial effusion. We also could not do a septal puncture initially and the attempts resulted in a septal dissection. Then IVC angiogram was done which showed the IVC is entering the RA in its middle one third (Figs 47.6A and B). Then the LA was entered through a PFO and the procedure was successfully completed.

Case II

30-year-old female was found to have the IVC crossing over to the left side in its mid segment and then recross to the right side and enter the usual position in RA (Fig. 47.7). Here we could track through the anomalous IVC and do the septal puncture and BMV without much difficulty.

▌ REFERENCES

1. Rawal J, Dahi S, Patel T, Shah S. Balloon mitral valvuloplasty using Inoue balloon catheter: the left femoral vein approach. Indian Heart J. 1996;48:531.
2. Patel TM, Dani SI, Rawal JR, Shah SC, Patel TK. Percutaneous transvenous mitral commissurotomy using Inoue balloon catheter: a left femoral vein approach. Cathet Cardiovasc Diagn. 1995;36(2):186–7.
3. Ebrahimi M, Eshraghi A. Percutaneus mitral balloon valvulotomy using left femoral vein; an unusual case. Int Cardiovasc Res J. 2013;7(2):75–6.
4. Ross J Jr, Braunwald E, Morrow AG. Transseptal left atrial puncture; new technique for the measurement of left atrial pressure in man. Am J Cardiol. 1959;3(5):653–5.
5. Ross J Jr, Braunwald E, Morrow AG. Left heart catheterization by the transseptal route: a description of the technique and its applications. Circulation. 1960;22: 927-34.
6. Agarwala MK, Singh M, Grover A, Varma JS. Balloon mitral valvotomy in pregnant patient with anomalous inferior vena cava. Asian Cardiovasc Thorac Ann. 1998;6:227-8.

Chapter 48

Retrograde Nontransseptal Balloon Mitral Valvuloplasty

Harikrishnan S, Arun Gopalakrishnan

▧ INTRODUCTION

Balloon mitral valvuloplasty (BMV) is currently a first line of treatment in suitable mitral stenosis patients.[1-2] It can be performed either through an antegrade or a retrograde approach. Former includes transseptal puncture followed by mitral dilatation using one of the various systems–Inoue balloon, double balloon system (DB), Cribier's metallic commissurotome and multi-track system.[3-6] Retrograde arterial access to mitral valve has the advantage of avoiding transseptal puncture but still has restricted applications in real world practise.

Indications

Retrograde arterial approach to mitral valve for valvotomy is preferred in following conditions:
- Failure to puncture the septum during antegrade approach
- Patients unsuitable for transseptal access due to anatomical deformities or prior interventional procedure (e.g. atrial septal defect device closure)
- Patient's preference in order to avoid left to right shunt resulting from antegrade approach.

Contraindications

Patients with concomitant aortic valve prosthesis cannot undergo mitral valvoplasty with retrograde approach.

Procedure

The first retrograde BMV, as described by Babic et al. in 1986, was not purely retrograde and required transseptal advancement of a guidewire inserted through the femoral vein, to be exteriorized and recovered through the femoral artery. Subsequently, the balloon was advanced retrogradely over the guidewire through the mitral valve.[7] In contrast, Buchler et al. and Ormes et al. described purely retrograde techniques for mitral dilation without transseptal catheterization, using a single balloon and DB, respectively.[8,9] Their techniques involved entering left atrium retrogradely with a Sones catheter and exchanging it with a long Teflon-coated wire over which balloon dilatation is performed. However, these approaches were adopted in isolated cases with no data on their feasibility in routine patients.

In 1990, Stefanadis C et al. described a novel method for left atrial retrograde catheterization which has been successfully used for BMV in large number of patients.[10] This technique utilizes a specially designed steerable left atrial catheter with external diameter of 8F or 9F.[11] The configuration of the tip of this catheter can be altered by external manipulation of steering arm. The steering arm consists of teflon-coated stainless steel wire that passes along the lumen of the catheter and emerges a short distance from the catheter tip and attached to the exterior of catheter close to its tip. Proximal end of the catheter has two system of hemostatic valves: steering arm passes through one of these and other is used for guidewire into catheter lumen.

Stepwise Approach for Retrograde Nontransseptal Balloon Mitral Valvuloplasty (RNBMV)

- Steerable left atrial (LA) catheter is inserted into left ventricular (LV) through femoral artery.
- Distal tip of catheter is formed by external manipulation to its desired configuration in LV apex so as to point towards mitral annulus. Catheter is then retracted until its tip reached a point immediately below mitral valve.
- A 0.038 inch J-guidewire is advanced through this catheter into LA and then exchanged with a stiffer guidewire using a pigtail catheter. Over this guidewire dilating balloon catheter (e.g. polyethylene single/double balloon, modified Inoue balloon) is advanced towards mitral valve for dilatation (Fig. 48.1).

Selecting Balloon Size in RNBMV

The main factors considered in selecting balloon size are mitral valve annulus and quality of mitral valve. In general, balloon of smaller size appear effective in retrograde approach as compared to transseptal method.[11] The optimal ratio of effective balloon dilating area (EBDA) and body surface area (BSA) is 2.7–3.8 cm^2/m^2. A gradual stepwise increase in balloon diameter can be done depending on the degree of residual stenosis and mitral regurgitation.

Special Tips and Tricks during RNBMV

- During manipulation, the tip of steerable left atrial catheter may get misplaced either towards ventricular outflow tract or free wall instead of mitral orifice. In former case, catheter is advanced a short distance towards the apex and rotated slightly clockwise and the curve is opened. While in the latter, catheter is rotated counter clockwise and the curve is slightly tightened.

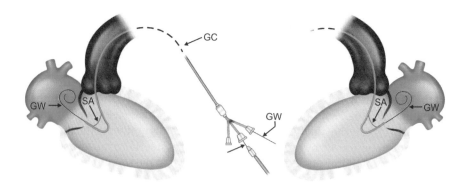

Fig. 48.1: Schematic representation of left atrial guiding catheter (GC) in RAO (left) and LAO (right) projection. By external manipulation of steering arm (SA), catheter's distal tip is directed towards mitral orifice. Guidewire (GW) is stabilized in LA. Balloon dilatation is done after exchanging guidewire with a stiffer wire

- To avoid damage to subvalvular apparatus, it is imperative that the guidewire should enter LA through true mitral orifice, avoiding entanglement in chordae or papillary muscle. The correct entry into LA is confirmed by unobstructed forward advancement of J-wire through catheter lumen. An additional safety check can be performed after introduction of stiff guidewire into LA by insertion of flow-directed catheter into the LV over it. The balloon is inflated with carbon dioxide in LV outflow tract and advanced towards mitral valve. Unobstructed movement of balloon signifies that guidewire has entered LA through true orifice and not involved with chordae.

Effectiveness of Retrograde Approach

Retrograde nontransseptal balloon mitral valvuloplasty (RNBMV) is associated with significant hemodynamic and functional improvement in mitral stenosis patients and appears to be noninferior to antegrade BMV. In the largest series of 438 patients, RNBMV immediately increased the mitral area from 1.0 ± 0.3 cm^2 to 2.1 ± 0.5 cm^2. This was associated with significant fall in pulmonary artery pressure and transmitral gradient which is maintained even on long-term follow-up.[13] However, the mean duration of RNBMV is slightly higher as compared to the usual antegrade approach which is partly accounted by the unfamiliarity of the approach in interventionalists. While RNBMV took 22 ± 14 (15–45) minutes from introduction of LA catheter to LV until removal of balloon guidewire, antegrade approach from positioning of Mullins sheath in superior vena cava to removal of slenderized Inoue balloon catheter was completed in 15 ± 8 (10–35) minutes ($p = 0.05$). The overall procedural success rate, however, is comparable in both approaches (93% vs 95%, p = ns).[14]

Complications

Since, RNBMV doesnot involve septal puncture, it is relatively free of complications like cardiac perforation, tamponade and post procedural left-right shunting (Table 48.1).[13,14] However, incidence of other complications are similar to antegrade approach.

Table 48.1: Complications after BMV in Retrograde and antegrade approach[14]

Complications	Inoue (Group 1) n = 1000	Retrograde approach (Group 2) n = 100	P value
Mitral regurgitation	140 (14%)	16 (16%)	NS
– Increase by 1 grade	40 (4%)	5 (5%)	NS
– Severe (≥ grade 3/4)			
Tamponade	20 (2%)	0%	NS
Atrial shunt (Qp/Qs ≥1.5/1)	25 (2.5%)	0%	
Local complications			
– Hematoma	5 (0.5%)	3 (3%)	<0.01
– Blood transfusion	0%	1 (1%)	<0.002
– Loss of femoral pulse	1 (0.1%)	2 (2%)	<0.001
Thromboembolism	1 (0.1%)	0%	NS
Conduction disturbances			
– Transient LBBB	0%	28 (28%)	<0.001
– Transient CHB	0%	2 (2%)	<0.001

a. *Mitral regurgitation (MR)*: The increase in MR grade by 1 is seen in approx 15–20% of patients with both approaches. EBDA/BSA, mitral valve rigidity and preprocedural MR are the most important predictors of post-RNBMV mitral regurgitation.[13]

b. *Intraventricular conduction abnormalities*: Transient disturbances in AV conduction like LBBB or complete heart block are commonly seen after RNBMV and they generally improve within 24 hours without any intervention.

c. *Bleeding and vascular complications*: Due to the arterial access local vascular complications like groin hematoma requiring blood transfusion and femoral artery embolism/occlusion are more common in retrograde approach.

◾ CONCLUSION

Retrograde arterial approach for BMV is as effective as the antegrade approach with added advantage of avoiding septal puncture and its associated complications. It can be a reliable alternative to the transseptal approach, thereby, broadening the application of percutaneous BMV.

REFERENCES

1. StefanLock JE, Khalilullah M, Shrivastava S, et al. Percutaneous catheter comissurotomy in rheumatic mitral stenosis. N Engl J Med. 1985;313:1515–8.
2. Nobuyoshi M, Hamasaki N, Kimura T Inoue K, et al. Indications, complications and short term clinical outcome of percutaneous transvenous mitral comissurotomy. Circulation. 1989;80:782–92.
3. Inoue K, Owaki T, Nakamura T, et al. Clinical application of transvenous mitral commissurotomy by a new balloon catheter. J Thorac Cardiovasc Surg. 1984;87:394–402.
4. Al Zaibag M, Ribeiro PA, Al Kasab S, et al. Percutaneous double-balloon mitral valvotomy for rheumatic mitral valve stenosis. Lancet. 1986;1:757–61.
5. Cribier A, Rath PC, Letac B. Percutaneous mitral valvotomy with a metal dilator Lancet. 1997;349:1667.
6. Bonhoeffer P, Piechaud JF, Sidi D, et al. Mitral dilatation with the multitrack system: an alternative approach. Catheter Cardiovasc Diagn. 1995;36:189–93.
7. Babic UU, Pejcic P, Djurisic Z, et al. Percutaneous transarterial balloon valvuloplasty for mitral valve stenosis. Am J Cardiol. 1986;57:1101–4.
8. Büchler JR, Fo SF, Braga SL, Sousa JE. Percutaneous mitral valvuloplasty in rheumatic mitral stenosis by isolated transarterial approach: A new and feasible technique. Jpn Heart J. 1987;28:791–98.
9. Orme EC, Wray RB, Mason JW. Balloon mitral valvuloplasty via retrograde left atrial catheterization. Am Heart J. 1989;117:680–83.
10. Stefanadis C, Kourouklis C, Stratos C, et al. Percutaneous balloon mitral valvuloplasty by retrograde left atrial catheterisation. Am J Cardiol. 1990;65:650.
11. Stefanadis C, Stratos C, Pitsavos C, et al. Retrograde nontransseptal balloon mitral valvuloplasty: Immediate results and long-term follow-up. Circulation 1992;85:1760–67.
12. Stefanadis C, Kourouklis C, Stratos C, et al. Retrograde left atrial catheterization with a new steerable cardiac catheter. Am Heart J. 1990;119:375–80.
13. Stefanadis C, Stratos C, Lambrou S, et al. Retrograde nontransseptal balloon mitral valvuloplasty: immediate results and intermediate long-term outcome in 441 cases—a multicenter experience. JACC. 1998; 32(4):1009–16.
14. Bahl VK, Chandra S, Jhamb DK, et al. Balloon Mitral Valvotomy: comparision between antegrade Inoue and retrograde transseptal techniques. European Heart J. 1997;18:1765–70.

Chapter 49

Percutaneous Mitral Valvotomy in Technically Challenging Situations

Harikrishnan S, Rohan Vijay Ainchwar

Even though PMV can be performed safely and easily in vast majority of cases, there may be situations where we encounter difficulties. This Chapter deals with such difficult situations which we face occasionally.

We encounter difficulties due to the morphology of the valve like calcium in the valve, eccentric orifice, or a too narrow valve orifice preventing entry of the balloon tip. Presence of thrombus in the left atrium or left atrial appendage (LA or LAA) is another challenging situation.

Difficulties arise due to unusual anatomy like aneurysmal left atrium, thick interatrial septum, septum bulging to the right atrium or the difficulty in accessing the heart due to vascular anomalies.

▓ CALCIFICATION OF THE VALVE

Calcification of the valve is known to give inadequate results and make the procedure prone to complications. The complications can be a tear of the valve, especially when the commissures are calcific leading to mitral regurgitation (MR) and the chance of embolization of the calcific material from the valve tissue.

When there is bicommissural calcification, BMV is contraindicated, as there is a high probability of leaflet tear with resultant acute severe MR. There are few reports of successful PMV in patients with severe calcific MS.[1-5] Recently, there was a report describing the successful performance of PMV in a patient with unicommissural calcium.[3] Tanaka et al. has reported the outcome of 13 patients with unicommissural calcium who underwent PMV.[6] The long-term outcomes of these patients with unilateral commissural calcification was similar to those who had no commissural calcium.[6]

Severe calcification seen on fluoroscopy (graded 1–4) is an indicator of poor outcome following PMV (Fig. 49.1).[6] Even in the presence of leaflet belly calcium, PMV can be considered if the commissures are free of calcium. But the results may not be as good as in noncalcified valves.

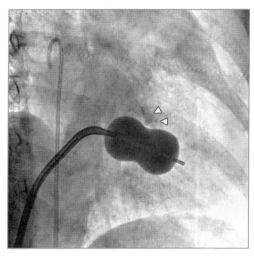

Fig. 49.1: PMV in a valve with unicommissural calcium (arrow heads). The mitral valve is seen with dense calcification confined to the lateral commissure, whereas the medial commissure is free of calcium. The Accura balloon is across the mitral valve with both the proximal and distal part of the balloon being inflated

LEFT ATRIAL THROMBI

Left atrial thrombi is usually a contraindication to PMV. But when the thrombi is localized to the LAA and organized, PMV can be performed by experienced operators. The detailed description of this topic is available in the Chapter on left atrial thrombus (Chapter 53).

DIFFICULTY AT THE GROIN PUNCTURE SITE

Problems of the access site may cause difficulties during PMV. A puncture through the inguinal ligament may not allow the passage of the septal dilator and the balloon. Then, it is advisable to obtain another puncture and proceed. Since, we are creating a large opening in the femoral vein, it is better to have the venous and arterial puncture at a little distance which will prevent the formation of an arteriovenous (AV) fistula. It is always advisable to avoid vertical puncture at the venous access, as this will cause difficulty in tracking the balloon.

Previous procedures in the groin may produce extensive fibrosis and will cause difficulty in tracking the balloon. Here making a good skin incision and creating a good track using a larger dilator will help to overcome the difficulties. This issue is common in the developing world where the patient may have to undergo the procedure many times due to restenosis.

The following steps are recommended to avoid difficulty at the groin. After septal puncture and insertion of the 0.025 pigtail-shaped guidewire into the left atrium, the sheath insertion site is dilated with an artery forceps along the guidewire.[7]

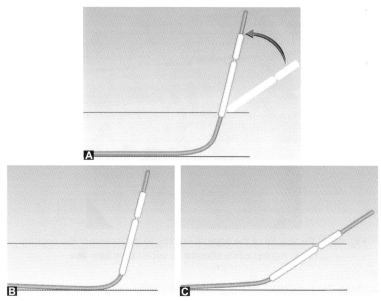

Fig. 49.2: Insertion of balloon catheter in the presence of marked resistance at the groin. (A) Guidewire is held taut by an assistant, and catheter is inserted into the vein at an angle of about 90°, (B) Catheter is advanced to the posterior venous wall, (C) Catheter in then tilted back to an acute angle and advanced over the wire (Artwork by courtesy of Dr Kanji Inoue)

If resistance is encountered in inserting the balloon, it is advised to insert the balloon assembly in a more vertical angle initially and then come back to a more horizontal alignment. During this maneuver, the assistant should keep the 0.025 pigtail wire taut (Fig. 49.2).

If resistance and difficulty in inserting the balloon or difficulty in manipulating the balloon is still encountered, the use of a 14 F sheath is recommended.

DIFFICULTY IN SEPTAL PUNCTURE, DILATATION AND BALLOON ENTRY

Large Left Atrium

Occasionally, we encounter very large LA especially in the developing world where the patients present very late. This will lead to technical difficulties in performing the procedure.

In a dilated and aneurysmal LA, the septum bulges into the right atrial side making the puncture difficult. The septum bulges anteriorly and inferiorly so that the puncture becomes technically challenging. Whenever we try to puncture, because of the vertical lie of the septum, the needle will go through the septum and will dissect it and not enter the LA (Fig. 49.3). When such a situation is encountered, there are two options:

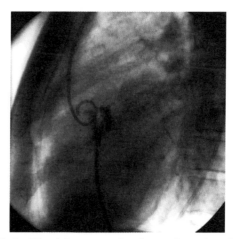

Fig. 49.3: Vertical lie of the septum leading to dissection of the septum (stain marks) while attempting septal puncture 📱◀

1. Increase the curvature of the Brockenbrough needle so that, it faces more posteriorly to enable the puncture.
2. Probing LA entry, Video 49.3.

   Probing is another technique used for LA entry. With the needle tip just kept inside the tip of the Mullins sheath or dilator, the whole assembly is used to probe the septum at the region of the fossa ovalis. This is by gently tenting the septum. When the needle and the sheath assembly slowly slide into the fossa and ultimately into the LA. In 50% of our cases, we are able to enter the LA by this technique. We always try this method in cases of bulging septum.

   Krishnamoorthy et al. has found that the procedure time and fluoroscopic time are less with the probing technique. He also reported that in 90% of the occasions, he could successfully enter the left atrium by probing. The left to right shunting through the iatrogenic ASD was also not significant following a "probing entry".[8]

Problems in Needle Entry into LA—Needle "Jerk"

In patients with thick septum, we may experience difficulty in advancing the Mullins sheath into the LA. The needle tip will be in the LA, as confirmed by contrast injection, but the rest of the system may not enter the LA with gentle pressure. If we use too much force, there is a danger that the needle will jerk and can hit and perforate the posterior LA wall.

In such situations, we withdraw the needle and redo the puncture at a different point in the septum. Another technique is to pass a thin wire like a PCI (coronary angioplasty 0.014 inch) guidewire through the needle and introduce it into the LA. Then even if we use little force to enter LA, it will not perforate the LA roof (Fig. 49.4).

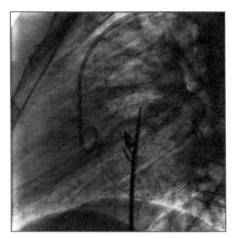

Fig. 49.4: Passage of a coronary angioplasty guidewire through the needle into the LA and coil in the LA. Over this wire the needle can be tracked into the LA without the needle "jerking" and hitting the posterior LA wall 🎥◀

■ DIFFICULTY IN NEGOTIATING THE ATRIAL SEPTUM

This is another area where we may face difficulty. After dilatation of the septum, while trying to pass the slenderized balloon into the LA, there may be difficulty in tracking it. This could be due to recoil of the puncture site or the problem of orientation (obliqueness) of the puncture site. This may be overcome by:
1. Dilatation of the septum with a larger dilator. Usually, we use a 14 F dilator, if we up size to 18 F dilator, we may be able to sort out this issue.
2. Changing the angle of entry—occasionally the puncture site may be oblique, preventing the passage of a slenderized balloon. In such a case, a change in angulation of the balloon assembly may help in easy passage. This is termed as the "screwdriver maneuver" where the balloon is rotated clockwise while being pushed across the septum.[7]

■ BALLOON CATHETER STUCK AT SEPTUM—SEPTAL CATCH

After the removal of the pigtail-shaped LA wire and the straightener, while trying to advance across the septum, the balloon may get stuck at the septum and not track forward towards the valve (Fig. 49.5). This situation is encountered not very infrequently.

This happens commonly during the second or subsequent dilatations. The catheter is placed deeply in the LA before the first dilatation, so this problem may not arise initially. During the first dilatation the catheter must have been inadvertently withdrawn towards the valve, which may "entrap" the catheter shaft.[7]

There are few methods to overcome this difficulty.
1. *Deep placement of the balloon catheter:* The problem of balloon "getting stuck" can be prevented to some extent by placing the balloon deep inside

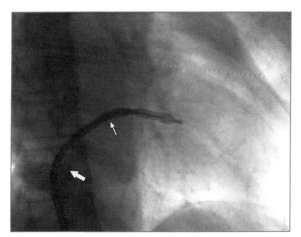

Fig. 49.5: Balloon stuck at the septum (thin arrow).
See the angulation in the shaft of the balloon (thick arrow)

the LA, with the tip medial to the mitral orifice. The balloon catheter usually get "stuck" when we try to advance it. When the catheter is deeply placed, we need only to withdraw it, which help in avoiding this problem.[7]

2. *Dilatation of the septum with a larger dilator*: Usually, we use a 14 F dilator, we can upgrade it to 18 F, which will create a larger hole in the septum.

3. Insert the stylet fully into the balloon to its tip, apply a clockwise twist to the stylet, directing the catheter posterolaterally. This will align it more or less perpendicular to the septal plane. Then the catheter can be advanced forward.

4. If the above maneuvers fail, the pigtail wire should be reintroduced into the left atrium and the balloon can be advanced forward and placed deep in the LA. Then the balloon can be withdrawn across the mitral valve.

5. This problem may be due to an oblique track created by the septal puncture, especially when the septum is thick. The oblique track may allow the passage of the balloon only in the posterosuperior direction and we may not be able to direct the balloon downwards towards the mitral valve. In such situations, we may have to resort to the so-called "hairpin loop" entry or a reverse loop entry.

Hairpin Loop Entry

Hairpin loop entry is a technique to overcome the problem of "stuck at septum" and also helpful in situations where there is difficulty in crossing the valve.

The balloon loop is pushed towards the LA roof (Figs 49.6A and B) till the tip of the balloon hits the floor of the LA near the mitral valve. Then the stylet is withdrawn from the balloon tip so that it takes an angulation and enters the mitral valve. Since, the proximal shaft of the balloon is directed posterosuperiorly, the catch at the septum will not hinder the forward movement of the balloon.

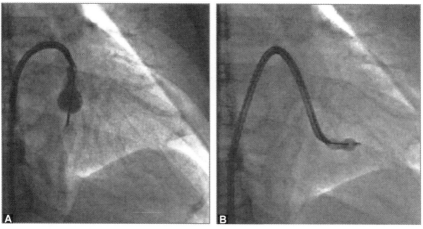

Figs 49.6A and B: Hairpin loop entry. (A) Pushing the balloon assembly towards the LA roof; (B) Directing the balloon towards the mitral valve by slightly withdrawing the stylet ▆◀

Reverse Loop Entry

Reverse loop entry is another technique which is used to overcome the problem of "stuck at septum". It can also be used when the septal puncture is low, and the balloon cannot be directed towards the mitral valve. Here the balloon shaft makes a loop in the anticlockwise fashion and crosses the mitral valve from the floor of the LA, almost like the "hairpin loop" entry (Fig. 49.7).

The stylet is rotated in the clockwise fashion for creating the reverse loop compared to the anticlockwise rotation used for the usual entry.

This technique is used when the balloon is stuck at the septum and also in a larger LA, where we are not able to enter the mitral valve in the usual manner.

Difficulty in Crossing the Valve

After the Inoue balloon catheter has been successfully introduced into the LA, the next hurdle in percutaneous balloon mitral valvuloplasty is to maneuver the Inoue balloon catheter through the stenotic orifice of the mitral valve.

The valve is usually crossed in the RAO 30° fluoroscopic view which displays the left ventricular long axis in profile. In patients with "giant" left atrium, lateral (90 degree) view may be better to cross the valve.

Sometimes difficulties may arise in crossing the mitral valve and make the conventional "direct entry" fail. Nonideal puncture sites, such as upward (cephalad), leftward (closer to the mitral valve), and very low punctures, are the major causes of failure to cross the mitral orifice with the conventional method.[7] Large atrium may also pose difficulty with this method.

Several maneuvers have been advocated to tackle this problem— changing the shape of the stylet, and different techniques of balloon entry—"catheter-sliding" method, "over-the-wire" method and "straight-balloon" technique are few of them.

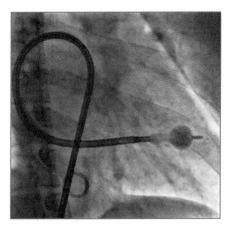

Fig. 49.7: Reverse loop entry. This is usually done in a roomy LA

TECHNIQUES FACILITATING ENTRY OF BALLOON ACROSS MITRAL VALVE

Changing the Shape of the Stylet

The stylet used for LV entry comes in a preformed "J" shape. Usually, a slight anterior curve is given to the stylet to facilitate LV entry.

If the septal puncture site is "high", i.e. above the arbitrary line of the aortic root, then the curve is made bigger. If the puncture site is low, then the curve is made shallower to allow LV entry. When the LA is dilated, the curve has to be made smoother and larger. When the LA is small, the curve needs to be made smaller (Fig. 49.8).

"Over-the-Wire" LV Entry

Over-the-wire entry can be done in many ways. The technique by Mehan and Meier is described below. The modification of this technique by Manjunath et al. and a detailed description of their "over-the-wire" technique is given in Chapter 42.

Using a Balloon Floatation Catheter

Following transseptal puncture, a balloon floatation catheter is introduced into the Mullins sheath and is directed into the LV. The Mullins sheath can be tracked over the balloon catheter into the LV, but sometimes the floatation catheter may not be able to support the Mullins sheath.

Once a good position of the sheath is attained in the LV, pigtail-shaped LA wire is introduced into the LV and the Inoue balloon is tracked across the mitral valve. The problem is that the pigtail-shaped LA wire will induce ventricular ectopics and even ventricular tachycardia (VT) which may be problematic.

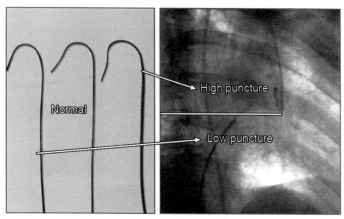

Fig. 49.8: Changing the shape of the stylet to facilitate crossing the mitral valve

Using a Judkins Right Coronary Catheter

Meier et al. used a 0.020 inch backup J-wire and a diagnostic right Judkins catheter to cross the mitral valve from the LA. They tracked the Mullins sheath over the RCA catheter and exchanged the backup wire for a 0.025 inch left atrial wire, over which the balloon was tracked (Figs 49.9A to C).

Direct Tracking of the Wire and Balloon

Sometimes the balloon may face the mitral valve orifice, but it may not track into LV. In such a situation, sometimes we will be able to pass a 0.35 Teflon guidewire into the LV and track the Inoue balloon across the mitral valve over-the-wire. We have done few cases like that successfully. There may be few ventricular ectopics, but it will usually be tolerable. Once the balloon has crossed, we can remove the wire and the balloon inflation is done (Fig. 49.10).

Manjunath et al.[9] reports that when compared to other "over-the-wire" methods, the simplified technique does not involve any additional accessories, such as backup guidewires, right Judkin's catheter, or balloon floatation catheter. Thus, additional expenses can be avoided. Since, the pigtail-shaped spring guidewire is directly introduced into LV through the Mullins sheath, multiple exchanges involved in the conventional over the wire methods can be avoided and the procedural time considerably reduced.

All their patients had ventricular ectopics and nonsustained VT, but reportedly these arrhythmias were well-tolerated.

As pointed out by Rajpal et al.[10] both the techniques described by Manjunath et al.[9] and Mehan et al.[11] carry the risk of inserting the guidewire between chordae tendinae. This could result in damage to the subvalvar apparatus on balloon inflation, thereby causing severe mitral regurgitation.

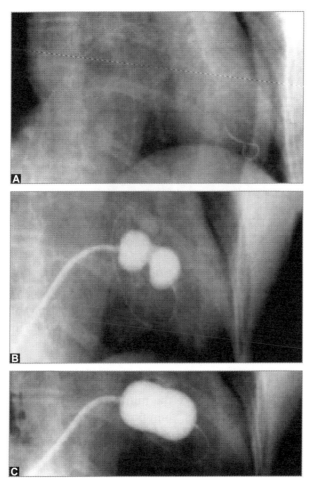

Figs 49.9A to C: Modified Inoue technique for percutaneous mitral balloon commissurotomy. (A) Steerable 0.020 inch backup guidewire introduced into the left ventricle through a diagnostic right Judkins coronary catheter; (B) Inoue balloon positioned across the stenosed mitral valve on the Inoue 0.025 inch pigtail wire placed in the left ventricle through the Judkins catheter previously advanced into the left ventricle over the 0.020 inch backup wire; (C) Balloon commissurotomy with the Inoue balloon supported by the 0.025 inch pigtail wire allowing for easy withdrawal and advancement of the balloon between inflations

Balloon Floatation Catheter and Wire in Aorta

Mehan and Meier have reported another technique to overcome the difficulty in crossing the mitral valve. Here the mitral valve is crossed with a balloon floatation catheter which is then advanced into the aorta. After this, a 0.021 inch long backup wire is placed in the descending aorta and the Inoue balloon is tracked over it.[11]

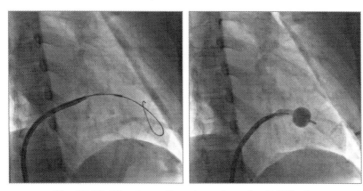

Fig. 49.10: Direct over-the-wire entry using 0.035 wire

Two-wire Technique

Rajpal and Joseph have described another over-the-wire technique.[10] This technique is to cross the mitral valve with a balloon floatation catheter and place a 0.035 inch backup valvuloplasty wire (Schneider, Minneapolis, MN) in the left ventricle (LV). When this wire is given a secondary bend in the stiff portion proximal to its distal soft part, it conforms to the anatomy of the heart and remains stable in the LV. The Mullins sheath can then be advanced into the LV over this wire. A 0.025 inch pigtail wire is introduced into the LV through the Mullins sheath side by side the 0.035 inch backup wire. Finally, the 0.035 inch wire and the Mullins sheath are removed and the Inoue balloon is introduced into the LV over the 0.025 inch wire.

It can be argued that the presence of two wires in the LV can be dangerous as it can lead onto perforation and arrhythmias.

Catheter Sliding Method[7]

The balloon is first directed towards the mitral valve by twisting the stylet counterclockwise, and then made more flexible by withdrawing the stylet out of the balloon segment. Then the balloon is slightly inflated and the inflation is maintained. Once the balloon is at the mitral orifice, cardiac contractions will cause the balloon segment to tilt upwards during systole. In diastole, the balloon segment aligns with the catheter shaft. Then the operator advances the catheter (only) forward (with the stylet kept fixed) during diastole to cross the valve. The stylet is then advanced to help align the catheter with the orifice-apex axis.[7]

Straight Balloon Technique

This technique is described by Tejus Patel et al.[12] The steps are as follows:
1. After the septal puncture and dilation, the Inoue balloon is placed in the left atrium (LA) over 0.025 inch pigtail wire.

2. The pigtail wire and slenderizing tube are removed, and the Inoue balloon is pushed slightly in, so as to keep its tip higher up and straight, pointing toward the LA appendage.
3. The J-stylet is negotiated up to the tip of the balloon making it point towards the mitral orifice.
4. The Inoue balloon, together with the J-stylet, is withdrawn slightly, bringing the tip of the balloon in coaxial alignment with the mitral orifice.
5. The Inoue catheter is pushed gently with the simultaneous counter-clockwise rotation of the J-stylet, leading to easy entry of the balloon across the mitral orifice.

Changing the Puncture Site

Once we have failed in all the above described techniques, we can puncture the septum at a new site and try again. The problem in obtaining another septal puncture is the anticoagulation status. The patient will already be on heparin. If it is not easy to get another puncture, it is better to postpone the procedure to another day.

▆ ENTRY OF BALLOON THROUGH THE SECONDARY ORIFICES

Another problem which we come across is that the balloon may track between the chordal structures and can lead to damage of the subvalvar apparatus and severe mitral regurgitation requiring emergency mitral valve replacement. This happens because the balloon is dilated between the chordal structures.

Fluoroscopic Pointers to the Entry through Secondary Orifices

1. The axis of the balloon catheter will deviate from the more horizontal valve orifice-apex axis to a more vertical orientation.
2. There will be no free movement of the partly inflated balloon, as the chordal structures restrict the movement.
3. Abnormal shapes of the balloon due to the restriction imposed by the chordal structures.

How to Overcome the Problem of Secondary Orifice Entry?

1. Never attempt to inflate the balloon if there is a doubt regarding inter-chordal entry. The inflation should be aborted and the balloon should be repositioned.
2. Crossing the mitral valve with a partly inflated balloon may help as the secondary orifices are usually smaller.
3. "Accordion maneuver" (Hung et al.):[7] This is done by simultaneously pushing the catheter and pulling the stylet in opposite directions to ensure that the partially inflated distal balloon slides freely along the orifice-apex axis.[7]

4. It is better to go fully to the apex and come back and dilate the valve. If the partly inflated balloon freely reaches the apex, we can be almost sure that the balloon has not tracked through the secondary orifices.
5. The "balloon impasse" phenomenon is discussed in Chapter 29.

FAILURE TO DILATE THE VALVE

In some cases, we may face difficulties in dilating the valve. This usually happens in a very fibrotic valve. To overcome such situations we can change the size of the balloon.

For example, a lower sized balloon at full capacity will produce more radial pressure than a larger balloon of the same size. This is because of the properties of the balloon as illustrated in the Figure 49.11. Here we can see that a 24 mm balloon at 24 mm will produce more radial pressure than 26 mm balloon at 24 mm (Fig. 49.11).

Another difficulty we face, is the inability to hold the balloon across the valve, during inflation. This usually happens after the initial dilation when the valve is partly open. In such situations, the over-the-wire technique allows the balloon to stay across the valve.

POPPING OF THE BALLOON BACK TO LEFT ATRIUM

This usually happens after one or two dilatations of the valve. When the valve is partly open, the valve orifice may be large enough to allow free passage of the inflated balloon across it. This is considered as a sign of success of PMV.

But this can happen in a partly inflated valve also. If this happens in a partly inflated valve, Hung et al. recommends the following technique to avoid this problem. The stylet is advanced far into the balloon segment to stiffen the catheter, and before the catheter is retracted to anchor the balloon at the orifice,

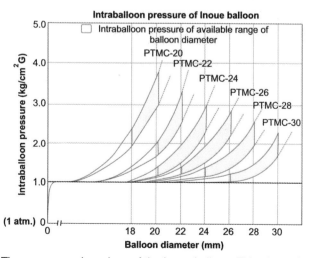

Fig. 49.11: The pressure volume loop of the Inoue balloon. This shows that a smaller balloon at full capacity can generate more radial pressure than a larger balloon (Published with permission from Toray Inc.)

the distal balloon is inflated to a diameter slightly larger than the previous one. As soon as the balloon assumes an hourglass configuration, the catheter is advanced slightly to prevent it from jerking out into the left atrium, and then the balloon is fully inflated.[7]

▮ SMALL LEFT ATRIUM

Patients with small-sized left atrium (Fig. 49.12)[13] can cause difficulties in performing PMV. Vijay Trehan et al. has described a case demonstrating all the problems associated with such a case[13] and they have described a new technique to successfully perform PMV.

The first hurdle they encountered was in tracking the stretched balloon across the atrial septum. The length of the stretched balloon was more than the vertical LA dimensions (Fig. 49.13A).[13] Hence, the whole length of the Inoue balloon in its low profile stretched position (with the stretcher fully advanced) could not be advanced into the LA (Fig. 49.13B). Taking the stretcher fully out resulted in a destretched and higher profile balloon getting trapped at the septal puncture site it not being able to advance over the coiled wire into the LA (Fig. 49.13B).

To overcome this difficulty, Trehan et al. kept the stretcher partially advanced so that the length of the now partly stretched slightly lower profile balloon was almost equal to the vertical dimension of the LA and then they could advance the balloon into the LA with its tip pointing upwards (Fig. 49.14).

Then the difficulty was in tracking the balloon across the mitral valve. The balloon catheter was getting "stuck" at the septum. So, they had to make two loops in the LA with the balloon (double loop technique) which made the balloon point towards the mitral orifice. Then they tracked the coiled wire and the balloon across the mitral valve and successfully completed the procedure (Figs 49.15A and B).[13]

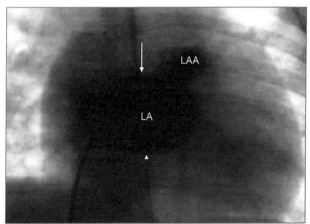

Fig. 49.12: Left atrial angiogram showing small left atrium
Abbreviations: LA, left atrium; LAA, left atrial appendage
(Published with permission Vijay Trehan et al. Difficult percutaneous transvenous mitral commissurotomy: A new technique for left atrium to left ventricular entry. Indian Heart J. 2004;56:158-62)

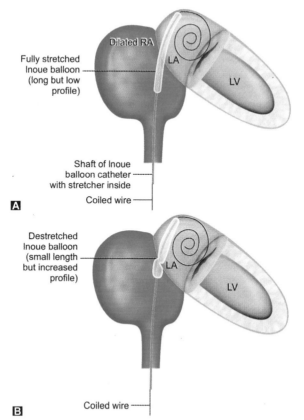

Figs 49.13A and B: Schematic diagram showing the difficulty of the stretched and nonstretched balloons to negotiate the septum
Abbreviations: LV, left ventricle, LA, left atrium
Published with permission Vijay Trehan et al. Difficult percutaneous transvenous mitral commissurotomy: A new technique for left atrium to left ventricular entry. Indian Heart J. 2004;56:158-62)

The "double loop" maneuver was possible in the patient described by Trehan et al. because of the small height of the patient, with enough length of the balloon shaft lying outside the body. This may not be possible in an adult patient. Another way of making the balloon free is to enlarge the atrial septal defect so as to allow free movement of the balloon across the septal puncture site, with the risk of residual left to right shunt.

■ PERCUTANEOUS MITRAL VALVOTOMY IN SMALL CHILDREN

Occasionally, we may come across small children with severe MS who may need PMV. There are few reports describing the procedure in such populations.[14-16] The problems which can arise are:
1. Requirement of general anesthesia.
2. Small-sized left atrium with its inherent problems as described in the previous section.

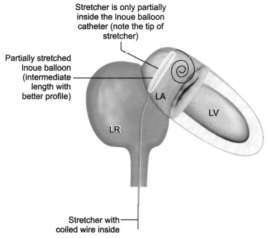

Fig. 49.14: Schematic showing the partially stretched balloon entering the LA without entrapment at the septum[13]
Abbreviations: LV, left ventricle, LA, left atrium

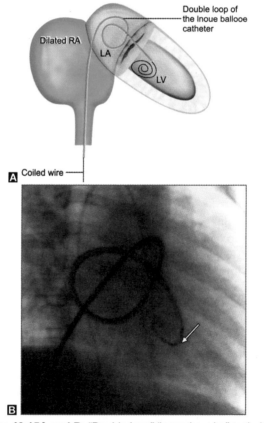

Figs 49.15A and B: "Double loop" "over-the-wire" technique
Abbreviations: LA, left atrium; LV, left ventricle (Published with permission Vijay Trehan et al. Difficult percutaneous transvenous mitral commissurotomy: A new technique for left atrium to left ventricular entry. Indian Heart J. 2004;56:158-62)

3. Transseptal puncture needs special care and may need the pediatric transseptal set.
4. In case the patient develops mitral regurgitation, getting an adequate-sized mitral valve prosthesis is also a problem.

◼ REFERENCES

1. Dugal JS, Jetley V, Sabharwal JS, Sofat S, Singh C. Life-saving PTMC for critical calcific mitral stenosis in cardiogenic shock with balloon impasse. Int J Cardiovasc Intervent. 2003;5(3):172–4.
2. Palacios IF, Lock JE, Keane JF, Block PC. Percutaneous transvenous balloon valvotomy in a patient with severe calcific mitral stenosis. J Am Coll Cardiol. 1986;7(6):1416–9.
3. Khandenahally SR, Dwarakaprasad R, Karur S, Bachahally KG, Panneerselvam A, Cholenahally NM. Balloon mitral valvotomy for calcific mitral stenosis. JACC Cardiovasc Interv. 2009;2(3):263–4.
4. Tuzcu EM, Block PC, Griffin B, Dinsmore R, Newell JB, Palacios IF. Percutaneous mitral balloon valvotomy in patients with calcific mitral stenosis: immediate and long-term outcome. J Am Coll Cardiol. 1994;23(7):1604–9.
5. Waller BF, VanTassel JW, McKay C. Anatomic basis for and morphologic results from catheter balloon valvuloplasty of stenotic mitral valves. Clin Cardiol. 1990;13(9):655–61.
6. Tanaka S, Watanabe S, Matsuo H, Segawa T, Iwama M, Hirose T, et al. Over 10 years clinical outcomes in patients with mitral stenosis with unilateral commissural calcification treated with catheter balloon commissurotomy: single-center experience. J Cardiol. 2008;51(1):33–41.
7. Hung JS, Lau KW. Pitfalls and tips in inoue balloon mitral commissurotomy. Cathet Cardiovasc Diagn. 1996;37(2):188–99.
8. Krishnamoorthy KM, Dash PK. Transseptal catheterization without needle puncture. Scand Cardiovasc J SCJ. 2001;35(3):199–200.
9. Manjunath CN, Srinivasa KH, Patil CB, Venkatesh HV, Bhoopal TS, Dhanalakshmi C. Balloon mitral valvuloplasty: our experience with a modified technique of crossing the mitral valve in difficult cases. Cathet Cardiovasc Diagn. 1998;44(1):23–6.
10. Rajpal KA, George J. Letter to the Editor, Catheterization and Cardiovascular Interventions. 1999;46:117–22.
11. Mehan VK, Meier B. Impossibility to cross a stenotic mitral valve with the Inoue balloon: success with a modified technique. Indian Heart J. 1994;46(1):51–2.
12. Patel TM, Dani SI, Chag MC, Shah SC, Shah UG, Patel TK. Crossing of mitral orifice with the inoue Balloon: the "straight-balloon" technique. Cathet Cardiovasc Diagn. 1996;37(2):231–2.
13. Trehan V, Mehta V, Mukhopadhyay S, Yusuf J, Kaul UA. Difficult percutaneous transvenous mitral commissurotomy: a new technique for left atrium to left ventricular entry. Indian Heart J. 2004;56(2):158–62.
14. Essop MR, Govendrageloo K, Du Plessis J, van Dyk M, Sareli P. Balloon mitral valvotomy for rheumatic mitral stenosis in children aged < or = 12 years. Am J Cardiol. 1993 Oct 1;72(11):850–1.
15. Kothari SS, Kamath P, Juneja R, Bahl VK, Airan B. Percutaneous transvenous mitral commissurotomy using Inoue balloon in children less than 12 years. Cathet Cardiovasc Diagn. 1998;43(4):408–11.
16. Krishnamoorthy KM, Tharakan JA. Balloon mitral valvulotomy in children aged < or = 12 years. J Heart Valve Dis. 2003;12(4):461–8.

Chapter 50

Left Atrial Appendage Occlusion and Percutaneous Mitral Valvotomy

Dale Murdoch, Darren Walters

■ BACKGROUND AND RATIONALE

Rheumatic heart disease is a major health burden worldwide, affecting 15–20 million people and causes up to 250,000 premature deaths annually.[1] Whilst primarily a disease of developing nations, acute rheumatic fever and rheumatic heart disease also occurs in affluent countries, particularly in underprivileged and indigenous populations. Improving living conditions, nutrition and access to improved medical prevention and treatment continue to change the epidemiology of the disease.

Whilst mitral incompetence is the most common valvular lesion in patients with rheumatic heart disease, mitral stenosis often develops as a result of persistent valvular inflammation leading to commissural fusion. Patients may present with a murmur (typically a loud first heart sound, opening 'snap' and low-pitched, decrescendo diastolic murmur), dyspnea or heart failure.

Atrial fibrillation (AF) often accompanies mitral pathology in rheumatic heart disease. Approximately 25% of patients with rheumatic heart disease have AF and 50–60% of cases of AF in India are related to rheumatic heart disease.[2] The etiology is multifactorial, with a number of potential contributing factors. Mitral stenosis (MS) results in left atrial hypertension and subsequent dilatation. These structural changes in the left atrium (LA) and pulmonary veins contribute to impaired atrial electrical conduction and the development of fibrillation. There is a strong correlation between increased left atrial size/volume and the presence of AF. Also, persistent rheumatic inflammation involves not only valvular tissue, but also the atrial myocardial tissue itself.[3] This leads to chronic histological change which further impedes electromechanical function and predisposes to AF.

The combined presence of MS and AF presents a number of challenging management considerations. Whilst balloon valvotomy or mitral valve surgery can be considered on their own merits for patients in sinus rhythm, the presence of AF adds complexity related to: (a) rhythm or rate control strategy, (b) stroke and systemic embolism risk, (c) the need for anticoagulation and management in the perioperative setting, and (d) short- and long-term bleeding and thrombosis risk. Patients with both MS and AF as a result of rheumatic heart disease have increased risk of thromboembolic stroke and systemic embolism compared to those with nonvalvular AF (NVAF).[1] If not treated with anticoagulation with a vitamin K antagonist, the annual risk of thromboembolism is 17–18%.[2] Whilst this seems alarmingly high, these estimates arise from highly-regarded observational studies, including the Framingham study.[4] This is in stark comparison to patients with nonvalvular AF, who typically have an annual risk of stroke of 2–12% if not anticoagulated. For patients with NVAF, stroke risk can be calculated via the CHADS2 or CHA2DS2-VASc scoring systems.[5,6] These useful clinical tools allow accurate estimation of thromboembolic risk and are routinely used to guide anticoagulation therapy for patients with AF. However, it is important to note that CHADS2 or CHA2DS2-VASc do not apply to patients with 'valvular' AF (i.e. significant mitral stenosis or regurgitation). It is, therefore, important to remember that rheumatic heart disease patients with AF routinely require anticoagulation regardless of the CHADS2 or CHA2DS2-VASc score.

Anticoagulation with a vitamin K antagonist (Coumadin or Warfarin) is recommended, with a target international normalized ratio (INR) of 2.5–3.5 for patients with rheumatic MS and 3.0–4.0 for patients with a mechanical mitral valve prosthesis.[2] Dose adjustment is necessary via careful monitoring of the INR. This can be troublesome due to the cost of monitoring and poor compliance, and even with good compliance many patients are frequently outside of the therapeutic range.[7] In various studies, time spent in the therapeutic range is only 55–64%. This compromises overall safety and efficacy, and new agents are now available which do not require monitoring of anticoagulation status. The so-called 'novel oral anticoagulants' (NOACs) have been approved for use in many countries following successful clinical trials comparing safety and efficacy. These agents include dabigatran (direct thrombin inhibitor), apixaban and rivaroxaban (direct Factor Xa inhibitors). Large clinical trials of the NOACs have excluded patients with rheumatic or valvular AF, and they are not indicated in this patient group. A massive left atrial thrombus has been reported in a patient with rheumatic MS and AF whilst anticoagulated with dabigatran.[8]

Anticoagulation therapy in patients at risk of thrombosis can be challenging. In addition to the problems discussed above relating to dose adjustment, INR monitoring and adherence, bleeding remains a significant concern for patients treated with vitamin K antagonists. Annual risk of bleeding whilst anticoagulated with a vitamin K antagonist is 2–5%, and the annual rate of intracranial hemorrhage is approximately 0.5%.[7] For these reasons, at least one-third of patients with atrial fibrillation who are at risk of thromboembolism are either not started on VKA therapy or discontinue the therapy once started.[9] This problem is compounded for rural and indigenous populations, who are at higher risk of rheumatic heart disease, but have poorer access to medical care and INR monitoring. A long-term study of Australian indigenous patients undergoing balloon mitral valvotomy found low rates of follow-up and poor compliance with warfarin therapy.[10] An audit of INR control in the Australian indigenous setting found patients on warfarin were in the target INR range only 45% of the time, well below the cited benchmark of 60%.[11]

A solution is therefore required for patients with AF and risk of stroke, but a contraindication to anticoagulation. Device-based closure of the left atrial appendage (LAA) is an emerging technology with promising results. The major rationale for the use of LAA closure devices is that 90% of thrombi found in patients with nonvalvular AF are in the LAA.[12] Also, echocardiographic evidence of slow flow or stasis in the left atrial appendage (low Doppler inflow velocities, spontaneous echocardiographic contrast) is associated with higher stroke rates in AF patients.[13]

The location of potential thrombus within the LA is important to consider, and there is some evidence to suggest the pattern of thrombus formation in patients with rheumatic heart disease/mitral stenosis is different. A transesophageal echocardiographic study conducted by Srimannarayana et al.[14] reported thrombus in 163 of 490 patients (33%) with rheumatic MS and AF, with 15% of all patients having thrombus in the LA body or LAA extending into the body of the LA. Fifty patients had repeat transesophageal echocardiography after 6 months of therapeutic anticoagulation. Whilst most of those with thrombus observed in the LAA had resolution at follow up (31 of 33), a significant number had thrombus in the body of the left atrium itself (17 patients, 34%), and this rarely resolved with 6 months of anticoagulation. It is important to recognize the additional pathology present in patients with AF and rheumatic heart disease. Firstly, not all will be suitable for device-based closure of the LAA due to the presence of thrombus in the left atrium or its appendage. Second, the propensity to form thrombus within the left atrium itself may make LAA closure a less effective therapy for the prevention of stroke. A patient with MS and a severely dilated LA may develop clot in the body of the atrium, which cannot be protected with a LAA closure device.

However, there remains an unmet clinical need for some patients with a strong contraindication to anticoagulation. Clinical tools, such as the HAS-BLED score may be used to identify patients with highest bleeding risk.[15] Those with prior intracranial, spinal or intraocular bleeding remain at risk of future events, whilst some patients flatly refuse vitamin K antagonist therapy despite medical advice. Others who may benefit most from this procedure are indigenous patients and those from rural and remote locations. Follow-up of these patients is challenging, and loss to follow-up can be associated with poor outcomes.[16] A single-visit device-based strategy may improve outcomes.

Left Atrial Appendage Occlusion Devices

A number of transcatheter LAA closure strategies are currently in development, clinical trials and routine clinical use. Efficacy of these devices is ultimately evaluated by prevention of stroke and systemic embolism. Anatomic closure of the LAA, as defined by noninvasive cardiac imaging, is frequently used as a surrogate endpoint. Due to significant anatomical variation of the left atrial appendage and differing designs of devices, complete anatomical closure is not always achieved. It remains to be seen whether small residual leaks will result in loss of clinical efficacy of the technology.[17] Safety considerations are also paramount, both at the time of implantation and long term. Procedural complications including pericardial effusion/tamponade, ischemic stroke, air embolism and access-site related bleeding are of particular concern, but appear to be less common with improved device design and operator experience.

The WATCHMAN (Boston Scientific, Natick, MA) device is a membranous cap over a self-expanding nitinol frame, which is delivered transvenously, via a transseptal puncture, through a 14Fr delivery sheath (Fig. 50.1). This device currently has the most robust clinical evidence, with two randomized clinical trials and a nonrandomized continuing-access registry. In the PROTECT-AF trial, patients with nonvalvular AF were randomized to the WATCHMAN device or vitamin K antagonist therapy. With the primary endpoint of cardiovascular death, any stroke or systemic embolism, the WATCHMAN device was noninferior after 1065 and 1588 patient-years of follow-up,[18] and became superior by 2621 patient-years of follow-up.[19] All-cause mortality was significantly lower in the group treated with the WATCHMAN device, and quality of life was also shown to improve. These favorable results are despite less-than-ideal safety outcomes. In PROTECT-AF, complications occurred in 8.7% of patients, with procedure related stroke in 1.1% and pericardial effusion requiring surgery or pericardiocentesis in 4.0%.[20]

However, safety outcomes have improved in subsequent studies, including the continued access registry of the PROTECT-AF trial and the randomized PREVAIL trial. In PREVAIL, 407 patients were randomized in a 2:1 manner to LAA occlusion with the WATCHMAN device or to warfarin therapy. The primary safety endpoint was met with an overall early safety event rate of 2.2% (pericardial effusion rate requiring intervention 1.9%) and noninferiority was shown for ischemic stroke prevention.[21]

The Amplatzer Cardiac Plug (St Jude Medical, Minneapolis, MN) is also a self-expanding nitinol device (Fig. 50.2). It is also delivered transvenously,

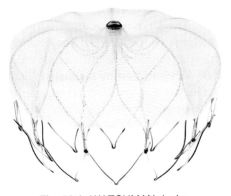

Fig. 50.1: WATCHMAN device

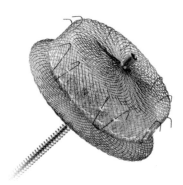

Fig. 50.2: Amplatzer cardiac plug

with a transseptal puncture and 9–13Fr delivery sheath. It has a distal lobe, a proximal disc, and polyester fabric in between. The distal lobe has anchors which secure the device within the LAA, whilst the proximal disc seals the LAA from the left atrial surface. Clinical data is limited to a number of observational studies, and the device is not currently approved for use in the United States of America. Initial data from the European postmarket registry reveals similar procedural success and complication rates to the WATCHMAN device.[22]

Other similar devices which are delivered via a transseptal puncture include the WaveCrest LAA occluder (Coherex Medical, Salt Lake City, UT) and the new LAmbre LAA occlude (Lifetech Scientific Corp., Shenzhen, China) (Fig. 50.3). The PLAATO system was the first transcatheter device developed for LAA closure, but is no longer in use.[20]

The Lariat device (SentreHeart, Redwood City, CA) utilizes a different approach for closure of the LAA and prevention of stroke (Fig. 50.4). Instead of occluding the appendage from within, it ligates and excludes the LAA from the outside, within the pericardial space. To achieve this, 'dry' pericardial puncture is performed and a 14Fr delivery sheath is advanced into the pericardial space. Transseptal puncture is also performed, and a magnet-tipped guidewire is advanced into the LAA. A complementary wire is advanced into the pericardium, and a magnetic connection is made. This allows the Lariat snare to be advanced over the pericardial wire and occlude the left atrial appendage at its origin. A specially-designed suture is deployed, and a drain is kept in the pericardium for at least 4–6 hours. Clinical experience with this device is limited, but it appears to provide high rates of anatomical closure of the LAA. Procedural complications are related to instrumentation of the pericardium and include tamponade/pericardial effusion, bleeding and pericarditis.

The morphology of the LAA is highly variable. A number of morphological descriptions of the LAA have been used, including 'chicken-wing', 'cauliflower', 'windsock' and 'cactus'. There is ongoing debate whether different shapes are

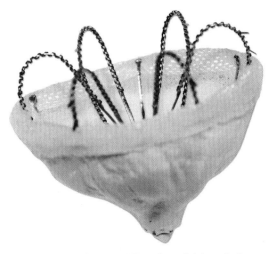

Fig. 50.3: Coherex WaveCrest LAA occluder

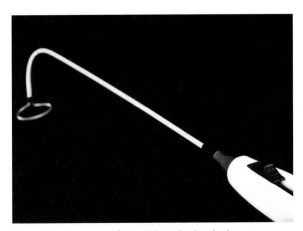

Fig. 50.4: SentreHeart Lariat device

related to higher stroke risk, but it seems a larger neck diameter and increased overall depth of the LAA are associated with a higher prevalence of prior stroke.[20] LAA morphology and size may make one device more suitable than another. For example, the Lariat procedure is contraindicated when the LAA diameter is greater than 40 mm, the appendage is posteriorly oriented or when there are lobes behind the pulmonary artery. For the WATCHMAN device, the length of the LAA must be greater than the ostium width; short and broad appendages may be difficult to treat. The WATCHMAN device is available in 5 sizes, whilst the Amplatzer Cardiac Plug comes in 8 different sizes. Computed tomography (CT), transesophageal or intracardiac echocardiography (TOE or ICE) and contrast-enhanced cineangiography can all be used to evaluate the size and morphology of the LAA, and a combination of cineangiography and TOE or ICE are recommended to guide the procedure in real-time.

Procedure

All procedures described above require femoral venous access and transseptal puncture, and thus may be combined with balloon mitral valvotomy (BMV).[23] The overall clinical utility and safety of this approach is currently unclear, as LAA occlusion is only approved for use in nonvalvular AF and application to patients with rheumatic heart disease is therefore off-label. This combined procedure may be most appropriate in patients with high stroke risk and a strong contraindication to long-term therapeutic anticoagulation. Interestingly, LAA occlusion devices are most commonly used by physicians for patients with nonvalvular AF and high bleeding risk or contraindication to warfarin, despite the only randomized evidence being in a patient population who were warfarin-eligibile.[20]

The procedure should be performed in a cardiac catheter laboratory or hybrid operating theatre with sterile equipment, fluoroscopy and transesophageal echocardiography capabilities. Whilst the procedure can be completed with procedural sedation, general anesthesia is advised. Transesophageal echocardiography (TEE) should be performed prior to the commencement of the procedure to confirm: (a) MS severity, (b) mitral valve suitability for balloon valvotomy, (c) LAA suitability for device-based closure and (d) absence of thrombus within the LA or LAA. Although performance of balloon mitral valvotomy has been described in patients with left atrial appendage thrombus,[24] this population is not suitable for LAA occlusion. All LAA occlusion procedures require direct instrumentation of the appendage, and this poses an unacceptably high risk of thromboembolism. Once the decision is made to proceed, femoral venous access can be gained.

Balloon mitral valvotomy can be performed in the standard fashion. The major consideration is the site of the transseptal puncture. The location of the puncture is vital for delivery and placement of the LAA occluder device, particularly for the WATCHMAN. Therefore, this takes precedence. The ideal interatrial septum puncture location is considered the mid to lower part of the posterior wall. For the WATCHMAN procedure, this allows direct access to the LAA with either a single curve or double curve access sheath. This may make balloon mitral valvotomy more difficult, but if the direct approach for crossing the mitral valve into the left ventricle is unsuccessful, other techniques such as the alternative loop method or catheter sliding method may facilitate success.[25] If LAA occlusion is to be performed with the LARIAT suture system, the position of the transseptal puncture may be less vital, as the magnet-tipped, steerable FindrWIRZ® guidewire system (SentreHeart, Redwood City, CA) is more maneuverable than a large delivery sheath.

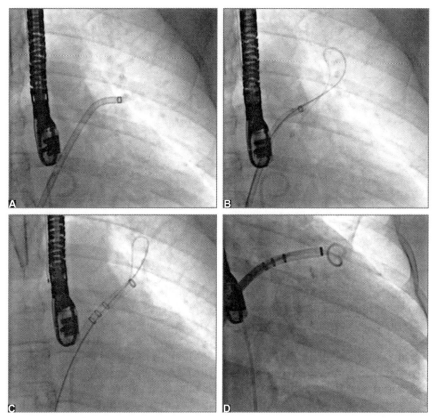

Figs 50.5A to D: The exchange procedure. After balloon mitral valvotomy, the Inoue balloon catheter was exchanged for an SL1 catheter (A). Via the SL1 catheter, a 0.035 in extra support wire was placed into the left upper pulmonary vein (B). Subsequently, a 14 Fr single-curve delivery catheter was passed over the wire (C). Finally, a 6 Fr pigtail catheter was delivered into the left atrium so that the left atrial appendage could be imaged (D)

Mitral valvotomy should be performed prior to LAA occluder device implantation in a combined procedure. There is potential for dislodgement and embolization of a previously placed occlusion device. Whilst the risk is low, particularly for well-anchored devices, such as the Amplatzer Cardiac Plug, repeated manipulation with an Inoue-balloon catheter within the left atrium has the potential to cause device embolization.

After mitral valvotomy, the exchange procedure requires careful consideration (Figs 50.5A to D). The Inoue balloon catheter can be exchanged for an 8Fr SL1 catheter, and a 0.035 in extrasupport wire placed into the left upper pulmonary vein. This maintains wire position across the interatrial septum. The delivery catheter can then be advanced over-the-wire. In the pictured example, a 14 Fr single-curve delivery catheter was used. Imaging of the LAA was performed with a 6 Fr pigtail catheter, before a 21mm WATCHMAN device was deployed (Figs 50.6A and B).

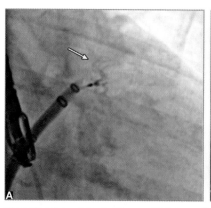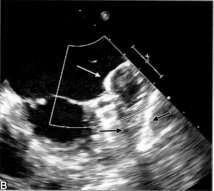

Figs 50.6A and B: A 21 mm Watchman® left atrial appendage (LAA) occluder device (white arrows) is seated in LAA (black arrows). The fluoroscopic image (A) is prior to deployment, while the TEE image (B) is after deployment

Summary and Future Directions

Patients with mitral stenosis and atrial fibrillation are at high risk of stroke and systemic embolism. There remains an unmet clinical need for patients who have contraindications to anticoagulation with warfarin or very high bleeding risk. A combined procedure involving balloon mitral valvotomy and left atrial appendage occlusion device implantation may reduce the risk of stroke by more than one mechanism.[21] The LAA occluder prevents thrombus formation in the appendage. Whilst this has been shown to prevent stroke in a nonvalvular AF population, we must exercise caution extending this mechanism to a rheumatic heart disease/valvular AF cohort. Balloon mitral valvotomy reduces stasis within the left atrium and may reduce thrombotic risk in this way. Relief of mitral stenosis also reduces left atrial enlargement, which is an independent risk factor for thromboembolism.[2] In addition, mitral valvotomy has been shown to reduce the hypercoagulable state associated with MS.[26]

As LAA device therapies evolve, procedural success will improve and we will learn new lessons from the nonvalvular AF population. No clinical trials have yet been conducted with LAA devices in a valvular heart disease cohort. An observational study or registry could be a first step. Currently, it is important to exercise caution in the MS patient population and combined mitral valvotomy and LAA occluder device therapy should be considered in the rare instance where conventional therapy is unsuitable.

▓ REFERENCES

1. Marijon E, Mirabel M, Celermajer DS, Jouven X. Rheumatic heart disease. Lancet. 2012;379:953–64.
2. Vora A. Management of atrial fibrillation in rheumatic valvular heart disease. Curr Opin Cardiol. 2006;21:47–50.
3. Alessandri N, Tufano F, Petrassi M, Alessandri C, Di Cristofano C, Della Rocca C, Gallo P. Atrial fibrillation in pure rheumatic mitral valvular disease is expression of

an atrial histological change. European Review for Medical and Pharmacological Sciences. 2009;13:431–42.

4. Kannel WB, Abbott RD, Savage DD, McNamara PM. Epidemiologic features of chronic atrial fibrillation. The Framingham Study. N Eng J Med. 1982;306:1018–22.

5. Gage BF, Waterman AD, Shannon W, Boechler M, Rich MW, Radford MJ. Validation of clinical classification schemes for preventing stroke: results from the National Registry of Atrial Fibrillation. JAMA. 2011;285:2864–70.

6. Lip GY, Nieuwlaat R, Pisters R, Lane DA, Crijns HJ. Refining clinical risk stratification for predicting stroke and thromboembolism in atrial fibrillation using a novel risk factor-based approach: the euro heart survey on atrial fibrillation. Chest. 2010;137:263–72.

7. Mearns ES, White CM, Kohn CG, Hawthorne J, Song JS, Meng J, et al. Quality of vitamin K antagonist control and outcomes in atrial fibrillation patients: a meta-analysis and meta-regression. Thromb J. 2014;12:14.

8. Luis SA, Poon K, Luis C, Shukla A, Bett N, Hamilton-Craig C. Massive left atrial thrombus in a patient with rheumatic mitral stenosis and atrial fibrillation while anticoagulated with dabigatran. Circ Cardiovasc Imaging. 2013;6:491–2.

9. Connolly SJ, Eikelboom J, Joyner C, et al. Apixaban in patients with atrial fibrillation. N Engl J Med. 2011;364:806–17.

10. McCann A, Walters DL, Aroney CN. Percutaneous mitral balloon commisurotomy in indigenous vs nonindigenous Australians. Heart, Lung and Circulation. 2008;17:200–5.

11. Pickering A, Thomas DP. An audit of INR control in the Australian indigenous setting. Aust Fam Physician. 2007;36:959–60.

12. Blackshear JL, Odell JA. Appendage obliteration to reduce stroke in cardiac surgical patients with atrial fibrillation. Ann Thorac Surg. 1996;61:755–9.

13. Zabalgoitia M, Halperin JL, Pearce LA, Blackshear JL, Asinger RW, Hart RG. Transesophageal echocardiographic correlates of clinical risk of thrombo-embolism in nonvalvular atrial fibrillation: Stroke prevention in atrial fibrillation III investigators. J Am Coll Cardiol. 1998;31:1622–26.

14. Srimannarayana J, Varma RS, Satheesh S, Anilkumar R, Balachander J. Prevalence of left atrial thrombus in rheumatic mitral stenosis with atrial fibrillation and its response to anticoagulation: a transesophageal echocardiographic study. Indian Heart J. 2003;55(4):358–61.

15. Pisters R, Lane DA, Nieuwlaat R, de Vos CB, Crijns HJ, Lip GY. A novel user-friendly score (HAS-BLED) to assess 1-year risk of major bleeding in patients with atrial fibrillation: the Euro Heart Survey. Chest. 2010;138:1093–100.

16. Matebele MP, Rohde S, Clarke A, Fraser JF. Cardiac surgery in indigenous Australians: early onset cardiac disease with follow-up challenges. Heart Lung Circ. 2014;23:566–71.

17. Viles-Gonzalez JF, Kar S, Douglas P, Dukkipati S, Feldman T, Horton R, et al. The clinical impact of incomplete left atrial appendage closure with the Watchman Device in patients with atrial fibrillation: a PROTECT AF (Percutaneous Closure of the Left Atrial Appendage Versus Warfarin Therapy for Prevention of Stroke in Patients with Atrial Fibrillation) substudy. J Am Coll Cardiol. 2012;59:923–9.

18. Reddy VY, Doshi SK, Sievert H, Buchbinder M, Neuzil P, Huber K, et al. PROTECT AF Investigators. Percutaneous left atrial appendage closure for stroke prophylaxis in patients with atrial fibrillation: 2.3-year follow-up of the PROTECT AF (Watchman Left Atrial Appendage System for Embolic Protection in Patients With Atrial Fibrillation) Trial. Circulation. 2013;127:720–9.

19. Reddy VY. Long term results of PROTECT AF: the mortality effects of left atrial appendage closure versus warfarin for stroke prophylaxis in AF. Paper presented at: Heart Rhythm Society Scientific Sessions; May 8–11, 2013.

20. Price MJ, Valderrabano M. Left atrial appendage closure to prevent stroke in patients with atrial fibrillation. Circulation. 2014;130:202-12.

21. Holmes DR, Kar S, Price MJ, Whisenant B, Sievert H, Doshi SK, et al. Prospective Randomized Evaluation of the Watchman Left Atrial Appendage Closure Device in Patients With Atrial Fibrillation Versus Long-Term Warfarin Therapy: The PREVAIL Trial. J Am Coll Cardiol. 2014;64:1–12.

22. Luis SA, Roper D, Incani A, Poon K, Haqqani H, Walters DL. Non-pharmacological therapy for atrial fibrillation: Managing the left atrial appendage. Cardiology Research and Practice. 2012;1-9.

23. Murdoch D, McAulay L, Walters DL. Combined percutaneous balloon mitral valvuloplasty and left atrial appendage occlusion device implantation for rheumatic mitral stenosis and atrial fibrillation. Cardiovasc Revasc Med. 2014;S1553-8389.

24. Manjunath CN, Srinivasa KH, Ravindranath KS, Manohar JS, Prabhavathi B, Dattatreya PV. Balloon mitral valvotomy in patients with mitral stenosis and left atrial thrombus. Catheter Cardiovasc Interv. 2009;74:653–61.

25. Hung JS, Lau KW. Pitfalls and tips in Inoue balloon mitral commissurotomy. Catheterization and Cardiovascular Diagnosis. 1996;37:188–99.

26. Chen MC, Wu CJ, Chang HW, Yip HK, Chen YH, Cheng CI, et al. Mechanism of reducing platelet activity by percutaneous transluminal mitral valvuloplasty in patients with rheumatic mitral stenosis. Chest. 2004;125:1629–34.

Chapter 51

Percutaneous Treatment of Lutembacher's Syndrome: Balloon Mitral Valvotomy and Device Closure of Atrial Septal Defect

Shiv Bagga, Saujatya Chakraborty, Ramalingam Vadivelu

▓ INTRODUCTION

The earliest description of Lutembacher's syndrome is found in a letter written by anatomist Johann Friedrich Meckel to Albert von Haller in 1750.[1] In 1811, Corvisart[2] described the association of atrial septal defect with mitral stenosis; and in 1916, Lutembacher[3] published the first comprehensive account of these two defects as a combination that has come to be called Lutembacher's syndrome. The current consensus is that Lutembacher's syndrome consists of a congenital defect in the atrial septum together with acquired mitral stenosis (MS).[4,5] The incidence of MS in patients with atrial septal defect (ASD) has been estimated at 4% and conversely, the incidence of ASD in patients with MS has been estimated at 0.6–0.7%.[6]

▓ PATHOPHYSIOLOGY

The hemodynamic features and natural history of this syndrome depends upon the interplay between the relative effects of ASD and MS.[6,7] It is well appreciated that the presence of an ASD impacts favorably on the natural history of MS. This is because the left atrium is decompressed into the right atrium, thus protecting the pulmonary vasculature from the deleterious effects of pulmonary venous hypertension. The same cannot be said about the hemodynamic consequences of the left to right shunt, which is accentuated. This leads to progressive right ventricular (RV) volume overload and RV dysfunction. Interestingly, development of Eisenmenger's syndrome or irreversible pulmonary vascular disease is very uncommon in the presence of a large ASD and high left atrial pressure because of MS.

▓ TREATMENT OF LUTEMBACHER'S SYNDROME

Lutembacher's syndrome, with its unfavorable long-term natural history[6] has traditionally been corrected by surgical treatment.[8] This commonly involves use of a median sternotomy to access the right atrium followed by replacement of the mitral valve. The ASD is then closed. The use of cardiopulmonary bypass, a longer duration of stay and slower recovery times are some of the drawbacks of this approach.

Due to widespread acceptance of transcatheter therapies for MS[9] and ASD[10] with its attendant safety, less morbidity and cosmetic advantage, percutaneous treatment for Lutembacher's syndrome seems an attractive and feasible alternative.[11]

■ PERCUTANEOUS TREATMENT OF LUTEMBACHER'S SYNDROME

The experience with transcatheter treatment of the Lutembacher's syndrome is limited to case reports only. The use of percutaneous treatment was first described by Ruiz et al.[12] in 1992. The authors combined umbrella closure of ASD with Lock's Clamshell occluder in conjunction with mitral and aortic balloon valvotomies as a palliative rescue procedure in a 43-year-old female with ASD, severe aortic and mitral stenosis and pulmonary hypertension. Unfortunately, that patient died suddenly at 8 weeks before surgical procedure could be undertaken. Subsequent reports demonstrated the feasibility of percutaneous balloon mitral valvuloplasty and ASD device closure using a variety of balloon catheter techniques and devices. The first successful definitive percutaneous treatment of Lutembacher's syndrome was reported by Joseph et al.[13] in 1999. They used the Amplatzer septal occluder (ASO) for ASD and the Joseph mitral balloon catheter for mitral valvuloplasty. Since then, several successful cases have been reported.[14-20]

Because of an excellent long-term follow-up data along with the safety and ease of usage, the Inoue balloon catheter technique has become the procedure of choice for percutaneous balloon mitral valvuloplasty.[21,22] The Joseph mitral balloon catheter (JOMIVA) is a simple over-the-wire mitral valvuloplasty balloon catheter, marketed only in India. It has got a comparable efficacy, safety and simplicity of use in comparison to Inoue balloon with an additional cost advantage.[23,24]

· The Amplatzer ASO, on the other hand, is a self-centering device with a high closure rate at mid and long-term follow-up.[25,26] The advantages of this device in comparison with other septal occluders include simple delivery system using smaller sized sheaths, easy retrievability and absence of sharp corners or spokes.

Preprocedural Planning

A comprehensive diagnostic evaluation is essential before embarking on a definitive treatment strategy. Two-dimensional transthoracic echocardiography (TTE) with color flow mapping (Figs 51.1A and B) and Doppler interrogation establishes the diagnosis of Lutembacher's syndrome, identify the location and size of the atrial septal defect and determine the degree of MS. Planimetry (Fig. 51.2) and the Doppler continuity equation are the preferred methods for an accurate assessment of the mitral valve orifice area as Doppler pressure half-time consistently overestimates the mitral valve

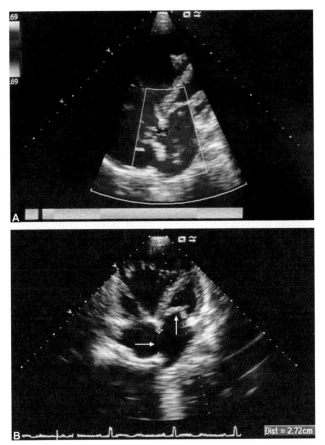

Figs 51.1A and B: Two-dimensional transthoracic echocardiogram with color flow mapping in apical four-chamber view showing a 27 mm atrial septal defect (horizontal arrow) and stenotic mitral valve (vertical arrow) with a significant left to right shunt across the atrial septal defect

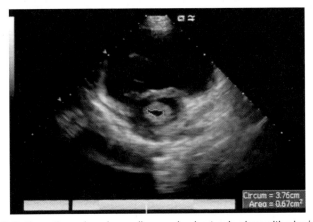

Fig. 51.2: Transthoracic echocardiogram in short axis view with planimetry, showing severe mitral stenosis with a mitral valve area of 0.67 cm² by planimetry

orifice area.[27] Transesophageal echocardiography (TEE) is used especially for proper sizing of the ASD and assessing its suitability for transcatheter device closure.

Though balloon sizing has been regarded as an integral part of transcatheter closure of ASDs,[28,29] there has been a recent trend towards transcatheter closure of these lesions without balloon sizing.[30-32] Though this is consequent to disadvantages of balloon sizing,[33-35] it may even be cost saving especially for developing countries. Selection of suitable device without balloon sizing is done by transthoracic, transesophageal or intracardiac echocardiography. As intracardiac echocardiography is relatively expensive for most patients to afford in developing countries, TTE, TEE offer convenient and accurate assessment of ASD sizing. TTE with its advantages of not requiring general anesthesia and the convenience of presenting multiplanar views of the heart can be sufficient for the assessment of the ASDs.[36-38] In addition, there is good linear correlation between TTE measurement of the defect and balloon-stretched diameter.[33,38,39] However, TTE is most efficient in predicting device size for defects smaller than 20 millimeters.[36] Defect sizing, based solely on TTE measurements (especially in adults) can lead to a serious judgemental error regarding device sizing with its attendant catastrophe of device embolization or malpositioning.[20]

TEE with its higher resolution is more appropriate for larger defects as the rims are usually weak, soft and floppy, and the measurement of accurate defect diameter might be a more challenging task with TTE. However, anatomical ASD diameter, measured with TEE using edge-to-edge defect borders still tends to underestimate the device size.[40] Hence, utilizing the procedural diameter measured using the maximal steadier rim border (thickness ≥2.5 mm) distance on TEE imaging as proposed by Carcagni and Presbitero[41] is recommended as it correlates well with stretched balloon diameter in adults. Adding 4-6 mm to TEE measured diameter gives a good estimate of the stretched diameter in most cases.[33,34,42,43]

In the present era, cardiac catheterization is rarely needed for the diagnosis of Lutembacher's syndrome, it is used more as an adjunct to the transcatheter treatment of this disease. In addition to identifying a significant oxygen step-up at the atrial level (Fig. 51.3), it is useful to quantify the severity of pulmonary arterial hypertension and the degree of left to right shunt based on calculation of systemic and pulmonary blood flows. In addition, careful measurement of the transmitral gradients (which are typically small) is essential for quantifying the severity of mitral valve disease (Fig. 51.4).[6]

Balloon Mitral Valvotomy in Lutembacher's Syndrome: Easier Said than Done

Over the years, development and refinement of catheter-based technologies has led to these techniques being used for treating structural and congenital heart diseases. Lutembacher's syndrome is one prototypical example of an entity which lends itself to catheter-based therapies. Percutaneous balloon mitral valvotomy (BMV) followed by ASD device closure is an elegant and

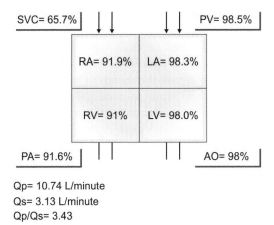

Qp= 10.74 L/minute
Qs= 3.13 L/minute
Qp/Qs= 3.43

PVR/SVR= 0.03

Fig. 51.3: Oximetry data in a patient with Lutembacher's syndrome showing a left to right shunt with significant oxygen step up at the atrial level

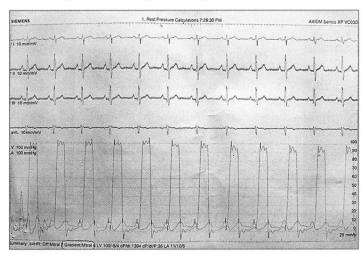

Fig. 51.4: Left atrial and left ventricular pressure tracings before mitral valvuloplasty in a patient with Lutembacher's syndrome, showing low left atrial pressure and transmitral gradients, in spite of significant mitral stenosis confirmed by planimetry on echocardiogram

efficacious way of managing this syndrome. However, growing experience with these techniques has fostered recognition of the unique set of problems that may be faced intra- and postprocedure. The interventional procedure unlike a case of isolated mitral stenosis; is not simply a combination of two simple procedures, BMV and ASD device closure). The coexisting structural anomalies with their secondary hemodynamic consequences, change the cardiac anatomy in a way that makes catheter manipulations complex.[19] In fact, none of the reported cases except for few recent ones,[19,20] have highlighted the challenges associated with simultaneous catheter-based treatment of this combination cardiac anomaly.

Contrary to the perception that presence of an ASD foregoes the need for atrial septal puncture and hence, simplifies balloon mitral valvuloplasty, the large septal defect provides excessive space for free floatation of the Inoue catheter which makes the balloon catheter unstable, posing technical difficulties in stabilizing it across the stenosed mitral valve. Attempting to cross mitral valve by standard Inoue method (counter clockwise rotation of Inoue balloon catheter) invariably leads to failure as instead of entering into left ventricle, the balloon jumps back towards the ASD and then into the right atrium and sometimes even the right ventricle. This happens because the shaft of the balloon catheter floats free in the space provided by ASD. This situation is unlike normal interatrial septum, which supports the catheter shaft, allowing it to maintain a curve and orienting balloon tip toward mitral valve. This warrants use of alternative methods for mitral valve crossing. Although, not described in the context of Lutembacher's syndrome, any of these can be tried according to operator's choice or multiple maneuvers can be tried if one is not successful. Some of the described methods are: Modified Inoue technique, use of balloon floatation catheters, modified over-the-wire (OTW) technique, and reshaping the stylet.

All of these variations involve an OTW technique have been described involving the use of back up valvuloplasty guidewire or 0.025 inch pigtail Inoue guidewire itself.[44-47] The underlying theme of all these methods is to cross the mitral valve with the help of a Judkins right catheter or balloon floatation or Mullins sheath and introducing wire into left ventricle (LV) or the aorta, overcoming the poor support due to septal defect and a small LV and passing the balloon over the wire into LV to accomplish mitral valve crossing. In addition, these techniques can be adapted to the varied hardware available at shelf.

Modified Inoue technique[44] involves placement of Judkins right coronary guide catheter in left atrium with its tip pointing towards mitral orifice. This is followed by crossing of mitral valve with a 0.020-inch backup valvuloplasty wire with a steerable J tip (Schneider, Minneapolis, MN) or a 0.032-inch exchange length J-tip guidewire,[35] which is later exchanged to a pigtail Inoue wire through the Judkins right catheter, already advanced in LV. This step is considered necessary to avoid chances of left ventricular perforation, which can occur while forcing balloon catheter over 0.032-inch J-tip wire.

Another described method[45] consists of advancing a balloon floatation catheter (Swan-Ganz) into left ventricle through mitral valve, maneuvering it into descending aorta through aortic valve, placing a 0.021-inch back-up valvuloplasty wire through this catheter into descending aorta, and advancing Inoue balloon catheter across mitral valve over the back-up wire.

Modified OTW technique[46] involves placing the 0.025-inch Inoue wire into left atrium through atrial septum; advancing Mullin's sheath over this wire; placing Mullin's sheath end hole near mitral orifice; and placement of Inoue pigtail wire directly into LV. The purported benefits of this simplified technique are that it does not involve use of any additional accessories, such as back-up guidewires, right Judkin's catheter, or balloon floatation catheters. Thus, additional expenses are avoided. The pigtail Inoue spring guidewire is directly introduced into left ventricle through the Mullin sheath. Thus, multiple exchanges involved in the earlier over-the-wire methods are avoided and the procedural time is considerably reduced. However, manipulation of pigtail wire through mitral valve might be difficult compared to that of a J-tip 0.032-inch guidewire as done in modified Inoue technique.

Another useful simple technique[47] is to cross the mitral valve with a balloon flotation catheter and place a 0.035 inch. back-up valvuloplasty wire (Schneider, Minneapolis, MN) in the left ventricle. When this wire is given a secondary bend in the stiff portion proximal to its distal soft part, it conforms to the anatomy of the heart and remains stable in the left ventricle. The Mullins sheath can then be advanced into the left ventricle over this wire. A 0.025-inch pigtail Inoue wire is introduced into the left ventricle through the Mullins sheath side by side the 0.035-inch back-up wire. Finally, the 0.035-inch wire and Mullins sheath are removed and the Inoue balloon is introduced into the left ventricle over the 0.025-inch wire.

Both modified Inoue technique[44] as well as modified over-the-wire technique[46] carry the risk of inserting the guidewire between chordae tendinae. This could result in damage of the subvalvular apparatus on balloon inflation, thereby causing severe mitral regurgitation. The balloon floatation variant techniques are safer in this regard and should be preferred. One needs to be careful while introducing the guidewire into the LV to ensure that the tip of the floatation catheter does not about the ventricular wall, and to ensure that the guidewire tip curls freely as it emerges from the catheter.

In one of the case reports,[20] described by the authors, multiple attempts with standard Inoue technique proved futile with repeated jumping of Inoue balloon back into the right atrium and right ventricle. Hence, an over-the-wire technique was adopted with the available hardware on shelf. The mitral valve was crossed using a balloon floatation catheter (Swan Ganz) and an Inoue wire was placed directly into the left ventricle. However, an attempt to introduce the Inoue balloon over the Inoue wire failed because of the inadequate support provided by a small left ventricular cavity as a result of left ventricular under filling consequent to significant mitral stenosis augmenting the left to right shunt across the ASD with enormous right ventricular volume overload. Modifying OTW technique, the mitral valve was recrossed with a balloon floatation catheter, parking an Inoue wire directly into the left ventricle. With Inoue wire in situ, the Swan Ganz catheter was removed and a Mullins Sheath was introduced into the left ventricle. Capitalizing on the adequate support provided by Mullins sheath, the Inoue wire was exchanged for a J tip Amplatz extra stiff wire. After removing the Mullins sheath, an Inoue balloon was carefully introduced into the left ventricle over the extra stiff wire. With Inoue balloon stabilized in the left ventricle cavity, the extra stiff wire was changed to Inoue wire as the latter provides better conformation to the left ventricle

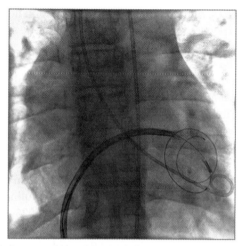

Fig. 51.5: Inoue balloon positioned in the left ventricular cavity over the Inoue wire after using an over-the-wire technique in a patient with Lutembacher's syndrome after unsuccessful mitral valve crossing with conventional method

anatomy in addition to providing safe support to Inoue balloon during mitral valvotomy. The mitral valve was successfully dilated using a 26 mm Inoue balloon with abolition of the transmitral gradient and a mitral valve area of 1.8 cm² (Fig. 51.5).

Issues with Device Closure of ASD

A diligent septal defect sizing using stop flow or procedural diameters on TEE as alluded to above is a key element in the success of percutaneous therapy of Lutembacher's syndrome. This is particularly relevant during transcatheter treatment for Lutembacher's syndrome, as unlike usual ASDs; post closure; one would expect the left atrial pressure to increase which is likely to dislodge the device which combined with an error in defect sizing can create a perfect setting for this catastrophe. TTE diameter measurements should not be relied upon except in a very young patient with small septal defect (<20 mm).

In case one does encounter this situation, the device can be retrieved successfully using percutaneous methods in majority of the cases.[20,48,49] Following device embolization, the safest method involves stabilizing the device with the bioptome to prevent further migration across the atrioventricular valves and snaring the device by catching the microscrew and withdrawing the whole device into the sheath.[20,50] Measures that facilitate entrance of the snared microscrew into the sheath include cutting a bevel at the tip of the sheath and rotating the sheath so it will engage the screw better.[49,50] In addition use of a stiff sheath (e.g. Cordis Brite Tip or Cook Flexor, Cook Cardiology, Bloomington, IN, USA) with the sheath size approximately two French sizes larger than the required implant sheath is recommended

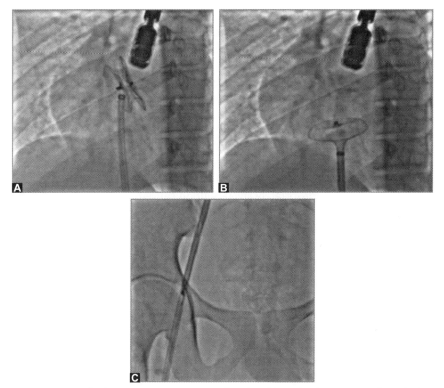

Figs 51.6A to C: Percutaneous retrieval of malpositioned atrial septal defect device under cinefluroscopic and transesophageal echocardiography guidance. (A) The right atrial disk microscrew mechanism being snared with a 1-cm Amplatz GooseNeck snare. (B) The device being pulled into the 12 French Amplatzer sheath with intentional bevel at the end. (C) Successful retrieval of the device from the right atrium into the inferior vena cava (causing the device to elongate) below the kidneys and through the femoral sheath

(Figs 51.6A to C).[20,50] It is important to understand that snaring the device in any location other than the microscrew will not permit the device to be pulled into the sheath.[50]

STEP-BY-STEP TECHNIQUE FOR PERCUTANEOUS THERAPY OF LUTEMBACHER'S SYNDROME

1. Preprocedural clinial history and examination, detailed TTE and TEE for delineating mitral valve disease severity as well as atrial septal defect sizing (Avoid TTE ASD sizing in adults).
2. Single or biplane cardiac catheterization laboratory.
3. Full range of device sizes, delivery and exchange systems.
4. Familiarity of operators with device retrieval techniques in case of embolization.
5. Working knowledge of various over-the-wire techniques with modification based on hardware available on shelf.

6. Preprocedure anticoagulation: Meaningful recommendations regarding specific anticoagulation or antiplatelet therapy after ASO remain controversial. Preferable to start dual antiplatelet (DAPT) 2–3 days before and continue DAPT for 6 months.

7. Right femoral arterial and venous access, heparin to achieve an activated clotting time of more than 200 seconds at the time of device deployment. Right and left heart catheterization with oximetry to confirm left to right shunt with step up at the atrial level and to quantify the severity of pulmonary arterial hypertension and the degree of left to right shunt based on calculation of systemic and pulmonary blood flows.

8. Mitral valve crossing using an over-the-wire technique.

9. BMV with an appropriately sized balloon catheter.

10. Assessment of pulmonary arterial pressure after BMV.

11. Device closure of ASD using stop flow balloon diameter and TEE guidance (Procedural diameter).

12. Electrocardiogram (ECG), chest roentgenogram (CXR) [posteroanterior and lateral (optional)] and a TTE with color Doppler to assess device position and resisdual shunt on postprocedure day 1.

13. No contact sports for 1 month postprocedure.

14. Antiplatelets and infective endocarditis prophylaxis for 6-12 months.

15. Recheck ECG, CXR and TTE/TEE 6 months postprocedure. Annual follow-up for first 2 years, then every 3–5 years depending on new symptoms.

The recommendations for use of antiplatelet therapy and follow up can vary based on institutional policy and have been extrapolated from data in the ASD device closure studies.

Limitations of Percutaneous Therapy for Lutembacher's Syndrome

With its attendant risk for restenosis following BMV, the presence of ASO in situ makes it undesirable to use transseptal approach for repeat BMV. The retrograde nontransseptal approach can be an alternative to surgery in this situation.[51]

■ CONCLUSION

Percutaneous interventional treatment of Lutembacher's syndrome is feasible, but can be complex, requiring alternative or modified methods for mitral valve crossing. In addition, a careful assessment of device size utilizing either TEE procedural diameter or conventional balloon sizing and choosing a larger device is highly recommended to prevent complications like device embolization. As this is a roadless traveled, prior anticipation of the difficulties to be encountered along with a skillful approach and familiarity of operators with device retrieval techniques improve the chances of success.

◼ REFERENCES

1. Wiedemann HR. Earliest description by Johann Friedrich Meckel, Senior (1750) of what is known today as Lutembacher syndrome (1916). Am J Med Genet. 1994;53:59-64.
2. Corvisart JN. Essai sur les maladies et les le'sions organiques de coeur et des gros vaisseaux. 2nd ed. Paris; 1811.
3. Lutembacher R. De la sténose mitrale avec communication interauriculaire. Arch Mal Coeur. 1916;9:237-60.
4. Gueron M, Gussarsky J. Lutembacher syndrome obsolete? A new modified concept of mitral disease and left-to-right at the level. Am Heart J. 1976;91:535.
5. Sambhi MP, Zimmerman HA. Pathologic physiology of Lutembacher syndrome. Am J Cardiol. 1958;2:681-6.
6. Bashi VV, Ravikumar E, Jairaj PS, Krishnaswami S, John S. Coexistent mitral valve disease with left-to-right shunt at the atrial level: clinical profile, hemodynamics, and surgical considerations in 67 consecutive patients. Am Heart J. 1987;114: 1406-14.
7. Goldfarb B, Wang Y. Mitral stenosis and left to right shunt at the atrial level: A broadened concept of the Lutembacher syndrome. Am J Cardiol. 1966;17:319-26.
8. John S, Munshi SC, Bhati BS, Gupta RP, Sukumar IP, Cherian G. Coexistent mitral valve disease with left-to-right shunt at the atrial level: Results of surgical treatment in 15 cases. J Thorac Cardiovasc Surg. 1970;60:174-87.
9. Carabello BA. Modern management of mitral stenosis. Circulation. 2005;112: 432-7.
10. Masura J, Gavora P, Podnar T. Long-term outcome of transcatheter secundum-type atrial septal defect closure using Amplatzer septal occluders. J Am Coll Cardiol. 2005;45:505-7.
11. Cheng TO. Coexistent atrial septal defect and mitral stenosis (Lutembacher syndrome): an ideal combination for percutaneous treatment. Cathet Cardiovasc Intervent. 1999;48:205-6.
12. Ruiz CE, Gamra H, Mahrer P, Allen JW, O'Laughlin MP, Lau FYK. Percutaneous closure of a secundum atrial septal defect and double balloon valvotomies of a severe mitral and aortic valve stenosis in a patient with Lutembacher's syndrome and severe pulmonary hypertension. Cathet Cardiovasc Diagn. 1992;25:309-12.
13. Joseph G, Rajpal KA, Kumar KS. Definitive percutanous treatment of Lutembacher's syndrome. Catheter Cardiovasc Interv. 1999;48:199-204.
14. Chua EM, Lee CH, Chow WH. Transcatheter treatment of case of Lutembacher syndrome. Catheter Cardiovasc Interv. 2000;50:68-70.
15. Aroney C, Lapanun W, Scalia G, Parsonage W. Transcatheter treatment of Lutembacher syndrome. Intern Med J. 2003;33:259-60.
16. Ahmed WH, Al-Shaibi KF, Chamsi-Pasha H, Abdelmenem A. Nonsurgical correction of Lutembacher syndrome. Saudi Med J. 2003;24:307-8.
17. Ledesma M, Martinez P, Cazares MA, Feldman T. Transcatheter treatment of Lutembacher syndrome: combined balloon mitral valvuloplasty and percutaneous atrial septal defect closure. J Invasive Cardiol. 2004;16:678-9.
18. CL Ho, Liang KW, Fu YC, Jan SL, Lin MC, Chi CS, Hwang B. Transcatheter therapy of Lutembacher syndrome. J Chin Med Assoc. 2007;70:253-6.
19. Bhambhani A, Somanath HS. Percutaneous treatment of Lutembacher syndrome in a case with difficult mitral valve crossing. J Invasive Cardiol. 2012;24:E54-56.

20. Velu V, Chakraborty S, Bagga S. Transcatheter therapy for Lutembacher's syndrome: The road less travelled. Ann Pediatr Cardiol. 2014;7:37–40.

21. Hernandez R, Bañuelos C, Alfonso F, Goicolea J, Fernández-Ortiz A, Escaned J, et al. Long-term clinical and echocardiographic follow-up after percutaneous mitral valvuloplasty with the Inoue balloon. Circulation. 1999;30;99:1580–6.

22. Chen CR, Cheng TO. Percutaneous balloon mitral valvuloplasty by the Inoue technique: a multicenter study of 4832 patients in China. Am Heart J. 1995;129(6):1197–203.

23. Joseph G, Chandy S, George P, George O, John B, Pati P, et al. Evaluation of a simplified transseptal mitral valvuloplasty technique using over-the-wire single balloons and complementary femoral and jugular venous approaches in 1407 consecutive patients. J Invasive Cardiol. 2005;17:132–8.

24. Routray SN, Mishra TK, Patnaik UK, Behera M. Percutaneous transatrial mitral commissurotomy by modified technique using a JOMIVA balloon catheter: a cost-effective alternative to the Inoue balloon. J Heart Valve Dis. 2004;13:430–8.

25. Masura J, Gavora P, Formanek A, Hijazi ZM.Transcatheter closure of secundum atrial septal defects using the new self-centering amplatzer septal occluder: initial human experience. Cathet Cardiovasc Diagn 1997;42:388–93.

26. Du ZD, Hijazi ZM, Kleinman CS, Silverman NH, Larntz K; Amplatzer Investigators. Comparison between transcatheter and surgical closure of secundum atrial septal defect in children and adults: results of a multicenter nonrandomized trial. J Am Coll Cardiol. 2002;5;39:1836–44.

27. Vasan RS, Shrivastava S, Kumar MV. Value and limitations of Doppler echocardiographic determination of mitral valve area in Lutembacher syndrome. J Am Coll Cardiol. 1992;20:1362–70.

28. Gu X, Han YM, Berry J, Myra Urness R, Amplatz K. A new technique for sizing atrial septal effects. Catheter Cardiovasc Interv. 1995;46:51–7.

29. Helgason H, Johansson M, Soderberg B, Eriksson P. Sizing of atrial septal defect in adults. Cardiology. 2005;104:1–5.

30. Zanchetta M. On-line intracardiac echocardiography alone for Amplatzer septal occluder selection and device deployment in adult patients with atrial septal defect. Int J Cardiol. 2004;95:61–8.

31. Amin Z, Daufors DA. Balloon sizing is not necessary for closure of secundum atrial septal defects. J Am Coll Cardiol. 2005;45:317.

32. Wang JK, Tsai SK, Lin SM, Chiu SN, Lin MT, Wu MH. Transcatheter closure of atrial septal defect without balloon sizing. Catheter Cardiovasc Interv. 2008;71:214–21.

33. Rao PS, Langhough R. Relationship of echocardiographic, shunt flow, and angiographic size to the stretched diameter of the atrial septal defect. Am Heart J. 1991;122:505–8.

34. Amin Z, Hijazi ZM, Bass JL, Cheatham JP, Hellenbrand WE, Kleinman CS. Erosion of secundum atrial septal defects: Review of registry of complications and recommendations to minimize future risk. Catheter Cardiovasc Interv. 2004;63:496–502.

35. Harikrishnan S, Narayanan NK, Sivasubramonian S. Sizing balloon-induced tear of the atrial septum. J Invasive Cardiol. 2005;17:546–7.

36. Li GS, Kong GM, Ji QS, Li JF, Chen YG, You BA, Zhang Y. Reliability of transthoracic echocardiography in estimating the size of Amplatzer septal occluder and guiding percutaneous closure of atrial septal defects. Chin Med J. 2008;121:973–6.

37. Sahin M, Ozkutlu S, Yıldırım I, Karagöz T, Celiker A. Transcatheter closure of atrial septal defects with transthoracic echocardiography. Cardiol Young. 2011;21:204–08.

38. Bartakian S, El-Said HG, Printz B, Moore JW. Prospective randomized trial of transthoracic echocardiography versus transesophageal echocardiography for assessment and guidance of transcatheter closure of atrial septal defects in children using the Amplatzer septal occluder. J Am Coll Cardiol Intv. 2013;6:974–80.
39. Godart F, Rey C, Francart C, Jarrar M, Vaksman G. Two dimensional echocardiographic and color doppler measurement of atrial septal defect and comparison with the balloon-stretched diameter. Am J Cardiol. 1993;72:1095–7.
40. Cook JC, Gelman JS, Richard WH. Echocardiologists' role in the deployment of the Amplatzer atrial septal occluder device in adults. J Am Soc Echocardiogr. 2001;14:588–94.
41. Carcagni A, Presbitero P. New echocardiographic diameter for Amplatzer sizing in adult patients with secundum atrial septal defect: Preliminary results. Catheter Cardiovasc Interv. 2004;62:409–14.
42. Walsh KP, Maadi IM. The Amplatzer septal occluder. Cardiol Young. 2000;10: 493–501.
43. Carlson KM, Justino H, OBrien RE, Dimas VV, Leonard GT Jr, Pignatelli RH, et al. Transcatheter atrial septal defect closure: Modified balloon sizing technique to avoid overstretching the defect and oversizing the Amplatzer septal occluder. Catheter Cardiovasc Interv. 2005;66:390–6.
44. Meier B. Modified Inoue technique for difficult mitral balloon commissurotomy. Cathet Cardiovasc Diagn. 1992;26:316–8.
45. Mehan VK, Meier B. Impossibility to cross a stenotic mitral valve with the Inoue balloon: Success with a modified technique. Indian Heart J. 1994;46:51–2.
46. Manjunath CN, Srinivasa KH, Patil CB, Venkatesh HV, Bhoopal TS, Dhanalakshmi C. Balloon mitral valvuloplasty: Our experience with a modified technique of crossing the mitral valve in difficult cases. Cathet. Cardiovasc. Diagn. 1998;44:23–6.
47. Abhaichand RK, Joseph G. Letter to the editor: Re Manjunath et al. Catheter Cardiovasc Interv. 1999;46:117.
48. Chessa M, Carminati M, Butera G, Bini RM, Drago M, Rosti L, et al. Early and late complications associated with transcatheter occlusion of secundumatrial septal defect. J Am Coll Cardiol. 2002;39:1061–5.
49. Levi DS, Moore JW. Embolization and retrieval of the amplatzer septal occluder. Catheter Cardiovasc Interv. 2004;61:543–7.
50. Tan CA, Levi DS, Moore JW. Embolization and transcatheter retrieval of coils and devices. Pediatr Cardiol. 2005;26:267–74.
51. Stefanadis C, Stratos C, Pitsavos C, Kallikazaros I, Triposkiadis F, Trikas A, et al. Retrograde nontransseptal balloon mitral valvuloplasty. Immediate results and long-term follow-up. Circulation. 1992;85:1760–7.

Chapter 52

Percutaneous Mitral Valvotomy in Mitral Restenosis

Krishnakumar Nair, Harikrishnan S

■ INTRODUCTION

Half a century back, an article in the "Circulation" categorically committed that restenosis of the mitral valve does not occur!![1] The article went on to state that the only cause of readherence of the valve commissures is a recrudescence of the rheumatic process.[1] But later reports showed that mitral restenosis following closed mitral valvotomy is a definite entity.[2-6] It was subsequently reported that restenosis could occur even within 1-year after successful percutaneous mitral valvotomy (PMV).[7,8] Cardiologists all over the world are now seeing a growing population of patients with mitral restenosis. Recognition of the natural history of this challenging condition and proper management is therefore important.

Many reported cases of restenosis were thought to represent merely unsuccessful valvotomies. However, hemodynamic studies indicate clearly that restenosis can take place in those patients in whom mitral valvotomy widened the orifice only slightly, as well as in those in whom the stenosis was nearly totally relieved.[9] It is important to distinguish between "true and false" restenosis. True restenosis refers to restenosis that occurs after one or both commissures have been fully split. False restenosis is not really restenosis. It is actually because the original procedure was inadequate, and neither commissure was fully split.[6]

■ DEFINITION

Post-PMV mitral restenosis is defined as a valve area <1.5 cm^2 or a $>50\%$ loss of the initial gain in valve area.[7,10] Chen et al. added reappearance of symptoms to this definition.[11] Our group has tended to use this definition because some restenosis may be silent. This definition itself is based on the definition of a successful PMV (post-PMV MVA ≥ 1.5 cm^2 and MR $\leq 2/4$) which itself is binary and arbitrary.[7] The incidence of restenosis has been reported to range from 4% to 39%[8,12-18] and progressive decrease of MVA overtime has been well-documented.[8,14]

The development of restenosis is time-dependent[14,19,20] which is represented in the wide range of reported restenosis incidence (from 4% to 39%) according to the different follow-up durations.[8,12-18]

PREVALENCE

The prevalence depends on the definition of restenosis and on the duration of follow-up. The frequency of restenosis is difficult to assess due to many issues. Restenosis is a broad term that embraces a mixture of inadequate results, errors in MVA determination, very early (within days) area loss, true restenosis and disease progression. The other problem is the definition of restenosis—it can be made on a clinical basis or in terms of mitral valve area, absolute valve area loss, percentage of valve area loss, or loss of the gain in valve area, or a combined definition including symptoms and mitral valve area.[11] In some studies, restenosis was found to be strongly associated with poor long-term functional results after good immediate results[21] and relatively sharp functional deterioration or progressive development of adverse clinical events 5 years after PMV.[22,23] However, restenosis may sometimes be silent too. With all these confounding factors, it is not surprising that restenosis rate after PMV has ranged from 3% to 70%[23,24] at 1 to 3 years, and restenosis definition in itself may play a major role in restenosis rate as will be clear from the studies quoted subsequently in the manuscript.

The reported rate of restenosis varies widely among series. In a post- PMV series, Chen et al.[25] reported a decrease in MVA of 0.2 cm^2 at 5 years and Treviño et al.[24] reported a decrease of 0.25 cm^2 at 3 years. In another study of 137 patients,[26] the restenosis rate was 28.3% after 4 years.

In a mid-term follow-up of PMV,[26] restenosis after percutaneous mitral balloon valvotomy, occurred in 28% of cases at 4 years. Other estimates say that restenosis may occur in 4% to as many as 40% of patients within 6 years following the procedure.[7,8,14,20,27-31] Hernandez's data[14] supports the fact that restenosis is rare within 3 years of the procedure in patients with a good mitral opening, but it increased over time, reaching 39% at 7 years. He observed that anatomical restenosis as determined by echocardiography was not always associated with recurrence of symptoms and the time to restenosis was difficult to determine clinically. However, approximately 7% to 21% of patients become symptomatic due to mitral restenosis on follow-up.[8,13,16,32-38] In another study, the incidence of reintervention has varied from 10% to 30%.[11]

Looking at restenosis free and event free survival, 2 studies reported similar results. The restenosis-free rates in Fawzy's study[39] of 78% at 10 years, 52% at 15 years and 26% at 19 years are in line with the rate of 66% at 10 years reported by Ben Farhat and colleagues[15] in a similar patient population (mean age, 33 ± 13 years).

PREDICTORS OF RESTENOSIS

As discussed earlier, interstudy comparisons are difficult because different definitions of restenosis were used. Analysis of data from Fawzy et al.[39] on clinical and echocardiographic follow-up (1.5–19 years) of 547 consecutive patients (mean age, 31.5 years) undergoing mitral balloon valvuloplasty found the restenosis rate lower in patients with Wilkins' score less than 8. Multivariate analysis also identified Wilkins echocardiographic score >8 and postprocedure valve area, and preexisting AF as predictors of restenosis.[39-42] In another study, the immediate post-PMV MVA >1.8 cm^2 was the most important independent continuous variable predicting the development of restenosis.[7] SJ Park[43] reported that the immediate success is related to clinical and echocardiographic characteristics of the patients, such as total echocardiographic score and pre-PMV MVA, but echocardiographic restenosis is more related to procedural variables, such as post-PMV MVA and development of commissural mitral regurgitation after PMV.

■ PATHOLOGY

The characteristic pathologic findings of mitral stenosis include thickening of the leaflets due to fibrosis and calcification, fusion of the commissures and shortening of the chordae tendineae[44] resulting in a narrow, funnel-shaped orifice.[40] PMV is an effective treatment for mitral stenosis because balloon dilatation makes slits in the commissures. Therefore, it seemed reasonable for early investigators to conclude that restenosis after PMV was due to recurrence of fusion.

Surprisingly, fusion was rarely seen in restenotic mitral valves on serial echocardiographic follow-up.[41] Additional evidence that fusion of commissures is not the main cause of restenosis following PMV was provided by a study which demonstrated that all the splits produced in the commissures after PMV were still present with restenosis.[44] In another study, end-stage rheumatic valvular disease in the leaflet and subvalvular fusion was the actual mechanism of restenosis as indicated by histologic absence of inflammation.[42] Similarly, a study on Japanese patients demonstrated with histologic and echocardiographic findings that restenosis is not due to recurrence of fusion in commissures, but is based on end-stage valvular disease, such as severe fibrosis and calcification.[44] These studies may suggest that the effect of the initial PMV is due to dissection of the fused commissures and that the second[44] PMV is mainly due to stretch of leaflet and relief of subvalvular stenosis.

The Wilkins echo score, which represents the degree of both leaflet and subvalvular disease,[42] deteriorated during the follow-up period in these patients indicating the progressive nature of the disease. Several studies have shown that repeat PMV is effective in patients with mitral valve restenosis if the Wilkins score is low,[45,46] which indicates low degree of leaflet pathology and subvalvular disease.

A study from Italy on mitral restenosis proposed two potential mechanisms of restenosis: (1) A more common slow process, due to turbulent flow-trauma on the mitral valve; (2) A rapid process that relates to valvulitis consequent to a subclinical occurrence of chronic rheumatic activity.[47,48]

MANAGEMENT

The options of these patients with restenosis are mitral valve replacement (MVR), or a repeat closed mitral valvotomy (CMV) or percutaneous mitral valvotomy. In a nonrandomized study published in 2007, patients with restenosis after PMV were treated either with repeat PMV or mitral valve replacement.[49] The outcomes were comparable, at least 4 years following either procedure. After 4 years, surgical treatment began to turn superior due to the fact that patients in the repeat PMV group needed another intervention (most commonly valve replacement). An estimated 9-year survival rate without an adverse event was 90.4% in the valve replacement group versus 36.0% in the PMV group.

Aslanabadi did a randomized comparison of MVR vs repeat PMV and found that the ten-year survival was significantly higher in re-PMV vs MVR (96% vs. 72.7%, $P<0.05$), but event-free survival was similar (52% vs. 50%, $P = 1.0$) due to high reintervention in the re-PBMV group (48% vs. 18.1%, $P = 0.02$).[50]

In the light of the data from these studies, and considering the factors discussed below, the main management option for restenosis in today's world remains PMV. Also the availability of surgery in the developing world, the costs and the problems associated with anticoagulation should also be taken into account.

Repeat PMV is the treatment of choice in young patients with favorable Wilkins score, especially those with minimal lesions in the subvalvular apparatus in whom the main mechanism of restenosis is likely bilateral commissural fusion.[51] A recent publication[27] suggests that patients with high echocardiographic scores (>7) are less likely to have long-term benefit and in such cases mitral valve surgery should be considered. Repeat PMV may be still be considered in patients with poor Wilkins score but as a palliative procedure, if they cannot undergo valve replacement due to comorbidities.

PMV for Restenosis Versus PMV for de novo Mitral Stenosis

In a study of the immediate and long-term outcome of redo percutaneous mitral valvuloplasty (PMV), Rifaie et al.[37] demonstrated that redo PMV can be safely performed in selected patients, with an immediate procedural success rate of 92.5%, an adequate final MVA comparable to that of first PMV (with a gain of MVA rather lower than that of initial PMV), a relatively low complication profile and a satisfactory long-term outcome.

Similar procedural success rate in restenosis was reported in by Iung et al.[46] and Pathan et al.[45] (91% and 75% respectively). In Iung's study consisting 53 patients with moderate lesions in the valve and the subvalvular apparatus, a good immediate result was observed in 91% of patients and the 5-years survival rate without a repeat intervention and the number of patients remaining in NYHA class I or II was 69%.[46] In an earlier work presented by Pathan et al.[45] good immediate outcome was achieved in 75% of 36 patients who underwent repeat PMV and the likelihood of survival at 3 years without an adverse event was 47.0%.

Another study demonstrated that immediate and late results of balloon valvuloplasty for patients who have mitral restenosis were slightly inferior compared to patients who underwent PMV as the initial procedure.[52]

However, patients with previous surgical and percutaneous valvuloplasty were not analyzed separately and the observed population was young, so the results cannot be extrapolated to older patients.

Overall, most series in PMV report a success rate of 80–95% in de novo mitral stenosis.[13,53] However, for PMV in mitral restenosis, success rate varies between 50% and 90%.[46,54-56] This lower success rate has been attributed to the higher age of the patients during the second procedure and higher Wilkins score.[55] The immediate success of PMV for mitral restenosis in our series was 59%,[57] which is lower than for de novo mitral stenosis.

Predictors of Success of PMV for Mitral Restenosis

In univariate analysis of an earlier study by our group, the major predictor of successful PMV for mitral restenosis was Wilkins score (P = 0.004). When we compared the Wilkins score between first and second procedure, the second procedure had higher score (6.31 ± 1.59 versus. 8.09 ± 1.43; P <0.0001). However, when we analyzed the results of percutaneous mitral valvotomy in patients with Wilkins score <8, the procedural success was 70.5% versus 43.5% for score >8.[57] The findings from other reports about mid-term follow-up after PMV for mitral restenosis were conflicting. In Iung et al. series,[58] valve anatomy was not a predictor of late outcome. However, the Wilkins score was an important determinant of outcome in other studies as reported by Serra et al.[59] Jang et al.[55] and Peixoto et al.[60] Young age in Rifae's series (mean age: 34.5 ± 7.2 years) was a known strong predictor of good immediate outcome of PMV.[21,33] In contrast, patients with atrial fibrillation were at a higher risk of poor outcome.[32,61]

Repeat Surgical Commissurotomy Versus PMV for Mitral Restenosis

There are no head to head comparisons of repeat surgical commissurotomy versus repeat balloon valvotomy for mitral restenosis, though there are reports of both procedures individually. Repeat surgical commissurotomy has an operative mortality of 2.5 to 10%, risk of systemic embolism ranging from 1% to 4%, and operative success and improvement in functional class in 50 to 85%.[62] Several studies have documented the feasibility of PMV for mitral restenosis in patients who have undergone surgical commissurotomy.[35,36,38,51,52,59-61] Following PMV for mitral restenosis, only one study showed a more rapid deterioration at 4 years than in patients without a history of prior commisurotomy.[58] Davidson et al.[63] have reported a 30-days mortality of 2% and a 6-months mortality of 6% in 133 patients who had undergone percutaneous mitral valvotomy after previous surgical commissurotomy.

Do Patients with Prior PMV Fare Better than Patients with Prior CMV at the Time of the Second Procedure?

In a patient with prior CMV, the concerns during PMV for mitral restenosis are the distorted cardiac anatomy because of ventriculotomy, amputated left atrial appendage and surgical adhesions.[57] There are no randomized or nonrandomized trials comparing PMV for mitral restenosis between postballoon mitral valvotomy patients and post-CMV patients, though there is follow-up data of both procedures individually. In a previously published work from our center,[57] PMV for mitral restenosis was a success in 59% patients (57.1% prior PMV, 59.3% prior CMV). The results were similar between both prior PMV and prior CMV groups, and the results were comparable to previous reports.[46,54-56] The combined end-point of mitral valve replacement (MVR), need for repeat PMV for mitral restenosis or death was higher in the prior CMV group (31.2% prior CMV, 7.1% prior PMV, P 5 0.027). Event-free survival at follow-up was lower in the prior CMV group (69% prior CMV, 92.8% prior PMV) mainly due to the higher need for MVR (11 versus. 0 patients, P < 0.03). The frequency of mitral regurgitation after PMV for mitral restenosis following CMV is the same as that following de novo PMV, in the published literature.[35,36,38,46,53-55,58,64,65] In conclusion, PMV in patients with mitral valve restenosis after a prior percutaneous valvuloplasty has lesser event rates compared to patients with restenosis after prior surgical commissurotomy.

Late Results and Event-Free Survival After PMV for Mitral Restenosis

In a report of 8-years follow-up of patients who underwent PMV for mitral restenosis, Iung et al.[46] have reported only 48% event-free survival. In Nair et al.'s series, the event-free survival at a mean follow-up of 3.47 + 2.07 years was 76%. Bouleti et al. analysed the long-term results of percutaneous mitral valvotomy performed for mitral restenosis after previous commissurotomy and PMC in 163 patients.[66] The found PMV provides good immediate result in most cases. Following that, one patient out of three remains free from surgery and one out of five has good functional results at 20 years.

Technical Considerations during PMV for Mitral Restenosis

The major technical issues in PMV for mitral restenosis are as follows:
1. *Septal puncture:* Residual opening in the interatrial septum from a previous PMV may facilitate entry into the left atrium. We have not faced any difficulties with supposedly fibrotic septum following multiple transseptal punctures. However, following multiple pulmonary vein isolation procedures for atrial fibrillation, operators have reported difficulty in septal puncture and have had to resort to radiofrequency energy application to get across the interatrial septum.
2. Mitral restenosis as we have discussed is generally noncommissural. The Wilkins' score is likely to be on the higher side in a restenotic valve. Mutiple slow dilatations may be needed to dilate the subvalvar region which is the

major site of stenosis. This may increase the risk of mitral regurgitation due to damage to subvalvar structure which may necessitate mitral valve replacement. "Better is the enemy of good" and we are more likely to accept a lesser result with no significant mitral regurgitation in a bad valve, rather than risk significant regurgitation in attempts to increase valve area.

3. Patients with restenosis are intuitively likely to be older and may have additional comorbidities which need to be tackled.

CONCLUSION

The "unnatural history" of treated mitral stenosis involves mitral restenosis. Understanding this and the factors responsible for this phenomenon may help in better management of these patients. An interventional technique like PMV for mitral restenosis is certainly much more desirable than a surgical procedure like MVR, which entails all the long-term complications of a prosthetic valve. This has to be looked at in the background of the developing world where this disease is much more common.

REFERENCES

1. Glover RP, Davila JC, O'Neill TJ, Janton OH. Does mitral stenosis recur after commissurotomy? Circulation. 1955;11(1):14–28.
2. McKusick VA. Rheumatic restenosis of mitral valve; report of a case with death almost five years after mitral valvulotomy. AMA Arch Intern Med. 1955; 95(4): 557–62.
3. Glenn F, Dineen P. Recurrent mitral stenosis; a case report. Ann Surg. 1956;143(3): 405–11.
4. E Donzelot CD. Reconstitution of a mitral stenosis after commissurotomy. Arch Mal Coeur Vaiss. 1953;46(4):300–9.
5. Morino F. Case of re-operation for recurrence of mitral stenosis. Minerva Med. 1955;46(84):1033–7.
6. Belcher JR. Restenosis of the mitral valve. Ann R Coll Surg Engl. 1979;61:258-64.
7. Song JK, Song JM, Kang DH, Yun SC, Park DW, Lee SW, et al. Restenosis and adverse clinical events after successful percutaneous mitral valvuloplasty: immediate postprocedural mitral valve area as an important prognosticator. Eur Heart J. 2009;30(10):1254–62.
8. Palacios IF, Block PC, Wilkins GT, Weyman AE. Follow-up of patients undergoing percutaneous mitral balloon valvotomy. Analysis of factors determining restenosis. Circulation. 1989;79(3):573–9.
9. Dubin AA, March HW, Cohn K, Selzer A. Longitudinal hemodynamic and clinical study of mitral stenosis. Circulation. 1971;44(3):381–9.
10. Abascal VM, Wilkins GT, O'Shea JP, Choong CY, Palacios IF, Thomas JD, et al. Prediction of successful outcome in 130 patients undergoing percutaneous balloon mitral valvotomy. Circulation. 1990;82(2):448–56.
11. Chen CR, Cheng TO, Chen JY, Huang YG, Huang T, Zhang B. Long-term results of percutaneous balloon mitral valvuloplasty for mitral stenosis: a follow-up study to 11 years in 202 patients. Cathet Cardiovasc Diagn. 1998;43(2):132–9.
12. Ben Farhat M, Ayari M, Maatouk F, Betbout F, Gamra H, Jarra M, et al. Percutaneous balloon versus surgical closed and open mitral commissurotomy: seven-year follow-up results of a randomized trial. Circulation. 1998;97(3):245–50.

13. Herrmann HC, Ramaswamy K, Isner JM, Feldman TE, Carroll JD, Pichard AD, et al. Factors influencing immediate results, complications, and short-term follow-up status after Inoue balloon mitral valvotomy: a North American multicenter study. Am Heart J. 1992;124(1):160-6.

14. Hernandez R, Bañuelos C, Alfonso F, Goicolea J, Fernández-Ortiz A, Escaned J, et al. Long-term clinical and echocardiographic follow-up after percutaneous mitral valvuloplasty with the Inoue balloon. Circulation. 1999;99(12):1580-6.

15. Ben-Farhat M, Betbout F, Gamra H, Maatouk F, Ben-Hamda K, Abdellaoui M, et al. Predictors of long-term event-free survival and of freedom from restenosis after percutaneous balloon mitral commissurotomy. Am Heart J. 2001;142(6):1072-9.

16. Vahanian A, Michel PL, Cormier B, Vitoux B, Michel X, Slama M, et al. Results of percutaneous mitral commissurotomy in 200 patients. Am J Cardiol. 1989;63(12):847-52.

17. Desideri A, Vanderperren O, Serra A, Barraud P, Petitclerc R, Lespérance J, et al. Long-term (9 to 33 months) echocardiographic follow-up after successful percutaneous mitral commissurotomy. Am J Cardiol. 1992;69(19):1602-6.

18. Lau KW, Ding ZP, Quek S, Kwok V, Hung JS. Long-term (36-63 month) clinical and echocardiographic follow-up after Inoue balloon mitral commissurotomy. Cathet Cardiovasc Diagn. 1998;43(1):33-8.

19. Kang DH, Park SW, Song JK, Kim HS, Hong MK, Kim JJ, et al. Long-term clinical and echocardiographic outcome of percutaneous mitral valvuloplasty: randomized comparison of Inoue and double-balloon techniques. J Am Coll Cardiol. 2000;35(1):169-75.

20. Wang A, Krasuski RA, Warner JJ, Pieper K, Kisslo KB, Bashore TM, et al. Serial echocardiographic evaluation of restenosis after successful percutaneous mitral commissurotomy. J Am Coll Cardiol. 2002;39(2):328-34.

21. Iung B, Garbarz E, Michaud P, Helou S, Farah B, Berdah P, et al. Late results of percutaneous mitral commissurotomy in a series of 1024 patients. Analysis of late clinical deterioration: frequency, anatomic findings, and predictive factors. Circulation. 1999;99(25):3272-8.

22. Pavlides GS, Nahhas GT, London J, Gangadharan C, Troszak E, Barth-Jones D, et al. Predictors of long-term event-free survival after percutaneous balloon mitral valvuloplasty. Am J Cardiol. 1997;79(10):1370-4.

23. Palacios IF, Sanchez PL, Harrell LC, Weyman AE, Block PC. Which patients benefit from percutaneous mitral balloon valvuloplasty? Prevalvuloplasty and postvalvuloplasty variables that predict long-term outcome. Circulation. 2002;105(12):1465-71.

24. Trevino AJ, Ibarra M, Garcia A, Uribe A, de la Fuente F, Bonfil MA, et al. Immediate and long-term results of balloon mitral commissurotomy for rheumatic mitral stenosis: comparison between Inoue and double-balloon techniques. Am Heart J. 1996;131(3):530-6.

25. Chen CR, Cheng TO, Chen JY, Zhou YL, Mei J, Ma TZ. Long-term results of percutaneous mitral valvuloplasty with the Inoue balloon catheter. Am J Cardiol. 1992;70(18):1445-8.

26. Langerveld J, Thijs Plokker HW, Ernst SM, Kelder JC, Jaarsma W. Predictors of clinical events or restenosis during follow-up after percutaneous mitral balloon valvotomy. Eur Heart J. 1999;20(7):519-26.

27. Chmielak Z, Klopotowski M, Kruk M, Demkow M, Konka M, Chojnowska L, et al. Repeat percutaneous mitral balloon valvuloplasty for patients with mitral valve restenosis. Catheter Cardiovasc Interv Off J Soc Card Angiogr Interv. 2010;76(7):986-92.

28. Fawzy ME, Shoukri M, Hassan W, Nambiar V, Stefadouros M, Canver CC. The impact of mitral valve morphology on the long-term outcome of mitral balloon valvuloplasty. Catheter Cardiovasc Interv Off J Soc Card Angiogr Interv. 2007;69(1):40–6.

29. Eid Fawzy M, Shoukri M, Hassan W, Badr A, Hamadanchi A, Eldali A, et al. Immediate and long-term results of percutaneous mitral balloon valvotomy in asymptomatic or minimally symptomatic patients with severe mitral stenosis. Catheter Cardiovasc Interv Off J Soc Card Angiogr Interv. 2005;66(2):297–302.

30. Chmielak Z, Kruk M, Demkow M, Kłopotowski M, Konka M, Ruzyłło W. Long-term follow-up of patients with percutaneous mitral commissurotomy. Kardiol Pol. 2008;66(5):525–530, discussion 531–32.

31. Cruz-Gonzalez I, Sanchez-Ledesma M, Sanchez PL, Martin-Moreiras J, Jneid H, Rengifo-Moreno P, et al. Predicting success and long-term outcomes of percutaneous mitral valvuloplasty: a multifactorial score. Am J Med. 2009;122(6):581.e11–19.

32. Cohen DJ, Kuntz RE, Gordon SP, Piana RN, Safian RD, McKay RG, et al. Predictors of long-term outcome after percutaneous balloon mitral valvuloplasty. N Engl J Med. 1992;327(19):1329–35.

33. Multicenter experience with balloon mitral commissurotomy. NHLBI balloon valvuloplasty registry report on immediate and 30-day follow-up results. The National Heart, Lung, and Blood Institute Balloon Valvuloplasty Registry Participants. Circulation. 1992;85:448–61.

34. Dean LS, Mickel M, Bonan R, Holmes DR Jr, O'Neill WW, Palacios IF, et al. Four-year follow-up of patients undergoing percutaneous balloon mitral commissurotomy. A report from the National Heart, Lung, and Blood Institute Balloon Valvuloplasty Registry. J Am Coll Cardiol. 1996;28(6):1452–7.

35. Iung B, Cormier B, Ducimetiere P, Porte JM, Nallet O, Michel PL, et al. Functional results 5 years after successful percutaneous mitral commissurotomy in a series of 528 patients and analysis of predictive factors. J Am Coll Cardiol. 1996;27(2):407–14.

36. Palacios IF, Tuzcu ME, Weyman AE, Newell JB, Block PC. Clinical follow-up of patients undergoing percutaneous mitral balloon valvotomy. Circulation. 1995;91(3):671–6.

37. Rifaie O, Ismail M, Nammas W. Immediate and long-term outcome of redo percutaneous mitral valvuloplasty: comparison with initial procedure in patients with rheumatic mitral restenosis. J Intervent Cardiol. 2010;23(1):1–6.

38. Turi ZG, Reyes VP, Raju BS, Raju AR, Kumar DN, Rajagopal P, et al. Percutaneous balloon versus surgical closed commissurotomy for mitral stenosis. A prospective, randomized trial. Circulation. 1991;83(4):1179–85.

39. Fawzy ME. Long-term results up to 19 years of mitral balloon valvuloplasty. Asian Cardiovasc Thorac Ann. 2009;17(6):627–33.

40. Gaasch WH, Folland ED. Left ventricular function in rheumatic mitral stenosis. Eur Heart J. 1991;12 Suppl B:66–9.

41. Saeki F, Ishizaka Y, Tamura T. Long-term clinical and echocardiographic outcome in patients with mitral stenosis treated with percutaneous transvenous mitral commissurotomy. Jpn Circ J. 1999 ;63(8):597–604.

42. Wilkins GT, Weyman AE, Abascal VM, Block PC, Palacios IF. Percutaneous balloon dilatation of the mitral valve: an analysis of echocardiographic variables related to outcome and the mechanism of dilatation. Br Heart J. 1988;60(4):299–308.

43. Park SJ, Kim JJ, Park SW, Song JK, Doo YC, Lee SJ. Immediate and one-year results of percutaneous mitral balloon valvuloplasty using Inoue and double-balloon techniques. Am J Cardiol. 1993;71(11):938–43.

44. Tsuji T, Ikari Y, Tamura T, Wanibuchi Y, Hara K. Pathologic analysis of restenosis following percutaneous transluminal mitral commissurotomy. Catheter Cardiovasc Interv Off J Soc Card Angiogr Interv. 2002;57(2):205–10.

45. Pathan AZ, Mahdi NA, Leon MN, Lopez-Cuellar J, Simosa H, Block PC, et al. Is redo percutaneous mitral balloon valvuloplasty (PMV) indicated in patients with post-PMV mitral restenosis? J Am Coll Cardiol. 1999;34(1):49–54.

46. Iung B, Garbarz E, Michaud P, Fondard O, Helou S, Kamblock J, et al. Immediate and mid-term results of repeat percutaneous mitral commissurotomy for restenosis following earlier percutaneous mitral commissurotomy. Eur Heart J. 2000;21(20):1683–9.

47. Nigri A, Alessandri N, Martuscelli E, Pizzuto F, Sardella G, Berni A, et al. Rheumatic fever recurrence: a possible cause of restenosis after percutaneous mitral valvuloplasty. Ital Heart J Off J Ital Fed Cardiol. 2001;2(11):845–7.

48. Rifaie O, Omar AMS, Abdel-Rahman MA, Raslan H. Does a chronic inflammatory state have a role in the development of mitral restenosis after balloon mitral valvuloplasty? Int J Cardiol. 2014;172(3):e417–418.

49. Kim J-B, Ha J-W, Kim J-S, Shim W-H, Kang S-M, Ko Y-G, et al. Comparison of long-term outcome after mitral valve replacement or repeated balloon mitral valvotomy in patients with restenosis after previous balloon valvotomy. Am J Cardiol. 2007;99(11):1571–4.

50. Aslanabadi N, Golmohammadi A, Sohrabi B, Kazemi B. Repeat percutaneous balloon mitral valvotomy vs. mitral valve replacement in patients with restenosis after previous balloon mitral valvotomy and unfavorable valve characteristics. Clin Cardiol. 2011;34(6):401–6.

51. Turgeman Y, Atar S, Suleiman K, Feldman A, Bloch L, Jabaren M, et al. Feasibility, safety, and morphologic predictors of outcome of repeat percutaneous balloon mitral commissurotomy. Am J Cardiol. 2005;95(8):989–91.

52. Fawzy ME, Hassan W, Shoukri M, Al Sanei A, Hamadanchi A, El Dali A, et al. Immediate and long-term results of mitral balloon valvotomy for restenosis following previous surgical or balloon mitral commissurotomy. Am J Cardiol. 2005;96(7):971–5.

53. ACC/AHA guidelines for the management of patients with valvular heart disease. A report of the American College of Cardiology/American Heart Association. Task Force on Practice Guidelines (Committee on Management of Patients with Valvular Heart Disease). J Am Coll Cardiol. 1998;32(5):1486–588.

54. Gupta S, Vora A, Lokhandwalla Y, Kerkar P, Gupta S, Kulkarni H, et al. Percutaneous balloon mitral valvotomy in mitral restenosis. Eur Heart J. 1996;17(10):1560–4.

55. Jang IK, Block PC, Newell JB, Tuzcu EM, Palacios IF. Percutaneous mitral balloon valvotomy for recurrent mitral stenosis after surgical commissurotomy. Am J Cardiol. 1995;75(8):601–5.

56. Ha JW, Shim WH, Yoon JH, Jang YS, Chung NS, Cho SY, et al. Percutaneous mitral balloon valvuloplasty in patients with restenosis after surgical commissurotomy: a comparative study. Yonsei Med J. 1993;34(3):243–7.

57. Nair K, Sivadasanpillai H, Sivasubramonium P, Ramachandran P, Tharakan JA, Titus T, et al. Percutaneous valvuloplasty for mitral valve restenosis: postballoon valvotomy patients fare better than postsurgical closed valvotomy patients. Catheter Cardiovasc Interv Off J Soc Card Angiogr Interv. 2010 Aug 1;76(2):174–80.

58. Iung B, Garbarz E, Michaud P, Mahdhaoui A, Helou S, Farah B, et al. Percutaneous mitral commissurotomy for restenosis after surgical commissurotomy: late efficacy and implications for patient selection. J Am Coll Cardiol. 2000;35(5):1295–302.

59. Serra A, Bonan R, Lefèvre T, Barraud P, Le Feuvre C, Leclerc Y, et al. Balloon mitral commissurotomy for mitral restenosis after surgical commissurotomy. Am J Cardiol. 1993;71(15):1311–5.

60. Peixoto EC, Peixoto RT, Borges IP, Oliveira PS, Labrunie M, Salles Netto M, et al. Influence of the echocardiographic score and not of the previous surgical mitral commissurotomy on the outcome of percutaneous mitral balloon valvuloplasty. Arq Bras Cardiol. 2001;76(6):473–82.

61. Iung B, Cormier B, Ducimetière P, Porte JM, Garbarz E, Michel PL, et al. 5 years results of percutaneous mitral commissurotomy. Apropos of a series of 606 patients; late results after mitral dilatation. Arch Mal Coeur Vaiss. 1996;89(12):1591–8.

62. Biswas B, Datta S, Dutta AL, Chakraborty A. Role of closed mitral commissurotomy for mitral restenosis. J Indian Med Assoc. 1999;97(7):255–8.

63. Davidson CJ, Bashore TM, Mickel M, Davis K. Balloon mitral commissurotomy after previous surgical commissurotomy. The National Heart, Lung, and Blood Institute Balloon Valvuloplasty Registry participants. Circulation. 1992;86(1):91–9.

64. Reyes VP, Raju BS, Wynne J, Stephenson LW, Raju R, Fromm BS, et al. Percutaneous balloon valvuloplasty compared with open surgical commissurotomy for mitral stenosis. N Engl J Med. 1994;331(15):961–7.

65. Fatkin D, Roy P, Morgan JJ, Feneley MP. Percutaneous balloon mitral valvotomy with the Inoue single-balloon catheter: commissural morphology as a determinant of outcome. J Am Coll Cardiol. 1993;21(2):390–7.

66. Bouleti C, Iung B, Himbert D, Brochet E, Messika-Zeitoun D, Détaint D, et al. Long-term efficacy of percutaneous mitral commissurotomy for restenosis after previous mitral commissurotomy. Heart Br Card Soc. 2013;99(18):1336–41.

Section 7

Long-term Outcome Following PMV

Chapter 53

Left Atrial Thrombosis in Rheumatic Mitral Stenosis

Sonny P Jacob

■ INTRODUCTION

Thrombus formation in the left atrium (LAT) is one of the major complications that occur frequently in rheumatic mitral valve disease especially in mitral stenosis (MS).[1] The incidence of LAT in MS ranges from 10 to 25%.[2] Most of the LAT occurs in the left atrial appendage (LAA) (Figs 53.1A to E).[3] LAT occurs in patients in atrial fibrillation (AF) and also in some who are in sinus rhythm (SR). In both these situations, LAA is large and has poor contractile function.[3,4]

The important predisposing factors implied for LA thrombus formation are older age, higher NYHA class, AF, severity and duration of MS, and presence of left atrial spontaneous echo contrast (LASEC).[5-12]

Development of AF is one of the strongest risk factors for the development of left atrial thrombus (LAT) in patients with MS.[9]

Chronic rheumatic disease results in LA dilatation and scarring, which causes multiple micro reentrant circuits in LA. This contributes to the development of AF and it further causes LA and LAA dilatation. AF also causes contractile dysfunction of LA and LAA. Both the above factors cause stagnation of blood and LAA behaves as an enlarged static pouch which predisposes to thrombus formation.[4,7,13] Longer duration of MS results in LA enlargement, which predisposes to the development of AF.[5] This may contribute to a higher incidence of LA thrombus.

LAT in MS can occur in patients in sinus rhythm also. The enlargement and contractile dysfunction of both LA and LAA contribute to thrombus formation.[3,10,13-17]

The shape of the left atrium also said to influence the development of thrombus in the left atrium in MS. A more spherical LA shape compared to an ellipsoidal shape was independently associated with an increased risk for embolic events suggesting increased chance of thrombus formation in the left atrium.[18]

The presence of LASEC is another important predictor of LAT in patients with MS.[1-3,5,10,12,19,20] The origin of LASEC is thought to be due to the stagnation of blood. This phenomenon is attributed to increased ultrasonic back scatter from aggregates of cellular components of blood in presence of stasis.[8] This is best visualized with transesophageal echocardiogram (TEE).[11] The major

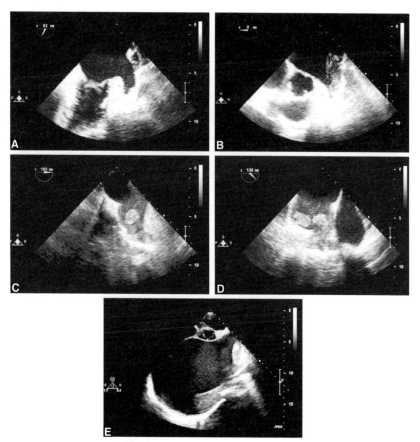

Figs 53.1A to E: Echocardiographic images demonstrating left atrial thrombi. (A to E) TEE images. (A) Normal left atrial appendage. (B) Left atrial appendage thrombus projecting into left atrial cavity. (C and D) Mobile thrombi in left atrial appendage. (E) TTE image showing a huge left atrium with large thrombi attached to the left atrial free wall

predisposing factors include AF, large LA, small mitral valve area (MVA) and absence of more than mild (>2+) mitral regurgitation (MR).[9]

The reported prevalence of LASEC was 55–100% in patients with LAT.[11] Regional coagulation activity is increased in LASEC no matter whether the patient is in SR or in AF.[17] It provides semiquantitative assessment of the stagnation of blood and also prothrombotic state in the LA. LASEC is graded from 0-4+ (Table 53.1).[7]

The presence of an echolucent area inside the thrombus or a "birdbeak sign" in TEE is considered as a marker of recent and growing thrombus and is considered as a contraindication for PMV (Figs 53.2 and 53.3).[21,22]

As mentioned above, the contractile dysfunction of LAA in MS with AF as well as in SR was reported by various investigators.[3] In one study, the mean LAA EF was 13.5 ±10.4% in patients with MS and AF vs 25.9 ± 12.9% in normal persons. The contractile dysfunction of LAA in MS patients in SR was impaired when compared to controls (29.5 ± 15% vs 58.1 ± 17.4%).[14,16] Another important parameter for assessment of LAA function is LAA emptying velocity which is impaired in patients with MS and AF.[13]

Table 53.1: Gradation of LASEC (Black et al. J. Am Coll Cardiol. 1991;18(2):398-404)

Grade 0	Absence of echogenicity -0
Grade 1+	Minimal echogenicity located in LAA detected transiently during cardiac cycle
Grade 2+	Mild to moderate intense swirling pattern
Grade 3+	Moderate dense swirling pattern in LAA detected constantly throughout the cardiac cycle
Grade 4+	Severe intense echogenicity and very slow swirling pattern LAA with similar intensity in LA main cavity[9]

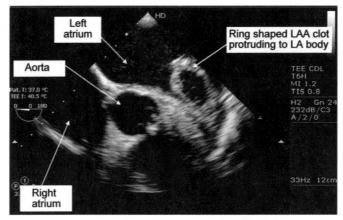

Fig. 53.2: Ring-shaped thrombus in LAA. Suggesting recently formed thrombi, a contra-indication for balloon valvotomy (Mahla et al. BMJ Case Reports 2013; doi:10.1136/bcr-2013-201108). (*Image Courtesy*: Dr CN Manjunath)

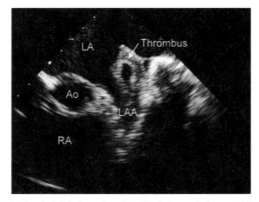

Fig. 53.3: Birdbeak sign in LAA thrombus in mitral stenosis imaged by transesophageal echocardiography—is considered as a marker of recent and growing thrombus; *Abbreviations*: LA, left atrium, LAA, left atrial appendage, RA, right atrium, Ao, aorta (Singla et al. BMJ Case Reports 2013; doi:10.1136/bcr-2013-010459) (*Image Courtesy:* Dr CN Manjunath)

A prospective study by Krishnamoorthy et al. has defined a clinical and echocardiographic model to predict the presence of left atrial thrombus in those undergoing PMV. In this study, they have highlighted that a subgroup of patients planning PMV need only transthoracic echo (TTE) to rule out LA/LAA thrombus. The TTE features which predicted absence of LAT included:

1. Age <28 year.
2. Absence of AF, CHF, LASEC or embolic phenomena.
3. LA dimension <4 cm, and
4. Wilkins score <7.[23]

Depending on the extent, LAT subdivided into three types:

Type I—Localized to LAA
Type II—Protruding beyond mouth of LAA
Type III—Extending into LA.

The reported incidence of the extent of thrombus in one study was 54.6% of Type I, 33.3% of Type II and 12% of Type III.[24]

There is another classification of LAT as given below (Fig. 53.4).

Left Atrial Thrombus—Types

Type Ia: LA appendage clot confined to appendage.
Type Ib: LA appendage clot protruding into LA cavity.
Type IIa: LA roof clot limited to a plane above the plane of fossa ovalis.
Type IIb: LA roof clot extending below the plane of fossa ovalis.
Type III: Layered clot over the interatrial septum (IAS).
Type IV: Mobile clot which is attached to LA free wall or roof or IAS.
Type V: Ball valve thrombus (Free Floating).

Resolution of LAT occurs with oral anticoagulation (OA).[1,2,19,24-33] Patients with smaller size of LAT and less severe LASEC have shown greater likelihood of the resolution of LA thrombus. There are many reports of successful balloon mitral valvuloplasty following resolution of LAT after varying periods of OA.[19] The overall resolution of LAT was reported to be 33.3% in 6 months with most of it occurring within 2 months. In a recent report from Jayadeva Institute, Bengaluru, only 53 out of 194 patients (27.3%) had LAT resolution following 8–12 weeks of adequate anticoagulation with international normalized ratio (INR) ranging from 2.5 to 3.5.

Apart from oral anticoagulation, the important prognostic factors which determine resolution of LAT are NYHA functional class and LAT area. Patients with lower NYHA class and smaller LAT area have better chance of thrombus resolution with anticoagulation.[5,23]

We routinely initiate OA on detection of LAT. INR is maintained at a level of 2.5–3 for 3 months and a repeat TTE is performed. If TTE does not reveal LAT, TEE is performed to confirm resolution of LAT. If TTE shows LAT, OA regimen is re-evaluated and intensified if needed and continued for another 3 months. If there is no resolution of LAT at 6 months of adequate anticoagulation, patients are referred for open mitral valvotomy (OMV)/mitral valve replacement (MVR). We have done a prospective evaluation of LAT in 54 patients and found that 50%

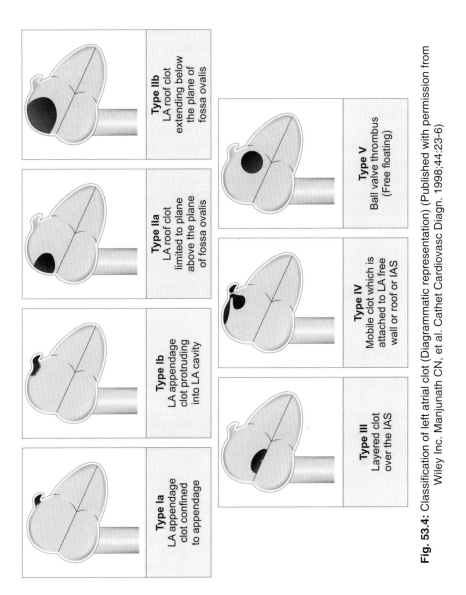

Fig. 53.4: Classification of left atrial clot (Diagrammatic representation) (Published with permission from Wiley Inc. Manjunath CN, et al. Cathet Cardiovasc Diagn. 1998;44:23-6)

of the patients had resolution of LA thrombus at 5 months of follow-up. The predictors of resolution of LAT were anticoagulation status, lower functional class, sinus rhythm and smaller sized LAT (Unpublished observations).

Balloon Valvotomy in Patients with LA Thrombus

PMV is reported to be performed successfully in patients after resolution of LAT.[19,24] There are reports of successful PMV in patients with persistent LAT. 108 patients with persistent LAT (Types Ia, Ib and IIa) underwent PMV successfully as reported by Manjunath et al.[23] In all the cases, a deliberate low IAS puncture was made (Figs 53.5A to D). Then the coiled LA wire was introduced into the left ventricle and optimal positioning was achieved in LV. Mullins septal dilator was introduced over this wire and septal dilatation was performed. Then the Accura balloon was inserted over the wire and the valve dilatation was performed. Since the balloon is tracked over-the-wire, LAA is totally excluded and the chance of clot dislodgement and embolization is minimized. In the 108 patients, only one had TIA 6 hours after the procedure. None of the others had any embolic events.[23]

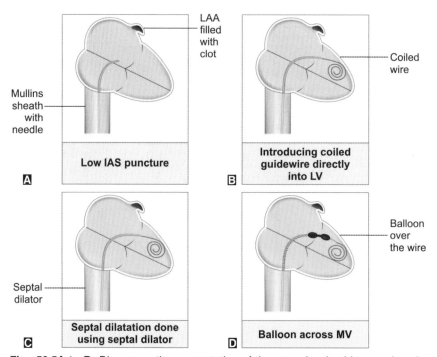

Figs 53.5A to D: Diagrammatic repesentation of the steps involved in over the wire technique (Published with permission from Wiley Inc. Manjunath CN, et al. Cathet Cardiovasc Diagn. 1998;44:23-6)

■ REFERENCES

1. Vigna C, de Rito V, Criconia GM, Russo A, Testa M, Fanelli R, et al. Left atrial thrombus and spontaneous echo-contrast in nonanticoagulated mitral stenosis. A transesophageal echocardiographic study. Chest. 1993;103(2):348–52.
2. Pytlewski G, Panidis IP, Combs W, McDonough MT. Resolution of left atrial thrombus with warfarin by transesophageal echocardiography before percutaneous commissurotomy in mitral stenosis. Am Heart J. 1994;128(4):843–5.
3. Hwang JJ, Li YH, Lin JM, Wang TL, Shyu KG, Ko YL, et al. Left atrial appendage function determined by transesophageal echocardiography in patients with rheumatic mitral valve disease. Cardiology. 1994;85(2):121–8.
4. Pollick C, Taylor D. Assessment of left atrial appendage function by transesophageal echocardiography. Implications for the development of thrombus. Circulation. 1991;84(1):223–31.
5. Silaruks S, Kiatchoosakun S, Tantikosum W, et al. A prognostic model for predicting the disappearance of left atrial thrombi among candidates for percutaneous transvenous mitral commissurotomy. J Am Coll Cardiol. 2002;39:886–91.
6. Chan SK, Kannam JP, Douglas PS, Manning WJ. Multiplane transesophageal echocardiographic assessment of left atrial appendage anatomy and function. Am J Cardiol. 1995;76(7):528–30.
7. Fatkin D, Kuchar DL, Thorburn CW, Feneley MP. Transesophageal echocardiography before and during direct current cardioversion of atrial fibrillation: evidence for "atrial stunning" as a mechanism of thromboembolic complications. J Am Coll Cardiol. 1994;23(2):307-16.
8. Fatkin D, Kelly RP, Feneley MP. Relations between left atrial appendage blood flow velocity, spontaneous echocardiographic contrast and thromboembolic risk in vivo. J Am Coll Cardiol. 1994;23(4):961–9.
9. Black IW, Hopkins AP, Lee LC, Walsh WF. Left atrial spontaneous echo contrast: a clinical and echocardiographic analysis. J Am Coll Cardiol. 1991;18(2):398–404.
10. Goswami KC, Yadav R, Rao MB, Bahl VK, Talwar KK, Manchanda SC. Clinical and echocardiographic predictors of left atrial clot and spontaneous echo contrast in patients with severe rheumatic mitral stenosis: a prospective study in 200 patients by transesophageal echocardiography. Int J Cardiol. 2000;73(3):273–9.
11. Fatkin D, Feneley M. Stratification of thromboembolic risk of atrial fibrillation by transthoracic echocardiography and transesophageal echocardiography: the relative role of left atrial appendage function, mitral valve disease, and spontaneous echocardiographic contrast. Prog Cardiovasc Dis. 1996;39(1):57–68.
12. Beppu S, Nimura Y, Sakakibara H, Nagata S, Park YD, Izumi S. Smoke-like echo in the left atrial cavity in mitral valve disease: its features and significance. J Am Coll Cardiol. 1985;6(4):744–9.
13. Daimee MA, Salama AL, Cherian G, Hayat NJ, Sugathan TN. Left atrial appendage function in mitral stenosis: is a group in sinus rhythm at risk of thromboembolism? Int J Cardiol. 1998;66(1):45–54.
14. Agmon Y, Khandheria BK, Gentile F, Seward JB. Echocardiographic assessment of the left atrial appendage. J Am Coll Cardiol. 1999;34(7):1867–77.
15. Agmon Y, Khandheria BK, Gentile F, Seward JB. Clinical and echocardiographic characteristics of patients with left atrial thrombus and sinus rhythm: experience in 20,643 consecutive transesophageal echocardiographic examinations. Circulation. 2002;105(1):27–31.

16. Al-Saady NM, Obel OA, Camm AJ. Left atrial appendage: structure, function, and role in thromboembolism. Heart Br Card Soc. 1999;82(5):547–54.
17. Peverill RE, Harper RW, Gelman J, Gan TE, Harris G, Smolich JJ. Determinants of increased regional left atrial coagulation activity in patients with mitral stenosis. Circulation. 1996;94(3):331–9.
18. Nunes MCP, Handschumacher MD, Levine RA, Barbosa MM, Carvalho VT, Esteves WA, et al. Role of LA shape in predicting embolic cerebrovascular events in mitral stenosis: mechanistic insights from 3D echocardiography. JACC Cardiovasc Imaging. 2014;7(5):453–61.
19. Silaruks S, Kiatchoosakun S, Tantikosum W, Wongvipaporn C, Tatsanavivat P, Klungboonkrong V, et al. Resolution of left atrial thrombi with anticoagulant therapy in candidates for percutaneous transvenous mitral commissurotomy. J Heart Valve Dis. 2002;11(3):346–52.
20. González-Torrecilla E, García-Fernández MA, Pérez-David E, Bermejo J, Moreno M, Delcán JL. Predictors of left atrial spontaneous echo contrast and thrombi in patients with mitral stenosis and atrial fibrillation. Am J Cardiol. 2000;86(5):529–34.
21. Mahla H, Bhat P, Bhairappa S, Manjunath CN. Ring-shaped thrombus in left atrial appendage: a contraindication for valvotomy. BMJ Case Rep. 2013;2013.
22. Singla V, Singh Y, Ravindranath SK, Manjunath CN. "Bird-beak sign" of left atrial thrombus: a guide to management. BMJ Case Rep. 2013;2013:bcr2013010459.
23. Manjunath CN, Srinivasa KH, Ravindranath KS, Manohar JS, Prabhavathi B, Dattatreya PV, et al. Balloon mitral valvotomy in patients with mitral stenosis and left atrial thrombus. Catheter Cardiovasc Interv Off J Soc Card Angiogr Interv. 2009;74(4):653–61.
24. Kandpal B, Garg N, Anand KV, Kapoor A, Sinha N. Role of oral anticoagulation and inoue balloon mitral valvulotomy in presence of left atrial thrombus: a prospective serial transesophageal echocardiographic study. J Heart Valve Dis. 2002;11(4):594–600.
25. Tsai LM, Hung JS, Chen JH, Lin LJ, Fu M. Resolution of left atrial appendage thrombus in mitral stenosis after warfarin therapy. Am Heart J. 1991;121(4 Pt 1):1232–4.
26. Kang DH, Song JK, Chae JK, Cheong SS, Hong MK, Song H, et al. Comparison of outcomes of percutaneous mitral valvuloplasty versus mitral valve replacement after resolution of left atrial appendage thrombi by warfarin therapy. Am J Cardiol. 1998;81(1):97–100.
27. Wolf PA, Dawber TR, Thomas HE Jr, Kannel WB. Epidemiologic assessment of chronic atrial fibrillation and risk of stroke: the Framingham study. Neurology. 1978;28(10):973–7.
28. Vincelj J, Sokol I, Jaksič O. Prevalence and clinical significance of left atrial spontaneous echo contrast detected by transesophageal echocardiography. Echocardiogr Mt Kisco N. 2002;19(4):319–24.
29. Kranidis A, Koulouris S, Filippatos G, Kappos K, Tsilias K, Karvounis H, et al. Mitral regurgitation protects from left atrial thrombogenesis in patients with mitral valve disease and atrial fibrillation. Pacing Clin Electrophysiol PACE. 2000;23(11 Pt 2):1863–6.
30. Buyukasic Y, Ileri M, Ozcebe OI, et al. Increased systemic coagulation activity in patients with rheumatic mitral stenosis: assessment of the clinical and echocardiographic determinents. Blood Coag Fibrinolysis. 1999;10(7):417–21.

31. Sananda K, Komaki S, Sannou K, et al. Significance of atrial fibrillation, left atrial thrombus and severity of stenosis for risk of systemic embolism in patients with mitral stenosis. J Cardiol. 1999;33(1):1–5.

32. Beppu S. Hypercoagulability in the left atrium: Part I: Echocardiography. J Heart Valve Dis. 1993;2(1):18–24.

33. Davison G, Greenland P. Predictors of left atrial thrombus in mitral valve disease. J Gen Intern Med. 1991;6(2):108–12.

Chapter 54

Comparison of Percutaneous Mitral Valvotomy and Surgical Mitral Commissurotomy

Sanjay G

■ INTRODUCTION

Subsequent to its introduction by Inoue et al. in 1984, percutaneous mitral valvotomy (PMV) has become the procedure of choice in management of selected patients with symptomatic mitral stenosis (MS).[1,2] Various studies and series have established the favorable outcomes of the procedure along with the safety of the procedure.[3-5] Still, surgical mitral commissurotomy is indicated in isolated pliable mitral stenosis in the presence of left atrial thrombus (open mitral commissurotomy—OMC) or an associated condition requiring surgical correction (e.g. significant aortic valve disease).

Studies Comparing the Techniques of Surgical Mitral Commissurotomy

Hickey et al. in a series of 339 patients has reported a 99.7% survival rate after surgical commissurotomy [both closed mitral commissurotomy (CMC), and OMC], and survival rates of 99%, 95%, 87% 59%, at 1, 5, 10 and 20 years respectively.[6] In a study by John et al. with follow-up of 24 years after CMC, the actuarial survival without the need to undergo another procedure was 94.0%, 89.4%, 85.0%, and 78.3% at 6, 12, 18, and 24 years, respectively. In the study by Hickey et al. after adjustment for risk factors, the survival did not differ between the surgical methods (CMC vs OMC). There was no predictor for early mortality. Old age, increased pulmonary vascular resistance, valve calcification and left ventricular dilatation predicted late mortality.[6] However, in a prospective randomized analysis of CMC versus OMC in patients with noncalcific mitral stenosis, the rates of surgical mortality, systemic embolism and surgically induced mitral regurgitation were similar between the groups. But OMC resulted in better mitral valve areas and better exercise hemodynamics.[7] Another study by Nakano et al.[8] concluded that OMC was the procedure of choice, given the favorable survival rates and freedom from reoperation.

Studies Comparing PMV and Surgical Commissurotomy

Early Studies

Randomized analysis and short-term follow-up of PMV (double balloon technique) versus CMC (Tubbs dilator, left ventriculotomy) by Turi et al.[9] during the early days of PMV revealed similar outcomes in both the groups with respect to postprocedure hemodynamics and mitral valve area. The procedure-related mitral regurgitation—both severe and moderate were similar between the groups. Another single center randomized study by Patel et al.[10] comparing PMV (single balloon) and CMC [digital exploration of mitral valve with transventricular Logan's dilator (Fig. 54.1)] reported no procedure related mortality and similar clinical improvement, but better mitral valve areas and exercise performance in patients undergoing PMV.

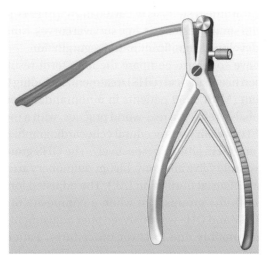

Fig. 54.1: The transventriculotomy dilator used for surgical mitral commissurotomy, popularly known as Tubbs dilator or Tubbs-Logan dilator was designed by Dr Andrew Logan and improved upon by Dr Oswold Tubbs

Intermediate and Late Follow-up Studies

A 7-year follow-up analysis of a randomized study comparing PMV (double balloon), OMC and CMC in pliable mitral valve stenosis by Ben Farhat et al. revealed better outcomes for PMV and OMC when compared with CMC.[11] Mitral valve area (Gorlin's method) increased much more after PMV (from $0.96 + 0.16$ to $2.26 + 0.4$ cm^2) and OMC (from $0.96 + 0.2$ to $2.26 + 0.4$ cm^2) than after CMC (from $0.96 + 0.2$ to $1.66 + 0.4$ cm^2). Residual MS was 0% after PMV or OMC and 27% after CMC. None of the groups had early or late mortality or thromboembolism. The authors reported less successful splitting of both commissures in the CMC group which might have accounted for the lesser immediate results achieved in the CMC group. At 7 years follow-up, the mitral valve area by echocardiography was equally higher in the PMV and OMC group when compared to CMC group. Restenosis (MVA < 1.5 cm^2) rate was 6.6% after PMV or OMC versus 37% after CMC. Freedom from reintervention was 90% after PMV, 93% after OMC, and 50% after CMC in this study. The mean preprocedural echocardiographic scores were not different between the groups and were 6, 6 and 6.1 in the PMV, OMC and CMC groups, respectively.

Another study comparing 7-year results of PMV and OMC[12] reported better functional recovery, better mitral valve area and lesser mitral regurgitation after OMC.

A long-term follow-up of a randomized study (mean follow-up 99 months) by Rifaie et al[13] comparing PMV (double balloon) and CMC in patients with pliable mitral valves reported similar immediate as well as long-term outcomes in both the groups. Mitral restenosis occurred in 26% in PMV group and 27.8% in CMC group with similar restenosis-free survival curves. None of the patients in either group developed significant mitral regurgitation.

Song et al. have sought to compare the long-term results of PMV (402 patients) and open heart surgical (OHS) treatment, including OMC and mitral valve replacement (MVR), 159 patients in a nonrandomized observational study, which probably reflects a real-world practice, with a median follow-up of 109 months.[14] The mean preprocedural echocardiographic scores were 7.3 and 9.6 in PMV and OHS groups, respectively. The OHS group patients were older, with unfavorable valve anatomy, higher pulmonary artery pressure and higher prevalence of atrial fibrillation (AF). The adjusted long-term survival was similar in both the groups. But when a composite of cardiovascular mortality, redo PMV and OHS was analyzed after adjustment, the OHS group performed better, mainly due to fewer procedures. Patients with higher echocardiographic scores and concomitant AF fared better with surgery (16% of the surgical candidates underwent Maze procedure). There was no difference in clinical events when patients with echocardiographic scores <8 in both the groups were compared.

▪ PMV VS SURGICAL COMMISSUROTOMY IN SPECIAL SITUATIONS

Pregnancy

Of the available studies cumulatively involving around 515 pregnant women who underwent PMV, procedural success was attained in about 98% patients, with one maternal death and 10 fetal mortalities (2%).[15] In an observational study comparing PMV and OMC, the fetal outcomes were better with PMV (fetal mortality of 6% in PMV group versus 33% in OMC group) with similar procedural success between the groups. Pavankumar et al. in their study of 126 pregnant women who underwent CMC reported full-term normal deliveries in 82% of the patients and 6% fetal loss.[16]

Calcific Mitral Valve

Heavily calcific valve with bicommissural calcification is best dealt with valve replacement. OMC has an advantage in view of the feasibility of debridement of the valve calcification. There is no direct comparison of PMV with surgical mitral commissurotomy in patients with lesser degrees of mitral valve calcification. Leaflet calcification was found to be a predictor of late mortality in the study by Hickey et al.[6] Another study by Detter et al. reported the association of higher late mortality as well as late reoperation risk with leaflet calcification.[17] Some studies have assessed the effect of fluoroscopic valve calcification on PMV.[18,19] As expected, these subset of patients with significantly calcified valves on fluoroscopy had poorer procedural outcome and in-hospital mortality.[19] The estimated 2-year survival was significantly lower for patients with calcified mitral valves than for those with noncalcified valves (80% vs 99%). Freedom from mitral valve replacement at 2 years was also significantly lower for patients with calcified valves (67% vs 93%).[20] In the study by Iung et al., for those patients who had a good immediate outcome, survival without reintervention at 8 years was 48 + 6% only, whereas, it was 40 + 5% for those who had a poor immediate outcome.[19]

Effect of commissural calcification was analyzed in an observational study, by Sutaria et al.[20] The authors classified commissural calcium from 0–3, with 0 being no calcium, 1 = calcification of one half of a commissure, 2 = full calcification of one commissure, 3 = full calcification of one and half of the other. They found that the PMV results were better among patients with echocardiographic score <8 and either grade 0 or grade 1 calcification. Significant mitral regurgitation occurred in 4.1% of patients with grade 2 or 3 calcification.

Mitral Restenosis

There are no direct head to head comparisons of PMV and surgical commissurotomy for mitral restenosis in the literature. The study by Nair et al.[21] reports procedural success of 59% for BMV in mitral restenosis as against 80-95% for PMV in de novo valves. Procedural successes varying from 50% to 90% have been reported in literature for PMV in restenosed mitral valves. There was no difference in outcome between the post-PMV restenosis versus post-surgical restenosis groups. The reported rates of severe mitral regurgitation after the PMV in the group of patients range from 2.5%–10%.[21] Repeat surgical commissurotomy has an operative mortality of 2.5%-10%, risk of systemic embolism ranging from 1% to 4%, and operative success and functional class improvement of 50–85%.[21]

▨ CONCLUSION

From what has been discussed above, it is evident that PMV is the procedure of choice for the management of uncomplicated and pliable mitral stenosis. Even in unfavorable situations, PMV has its place in the treatment of the disease, especially in the developing world, where facilities for MVR are limited and also where problems of anticoagulation are common. PMV may have an advantage over CMC and may be on par with OMC for a pliable valve. It is a better option than surgical mitral commissurotomy in pregnant patients. In the presence of LA thrombus, OMC is the procedure of choice for a pliable valve.

■ REFERENCES

1. Inoue K, Owaki T, Nakamura T, Kitamura F, Miyamoto N. Clinical application of transvenous mitral commissurotomy by a new balloon catheter. J Thorac Cardiovasc Surg. 1984;87(3):394–402.
2. Palacios IF. Farewell to surgical mitral commissurotomy for many patients. Circulation. 1998;97(3):223–6.
3. Palacios IF, Tuzcu ME, Weyman AE, Newell JB, Block PC. Clinical follow-up of patients undergoing percutaneous mitral balloon valvotomy. Circulation. 1995;91(3):671–6.
4. Multicenter experience with balloon mitral valvuloplasty registry report on immediate and 30-day follow-up results. The national heart, lung, and blood institute balloon valvuloplasty registry participants. Circulation 1992;85:448-61.
5. Iung B, Garbarz E, Michaud P, Helou S, Farah B, Berdah P, et al. Late results of percutaneous mitral commissurotomy in a series of 1024 patients. Analysis of late clinical deterioration: frequency, anatomic findings, and predictive factors. Circulation. 1999;99(25):3272–8.
6. Hickey MS, Blackstone EH, Kirklin JW, Dean LS. Outcome probabilities and life history after surgical mitral commissurotomy: implications for balloon commissurotomy. J Am Coll Cardiol. 1991;17(1):29–42.
7. Ben Farhat M, Boussadia H, Gandjbakhch I, Mzali H, Chouaieb A, Ayari M, et al. Closed versus open mitral commissurotomy in pure noncalcific mitral stenosis: hemodynamic studies before and after operation. J Thorac Cardiovasc Surg. 1990;99(4):639–44.
8. Nakano S, Kawashima Y, Hirose H, Matsuda H, Shirakura R, Sato S, et al. Reconsiderations of indications for open mitral commissurotomy based on pathologic features of the stenosed mitral valve. A 14-year follow-up study in 347 consecutive patients. J Thorac Cardiovasc Surg. 1987;94(3):336–42.
9. Turi ZG, Reyes VP, Raju BS, Raju AR, Kumar DN, Rajagopal P, et al. Percutaneous balloon versus surgical closed commissurotomy for mitral stenosis. A prospective, randomized trial. Circulation. 1991;83(4):1179–85.
10. Patel JJ, Shama D, Mitha AS, Blyth D, Hassen F, Le Roux BT, et al. Balloon valvuloplasty versus closed commissurotomy for pliable mitral stenosis: a prospective hemodynamic study. J Am Coll Cardiol. 1991;18(5):1318–22.
11. Ben Farhat M, Ayari M, Maatouk F, Betbout F, Gamra H, Jarra M, et al. Percutaneous balloon versus surgical closed and open mitral commissurotomy: 7-year follow-up results of a randomized trial. Circulation. 1998;97(3):245–50.
12. Cotrufo M, Renzulli A, Ismeno G, Caruso A, Mauro C, Caso P, et al. Percutaneous mitral commissurotomy versus open mitral commissurotomy: a comparative study. Eur J Cardio-Thorac Surg Off J Eur Assoc Cardio-Thorac Surg. 1999;15(5):646–651; discussion 651–652.
13. Rifaie O, Abdel-Dayem MK, Ramzy A, Ezz-El-Din H, El-Ziady G, El-Itriby A, et al. Percutaneous mitral valvotomy versus closed surgical commissurotomy. Up to 15 years of follow-up of a prospective randomized study. J Cardiol. 2009;53(1):28–34.

14. Song J-K, Kim M-J, Yun S-C, Choo SJ, Song J-M, Song H, et al. Long-term outcomes of percutaneous mitral balloon valvuloplasty versus open cardiac surgery. J Thorac Cardiovasc Surg. 2010;139(1):103–10.

15. Hameed AB, Mehra A, Rahimtoola SH. The role of catheter balloon commissurotomy for severe mitral stenosis in pregnancy. Obstet Gynecol. 2009;114(6):1336–40.

16. Pavankumar P, Venugopal P, Kaul U, Iyer KS, Das B, Sampathkumar A, et al. Closed mitral valvotomy during pregnancy. A 20-year experience. Scand J Thorac Cardiovasc Surg. 1988;22(1):11–5.

17. Detter C, Fischlein T, Feldmeier C, Nollert G, Reichenspurner H, Reichart B. Mitral commissurotomy, a technique outdated? Long-term follow-up over a period of 35 years. Ann Thorac Surg. 1999;68(6):2112–8.

18. Iung B, Garbarz E, Doutrelant L, Berdah P, Michaud P, Farah B, et al. Late results of percutaneous mitral commissurotomy for calcific mitral stenosis. Am J Cardiol. 2000;85(11):1308–14.

19. Tuzcu EM, Block PC, Griffin B, Dinsmore R, Newell JB, Palacios IF. Percutaneous mitral balloon valvotomy in patients with calcific mitral stenosis: immediate and long-term outcome. J Am Coll Cardiol. 1994;23(7):1604–9.

20. Sutaria N, Northridge DB, Shaw TR. Significance of commissural calcification on outcome of mitral balloon valvotomy. Heart Br Card Soc. 2000;84(4):398–402.

21. Nair K, Sivadasanpillai H, Sivasubramonium P, Ramachandran P, Tharakan JA, Titus T, et al. Percutaneous valvuloplasty for mitral valve restenosis: Postballoon valvotomy patients fare better than postsurgical closed valvotomy patients. Catheter Cardiovasc Interv. 2010;76(2):174–80.

Chapter 55

Mitral Regurgitation Following Percutaneous Mitral Valvotomy

Rachel Daniel, Anees Thajudeen

Since commissural splitting is the main mechanism by which the mitral valve area increases after percutaneous mitral valvotomy (PMV), mitral regurgitation (MR) is a common accompaniment following PMV. MR occurs in up to 50% patients after PMV, but in most cases the regurgitation is mild and produced by complete commissurotomy, which only minimally detracts from the hemodynamic improvement provided by the relief of mitral valve obstruction. But sometimes damage to the mitral valve apparatus during valve dilatation leads to significant mitral regurgitation. This includes valve tear, chordal rupture, valve rupture and avulsion from the mitral annulus.

■ MECHANISM OF MITRAL REGURGITATION FOLLOWING PMV

Post-PMV MR most commonly occurs at the site of successful commissural split.[1,2] Commissural MR, and the less frequently occurring anterior mitral leaflet (AML) prolapse is usually mild and of no clinical consequence.[2]

The mechanism of production of moderate MR is the same which increases mitral valve area (MVA) after PMV, i.e. splitting of tissues along the planes of the commissures.[3] Krishnamoorthy et al.[4] who followed up 590 patients, reported that stretching of the mitral valve annulus due to PMV is not likely to be a contributory factor as the size of the annulus was the same before and after PMV. In addition, they pointed out the fact that the degree of MR did not decrease within 24 hours after PMV points against annular stretching being a significant cause of MR. In contrast, severe MR following PMV is an unpredictable event[2] and is almost always due to noncommissural tearing of the anterior or posterior mitral leaflet with disruption of the valve mechanism, and less frequently, due to damage to the subvalvular apparatus, mainly chordal rupture.[5] In Manjunath series of 3855 patients[6] severe MR requiring emergency MVR (1.3%) was secondary to anterior mitral leaflet tear (72%), paracommissural tear with annular involvement (14%), posterior mitral leaflet tear (10%) and chordal tear (4%). The influence of mitral anatomy in the development of MR is still controversial and studies have failed to identify patients who subsequently developed severe MR.[5] The widely accepted

Wilkins score, although useful in patient selection for PMV and to predict the procedural success, it has been unable to predict the development of severe MR.[6,7]

With increasing experience, individuals with a valve score >8 are being frequently taken up for PMV, with acceptable symptomatic relief and hemodynamic improvement. In young adults with noncalcified MS, in addition to morphological features, none of the technical or patient characteristics studied predicted the development of MR after balloon dilatation.[8] Of all the morphological characteristics assessed by 2D-Trans Thoracic Echo, submitral disease was likely to be underestimated.

However, this cannot be the only explanation for severe MR, as many patients with significant subvalvular pathology achieve a satisfactory result with PMV. The rheumatic affection of mitral valve is not uniform. Certain areas like commissures, which normally yield to balloon pressure, may be more fibrosed and rigid and in these circumstances, areas with lesser resistance give way resulting in severe MR. Hence, a relatively thin and pliable anterior mitral leaflet becomes susceptible for tear, which is the most common etiology for severe MR.[6]

Nevertheless, certain factors have shown to be associated with the development of severe mitral regurgitation. They are: (1) mitral leaflets with nonuniform thickness, thick areas coexisting with more normal or even thin areas; (2) severe subvalvular pathology—severe and extensive fusion, thickening and foreshortening of subvalvular structures; (3) bilateral or unilateral commissural and paracommissural fibrocalcific dystrophy.[5]

Commissural and paracommissural fibrocalcific dystrophy are sites of greater resistance that hinder commissural splitting, leading to delivery of the balloon pressure to the areas with lesser resistance like the AML, which can "give way" causing it to tear.[6,9] The posterior leaflet is often rolled up and thickened, whereas a more pliable anterior leaflet becomes vulnerable (Figs 55.1 and 55.2). In the case of severely thickened and foreshortened subvalvular structures, an excessive tension might be transmitted at the insertion site of the

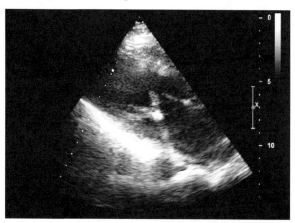

Fig. 55.1: Echocardiographic picture (PLAX view) showing tear of AML

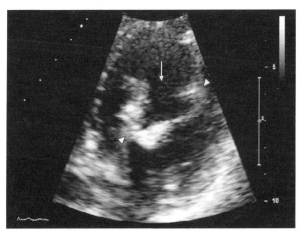

Fig. 55.2: Echocardiographic picture: Short axis view showing tear of AML.
Note the intact commissures (arrowheads)

chordae in the leaflet, which produces a leaflet tear extending from the insertion point of the leaflet to the mitral annulus. The thickening and shortening of subvalvular structures is often underestimated by echocardiography.[5] The "string-plucking effect" leading to chordal rupture and severe MR has also reported[10] (Figs 55.3A to D). Other mechanisms noted are paracommissural tears and rupture of the papillary muscle.[11]

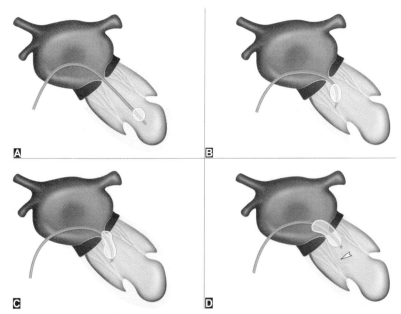

Figs 55.3A to D: The "string-plucking effect" leading to chordal rupture and severe MR
(Published with permission from Chern et al. Catheter Cardiovasc Interv. 1999;47(2):213–7)

■ INCIDENCE

The incidence of significant MR (MR 3+ or more) varied in different reports—7.5% (North American Inoue Balloon Investigators[3]), 12.4% Kim et al.[12] (long-term follow-up of 380 patients following PMV for 8 years) and 17% by Essop et al.[2]

In a series of 3650 patients from India, severe MR occurred in 120 patients (3.3%), of whom 66 (1.8%) required urgent mitral valve replacement (MVR). Echocardiography in these latter patients showed leaflet rupture in 48 (72.7%), chordal rupture in 12 (18.2%) and excessive commissural tear in six (9.1%). The same group reported that moderate MR was seen in 188 cases (5.1%), with predominant causative mechanisms of excessive commissural tear in 120 (63.8%) and chordal rupture in 68 (36.2%).[13] Chen et al. in the largest series on PMV from China reported an incidence of 1.4% of severe MR from a series of 4832 patients.[14] severe MR requiring emergency MVR was 1.3%[6] by Manjunath et al. and 1.6–3% by Fawzy et al.[15]

Both the Inoue and double-balloon techniques which obtained a similar extent of commissurotomy, was noted to produce a similar incidence of MR.[16] In a randomized comparison of Cribier's metallic commissurotome with Inoue balloon, Bhat et al. found both techniques resulted in similar grades of MR postprocedure.[17] There are some echocardiographic criteria which can predict the development of MR. The scoring system when used, found that a score of 10 or more predicted a higher chance of development of severe MR with a sensitivity of 90% and a specificity of 97% were obtained[18] (Table 55.1).

Table 55.1: Echocardiographic score for severe mitral regurgitation after percutaneous mitral valvulotomy

I-II. Valvular thickening (score each leaflet separately)
1. Leaflet near normal (4–5 mm) or with only a thick segment
2. Leaflet fibrotic and/or calcified evenly; no thin areas
3. Leaflet fibrotic and/or calcified with uneven distribution; thinner segments are mildly thickened (5–8 mm)
4. Leaflet fibrotic and/or calcified with uneven distribution; thinner segments are near normal (4–5 mm)

III. Commissural calcification
1. Fibrosis and/or calcium in only one commissure
2. Both commissures mildly affected
3. Calcium in both commissures, one markedly affected
4. Calcium in both commissures, both markedly affected

IV. Subvalvular disease
1. Minimal thickening of chordal structures just below the valve
2. Thickening of chordae extending up to one-third of chordal length
3. Thickening to the distal third of the chordae
4. Extensive thickening and shortening of all chordae extending down to the papillary muscle

The total score is the sum of these echocardiographic features (maximum 16) (Reprinted with permission from Elsevier, Padial, et al. J Am Coil Cardiology. 1996;27:1225–31)

CLINICAL COURSE OF MR

Following acute MR, the clinical manifestations were hypotension (72%), hypoxia (64%), orthopnea (14%), and pulmonary edema (12%).[6] A major hemodynamic distinction between MR in the setting of post-PMV from other causes of acute MR relates to differences in LA compliance. Hence, hemodynamic impact of severe MR following PMV will predominantly manifest in the form of low cardiac output.[2] The clinical outcome of patients with significant MR after PMV varied according to the mechanism of MR, which can be easily assessed by echocardiography immediately after PMV. The natural history can be divided as those having moderate MR due to excessive commissural split and those with severe MR.

Mechanisms of Reduction in MR

Four mechanisms have been postulated:[19]
1. Reversible mitral valve stretching by PMV.
2. Better leaflet coaptation following balloon dilation of the stenotic mitral valve.
3. Fibrosis and healing of the end of the commissures which may diminish MR which has resulted from excessive commissural splitting; and
4. Improvement in transient papillary muscle dysfunction caused by balloon trauma to the papillary muscles at the time of PMV.

Contrary to the belief 'MR begets more MR', none of the patients with moderate MR in the series reported by Krishnamoorthy et al. had increase in the degree of MR on follow-up.[4] They attributed the 76.2% decrease in the degree of MR in their series to the partial refusion and healing of the split commissures of the mitral valve. They cited the slight decrease in MVA on serial follow-up in their patients to support this hypothesis. The alternative explanations are: (1) The delayed recoil of the stretched mitral valve annulus, and (2) The improvement in the transient papillary muscle dysfunction (due to edema) caused by balloon trauma during PMV.[20,21]

While annular stretching and papillary muscle dysfunction are reversible over a short-term, excessive commissural splitting is reversible only over a long-term. Thus, the reduction in the severity of moderate MR, usually occurs over a prolonged period. It occurred over 1 year in one-fourth of the 590 patients reported by Krishnamoorthy et al.[4] Gradual resolution of MR has also been noticed in other studies-up to 9 months or upto one year.[20,23] So in view of this, MR warrants a long period of follow-up.

All this data shows that patients with moderate MR can be closely followed up. Acute MR in patients accustomed to chronic pulmonary venous hypertension, as in patients undergoing PMV, is better tolerated than in those without underlying pulmonary venous hypertension.[22] In addition, preexisting pulmonary artery hypertension and a larger LA size helps these patients to tolerate the acute hemodynamic insult better (Fig. 55.4). Even the patients with persistent moderate MR at 1-year showed symptomatic improvement.[4,22]

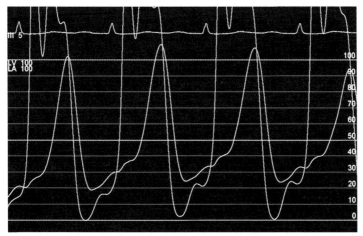

Fig. 55.4: Hemodynamic tracing in a patient who developed severe MR due to tear of AML following PMV. Note the huge "V" wave measuring more than 100 mm Hg

Kim et al.[9] noted the 8-year event-free survival rate was significantly lower in patients with significant MR than in those without (47 ± 8% versus 83 ± 3%, P<0.001) and significantly higher in patients with commissural versus noncommissural MR (63±11% versus 29 ± 11%, P<0.001). Of the 47 patients with significant MR, who were followed up for 74 ± 29 months, 19 patients (40%) underwent mitral valve replacement, and 28 patients (60%) received medical treatment only. Patients with commissural MR had a significantly lower rate of mitral valve replacement than patients with noncommissural MR (15% versus 70%, P<0.001).

Kaul et al.[13] who followed up 3650 patients following PMV, reported that 54 patients (1.5%) who developed severe MR were followed with medical treatment. Echocardiography in these patients revealed chordal rupture in 40 (74.1%) and excessive commissural tear in 14 (25.9%). Follow-up data of these patients showed that 60% required MVR at a median follow-up of 24 months and 40% remained relatively stable with NYHA class II symptoms on follow-up. Three clinical and echocardiographic variables were useful for predicting the likelihood of MVR for significant MR developing after PMV.[9]

1. Atrial fibrillation
2. Noncommissural MR
3. Higher mean mitral gradient immediately after PMV.

From these data we can reach the following consensus—Almost all valve tears will require emergency surgery. Those patients with MR due to chordal rupture and excessive commissural split, if hemodynamically stable can be followed up closely. Majority of them will end up in MVR, but 20–40% of them can be closely followed up, and may not need MVR. Moderate MR is almost always due to excessive commissural split. Almost all of them have very good prognosis and in majority, there is a slow decrease in MR.

▓ SURGICAL MANAGEMENT OF MR FOLLOWING PMV

In severe MR following PMV, the mortality is significantly high when time interval to surgery is more than 24 hours, cause being multiorgan dysfunction secondary to low cardiac output.[6] Hence, it is extremely important that patients with severe MR are taken up for surgery at the earliest, before the vicious cycle and consequences of low output manifest.

This is discussed in detail in the Chapter 19.

KEYPOINTS

- Significant mitral regurgitation following PMV occurs due to varying mechanisms.
- MR regresses in a significant number of patients on follow-up.
- Watchful waiting is only required in the majority of patients with moderate MR.
- Identifying patients who have significant damage to the valve apparatus and sending them for MVR is important.

▓ CONCLUSION

The development of significant MR does not necessarily mean failure of PMV or a grave prognosis. Clinical tolerance to the acute MR is variable, with some patients requiring emergency surgery and others not needing it and some patients experiencing a decrease in MR severity overtime. All these findings suggest that significant MR is a heterogeneous disease entity in terms of mechanisms and its clinical impact on the natural course after PMV.

▓ REFERENCES

1. Vahanian A, Iung B, Cormier B. Mitral valvuloplasty. In: Topol EL (Ed). Textbook of Interventional Cardiology. 4th edn. Philadelphia: W B Saunders; 2003. pp. 921–40.
2. Essop MR, Wisenbaugh T, Skoularigis J, Middlemost S, Sareli P. Mitral regurgitation following mitral balloon valvotomy. Differing mechanisms for severe versus mild-to-moderate lesions. J Heart Valve Dis. 1991;84:1669-79.
3. Herrmann HC, Lima JC, Feldman T, Chisholm R, Isner J, Neill WO, et al. Mechanism and outcome of severe mitral regurgitation after Inoue balloon valvuloplasty. J Am Coll Cardiol. 1993;22(3):783–9.
4. Krishnamoorthy KM, Radhakrishnan S, Shrivastava S. Natural history and predictors of moderate mitral regurgitation following balloon mitral valvuloplasty using Inoue balloon. International Journal of Cardiology. 2003; 87:31-6.
5. Hernandez R, Macaya C, Banuelos C, Alfonso F, et al. Predictors, mechanisms and outcomes of severe mitral regurgitation complicating percutaneous mitral valvotomy with Inoue balloon. Am J Cardio. 1992; 70:1169-74.
6. Nanjappa MC, Ananthakrishna R, Hemanna setty SK. Acute severe mitral regurgitation following balloon mitral valvotomy: Echocardiographic features, operative findings, and outcome in 50 surgical cases Catheterization and Cardiovascular Interventions. 2013 81:603–8 .
7. Rodriguez L, Monterroso VH, Abascal VM, King ME, O'Shea JP, Palacios IF, et al. Does asymmetric mitral valve disease predict an adverse outcome after

percutaneous balloon mitral valvotomy? An echocardiographic study. Am Heart J. 1992;123:1678–82.

8. Nair M, Agarwala R, Kalra GS, Arora R, Khalilullah M. Can mitral regurgitation after balloon dilatation of the mitral valve be predicted ? Br Heart J. 1992;67:442–4.

9. Varma PK, Theodore S, Neema PK, Ramachandran P, Sivadasanpillai H, Nair KK, et al. Emergency surgery after percutaneous transmitral commissurotomy: Operative versus echocardiographic findings, mechanism of complications and outcomes. J Thorac Cardiovasc Surg. 2005;130: 772–6.

10. Chern MS, Chang HJ, Lin FC, Wu D. String-plucking as a mechanism of chordal rupture during balloon mitral valvuloplasty using Inoue balloon catheter. Catheter Cardiovasc Interv. 1999;47(2):213–7.

11. Acar C, Deloche A, Tibi PR, Jabara V, Chachques JC, Fabiani JN, et al. Operative findings after percutaneous mitral dilation. Ann Thorac Surg. 1990; 49:959–63.

12. Mi-Jeong Kim, Jae-Kwan Song, Jong-Min Song, Duk-Hyun Kang, Young-Hak Kim, Cheol Whan Lee, et al. Long-term outcomes of significant mitral regurgitation after percutaneous mitral valvuloplasty. Circulation. 2006;114:2815–22.

13. Kaul UA, Singh S, Kalra GS, Nair M, Mohan JC, Nigam M, et al. Mitral regurgitation following percutaneous transvenous mitral commissurotomy: a single-center experience. J Heart Valve Dis. 2000;9(2):262–6; discussion 266–8.

14. Chen C, Cheng TO. For the Multicenter Study Group: Percutaneous balloon mitral valvuloplasty using Inoue technique: a multicenter study of 4832 patients in China. Am Heart J. 1995;129:1197-204.

15. Fawzy ME. Percutaneous mitral balloon valvotomy. Catheter Cardiovasc Interv. 2007;69:313-21.

16. Duk-Hyun Kang, Seong-Wook Park, Jae-Kwan Song, Hyun-Sook Kim, Myeong-Ki Hong, Jae-Joong Kim, et al. Long-term clinical and echocardiographic outcome of percutaneous mitral valvuloplasty. Randomized comparison of Inoue and double-balloon techniques. J Am Coll Cardiol. 2000;35:169-75.

17. Bhat A, Harikrishnan S, Tharakan JM, Titus T, Kumar VK, Sivasankaran S, et al. Comparison of percutaneous transmitral commissurotomy with Inoue balloon technique and metallic commissurotomy: immediate and short-term follow-up results of a randomized study. Am Heart J. 2002;144(6):1074–80.

18. Padial LR, Freitas N, Sagie A, Newell JB, Weyman AE, Levine RA, et al. Echo-cardiography can predict which patients will develop severe mitral regurgitation after percutaneous mitral valvulotomy. J Am Coll Cardiol. 1996;27(5):1225–31.

19. Tsung O Cheng. Mechanism of spontaneous diminution of mitral regurgitation following percutaneous mitral valvuloplasty with the Inoue balloon. International Journal of Cardiol. 2004;93:329.

20. Roth RB, Block PC, Palacios IF. Mitral regurgitation after percutaneous mitral valvuloplasty: Predictors and follow-up. Cathet Cardiovasc Diagn. 20 (1990). pp.17–21.

21. Palacios IF, Block PC, Wilkins GT, Weyman AE. Follow-up of patients undergoing balloon mitral valvotomy: analysis of factors determining restenosis. Circulation. 79 (1989). pp. 573–9.

22. Harrison JK, Wilson JS, Hearne SE, Bashore TM. Complications related to percutaneous transvenous mitral commissurotomy. Cathet Cardiovasc Diagn. 1994; suppl 2:52-60.

23. Pan JP, Lin SL, Go JU, Hsu TL, Chen CY, Wang SP, et al. Frequency and severity of mitral regurgitation 1 year after balloon mitral valvuloplasty. Am J Cardiol. 67 (1991). pp. 264–8.

Chapter 56

Atrial Septal Defects Following Percutaneous Mitral Valvotomy

Harikrishnan S, Kiron Sukulal

In percutaneous mitral valvotomy, often the procedure is done through the transseptal approach in which the septum is punctured and later dilated with a 12–14 French dilator to facilitate passage of the balloon. This occasionally leaves a defect in the atrial septum—iatrogenic ASD or iASD.

In a review series of 10 publications on iatrogenic ASDs, Mc Ginty et al.[1] found that the immediate postprocedural incidence of iASD was as high as 87%, with decreased incidence of residual iASD detected over time. At 18 months of follow-up, up to 15% of iASD cases persisted. Residual iASDs were not associated with clinical sequelae of embolism, cyanosis, or right heart failure.[1]

Korkmaz et al. in a study of patients who had PMV, concluded that the presence of persistent iatrogenic atrial septal defects might not be predicted from echocardiographic or demographic data in patients undergoing percutaneous mitral balloon valvuloplasty. Fortunately, these defects are small in size and low in shunt ratio. They appear not to be associated with serious long-term outcomes.[2]

The incidence of left to right shunting through this iatrogenic ASD has been reported to vary from 16% to 89% depending on the modality used to detect this.[3-5] The defects seem to close spontaneously or the magnitude of the shunt comes down.[6] Smith et al. in a series reporting the data of 30 patients who underwent mitraclip repair, suggested that increased LA pressure may be a mechanism for persistent iASD.[7]

These iatrogenic ASDs invariably shunt from left to right with very little chance of right to left shunt as reported in the literature (Fig. 56.1).[8] In a series of 253 patients who underwent transseptal catheterization using a 12 F sheath (similar to the size of the Inoue balloon), Singh et al. found that the interatrial shunting was predominantly left-to-right when an iASD was present. There was no significant difference in the rate of stroke and/or systemic embolism during the follow-up period in patients with or without iASD.[9]

The left to right shunting especially in the case of PMV is because there will be some gradient persisting across the mitral valve leading to high left atrial pressure which leads to a left to right shunt. The left to right shunt can increase in the presence of mitral regurgitation (Fig. 56.2). One exception to

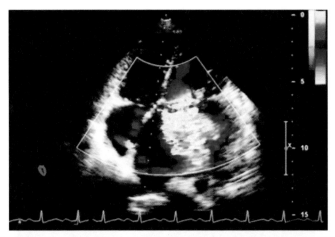

Fig. 56.1: Left to right shunt through the iatrogenic ASD following PMV

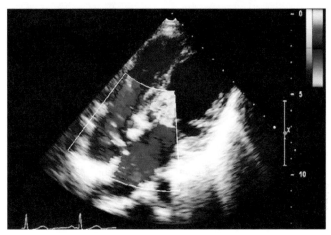

Fig. 56.2: Moderate-to-severe MR following PMV.
ASD shunting left to right is seen

the situation is the presence of severe tricuspid regurgitation which can lead to a higher pressure in the right atrium leading to right to left shunt.[10]

Rarely right to left shunts can occur through the iatrogenic ASD with embolic complications. Harikrishnan et al. has reported a 45-year-old female who presented with transient ischemic attack 4 months following PMV. She was found to have an iatrogenic ASD probably thought to be responsible for the right to left shunt. During TEE, she was found to have intermittent right to left shunt in between continuous L–R shunt (Fig. 56.3). She was in sinus rhythm and mitral stenosis was only mild and she did not have significant tricuspid regurgitation.[11]

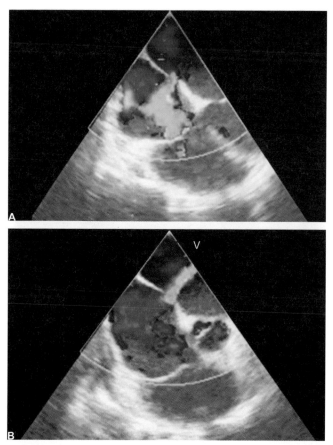

Figs 56.3A and B: TEE images showing left to right shunt (A) and transient right to left shunt a few moments later (B) (Published with permission from Harikrishnan S et al. J Am Soc Echocardiogr. 2005;18:183-4)

Abernethy et al. reported a case of a 45-year-old woman who underwent successful percutaneous mitral balloon valvuloplasty for rheumatic mitral valve stenosis, but had an immediate postprocedural course complicated by refractory migraine headaches. Interestingly, resolution of her headaches coincided with the spontaneous closure of the interatrial communication created during valvuloplasty. This suggests interatrial flow as an important trigger for migraine headaches in this patient.[12]

There is controversy about the initiation of OAC in patients with persistent ASD and demonstrable right to left shunt. Since patients in AF will be on anticoagulants, the patients in SR and persistent large ASDs are the patient group in question. We require more data to get an answer to this question.[13]

REFERENCES

1. McGinty PM, Smith TW, Rogers JH. Transseptal left heart catheterization and the incidence of persistent iatrogenic atrial septal defects. J Intervent Cardiol. 2011;24(3):254–63.
2. Korkmaz S, Demirkan B, Guray Y, Yilmaz MB, Sasmaz H. Long-term follow-up of iatrogenic atrial septal defect: after percutaneous mitral balloon valvuloplasty. Tex Heart Inst J Tex Heart Inst St Lukes Episcop Hosp Tex Child Hosp. 2011;38(5):523–7.
3. Arora R, Jolly N, Kalra GS, Khalilullah M. Atrial septal defect after balloon mitral valvuloplasty: a transesophageal echocardiographic study. Angiology. 1993;44(3):217–21.
4. Casale P, Block PC, O'Shea JP, Palacios IF. Atrial septal defect after percutaneous mitral balloon valvuloplasty: immediate results and follow-up. J Am Coll Cardiol. 1990;15(6):1300–4.
5. Arora R, Trehan V. Iatrogenic atrial septal defect following balloon mitral valvuloplasty. Indian Heart J. 1996;48(1):19–22.
6. Cequier A, Bonan R, Serra A, Dyrda I, Crépeau J, Dethy M, et al. Left-to-right atrial shunting after percutaneous mitral valvuloplasty. Incidence and long-term hemodynamic follow-up. Circulation. 1990;81(4):1190–7.
7. Smith T, McGinty P, Bommer W, Low RI, Lim S, Fail P, et al. Prevalence and echocardiographic features of iatrogenic atrial septal defect after catheter-based mitral valve repair with the MitraClip system. Catheter Cardiovasc Interv Off J Soc Card Angiogr Interv. 2012;80(4):678–85.
8. Kronzon I, Tunick PA, Goldfarb A, Freedberg RS, Chinitz L, Slater J, et al. Echocardiographic and hemodynamic characteristics of atrial septal defects created by percutaneous valvuloplasty. J Am Soc Echocardiogr Off Publ Am Soc Echocardiogr. 1990;3(1):64–71.
9. Singh SM, Douglas PS, Reddy VY. The incidence and long-term clinical outcome of iatrogenic atrial septal defects secondary to transseptal catheterization with a 12F transseptal sheath. Circ Arrhythm Electrophysiol. 2011;4(2):166–71.
10. Lai LP, Shyu KG, Hsu KL, Chiang FT, Tseng CD, Tseng YZ. Bidirectional shunt through a residual atrial septal defect after percutaneous transvenous mitral commissurotomy. Cardiology. 1993;83(3):205–7.
11. Harikrishnan S, Titus T, Tharakan JM. Septal defects after percutaneous mitral valvotomy—all are not innocent. J Am Soc Echocardiogr Off Publ Am Soc Echocardiogr. 2005;18(2):183–4.
12. Abernethy A, Ruiz-Rodriguez E, Krasuski RA. Migraine headaches following mitral valvuloplasty: Koch's postulates finally satisfied? J Invasive Cardiol. 2013;25(6):E120–123.
13. Harikrishnan S, Nair K, Tharakan J. Persisting iatrogenic atrial septal defect after transseptal procedures--what should be done? Am Heart J. 2007;153(3):e9; author reply e11.

Chapter 57

Pulmonary Hypertension in Rheumatic Mitral Stenosis— Influence of Percutaneous Mitral Valvotomy

Harikrishnan S, Chandrasekharan C Kartha

■ INTRODUCTION

Rheumatic heart disease (RHD) continues to be a major public health problem in the developing world.[1] RHD occurs as a sequel to an autoimmune response of cardiac tissues to *Streptococcus* throat infection. Common clinical manifestations of RHD are secondary to chronic valvulitis that leads to mitral, aortic, or tricuspid valve deformities.

Pulmonary hypertension (PH) is known to complicate both aortic and mitral valve disease.[2-4] It is reported to occur in about 70% of patients with RHD[5] and is a prognostic variable affecting the course of the disease.[4,6,7] In this review, we will discuss the clinical implications of pulmonary hypertension in mitral stenosis (MS) and the effect of percutaneous mitral valvotomy (PMV). Pulmonary hypertension associated with left heart disease is classified under Group II in the WHO classification.

Pathogenesis of PH in RHD

The left-sided rheumatic valvular pathology over a period of time results in pulmonary venous hypertension followed by pulmonary arterial hypertension (Fig. 57.1). Compared to patients with primary forms of PHT, those secondary to valvular heart disease (VHD) have significantly elevated pulmonary artery pressure and pulmonary vascular resistance, but lesser cardiac output.[8]

Evaluation of PH in RHD

In addition to the findings of valvular lesions, clinical examination in patients with PH may reveal left parasternal lift, loud pulmonary component of the second heart sound and the murmur of tricuspid regurgitation. Chest Roentgenogram may show dilated pulmonary arteries (Fig. 57.2). ECG may show right ventricular hypertrophy and right atrial enlargement (Fig. 57.3).

This article is modified with permission from Medknow Publications, Bombay, India from the article, S Harikrishnan, Chandrasekharan C Kartha. Pulmonary hypertension in rheumatic heart disease, PVRI Review. 2011;1(1):13-17.

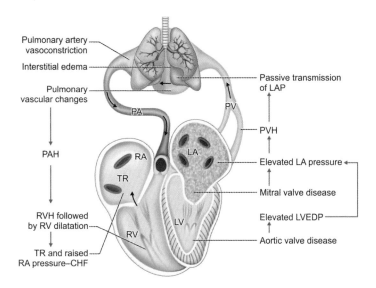

Fig. 57.1: Pathophysiology of PHT in valvular heart disease

Abbreviations: LV, left ventricle; LVEDP, left ventricular end-diastolic pressure; LA, left atrial; PVH, pulmonary venous hypertension; LAP, left atrial pressure; PV, pulmonary veins; PA, pulmonary artery; PAH, pulmonary arterial hypertension; RVH, right ventricular hypertrophy; RV, right ventricular; TR, tricuspid regurgitation; RA, right atrium; CHF, congestive heart failure) (Published with permission from Medknow Publications, Bombay, India from the article, S Harikrishnan, Chandrasekharan C Kartha, Pulmonary hypertension in rheumatic heart disease, PVRI Review. 2011;1(1):13–17

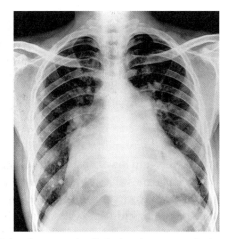

Fig. 57.2: Left atrial enlargement, dilated pulmonary arteries, pulmonary venous hypertension, pulmonary hemosiderosis seen in the chest X-ray of a patient with severe MS (Published with permission from Medknow Publications, Bombay, India from the article, Harikrishnan S et al. PVRI Review. 2011;1(1):13–17)

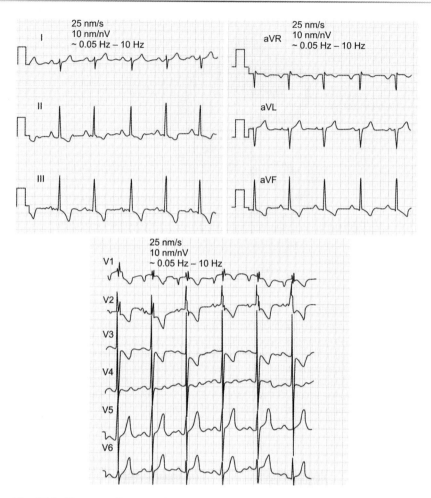

Fig. 57.3: Electrocardiogram of a patient with Juvenile MS. Biatrial enlargement, right axis deviation, incomplete right bundle branch block and right ventricular hypertrophy can be seen (Published with permission from Medknow Publications, Bombay, India from the article, Harikrishnan S et al. PVRI Review. 2011;1(1):13–17)

Echocardiography is the primary modality to assess PH in MS. It has the convenience of easy availability and lower costs. It has also got the advantage that, simultaneous assessment of the valves, chambers and ventricular function is possible. With echocardiography we can assess the size of the right ventricle and also the ventricular function. Indirect assessment of pulmonary artery pressure can be obtained from the jet of tricuspid regurgitation (Fig. 57.4) and also from the peak pulmonary regurgitation pressure.[9] Pulmonary artery systolic pressure lesser than 50 mm Hg is defined as moderate and greater than 50 is termed severe PH.[10]

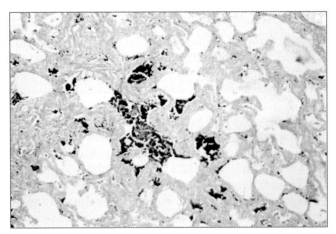

Fig. 57.4: Photomicrograph of hemosiderosis in lung tissue in a patient with mitral stenosis—Prussian Blue stain X200 (Published with permission from Medknow Publications, Bombay, India from the article, Harikrishnan S et al. PVRI Review. 2011;1(1):13–17)

But we should realize the fact that, due to its complex shape and orientation it is difficult to evaluate the right ventricle using a two-dimensional (2D) cross-sectional imaging modality like echocardiography. Cardiovascular magnetic resonance imaging (CMR) is a virtually three-dimensional (3D) tomographic technique which has entered the mainstream of clinical cardiovascular imaging over the last decade.

Compared to other imaging methods, CMR allows the accurate quantification of RV volumes, myocardial mass, and transvalvular flow with the added benefit of tissue characterization and without the use of ionizing radiation.[11,12] With CMR it will be possible to confirm the increased RV mass in patients with PH. Myocardial delayed contrast enhancement occurs frequently in patients with severe symptomatic pulmonary artery hypertension and is inversely related to measures of right ventricular systolic function.[13]

The role of CMR as a tool to evaluate RV morphology and function in patients with PH is increasingly being recognized. It can also be used as a tool to follow-up patients with PH.[10]

CT imaging can be useful in a variety of selected situations, when there is need for cross-sectional imaging in patients with pacemakers and old generation mechanical heart valves that preclude MR.

The other modality to assess PH in RHD is cardiac catheterization. But the problem is the availability, costs, radiation and expertise to perform accurate assessment of intracardiac pressures. We should also realize the limitation of cineangiogram in assessing RV function.

So among the modalities available for assessment of PH in RHD, echocardiography may have an edge over CMR and catheterization, taking into account the costs and availability in developing countries where the problem of RHD is endemic.

PH IN RHEUMATIC MITRAL VALVE DISEASE

Pulmonary hypertension, a frequent complication of rheumatic mitral valve disease[14] is known to be associated with both rheumatic mitral valve stenosis (MS) and mitral regurgitation[5] (MR). PH influences the natural history of the disease, affects the response to treatments and also the postintervention prognosis.[6,7]

Pulmonary hypertension in patients with rheumatic mitral valve stenosis is often out of proportion to the degree of left atrial hypertension.[14] The main mechanisms contributing to the development of pulmonary hypertension in patients with MS is given in Table 57.1 and illustrated in Figure 57.1.

All the above-mentioned factors protect the pulmonary capillaries from the surge of blood passing into them during physical activity and thus, from developing pulmonary congestion. As pulmonary hypertension progressively increases, right ventricular dilation, and congestive heart failure (CHF) ensue. RV dilatation can lead to the development of functional tricuspid regurgitation, which will worsen congestive heart failure.

Paul Wood[2] noted that severe PH was associated with both moderately severe and severe MS. Fawzy[14] and Rebeiro[15] pointed out that there is another group of patients with severe MS, yet only a mild increase in pulmonary arterial pressure. The reasons for the nondevelopment of PH in such instances are not clear.[16] No significant relation between left atrial size and pulmonary artery pressure (PAP) has been noted.[16] There is a view that left atrial enlargement may "cushion of" the sequelae of increase in pressure.[16]

Pulmonary hypertension in rheumatic mitral stenosis adversely affects long-term prognosis.[6,7] Bahl et al.[17] and Krishnamoorthy[18] et al. have observed that PH is an indicator of disease severity in patients with MS (Table 57.2). Chronicity of the disease process as indicated by the presence of severe fibrosis[16] and atrial fibrillation (AF)[18] is important in the development of reactive PH.[16]

Pathological Findings

The pathological changes in lungs in rheumatic mitral stenosis include prominent vascular and parenchymal changes. Pulmonary veins develop muscular media. Moderate to marked medial hypertrophy is seen in medium-sized branches of the pulmonary arteries. Dilation lesions and plexiform lesions

---

Table 57.1: Mechanisms responsible for the development of PH in valvular heart disease

1. Passive retrograde transmission of elevated left atrial and pulmonary venous pressure into the pulmonary arterial vasculature

2. Reactive pulmonary arteriolar vasoconstriction induced by pulmonary venous hypertension[22,23]—typically occurring when the left atrial pressure (LAP) is chronically elevated to more 20 mm Hg[16]

3. Interstitial edema

4. Induced morphological changes in the pulmonary vasculature[14,24]

Table 57.2: Features indicating severity of disease in patients with mitral valve disease complicated by PHT

1. Severe subvalvular pathology
2. Higher symptom status
3. Higher transmitral valve gradients
4. Smaller mitral valve area
5. Higher pulmonary vascular resistance (PVR)
6. Higher Wilkins' echocardiographic score
7. More fibrotic valves (poor splitability during BMV as indicated by the need for larger balloons)
8. Higher residual gradients and smaller mitral valve area despite normalized left atrial pressure after BMV
9. A higher incidence of atrial fibrillation

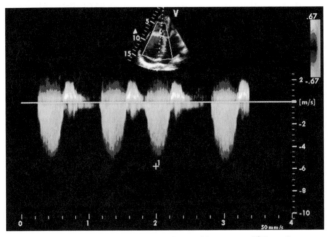

Fig. 57.5: Echocardiographic picture of a patient with severe MS and severe PHT. The estimated RV systolic pressure—measured from tricuspid regurgitation jet is 133 mm Hg (Published with permission from Medknow Publications, Bombay, India from the article, S Harikrishnan et al. PVRI Review. 2011;1(1):13–17)

are rarely reported in rheumatic MS. Tandon[19] and Chopra[20] et al. have reported such lesions in 4% of their autopsy studies conducted at New Delhi, India. Mubeen[21] et al. recently reported that pulmonary vascular changes do not go beyond grade 3 (Heath and Edwards) in RHD. The most striking parenchymal change is the prominent smooth muscle layers in the bronchoalveolar walls. The extent and severity of both vascular and parenchymal changes are more marked in juvenile patients. Hemosiderosis may be visible in long standing disease (Fig. 57.5).

Treatment Options and Effect of Treatments

Patients with mitral valvular disease and PH are started on heart-rate reducing drugs (beta-blockers or calcium channel blockers) and diuretics once they become symptomatic. The reduction in heart rate will indirectly bring down the PAP by lessening the transmitral valve gradient. Digoxin is traditionally prescribed in developing countries for dilated and failing RV which pumps against a hypertensive pulmonary vascular bed. However, there are no major studies addressing the role of digoxin in RHD.

Pulmonary hypertension usually regresses once the gradient across the mitral valve is relieved by either mitral valve replacement (MVR)[25,26] or valvotomy.[15-18,24] Hemodynamic studies in patients who underwent MVR have demonstrated a reversibility of pulmonary arterial hypertension.[25]

Balloon mitral valvotomy (BMV) has now become the treatment of choice in patients with pliable mitral valve. Nevertheless, BMV is reportedly to be technically difficult in patients with PH[27] (Table 57.3). The presence of significant PH is an indication to perform BMV in patients with moderate or severe MS[9] as per the latest recommendation by AHA (Table 57.4).

Balloon mitral valvotomy is found to give excellent and comparable results in all grades of PH.[14,28] Bahl[17] et al. found similar efficacy in patients with suprasystemic PA pressure and in those with lesser grades of PH. It is noteworthy that another Indian study found that mitral valve area after BMV remained lesser in patients with severe PH despite a greater absolute decrease in pulmonary artery pressures and resistance.[18]

Table 57.3: Technical challenges for performing BMV in MS and PH[27]

1. Less tolerance to the stress of the procedure because of the precarious hemo-dynamics
2. Transseptal puncture being difficult given the larger right sided chambers
3. Tighter stenosis, leading to difficulty for the balloon to cross the valve
4. Susceptibility to tearing of the valve and development of mitral regurgitation

Table 57.4: AHA 2008 recommendation for BMV in patients with PH[10]

Class I
Percutaneous mitral balloon valvotomy is effective for asymptomatic patients with moderate or severe MS and valve morphology that is favorable for percutaneous mitral balloon valvotomy who have pulmonary hypertension (pulmonary artery systolic pressure greater than 50 mm Hg at rest or greater than 60 mm Hg with exercise) in the absence of left atrial thrombus or moderate to severe MR. (*Level of Evidence*: C)
Class IIB
Percutaneous mitral balloon valvotomy may be considered for symptomatic patients (NYHA functional class II, III, or IV) with MV area greater than 1.5 cm² if there is evidence of hemodynamically significant MS based on pulmonary artery systolic pressure greater than 60 mm Hg, pulmonary artery wedge pressure of 25 mm Hg or more, or mean MV gradient greater than 15 mm Hg during exercise. (*Level of Evidence*: C)

◼ EFFECT OF BALLOON MITRAL VALVOTOMY ON PH

Fawzy[14] and others[15-18,24] have shown that in patients with mild PH, the pulmonary artery systolic pressure (PASP) and the pulmonary vascular resistance (PVR) decreased to normal or near-normal levels immediately after a successful BMV. On the contrary, in patients with moderate or severe pulmonary hypertension[14] despite greater absolute and relative reductions, PASP and PVR remained significantly elevated.

Analyzing the hemodynamic data at 3 and 12 months following BMV, Dev and Shrivastava[29] concluded that passive pulmonary hypertension regressed immediately after BMV, and was equivalent to reduction in pulmonary capillary wedge pressure. Pulmonary artery pressure decreased steadily over one week and that reduction temporally coincided with the decrease in PVR. Most of the reduction in PVR occurred in the first week following BMV, following which reductions were very minimal.[29] On the contrary, Umesan[29] and Fawzy[14] et al. (at follow-up of 33 months and 4 years respectively) found a sustained fall in pulmonary artery pressure following BMV.

Two of the three major factors responsible for PH in mitral stenosis—left atrial hypertension and pulmonary arteriolar constriction are reversible. Left atrial hypertension related PH regresses immediately after BMV. PHT contributed by PVR or pulmonary vasoconstriction decreases slowly on follow-up. Pulmonary vascular disease, the irreversible component is the one that leads to "fixed VR".[18,24]

Krishnamoorthy et al. found the gain in mitral valve area was not predictive of decrease in mean PAP.[18] Lack of association between relief of mitral obstruction and improvement in pulmonary hemodynamics is reported by others as well.[16,30]

Fawzy[31] found that on follow-up, the PAP and PVR normalized in many patients who had optimal BMV results. In contrast, no such improvement was noted in patients with suboptimal BMV results (MVA <1.5 cm^2 or MR grade >2). Occurrence or worsening of the degree of mitral regurgitation following BMV is a factor, which can cause a gradual increase in PVR over the next 3–12 months following BMV.[26] Presence of significant shunt through an iatrogenic ASD is another factor that may retard the regression of PH following a successful BMV. Development of restenosis could lead to the return of pulmonary pressure even to the premitral valve dilatation values.[18,32]

Despite adequate relief of mitral valve obstruction, persistently abnormal PVR, in the absence of restenosis or other significant valvular or myocardial diseases, is attributed to fixed PVR. Since patients with fixed PVR have a poorer prognosis than those with normalized PVR,[33] identification of such patients are important.

Gamra[24] found that persistently abnormal PVR could be predicted by baseline clinical and hemodynamic characteristics. PVR was most likely to remain abnormal in older patients and in those with the pre-BMV characteristics, such as higher Wilkins' echo score, smaller mitral valve area and higher mean pulmonary artery pressure. The presence of a pulmonary bed gradient (mean pulmonary artery pressure—mean left atrial pressure >12 mm Hg), shown to be an indicator of reactive pulmonary hypertension is a useful predictor of persistently high PVR. To prevent the fixed PVR stage, an early intervention, as recommended by Pan et al.[34] and by Ribeiro[15] et al. would be justified. It is reported that assessing the response of pulmonary artery pressure to inhalation of nitric oxide during cardiac catheterization can be useful to divorce fixed from reversible pulmonary hypertension.[23]

Juvenile Mitral Stenosis

In developing countries like India, 25% of the patients with MS are less than of 20 years of age. Roy et al.[35] named this entity as juvenile mitral stenosis. The characteristic features are gross pulmonary vascular changes leading to severe pulmonary artery hypertension and critical stenosis of the mitral valve with normal cardiac output.[36] In a cohort of 1112 patients with juvenile MS, Roy et al.[36] found that 70% had moderate or severe pulmonary hypertension. Lung biopsy revealed grade III/IV changes of pulmonary hypertension in pulmonary arteries, with muscle bands in the terminal bronchi. In a group of patients undergoing BMV, Joseph[37] et al. reported that children were found to have higher pulmonary artery pressure compared to adults.

Juvenile patients with MS have good outcomes following closed mitral valvotomy (CMV)[38] and BMV.[37,39] Both after CMV and BMV early and sustained drop in PAP on follow-up have been observed.[40,41]

PERSISTENT PULMONARY ARTERY HYPERTENSION FOLLOWING PMV

Persistent pulmonary artery hypertension (PPAH) [defined by pulmonary artery systolic pressure (PASP) of ≥ 40 mm Hg at one year following BMV] was seen in 40% patients as reported from SCTIMST by Nair et al. in a series of 701 patients.[42] Patients with PPAH were older, sicker, and had advanced mitral valve disease. Those patients had higher incidence of restenosis and need for reinterventions on long-term follow-up. PPAH represents an advanced stage of rheumatic valve disease and indicates chronicity of the disease, which may be the reason for the poorer prognosis of these patients. Patients with PPAH requires intense and more frequent follow-up.

■ CONCLUSION

Pulmonary hypertension is a very common accompaniment of rheumatic valvular heart disease. It is a prognostic variable affecting the natural history of the disease in patients with mitral valve stenosis. It affects the response to balloon mitral valvotomy. PH also influences the postintervention prognosis.

■ REFERENCES

1. Rheumatic fever and rheumatic heart disease. World Health Organ Tech Rep Ser. 2004;923:1–122.
2. Wood P. An appreciation of mitral stenosis. Br Med J. 1954;i:1051–63 and 1113–24.
3. Evans W, Short DS. Pulmonary hypertension in mitral stenosis. Br Heart J. 1957;19(4):457–72.
4. Malouf JF, Enriquez-Sarano M, Pellikka PA, Oh JK, Bailey KR, Chandrasekaran K, et al. Severe pulmonary hypertension in patients with severe aortic valve stenosis: clinical profile and prognostic implications. J Am Coll Cardiol. 2002;40(4):789–95.

5. Sani MU, Karaye KM, Borodo MM. Prevalence and pattern of rheumatic heart disease in the Nigerian savannah: an echocardiographic study. Cardiovasc J Afr. 2007;18(5):295-9.

6. Walston A, Peter RH, Morris JJ, Kong Y, Behar VS. Clinical implications of pulmonary hypertension in mitral stenosis. Am J Cardiol. 1973;32(5):650-5.

7. Ward C, Hancock BW. Extreme pulmonary hypertension caused by mitral valve disease. Natural history and results of surgery. Br Heart J. 1975;37(1):74-8.

8. Radulescu D, Pripon S, Duncea C, Constantea NA, Gulei I. Conventional radiology and right heart catheterization in estimating primary pulmonary hypertension and pulmonary hypertension secondary to left-sided valvular disease. Acta Medica Indones. 2008;40(1):24-8.

9. McLure LER, Peacock AJ. Imaging of the heart in pulmonary hypertension. Int J Clin Pract Suppl. 2007;(156):15-26.

10. Bonow RO, Carabello BA, Chatterjee K, de Leon AC Jr, Faxon DP, Freed MD, et al. 2008 Focused update incorporated into the ACC/AHA 2006 guidelines for the management of patients with valvular heart disease: a report of the American College of Cardiology/American Heart Association Task Force on Practice Guidelines (Writing Committee to Revise the 1998 Guidelines for the Management of Patients With Valvular Heart Disease): endorsed by the Society of Cardiovascular Anesthesiologists, Society for Cardiovascular Angiography and Interventions, and Society of Thoracic Surgeons. Circulation. 2008;118(15):e523-661.

11. Marcu CB, Beek AM, Van Rossum AC. Cardiovascular magnetic resonance imaging for the assessment of right heart involvement in cardiac and pulmonary disease. Heart Lung Circ. 2006;15(6):362-70.

12. Benza R, Biederman R, Murali S, Gupta H. Role of cardiac magnetic resonance imaging in the management of patients with pulmonary arterial hypertension. J Am Coll Cardiol. 2008;52(21):1683-92.

13. McCann GP, Gan CT, Beek AM, Niessen HWM, Vonk Noordegraaf A, van Rossum AC. Extent of MRI delayed enhancement of myocardial mass is related to right ventricular dysfunction in pulmonary artery hypertension. AJR Am J Roentgenol. 2007;188(2):349-55.

14. Fawzy ME, Hassan W, Stefadouros M, Moursi M, El Shaer F, Chaudhary MA. Prevalence and fate of severe pulmonary hypertension in 559 consecutive patients with severe rheumatic mitral stenosis undergoing mitral balloon valvotomy. J Heart Valve Dis. 2004;13(6):942-47; discussion 947-48.

15. Ribeiro PA, al Zaibag M, Abdullah M. Pulmonary artery pressure and pulmonary vascular resistance before and after mitral balloon valvotomy in 100 patients with severe mitral valve stenosis. Am Heart J. 1993;125(4):1110-4.

16. Otto CM, Davis KB, Reid CL, Slater JN, Kronzon I, Kisslo KB, et al. Relation between pulmonary artery pressure and mitral stenosis severity in patients undergoing balloon mitral commissurotomy. Am J Cardiol. 1993;71(10):874-8.

17. Bahl VK, Chandra S, Talwar KK, Kaul U, Sharma S, Wasir HS. Balloon mitral valvotomy in patients with systemic and suprasystemic pulmonary artery pressures. Cathet Cardiovasc Diagn. 1995;36(3):211-5.

18. Krishnamoorthy KM, Dash PK, Radhakrishnan S, Shrivastava S. Response of different grades of pulmonary artery hypertension to balloon mitral valvuloplasty. Am J Cardiol. 2002;90(10):1170-3.

19. Tandon HD, Kasturi J. Pulmonary vascular changes associated with isolated mitral stenosis in India. Br Heart J. 1975;37(1):26-36.

20. Chopra P, Bhatia ML. Chronic rheumatic heart disease in India: a reappraisal of pathologic changes. J Heart Valve Dis. 1992;1(1):92-101.

21. Mubeen M, Singh AK, Agarwal SK, Pillai J, Kapoor S, Srivastava AK. Mitral valve replacement in severe pulmonary arterial hypertension. Asian Cardiovasc Thorac Ann. 2008;16(1):37–42.

22. Wood P, Besterman EM, Towers MK, Mcilroy MB. The effect of acetylcholine on pulmonary vascular resistance and left atrial pressure in mitral stenosis. Br Heart J. 1957;19(2):279–86.

23. Mahoney PD, Loh E, Blitz LR, Herrmann HC. Hemodynamic effects of inhaled nitric oxide in women with mitral stenosis and pulmonary hypertension. Am J Cardiol. 2001;87(2):188–92.

24. Gamra H, Zhang HP, Allen JW, Lou FY, Ruiz CE. Factors determining normalization of pulmonary vascular resistance following successful balloon mitral valvotomy. Am J Cardiol. 1999;83(3):392–5.

25. Braunwald E, Braunwald NS, Ross J Jr, Morrow AG. Effects of mitral-valve replacement on the pulmonary vascular dynamics of patients with pulmonary hypertension. N Engl J Med. 1965;273:509–14.

26. Zener JC, Hancock EW, Shumway NE, Harrison DC. Regression of extreme pulmonary hypertension after mitral valve surgery. Am J Cardiol. 1972;30(8):820–6.

27. Wisenbaugh T, Essop R, Middlemost S, Skoularigis J, Röthlisberger C, Skudicky D, et al. Effects of severe pulmonary hypertension on outcome of balloon mitral valvotomy. Am J Cardiol. 1992;70(7):823–5.

28. Umesan CV, Kapoor A, Sinha N, Kumar AS, Goel PK. Effect of Inoue balloon mitral valvotomy on severe pulmonary arterial hypertension in 315 patients with rheumatic mitral stenosis: immediate and long-term results. J Heart Valve Dis. 2000;9(5):609–15.

29. Dev V, Shrivastava S. Time course of changes in pulmonary vascular resistance and the mechanism of regression of pulmonary arterial hypertension after balloon mitral valvuloplasty. Am J Cardiol. 1991;67(5):439–42.

30. Block PC, Palacios IF. Pulmonary vascular dynamics after percutaneous mitral valvotomy. J Thorac Cardiovasc Surg. 1988;96(1):39–43.

31. Fawzy ME, Mimish L, Sivanandam V, Lingamanaicker J, Patel A, Khan B, et al. Immediate and long-term effect of mitral balloon valvotomy on severe pulmonary hypertension in patients with mitral stenosis. Am Heart J. 1996;131(1):89–93.

32. Levine MJ, Weinstein JS, Diver DJ, Berman AD, Wyman RM, Cunningham MJ, et al. Progressive improvement in pulmonary vascular resistance after percutaneous mitral valvuloplasty. Circulation. 1989;79(5):1061–7.

33. Emanuel R. Valvotomy in mitral stenosis with extreme pulmonary vascular resistance. Br Heart J. 1963;25(1):119–25.

34. Pan M, Medina A, Suarez de Lezo J, Romero M, Hernandez E, Segura J, et al. Balloon valvuloplasty for mild mitral stenosis. Cathet Cardiovasc Diagn. 1991;24(1):1–5.

35. Roy SB, Bhatia ML, Lazaro EJ, Ramalingaswami V. Juvenile mitral stenosis in India. Lancet. 1963;2(7319):1193–5.

36. Roy SB. Proceedings: Challenge of juvenile mitral stenosis in India. Jpn Circ J. 1975;39(2):198.

37. Joseph PK, Bhat A, Francis B, Sivasankaran S, Kumar A, Pillai VR, et al. Percutaneous transvenous mitral commissurotomy using an Inoue balloon in children with rheumatic mitral stenosis. Int J Cardiol. 1997;62(1):19–22.

38. Dias F, Fletcher AG Jr, Mody SM, Padhi RK. Closed valvotomy in juvenile mitral stenosis. Can Med Assoc J. 1968;99(15):746–51.

39. Fawzy ME, Stefadouros M, El Amraoui S, Osman A, Ibrahim I, Nowayhed O, et al. Long-term (up to 18 years) clinical and echocardiographic results of mitral balloon valvuloplasty in children in comparison with adult population. J Intervent Cardiol. 2008;21(3):252–9.

40. Fawzy ME, Stefadouros MA, Hegazy H, Shaer FE, Chaudhary MA, Fadley FA. Long-term clinical and echocardiographic results of mitral balloon valvotomy in children and adolescents. Heart Br Card Soc. 2005;91(6):743–8.

41. Harikrishnan S, Nair K, Tharakan JM, Titus T, Kumar VK, Sivasankaran S. Percutaneous transmitral commissurotomy in juvenile mitral stenosis—comparison of long-term results of Inoue balloon technique and metallic commissurotomy. Catheter Cardiovasc Interv. 2006;67(3):453–9.

42. Nair KKM, Pillai HS, Titus T, Varaparambil A, Sivasankaran S, Krishnamoorthy KM, et al. Persistent pulmonary artery hypertension in patients undergoing balloon mitral valvotomy. Pulm Circ. 2013;3(2):426–31.

Chapter 58

Long-term Follow-up of Patients Undergoing Percutaneous Mitral Valvotomy

Rachel Daniel

■ INTRODUCTION

Several prospective studies have demonstrated the efficacy of PMV and found it to be comparable or better than surgical commissurotomy in terms of improvement in hemodynamics and betterment of functional status.[1]

Restenosis rates were also comparable between the two treatment modalities (25% in PMV and 27% in Closed surgical commissurotomy) at up to 15 years of follow-up.[2] Event-free survival after successful PMV ranges from 30% to 70% after 10–20 years, depending on patient characteristics.[3-5] Long-term results can be predicted by preoperative valve morphology and clinical characteristics, and the quality of the immediate results.[3,4,6] So the selection of patients for the procedure becomes of utmost importance.

Factors Affecting Long-term Prognosis after PMV

The major factors are:
1. Immediate postprocedure valve area and transvalvular gradients
2. Age
3. Unfavorable valve anatomy (Wilkins echocardiographic score >8)
4. History of previous commissurotomy
5. High NYHA class
6. Atrial fibrillation
7. Pulmonary hypertension
8. Severe tricuspid regurgitation
9. Increase in mitral regurgitation by two grades following PMV.

Symptom Benefit Following PMV

Symptomatic improvement occurs almost immediately after a successful PMV, although objective measurement of maximum oxygen consumption may continue to improve over several months owing to the gradual improvement in skeletal muscle metabolism.[7] Patients with Wilkins echocardiographic scores <8 had significantly greater actuarial survival, freedom from mitral valve replacement (MVR), and event-free survival rates than those patients with echocardiographic scores >8.[8]

Recurrent symptoms after successful surgical commissurotomy have been reported to occur in as many as 60% of patients after 9 years; however, restenosis accounts for symptoms in fewer than 20% of patients.[9] Patients undergoing balloon mitral valvotomy with an unfavorable MV morphology have a higher incidence of recurrent symptoms at 1- to 2-year follow-up due to either an initial inadequate result or restenosis.[10]

Reasons for the Recurrence of Symptoms Following PMV

The main reasons for the recurrence of symptoms following PMV are:
1. Valve restenosis
2. Progressive MR
3. Development/worsening of disease in other valves
4. Coronary artery disease
5. Nonregression of PH and related complications
6. Progression of PAH/TR
7. LV dysfunction
8. Atrial fibrillation.

Thus, in patients presenting with symptoms late after PMV, a comprehensive evaluation is required to look for all the above causes.

Effect of Atrial Fibrillation

See Chapter 45 on Atrial Fibrillation.

Effect of Mitral Regurgitation

See Chapter 55 on Mitral Regurgitation.

Clinical Course of Tricuspid Regurgitation

Patients with MS requiring PMV often have a degree of concomitant TR. Although most TR regressed immediately after the procedure, significant TR after successful PMV in patients with MS is not uncommon long after PMV. Tricuspid regurgitation did not improve in 49–80% of the patients with moderate or severe TR after successful mitral balloon valvotomy.[11]

Tricuspid regurgitation was more likely to improve in patients with the following characteristics:
1. Younger age
2. Functional (as opposed to organic) TR
3. Smaller MV area, preprocedure
4. Significant relief of pulmonary hypertension after valvotomy
5. Absence of AF.

Song et al.[12] compared PMV and surgical treatment (MV surgery and TV repair) in 92 patients with MS and severe TR. Although event-free survival was not different in this relatively small retrospective study, patients in the surgical group were older and had more AF and a higher MV score. Event-free survival at 7 years, however, was significantly better in the subgroup of patients with AF who had surgery mainly due to heart failure events secondary to TR in the valvotomy group. Furthermore, 98% of the patients in the surgical group were free of TR of grade 2 or more, compared to 46% of the patients who had PMV.

In 12 years' follow-up of one center prospective registry of 299 patients with symptomatic MS who underwent successful PMV, Lee et al.[13] found that the cumulative incidence of significant TR increased time-dependently (9.4%, 19.8% and 35.2% at 8, 12 and 18 years of follow-up, respectively). Pre-PMV AF, significant TR, MV restenosis were found to be the three factors predicting significant TR (re)development long after successful PMV.

Once significant late TR develops, quality of life and prognosis of patients worsen, even in the absence of LV dysfunction or pulmonary hypertension. Management of such patients is challenging because advanced right ventricular dysfunction frequently coexists.

TV annular dilatation, often seen in patients with significant TR before PMV, is considered the most important contributor to the development of late TR. A continuous subclinical interaction between AF and tricuspid annular dilatation after successful PMV could cause TR to progress gradually with time.

The gradual but progressive increase in the hemodynamic burden induced by MV restenosis may lead to atrial enlargement with concomitant tricuspid annular dilatation and AF, all of which are generally accepted as the most important substrates of TR (re)development. Thus, the prevention of MV restenosis is an important therapeutic strategy to prevent late TR (re)development.

■ MITRAL RESTENOSIS AND LONG-TERM OUTCOME

See Chapter 52 on Restenosis.

■ FOLLOW-UP AND MANAGEMENT OF PATIENTS AFTER PMV

The management of patients after successful PMV is similar to that of the asymptomatic patient with MS. An echocardiogram should be performed after the procedure to obtain a baseline measurement of postprocedure hemodynamics and to exclude significant complications, such as MR, LV dysfunction, or atrial septal defect.

This echocardiographic evaluation should be performed at least 48–72 hours after the procedure, because acute changes in atrial and ventricular compliance immediately after the procedure affect the reliability of pressure half-time method of calculation of valve area.

Clinical examination including physical examination, chest X-ray, and ECG should be performed at yearly intervals in patients who remains asymptomatic or minimally symptomatic.

If the patient is in AF or has a history of AF, anticoagulation is recommended. Anticoagulant therapy with a target INR in the upper half of the range 2 to 3 is indicated in patients with either permanent or paroxysmal AF.

Mitral Stenosis and Sinus Rhythm

In patients of sinus rhythm, anticoagulation is mandatory when there has been prior embolism or when a thrombus is present in the left atrium[14] (recommendation Class I, level of evidence C). Anticoagulation is also recommended when TEE shows dense spontaneous echo contrast or an enlarged left atrium (M mode diameter >50 mm or LA volume 60 ml/m^2)[14,15] (Recommendation Class IIa, level of evidence C) .

Mitral Stenosis and Atrial Fibrillation

In patients with a history of atrial fibrillation, heparin should be continued and warfarin should be restarted following PMV. Heparin is continued until the INR is in range. In patients without history of embolism, anticoagulation is recommended with an INR of 2.0–3.0. In patients with history of prior embolism, combined therapy with aspirin 150 mg and anticoagulation with an INR of 2.0–3.0 is recommended.

■ INFECTIVE ENDOCARDITIS PROPHYLAXIS

The AHA recommendation 2007,[16] 2009[17] and ESC guidelines[18] limited the indication for antibiotic prophylaxis to patients with the highest risk of IE undergoing the highest risk procedures.

Rheumatic heart disease (RHD) is not in the list of cardiac conditions for IE prophylaxis. But this recommendation needs to be tailored to the situation in developing countries like India. RHD is still the most common underlying condition predisposing to endocarditis, in developing countries.[19-21]

Steckelberg and Wilson[22] reported that per 10,000 patient years, the lifetime risk (380–440) for RHD was similar to that (308–383) for patients with a mechanical or bioprosthetic cardiac valve.

Australian guidelines[23] still consider indigenous Australian patients with rheumatic heart disease a special population at high risk (Infective Endocarditis Prophylaxis Expert Group, 2008).

All dental procedures that involve manipulation of gingival tissue or the periapical region of teeth or perforation of the oral mucosa, IE prophylaxis is reasonable in the developing country situation. The opponents to this view says that bacteremia can occur during routine brushing of the teeth. However, the general role of prevention of endocarditis is still very important in all patients with MS including good oral hygiene and aseptic measures during catheter manipulation or any invasive procedure, in order to reduce the rate of healthcare-associated infective endocarditis (IE).

Antibiotic prophylaxis solely to prevent IE is not recommended for genitourinary or gastrointestinal tract procedures. Respiratory tract procedures with mucosal injury is also included in the select list.

Antibiotics for prophylaxis should be administered as a single dose before the procedure (Table 58.1). If the antibiotic was not inadvertently administered before the procedure, it should be administered up to 2 hours following the procedure.

In RHD patients on penicillin prophylaxis, the provider should select either clindamycin, azithromycin, or clarithromycin for IE prophylaxis. Patients who take oral penicillin for secondary prevention of rheumatic fever or for any other purposes are likely to have viridans group streptococci in their oral cavity that are relatively resistant to penicillin or amoxicillin. Because of possible cross-resistance of viridans group streptococci with cephalosporins, this class of antibiotics also should be avoided.

Despite marked changes in IE prevention guidelines that were published by the AHA in 2007 that restricted antibiotic prophylaxis, follow-up studies [24-26] proved that the incidence of Viridans Group Streptococci IE after publication of these guidelines did not increase.

Table 58.1: Regimens for infective endocarditis prophylaxis prior to a dental procedure[28]

Regimen: Single dose 30–60 minutes before procedure			
Situation	*Agent*	*Adult*	*Children*
Oral	Amoxicillin	2 g	50 mg/kg
Unable to take oral medication	Ampicillin	2 g/IM or IV	50 mg/kg IM or IV
OR			
	Cefazolin or ceftriaxone	1 g IM or IV	50 mg/kg IM or IV
Allergic to penicillins or ampicillin-oral	Cephalexin	2 g	50 mg/kg
OR			
	Clindamycin	600 mg	20 mg/kg
OR			
	Azithromycin or clarithromycin	500 mg	15 mg/kg
Allergic to penicillins or ampicillin and unable to take oral medication	Cefazolin or ceftriaxone		
OR			
	Clindamycin	600 mg IM or IV	20 mg/kg IM or IV

Rheumatic Fever Prophylaxis

The duration of secondary prophylaxis for prevention of recurrence of rheumatic fever for post-PMV patients is preferably lifelong.[27,29] As per the AHA recommendation 2009,[28] the following drugs can be used for secondary prophylaxis (Table 58.2).

When symptoms recur on follow-up, 2D and Doppler echocardiography should be performed to evaluate the MV hemodynamics and pulmonary artery pressure and to rule out significant MR or a left-to-right shunt. As with all patients with MS, exercise hemodynamics may be indicated in the patient with a discrepancy in clinical and hemodynamic findings.

Table 58.2: Secondary prevention of rheumatic fever (prevention of recurrent attacks)

Agent	Dose	Mode	Rating
Benzathine penicillin G	600000 U for children ≤ 27 kg (60 lb). 1200000 U for those > 27 kg (60 lb) every 4 weeks*	Intramuscular	IA
Penicillin V	250 mg twice daily	Oral	IB
Sulfadiazine	0.5 gm once daily for patients ≤ 27 kg (60 lb). 1.0 gm once daily for patients > 27 kg (60 lb)	Oral	IB
For individuals allergic to penicillin and sulfadiazine Macrolide or azalide	Variable	Oral	IC

Rating indicates classification of recommendation and LOE (e.g. IA indicates class L, LOE A).
*In high-risk situation, administration every 3 weeks is justified and recommended.
(See discussion of high-risk situations in the text).

Diuretics or long acting nitrates transiently ameliorate dyspnea. Beta-blockers or heart-rate regulating calcium channel blockers are useful to slow the heart rate and can greatly improve exercise tolerance by prolonging diastole and increasing the time available for LV filling via the stenosed valve.

Repeat PMV can be performed in those patients who develop restenosis with symptoms, following PMV. The results of these procedures are adequate in many patients but may be less satisfactory than the overall results of initial valvotomy, because there is usually more valve deformity, calcification, and fibrosis than with the initial procedure. Result of re-PMV is better if the predominant mechanism is commissural refusion[30] and in cases with an initially successful PMV if restenosis occurs after several years.

In patients with incomplete commissural fusion, repeat PMV might end in suboptimal results.[31] In cases without any commissural fusion, MS could be due to a rigid valve or subvalvular apparatus, and therefore repeat PBMV should be considered as contraindicated.

Mitral valve replacement should be considered in those patients with valves not suitable for a re-PMV or a failed PMV.

REFERENCES

1. Reyes VP, Raju BS, Wynne J, et al. Percutaneous balloon valvuloplasty compared with open surgical commissurotomy for mitral stenosis. N Engl J Med. 1994;331:961-7.
2. Osama Rifaie, M Khairy Abdel-Dayem, Ali Ramzy, Hassan Ezz-El-din, Galal El-Ziady, Adel El-Itriby, et al. Percutaneous mitral valvotomy versus closed surgical commissurotomy. Up to 15 years of follow-up of a prospective randomized study. Journal of Cardiology. 2009;53:28-34.
3. Bouleti C, Iung B, Laoue'nan C, Himbert D, Brochet E, Messika-Zeitoun D, et al. Late results of percutaneous mitral commissurotomy up to 20 years. Development and validation of a risk score predicting late functional results from a series of 912 patients. Circulation. 2012;125:2119-27.
4. Fawzy ME, Shoukri M, Al Buraiki J, Hassan W, El Widaa H, Kharabsheh S, et al. Seventeen years' clinical and echocardiographic follow up of mitral balloon valvuloplasty in 520 patients, and predictors of long-term outcome. J Heart Valve Dis. 2007;16:454-60.
5. Kim MJ, Song JK, Song JM, Kang DH, Kim YH, Lee CW, et al. Long-term outcomes of significant mitral regurgitation after percutaneous mitral valvuloplasty. Circulation. 2006;114:2815-22.
6. Song JK, Song JM, Kang DH, Yun SC, Park DW, Lee SW, et al. Restenosis and adverse clinical events after successful percutaneous mitral valvuloplasty: immediate post-procedural mitral valve area as an important prognosticator. Eur Heart J. 2009;30:1254-62.
7. Yasu T, Katsuki T, Ohmura N, et al. Delayed improvement in skeletal muscle metabolism and exercise capacity in patients with mitral stenosis following immediate hemodynamic amelioration by percutaneous transvenous mitral commissurotomy. Am J Cardiol. 1996;77:492-7.
8. Igor F Palacios, Murat E Tuzcu, Arthur E Weyman, John B Newell, Peter C Block. Clinical follow-up of patients undergoing percutaneous mitral balloon valvotomy. Circulation. 1995;91:671-6.
9. Higgs LM, Glancy DL, O'Brien KP, Epstein SE, Morrow AG. Mitral restenosis: an uncommon cause of recurrent symptoms following mitral commissurotomy. Am J Cardiol. 1970;26:34-7.
10. Abascal VM, Wilkins GT, Choong CY, et al. Echocardiographic evaluation of mitral valve structure and function in patients followed for at least 6 months after percutaneous balloon mitral valvuloplasty. J Am Coll Cardiol. 1988;12:606-15.
11. Hannoush H, Fawzy ME, Stefadouros M, Moursi M, Chaudhary MA, Dunn B. Regression of significant tricuspid regurgitation after mitral balloon valvotomy for severe mitral stenosis. Am Heart J. 2004;148:865-70.
12. Song H, Kang DH, Kim JH, et al. Percutaneous mitral valvuloplasty versus surgical treatment in mitral stenosis with severe tricuspid regurgitation. Circulation. 2007;116:I246-50.
13. Seung-Pyo Lee, Hyung-Kwan Kim,Kyung-Hee Kim, Ji-Hyun Kim, Hyo Eun Park, Yong-Jin Kim et al. Prevalence of significant tricuspid regurgitation in patients with successful percutaneous mitral valvuloplasty for mitral stenosis: results from 12 years' follow-up of one centre prospective Registry. Heart. 2013;99:91-97 .
14. ESC/EACTS Guidelines on the management of valvular heart disease (version 2012) .
15. Keenan NG, Cueff C, Cimadevella C, Brochet E, Lepage L, Detaint D, et al. Usefulness of left atrial volume versus diameter to assess thromboembolic risk in mitral stenosis. Am J Cardiol. 2010;106:1152-56.

16. Wilson W, Taubert KA, Gewitz M, et al. Prevention of infective endocarditis. Guidelines from the American Heart Association. A guideline from the American Heart Association Rheumatic Fever, Endocarditis, and Kawasaki Disease Committee, Council on Cardiovascular Disease in the Young, and the Council on Clinical Cardiology, Council on Cardiovascular Surgery and Anesthesia, and the Quality of Care and Outcomes Research Interdisciplinary Working Group. Circulation. 2007;116:1736–54.

17. Rick A Nishimura, Blase A, Carabello, et al. ACC/AHA 2008 Guideline Update on Valvular Heart Disease: Focused Update on Infective Endocarditis. Journal of the American College of Cardiology. 2008;52:676–85.

18. ESC Guidelines on the prevention, diagnosis, and treatment of infective endocarditis (new version 2009).

19. Tleyjeh IM, Steckelberg JM, Murad HS, et al. Temporal trends in infective endocarditis: a population-based study in Olmsted County, Minnesota. JAMA. 2005;293(24):3022–8.

20. Nkomo VT. Epidemiology and prevention of valvular heart disease and infective endocarditis in Africa. Heart. 2007;93:1510–19.

21. Carapetis JR. Rheumatic heart disease in Asia. Circulation. 2008;118:2748–53.

22. Steckelberg JM, Wilson WR. Risk factors for infective endocarditis. Infect Dis Clin North Am. 1993;7(1):9–19.

23. Infective Endocarditis Prophylaxis Expert Group (2008). Prevention of Endocarditis 2008 update from Therapeutic Guidelines: Antibiotic Version 13, and Therapeutic Guidelines: Oral and Dental Version 1. Therapeutic Guidelines Limited: Melbourne.

24. Daniel C, DeSimone, Imad M Tleyjeh, Daniel D, Correa de Sa, Nandan S, et el. Mayo Cardiovascular Infections Study Group. Incidence of Infective Endocarditis Caused by Viridans Group Streptococci Before and After Publication of the 2007 American Heart Association's Endocarditis Prevention Guidelines. Circulation. 2012;126:60-64.

25. Xavier Duval, François Delahaye, François Alla, Pierre Tattevin, Jean-François Obadia, Vincent Le Moing, et al. Christophe Strady, Catherine Chirouze, Michelle Bes, Emmanuelle Cambau, on behalf of the AEPEI Study Group. Temporal Trends in Infective Endocarditis in the Context of Prophylaxis Guideline Modifications: Three Successive Population-Based Surveys. J Am Coll Cardiol. 2012;59:1968–76.

26. Thornhill MH, Dayer MJ, Forde JM, et al. Impact of the NICE guideline recommending cessation of antibiotic prophylaxis for prevention of infective endocarditis: before and after study. BMJ. 2011;342:d2392.

27. WHO Technical report series – Rheumatic fever and rheumatic heart disease, 2004.

28. Gerber MA, Baltimore RS, Eaton CB, et al. Prevention of rheumatic fever and diagnosis and treatment of acute streptococcal pharyngitis. Circulation. 2009;119:1541-51.

29. ESC/EACTS Guidelines on the management of valvular heart disease (version 2012).

30. Fawzy ME, Hassan W, Shoukri M, Al Sanei A, Hamadanchi A, El Dali A, et al. Immediate and long-term results of mitral balloon valvotomy for restenosis following previous surgical or balloon mitral commissurotomy. Am J Cardiol. 2005;96:971–75.

31. Turgeman Y, Atar S, Suleiman K, Feldman A, Bloch L, Jabaren M, Rosenfeld T. Feasibility, safety, and morphologic predictors of outcome of repeat percutaneous balloon mitral commissurotomy. Am J Cardiol. 2005;95:989–91.

Chapter 59

Setting A New PMV Program

Ajeet Arulkumar, Harikrishnan S

▮ INTRODUCTION

Percutaneous mitral valvuloplasty (PMV) is usually performed in a limited number of tertiary care centers. This chapter is dedicated to the issues and concerns that have to be considered while setting the program for the first time in a new center. The chapter concludes with precautions which a relatively inexperienced operator must take when he is attempting the initial few PMV cases.

The center contemplating to start the program should have a good number of patients with rheumatic heart disease (RHD), experienced personnel, on site cardiac surgery back up and all necessary hardware.

Percutaneous mitral valvuloplasty program usually runs in two scenarios, one in a developed country where the cases are occasional and one or two experienced operators perform the cases. The second scenario is in a developing country where the cases are plenty and there are many operators who all are well-experienced. The cathlab staff and the set-up will also differ with regard to their experiences in these two contrasting scenarios.

Setting up a PMV program requires careful planning and utilization of resources. Cost is an important concern as the program when it established in a developing country. The main components of the program include personnel, hardware and supporting staff.

Personnel

Percutaneous mitral valvuloplasty is a relatively complex procedure, requiring considerable skill. Like all surgical procedures, the success of the procedure depends on a team approach. The physician should ensure that all team members know their roles, so that the procedure is smooth and successful. A brief description of the various personnel is described below.

Physicians with Adequate Training

A fully competent and trained cardiologist who can independently perform PMV and handle its complications is the central component of the PMV program. Physician experience is directly proportional to the outcome of the procedure.[1-3]

Transseptal puncture alone requires significant training and the learning curve can be quite steep. Unfortunately, even though there are centers which perform good number of PMV in developing countries, there are no organized fellowships or training programs in many countries.

The physician should be able to recognize complications in an early stage itself and treat them. For example, chest pain and hypotension after trans-septal puncture should make the interventionist suspect cardiac tamponade. If identified early and treated effectively, the otherwise fatal outcome can be prevented.

The physician should also be able to perform the procedure in high risk patients like pregnant patients, kyphoscoliosis, bulging IAS which require expertize and skills.

Nursing Staff

In many developing countries, the Cath Lab Scrub Nurses take the role of the second operator. Hence, it is imperative that they are well trained especially in handling the hardware. PMV hardware is very much different from the much more commonly performed coronary interventions. Therefore, unless specifically trained for PMV, nurses assisting these procedures may unintentionally damage the hardware (E.g. Bending the LA entry wire, Balloon etc.).

Cath Lab Technicians

In India, the preparation of the balloon and other hardware is usually done by trained cath-lab technicians. They also assist the physician in Echocardiography during the procedure.

The resterilization of the hardware is done by the cath-lab technicians. This job requires expertize since careless handling of the balloon leads to damage and can lead to many complications on reuse.

Equipment

Cath Lab

Standard cath lab is suitable for PMV. Biplane fluoroscopy, if available may be helpful in septal puncture and also in entry of balloon into the left ventricle. Special protective lead shields should be available for pregnant patients.

Septal Puncture/Balloon

The center performing PMV must have at least 2 or 3 sets of septal puncture hardware and balloon kits in different sizes. It is better to have a hardware supplied by a single manufacturer, otherwise it will lead to confusion as majority of the hardware are reused and packaged separately in India. For example, the stretching tube of ACCURA balloon, although externally similar, is slightly different from INOUE and cannot be interchanged.

Pressure Transducers, Pulse Oximeter, Blood Gas Analyzer

Ideally, the cath lab requires two similarly calibrated pressure transducers. The tubing which connects the patient and each of the transducers should be of the same size and diameter. Otherwise, comparison of simultaneous left atrial and left ventricular pressure will give erroneous values.

Both transducers should be calibrated using the same equipment and zeroed at the same height during the procedure.

Percutaneous mitral valvuloplasty also can be done using a single pressure transducer if two transducers are not available. Here the left atrial and left ventricular pressure has to be recorded sequentially and the tracings should be superimposed to calculate the mitral valve area.

As in coronary interventions, continuous monitoring of oxygen saturation by pulse oximeter should be available in the lab and this has been found helpful in detecting early pulmonary edema.

A basic hemodynamic study must be done before and after the procedure. This requires a blood gas analyzer or hemoximeter.

Echocardiographic Monitoring

Echocardiographic evaluation is the essential imaging modality in a PMV program. It is used during all stages of PMV—prior to PMV, periprocedural period and also postprocedure. Most of the evaluation can be done by TTE. However, ruling out clot in LA/LAA requires a detailed transesophageal echo (TEE) evaluation.

Transthoracic echocardiogram (TTE) will assess commissural fusion, commissural calcium and assessment of MR by color flow which is crucial in selecting patients for PMV. The standard procedure followed in all PMV labs is to proceed to the final diameter of the balloon by giving serial dilatations. Periprocedural echocardiography must be used in assessing the adequacy of commissural split and the degree of MR after each balloon dilatation. Increase in MR of two grades is an indication to stop the PMV procedure.

Transthoracic echocardiogram will also help in locating the valve orifice when the operator faces difficulties in entering the mitral valve. Assessment of complications also is done by echocardiography. Pericardial effusion and tamponade is essentially diagnosed and confirmed by echocardiography.

Resterilization Facility

Details of resterilization system are given in chapter 28.

Supporting Team

Surgical Standby

Back-up of an on-site surgical team is an important component of a successful and safe PMV program. Valve tear and severe MR and cardiac tamponade not responding to pericardial aspiration are the two most common situations where immediate surgical support is required.

Other situation where surgical support is required is femoral arterial thrombosis which requires embolectomy. Non-yielding valves requires elective OMV/MVR.

Anesthesia

Support of the anesthetists is also important in any PMV program. Patients may develop acute pulmonary edema, if atrial fibrillation with fast ventricular rate or acute MR develops during the procedure. In such cases, anesthesia support in intubating, ventilating and shifting the patient to the surgical theater is required.[4,5]

A successful PMV program is always a team work. Selecting suitable patients and performing the procedure by an experienced operator make the procedure safe and effective. A good and understanding support from the surgical and anesthetic team will make the program a very successful one.

▓ REFERENCES

1. Rihal CS, Nishimura RA, Holmes DR Jr. Percutaneous balloon mitral valvuloplasty: the learning curve. Am Heart J. 1991;122(6):1750–6.
2. Sanchez PL, Harrell LC, Salas RE, Palacios IF. Learning curve of the Inoue technique of percutaneous mitral balloon valvuloplasty. Am J Cardiol. 2001;88(6):662–7.
3. Hung JS, Lau KW, Lo PH, Chern MS, Wu JJ. Complications of Inoue balloon mitral commissurotomy: impact of operator experience and evolving technique. Am Heart J. 1999;138(1 Pt 1):114–21.
4. Tempe DK, Gupta B, Banerjee A, Virmani S, Datt V, Marwah C, et al. Surgical interventions in patients undergoing percutaneous balloon mitral valvotomy: a retrospective analysis of anaesthetic considerations. Nn Card Anaesth. 2004;7(2):129–36.
5. Tempe DK, Mehta N, Mohan JC, Tandon MS, Nigam M. Emergency mitral valve replacement for traumatic mitral insufficiency following balloon mitral valvotomy: an early haemodynamic study. Ann Card Anaesth. 1998;1(2):49–55.

INDEX

Page numbers followed by *f* refer to figure and *t* refer to table